HISTORY, PHILOSOPHY AND SOCIOLOGY OF SCIENCE

SOCIOLOGY OF SCIENCE

Classics, Staples and Precursors

HISTORY, PHILOSOPHY AND SOCIOLOGY OF SCIENCE

Classics, Staples and Precursors

Selected By

YEHUDA ELKANA
ROBERT K. MERTON
ARNOLD THACKRAY
HARRIET ZUCKERMAN

SCIENCE
MEDICINE AND
HISTORY

Collected and Edited by

E. ASHWORTH UNDERWOOD

VOLUME ONE

ARNO PRESS

A New York Times Company

New York – 1975

Reprint Edition 1975 by Arno Press Inc.

Reprinted from a copy in
  The Princeton University Library

HISTORY, PHILOSOPHY AND SOCIOLOGY OF SCIENCE:
Classics, Staples and Precursors
ISBN for complete set: 0-405-06575-2
See last pages of this volume for titles.

Manufactured in the United States of America

————◆————

Library of Congress Cataloging in Publication Data
Underwood, Edgar Ashworth.
    Science, medicine, and history.

    (History, philosophy and sociology of science)
    Reprint of the 1953 ed. published by Oxford Univer-
sity Press, London.
    Written in honour of Charles Singer.
    1. Medicine--History--Addresses, essays, lectures.
2. Science--History--Addresses, essays, lectures.
3. Singer, Charles Joseph, 1876-1960. I. Singer,
Charles Joseph, 1876-1960. II. Title. III. Series.
[DNLM: 1. History of medicine--Essays. 2. Science
--History--Essays. WZ5 U56s 1953a]
R111.S54 1975   610   74-26300
ISBN 0-405-06624-4

SCIENCE
MEDICINE AND
HISTORY

PLATE I

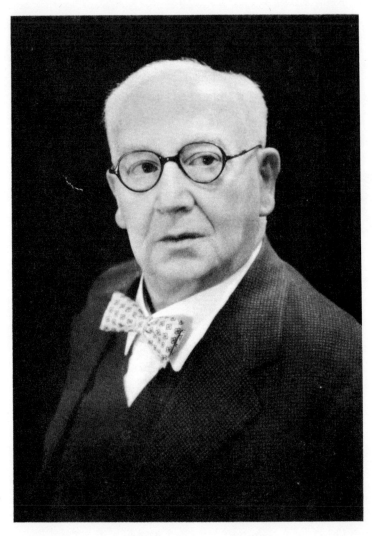

(Photograph by Negus, St. Austell, February 1953)

SCIENCE
MEDICINE AND
HISTORY

ESSAYS ON THE
EVOLUTION OF SCIENTIFIC THOUGHT
AND MEDICAL PRACTICE

written in honour of

CHARLES SINGER

Collected and Edited by

E. ASHWORTH UNDERWOOD

VOLUME ONE

GEOFFREY CUMBERLEGE

OXFORD UNIVERSITY PRESS

LONDON   NEW YORK   TORONTO

1953

*Oxford University Press, Amen House, London E.C.*4

GLASGOW   NEW YORK   TORONTO   MELBOURNE   WELLINGTON
BOMBAY   CALCUTTA   MADRAS   KARACHI   CAPE TOWN   IBADAN

Geoffrey Cumberlege, Publisher to the University

Printed in Great Britain by Taylor & Francis, Ltd. London

CHARLES SINGER

A Biographical Note

CHARLES JOSEPH SINGER was born in Camberwell on 2 November 1876. From his earliest years he lived in an atmosphere of scholarship, for his father, the Rev. Simeon Singer, was a Hebrew scholar of international reputation, in addition to being learned in the classical tongues. He is still well remembered as the author of the standard English translation of the Hebrew liturgy. Charles Singer received most of his early education at the City of London School, which then had the redoubtable Edwin Abbott as its headmaster. He left there in 1892, and after spending a year at a tutorial college with a view to matriculation, he entered University College, London, as a medical student in September 1893. After a year he transferred to the Faculty of Sciences, with the intention of reading biology instead of medicine. From the stimulating lectures of Weldon in zoology and F. W. Oliver in botany dates his intense interest in these subjects. To this day he regrets that he was never a professional biologist. As a result of a strange chance he was invited by the President of Magdalen College, Oxford, to enter for a scholarship there. He was successful, and he spent the three years from 1896 to 1899 at Oxford. There he graduated B.A. with a second class in zoology in 1899: there were no firsts in that year. He then decided to adopt the profession of medicine, and in October 1899 he began his strictly medical studies at St. Mary's Hospital, Paddington, where his chief teachers were the younger Augustus Waller for physiology, Almroth Wright for pathology, Pepper and William Collier for surgery, and W. B. Cheadle and Arthur Luff for medicine.

Charles Singer qualified M.R.C.S., L.R.C.P. in October 1903, and on the same day he accepted the post of medical officer to an expedition under Sir John Harrington for the delimitation of the Abyssinian frontier with the Sudan. On the outward journey he had time to make a full inspection of the accessible antiquities in Egypt and Nubia. The biological specimens which he collected on that expedition are now in the British Museum (Natural History). After his return Singer wrote an article on some interesting medical cases which he had encountered. This was his first published paper [No. 1]*. On his way home from Abyssinia he visited some of the classical sites in Greece and Sicily.

Singer then settled down to professional work with resident posts at St. Mary's Hospital, and a year at the Sussex County Hospital at Brighton. He had meanwhile graduated M.B. at Oxford (1905). He next took a post in the Government General Hospital at Singapore, and he did not return to London until the summer of 1908. After a six-months' appointment as resident anaesthetist at St. Mary's Hospital be began consulting practice, and at the same time held posts as clinical assistant to Sir William Willcox at the Great Northern Hospital, to G. F. Still at Great Ormond Street, and as medical registrar at the Cancer Hospital in Fulham Road. In 1909 he was appointed

---

* Figures in square brackets refer to the bibliography of his writings at the end of this work.

physician to the Dreadnought Seamen's Hospital, and this post he retained—along with his post at the Cancer Hospital—until he left London for Oxford in 1914.

During these five formative years Singer had considerable experience of medical cases, and he devised what was probably the first portable apparatus for obtaining a graphic record of the blood-pressure [No. 3]. He also developed his inherent interest in laboratory research. At the Cancer Hospital he had as senior colleagues E. M. Kettle, E. W. R. Nicholson, and S. B. Schryver. With the latter he carried out an extensive research into the gastric juice in carcinoma of the stomach [Nos. 9, 12]. He had already done pioneer statistical work on the duration of cancer of the external surface of the body, in which graphs were used to illustrate the age incidence of oral carcinoma in relation to the age constitution of the population [No. 4].

The year 1910 was eventful in Singer's life, for on 17 July he married Dorothea Waley Cohen, who was before long to establish in her own right an international reputation for her work on medical, alchemical and scientific manuscripts. In 1912 Singer suddenly felt dissatisfied with his knowledge of scientific German, and within a week or so he and his wife had let their house in London and were installed at Heidelberg, where Singer did cancer research for eight months in Czerny's laboratory. He had already discovered a worm in a cancerous growth in a rat's stomach—actually in the same week in which Fibiger published his discovery—and had worked much with a transplantable sarcoma in a rat's uterus. Some of these investigations were reported to the International Congress of Medicine which met in London in 1913. Singer was therefore a busy hospital physician, consultant, and laboratory worker when, in the spring of 1914, there came a fateful telephone call from Sir William Osler at Oxford which virtually determined the course of his life. Osler offered him the Philip Walker Studentship in Pathology at £250 a year: the pathological duties were to be minimal, and the rest of his time was to be devoted to history. Singer accepted at once. At thirty-eight he had virtually burnt his boats and had taken the first step to becoming a professional historian.

It will be obvious that such an enlightened judge of men as Osler did not make this offer without good reason. Singer had long had a general interest in the history of medicine, but he can date his practical interest to an evening in the late summer of 1910, when he picked up for a few pence in Church Street, Kensington, a copy of Benjamin Marten's *New Theory of Consumptions*. He was entranced to find that Marten had anticipated the germ theory. The papers which Singer wrote in 1911 on this work [Nos. 5, 6] were his first historical writings. Then followed his historical notes on tropical diseases [No. 8], and his important work with Dorothea Singer on the *contagium vivum* [No. 11]. He had meanwhile become interested in St. Hildegard of Bingen, and at home, during his residence in Heidelberg, and on two subsequent visits to Germany he worked on Hildegard manuscripts. On the second of these visits (1914) he and Mrs. Singer just succeeded in escaping into Holland on 3 August; on the following day Great Britain declared war on Germany. But Singer's heavy luggage, with the Hildegard article on which he had worked for two years, had to be left behind. Later on he re-wrote it. His work on Hildegard [No. 32] established migraine as one of the physical bases of mystical visions.

Singer was commissioned in the R.A.M.C. in the early autumn of 1914, and he was demobilized in November 1918. In the spring of 1915 he was sent to Malta, and while there he did archaeological work with the Hon. T. Zammit which was published some years later [No. 121]. He was transferred to Salonika in January 1916 and there he remained for nearly two years. There he prosecuted studies in Byzantine Greek which led to an interesting publication [No. 42]. Singer had a great deal of material on hand when war broke out, so that with the help of Dorothea Singer he was able to complete much of this work from the material and photographs which she sent out to him. His first book, the *Cures of the Diseased* [No. 23], was published while he was at Chatham. Dorothea Singer rendered him invaluable assistance by seeing through the press the first volume of his *Studies* [No. 31], which was published while he was on active service (1917).

Singer had been a member of the History Section of the Royal Society of Medicine from its inception, and he read his first paper to the section on 9 November 1913 [No. 19]. He was then put on the Council, and from 1916 to 1919 he acted as an honorary secretary. He was president of the section from 1920 to 1922, and for twenty-three years (1918 to 1941) he was editorial representative.

Back at Oxford after the war, Singer was made lecturer on the history of biology. On his arrival there in 1914 he and his wife had thrown themselves with characteristic energy into a scheme to establish a History of Science Room in the Radcliffe Camera, in which interested workers could carry on their researches without interruption. Dorothea Singer had kept this scheme going during the war years. They had presented many books, and out of their own income had contributed materially to the annual cost. But soon after Singer's return he found that altered circumstances, and especially the death of Osler, made it more difficult to obtain the necessary facilities. In 1920 he was offered a post at University College, London, as lecturer on the history of medicine, with a seat on the professorial board from the start. This he accepted, and in the autumn of that year he removed to London. His first courses of lectures were given in the session 1920–21. Meanwhile, he continued with his Oxford lectures, and he did not resign his post there until the summer of 1921.

There is no doubt that Singer left Oxford with disappointment in his heart at the apathy which he thought had been shown to his subjects. As the years passed Oxford made amends. In 1922 A. C. Clark, who was then professor of Latin, suggested to Singer that he should submit his Hildegard study and certain other writings for the degree of Doctor of Letters. The degree was awarded in the same year. In 1936 Oxford University conferred upon him the honorary degree of Doctor of Science. Three years ago he received the honour which has perhaps gratified him most—the Honorary Fellowship of Magdalen, his old college. Singer is probably the only man living who holds the Oxford doctorates in the three faculties of medicine, science, and letters.

Installed in his new post, Singer found himself in the wonderfully stimulating atmosphere of University College during the early 1920's. There were Bayliss and Starling—very complementary in their differences—F. G. Donnan, Jack Drummond, and G. D. Thane, who, though he had retired from his chair and had taken up the post of Inspector of Anatomy, was a frequent visitor.

Singer had the greatest respect for Karl Pearson, W. P. Ker, R. W. Chambers and A. F. Pollard. He learned much from Flinders Petrie, and he was on terms of intimate friendship with H. E. Butler and J. H. G. Grattan. With the latter he studied Anglo-Saxon from the start; the result was Singer's classical paper to the British Academy [No. 58], and their recent joint publication of the text of *Lacnunga* [No. 368]. Perhaps Singer's greatest debt was to Arthur Platt, the professor of Greek, with whom he went through the Hippocratic Collection in great detail.

These were halcyon years, with one book following another in rapid succession. Singer had already written on medieval and Renaissance anatomy [see e.g. No. 31 (iii)], and from 1923 onwards his interest in this subject was intensified. In 1923 and 1924 he gave the FitzPatrick Lectures on the evolution of anatomy at the Royal College of Physicians, and in 1925 they were published [No. 132]. About the same time there appeared his important books on the Mundinus texts [Nos. 117, 130]. His first paper on the origin of the herbal was published in 1923 [No. 104], and four years later his classical contribution to this subject appeared in the *Journal of Hellenic Studies* [No. 158]. From this period, too, date his early contributions to the relations between religion and science, a subject in which he had shown interest for many years.

In 1929 Singer received an invitation to give the first course of Noguchi Lectures at the Johns Hopkins University, and to act as visiting professor to the University of California. He and Mrs. Singer sailed in June 1930. On arrival at New York Singer lectured at Columbia, and met 'Popsy' Welch for the first time. Lecturing *en route* the Singers continued their journey to the Huntington Library at Passadena, where Welch joined them. There the Singers had been invited to examine some early printed books and alchemical manuscripts for two or three weeks. They then proceeded to Berkeley, where they remained for three months. During this time Singer delivered about fifty lectures on the history of science while Dorothea initiated the uninitiated into the mysteries of palaeography. Mid-September saw them back in London again.

During the session 1930–31 Singer was elected professor of the history of medicine at University College. The appointment gave him great satisfaction, since it marked a further step in the official recognition of his subject. It should be said, however, that the chair, like the lectureship which he held until then, was honorary, and was in essence a recognition by the University of Singer's own great contributions to scholarship.

The invitation to act again as visiting professor at Berkeley for the first six months of 1932 was received in the summer of 1931. At the end of November Singer left England with his family. After a wonderful month in Jamaica they sailed through the Panama Canal and up the west coast of America to San Francisco. By the first week of January they were installed at Berkeley, and the invitation was soon extended to cover the whole year. While he was travelling during the Easter vacation Singer unfortunately contracted pneumonia, and this illness interfered slightly with his lectures during the summer term. About Christmas time they left for home—on a voyage which was to last four months, and to include prolonged stays in Malaya and Ceylon. The fact that Singer was invited so soon to return to Berkeley demonstrates the success of his first visit. The respect and affection with which his name is held in California is evidence of the good seed which he sowed during his second period as visiting professor.

Soon after his return to London Singer decided that he would not again risk living in the fogs of that city during the winter. Cornwall was the obvious solution, since he loved that county, and had indeed done some of his best work there. He and his wife finally decided on 'Kilmarth', a fine old house overlooking the sea between Par and Fowey. By December they had obtained possession, and they moved in during February 1934. From then until the outbreak of war Singer had rooms in London in the autumn and summer terms, during which he gave his lectures at University College. In 1933, the tragic events in Germany came as a shock to his estimate of man. He helped to found the Society for the Protection of Science and Learning, and much of his time during the next two years was devoted to the rescue and succour of victims of Nazi oppression. He retired from his chair in 1942, and the title of Professor Emeritus was conferred on him. In 1950 he was elected Fellow of University College.

From his early years as a historian Singer had been widely known—both for his writings and in person—to historians all over the world. In 1922 he was president of the Third International Congress of the History of Medicine which met in London in that year; and in 1931 he was president of the Second International Congress of the History of Science and Technology, also in London. In the years 1928 to 1931 he served as president of the Académie Internationale d'Histoire des Sciences, and from 1947 to 1950 he was the first president of the International Union for the History of Science. After the war there was a strong movement for the foundation of a British Society for the History of Science, and in this Singer played an important role. In the years 1946 to 1948 he was the first president of the new society. In 1948 he was elected an Honorary Fellow of the Royal Society of Medicine.

Even those who know Singer and his writings intimately may perhaps be astonished at the number of unsigned articles which are revealed in his bibliography. Many of these articles contain critical material of some importance. This is specially so in respect of the numerous essay-reviews which he has written for the *Times Literary Supplement*. His first connexion with that journal dates from 10 June 1921, when he was entrusted with the review of Sir Clifford Allbutt's *Greek Medicine in Rome* [No. 78].

The post-war period has been a remarkable Indian summer in Singer's literary and research activities. Since 1945 he has published four major new works, and two others are in the press. This takes no account of the monumental History of Technology, which was his conception and of which he is joint-editor. The first volume of this work—which will be published in five volumes—is already in the press. Such activity would do the greatest credit to any younger man. It is a tribute to the persistence of an enquiring mind and to the wonderful library and research facilities which Singer, with the assistance of his wife, has built up at 'Kilmarth'.

E. A. U.

CONTRIBUTORS

JAMES JOHNSTON ABRAHAM, C.B.E., D.S.O., M.A., Litt.D., M.D., F.R.C.S. Consulting Surgeon, Princess Beatrice Hospital and London Lock Hospitals. Thomas Vicary Lecturer, Royal College of Surgeons, 1943. Orator, Medical Society of London, 1946. Lloyd Roberts Lecturer, 1948.

AGNES ARBER, M.A., D.Sc., F.L.S., F.R.S. Fellow of University College, London. Linnean Medal, 1948. Writer on botany and the history of botany.

HENRY PETER BAYON, M.D., Ph.D. H. G. Plimmer Fellow in Animal Pathology, University of Cambridge. Formerly member of the Commission for the Study of Trypanosomiasis in Uganda, and research bacteriologist to the Union of South Africa. Writer on Harvey and other aspects of medical history.†

WILLIAM JOHN BISHOP, F.L.A. Librarian of the Wellcome Historical Medical Library, London. Formerly Sub-Librarian of the Royal Society of Medicine.

WILFRID BONSER, B.A., Ph.D., F.R.A.I., F.L.A. Formerly Librarian of the University of Birmingham. Writer on Anglo-Saxon magic and medicine.

DONALD CAMPBELL, B.Sc., M.R.C.P., L.A.H. Author of works on Arabian medicine.†

ARTURO CASTIGLIONI, M.D. Fermerly head of the sanitary service of the Lloyd-Triestino and Italian lines. Formerly Professor of the History of Medicine in the University of Padua, and Lecturer on the History of Medicine at Yale University. Noguchi Lecturer, Johns Hopkins University, 1933. Elected in 1932 an Honorary Member of the History of Medicine Section of the Royal Society of Medicine.†

ALEXANDER JAMES EDWARD CAVE, M.D., D.Sc., F.L.S., F.Z.S., F.R.A.I. Professor of Anatomy in the University of London (St. Bartholomew's Hospital Medical College). Formerly Assistant Conservator of the Museum, and Professor of Human and Comparative Anatomy, Royal College of Surgeons.

ALEXANDER POLYCLEITOS CAWADIAS, O.B.E., M.D., F.R.C.P. Knight Commander of the Royal Greek Order of the Phoenix. Emeritus Professor of Medicine in the University of Athens. Thomas Vicary Lecturer, Royal College of Surgeons, 1941. President of the History of Medicine Section, Royal Society of Medicine, 1937-9.

VERE GORDON CHILDE, D.Litt., D.Sc., F.B.A., F.R.A.I., F.S.A. Professor of Prehistoric European Archaeology, and Director of the Institute of Archaeology, University of London. Rhind Lecturer, Society of Antiquaries of Scotland, 1944.

FRANCIS JOSEPH COLE, D.Sc., F.R.S. Emeritus Professor of Zoology, University of Reading. Special University Lecturer in the History and Philosophy of Science, University of London, 1925, 1929-30, 1949. Wilkins Lecturer, Royal Society, 1950. Author of works on the history of zoology and of comparative anatomy.

† indicates deceased.

SIR VINCENT ZACHARY COPE, B.A., M.D., M.S., F.R.C.S. Consulting Surgeon to St. Mary's Hospital, Paddington. Thomas Vicary Lecturer, Royal College of Surgeons, 1952. Formerly President, Lettsomian Lecturer and Orator, Medical Society of London. Elected in 1951 an Honorary Fellow of the Royal Society of Medicine.

GEORGE WASHINGTON CORNER, A.B., M.D., D.Sc. Director of the Department of Embryology, Carnegie Institute of Washington. Thomas Vicary Lecturer, Royal College of Surgeons, 1936. Terry Lecturer, Yale University, 1944.

ARMANDO CORTESÃO. Formerly Lecturer on Cartography, University of Lisbon and Counsellor in the Natural Sciences Division in UNESCO. Writer on the science of navigation and the history of astronomy.

STEVENSON LYLE CUMMINS, C.B., C.M.G., M.D., LL.D., D.T.M. & H. Officier de la Légion d'Honneur. Formerly David Davies Professor of Tuberculosis, Welsh National School of Medicine, and Director of Research to the King Edward VII Welsh National Memorial Association. Col. A.M.S., Professor of Pathology, R.A.M.C. College.†

CYRIL DEAN DARLINGTON, D.Sc., F.R.S. Professor of Botany in the University of Oxford. Formerly Director of the John Innes Horticultural Institution.

WARREN ROYAL DAWSON, F.R.S.E., F.R.S.L., F.S.A. Honorary Fellow of the Imperial College of Science, and of the Medical Society of London. Honorary Member of the Egyptian Exploration Society. Frazer Lecturer, University of Glasgow, 1936.

GAVIN RYLANDS DE BEER, M.A., D.Sc., F.R.S., Hon.D.-ès-L. Director of the British Museum (Natural History). Formerly Professor of Embryology at University College, London. President of the Linnean Society, 1946–9.

PAUL DELAUNAY, M.D. Ancien interne des hôpitaux de Paris. Elected in 1940 an Honorary Member of the History of Medicine Section of the Royal Society of Medicine. Formerly President of the Société Française d'Histoire de la Médecine. Author of works on Belon, and on post-medieval French medicine.

HERBERT DINGLE, D.Sc., A.R.C.S. Professor of the History and Philosophy of Science, University College, London. Formerly Professor of Natural Philosophy, Imperial College of Science and Technology. President of the Royal Astronomical Society, 1951–2.

CYRIL LLOYD ELGOOD, M.A., M.D., F.R.C.P. Consulting Physician to the Government of Cyrenaica. Author of works on Persian medicine.

BENJAMIN FARRINGTON, M.A. Professor of Classics at University College, Swansea. Writer on science in the ancient world.

MAX HAROLD FISCH, A.B., Ph.D. Professor of Philosophy in the University of Illinois, Urbana. Formerly Assistant Professor at Western Reserve University, Cleveland. Author of works on Vico, etc.

HERBERT JOHN FLEURE, M.A., D.Sc., LL.D., Sc.D., F.R.S. Commandeur de l'ordre de Leopold (Belgium). Formerly Professor of Geography in the University of Manchester. President of the Royal Anthropological Institute, 1945-7, of the Folk-Lore Society, 1947-8, and of the Geographical Association, 1940. Tallman Visiting Professor, Bowdoin College, Maine, 1944-5. Visiting Professor in Egypt, 1949, 1950. J. G. Frazer Memorial Lecturer, Oxford, 1947. Honorary editor of *Geography*, 1917-47.

KENNETH JAMES FRANKLIN, M.A., D.M., D.Sc., F.R.C.P., F.Z.S. Professor of Physiology in the University of London (St. Bartholomew's Hospital Medical College). Visiting Professor of Physiology, University of Illinois, 1951-2.

KURT VON FRITZ, Ph.D. Professor of Greek and Latin at Columbia University, New York. Formerly Professor of Greek, University of Rostock. Writer on Greek philosophy and other classical studies.

JOHN FARQUAR FULTON, M.A., Ph.D., D.Sc., LL.D. Honorary Officer, Order of the British Empire. Professor of the History of Medicine, and formerly Sterling Professor of Physiology, Yale University. Elected in 1940 an Honorary Member of the History of Medicine Section of the Royal Society of Medicine. Heath Clark Lecturer, University of London, 1947. William Withering Lecturer, University of Birmingham, 1948. Editor of the *Journal of the History of Medicine and Allied Sciences*.

IAGO GALDSTON, B.S., M.D. Secretary of the Medical Information Bureau, New York Academy of Medicine. Consultant, National Tuberculosis Association.

GEORGE ERNEST GASK, C.M.G., M.A., F.R.C.S., F.A.C.S. Officier de la Légion d'Honneur. Emeritus Professor of Surgery in the University of London (St. Bartholmew's Hospital). Thomas Vicary Lecturer, Royal College of Surgeons, 1930. Special Hunterian Lecturer, Royal College of Surgeons, 1937.†

OTTO CHARLES GLASER, A.B., Ph.D. Harkness Professor of Biology, Amherst College, Massachusetts. Writer on developmental physiology and growth.†

EDGAR GOLDSCHMID, Dr. med. Formerly Professor of Pathology in the University of Frankfort-on-Main (1922-33), and Lecturer on the History of Medicine in the University of Lausanne (1933-51). Writer on the history of pathology and of pathological illustration.

RICHARD BENEDICT GOLDSCHMIDT, Ph.D., M.D., D.Sc. Emeritus Professor of Zoology, University of California, Berkeley. Formerly Director of the Kaiser Wilhelm Institute for Biological Research, Berlin. Silliman Lecturer, Yale University, 1939-40.

MAJOR GREENWOOD, D.Sc., F.R.C.P., F.R.S. Emeritus Professor of Epidemiology and Vital Statistics in the University of London. President of the Royal Statistical Society. Herter Lecturer, Johns Hopkins University, Baltimore, 1931. FitzPatrick Lecturer, Royal College of Physicians, 1941-3. Heath Clark Lecturer, University of London, 1946.†

SIR RICHARD ARMAN GREGORY, Bart., D.Sc., LL.D., F.R.A.S., F.R.S. Emeritus Professor of Astronomy, Queen's College, London. President of the British Association for the Advancement of Science, 1940–6. Editor of *Nature*, 1919–39.†

ANDREAS FREDRIK GRÖN, M.D. Formerly a specialist in dermatology in Oslo. Author of works on Nordic medicine, and joint editor of " The History of Medicine in Norway ", published in Norwegian in 1936.†

DOUGLAS GUTHRIE, M.D., F.R.C.S.(Ed.), F.R.S.(Ed.). Lecturer on the History of Medicine, University of Edinburgh. Consulting Surgeon, Edinburgh Royal Hospital for Sick Children. President, Scottish Society of the History of Medicine. Curator of the Royal Society of Edinburgh. Author of works on the history of medicine.

AAGE GUDMUND HATT, Ph.D. Fellow of the Royal Society of Copenhagen. Formerly Professor of Cultural Geography in the University of Copenhagen. Author of works on anthropology.

SIR GEOFFREY JEFFERSON, C.B.E., M.S., LL.D., F.R.C.S., F.R.C.P., F.R.S. Emeritus Professor of Neuro-Surgery in the University of Manchester. Honorary Neurological Surgeon, Manchester Royal Infirmary. Lister Medallist, Royal College of Surgeons, 1948.

CLAUDE JENKINS, M.A., D.D., F.S.A. Canon of Christ Church, and Regius Professor of Ecclesiastical History in the University of Oxford. Formerly Professor of Ecclesiastical History and Reader in Greek and Latin Palaeography, University of London.

FRANCIS RARICK JOHNSON, M.A., Ph.D. Professor of English, Stanford University, California. Visiting Professor, University of California, 1939. Visiting Professor, Claremont College, 1948. Author of works on medieval astronomy, etc.

WILLIAM HENRY SAMUEL JONES, M.A., Litt.D., F.B.A. Hon. Fellow of St. Catherine's College, Cambridge. Elected in 1921 an Honorary Member of the History of Medicine Section of the Royal Society of Medicine. Translator of Hippocrates and Pliny.

EDWARD BELL KRUMBHAAR, A.B., M.D., Ph.D. Emeritus Professor of Pathology, University of Pennsylvania. Elected in 1944 an Honorary Fellow of the Royal Society of Medicine. Editor of the *American Journal of the Medical Sciences* and of the ' Clio Medica ' series.

ARMAND DONALD LACAILLE, M.A., B.-ès-L., F.S.A., F.M.A. Member of the scientific staff of the Wellcome Historical Medical Museum, London. Archaeologist and writer on the Stone Age, palaeontology, and ecclesiology.

SANFORD VINCENT LARKEY, M.A., M.D. Librarian, Welch Medical Library, Johns Hopkins University, Baltimore. Formerly Assistant Professor of the History of Medicine, University of California.

CHAUNCEY DEPEW LEAKE, Litt.B., M.S., Ph.D. Executive Director of the Medical Branch, University of Texas, Galveston. Formerly Professor of Pharmacology in the University of California. Logan Clendenning Lecturer, University of Kansas, 1951. President of the History of Science Society, 1936–9.

WILLIAM RICHARD LEFANU, M.A., F.L.A. Librarian of the Royal College of Surgeons. Thomas Vicary Lecturer, Royal College of Surgeons, 1951.

LILIAN LINDSAY, C.B.E., LL.D., M.D.S., F.D.S., H.D.D., F.S.A. Honorary Librarian, British Dental Association. C. E. Wallis Lecturer, Royal Society of Medicine, 1933. Northcroft Lecturer, British Society for the Study of Orthodontics, 1948. President of the British Dental Association, 1946–7. President of the History of Medicine Section, Royal Society of Medicine, 1950–2.

ESMOND RAY LONG, A.B., Ph.D., M.D., Sc.D. Director of the Henry Phipps Institute for the Study, Treatment and Prevention of Tuberculosis, Philadelphia, and Professor of Pathology in the University of Pennsylvania. Member of the National Research Council. President of the National Tuberculosis Association, 1936–7, and of the American Association of Pathologists and Bacteriologists, 1936–7.

GINO LORIA, Dr. maths. Emeritus Professor of Higher Geometry in the University of Genoa. President of the Académie Internationale d'Histoire des Sciences, 1929. Formerly joint-editor of the *Bolletino Matematico*. Author of works on the history of mathematics.

HENRY FREDERICK LUTZ, Ph.D., D.D. Professor of Assyriology and Egyptology, University of California. Author of works on the philology, archaeology and history of the ancient Near-East.

DOUGLAS MCKIE, Ph.D., D.Sc. Reader in the History of Science in the University of London (University College). Joint-editor of *Annals of Science*. Author of works on Lavoisier and the history of science.

SIR ARTHUR SALUSBURY MACNALTY, K.C.B., M.A., M.D., F.R.C.P., F.R.C.S., Hon.F.R.S.(Ed.). Fellow of University College, London. Editor-in-chief, Official Medical History of the Second World War. Formerly Chief Medical Officer of the Ministry of Health. Thomas Vicary Lecturer, Royal College of Surgeons, 1945; FitzPatrick Lecturer, Royal College of Physicians, 1946–7. President of the History of Medicine Section, Royal Society of Medicine, 1945–7.

RALPH HERMAN MAJOR, A.B., M.D., LL.D. Professor of Internal Medicine, and formerly Professor of Pathology, University of Kansas. Author of works on historical subjects.

CLAUDIUS FRANCIS MAYER, A.B., M.D. Editor of the *Index-Catalogue* of the Surgeon-General's Library since 1932. Writer on medieval, Arabian and Renaissance medicine, medical nomenclature, and methods of medical research.

ARTHUR WILLIAM MEYER, B.S., M.D. Emeritus Professor of Human Anatomy in Stanford University, California. Writer on the history of embryology.

GENEVIEVE MILLER, M.A. Formerly Assistant in the Institute of the History of Medicine, Johns Hopkins University, Baltimore, and associate editor of the *Bulletin of the History of Medicine*, 1944–8.

MONTAGUE FRANCIS ASHLEY MONTAGU, Ph.D. Chairman, Department of Anthropology, Rutgers University, New Brunswick, N.J. Formerly Associate Professor of Anatomy, Hahnemann Medical College, Philadelphia. Visiting Lecturer, Department of Social Science, Harvard University, 1945.

HERNANI BASTOS MONTEIRO, Doutor em Medicina. Professor of Anatomy and Director of the Institute of Anatomy in the University of Oporto, Portugal. Honorary Professor of the University of Santiago de Compostela, Spain. Writer on the works of Vesalius and on the history of Portuguese surgery.

LESLIE THOMAS MORTON, F.L.A. Information Officer, *British Medical Journal*. Formerly Librarian of the Medical Department, The British Council. Editor of Garrison-Morton, *Medical Bibliography*.

JOSEPH NEEDHAM, M.A., Ph.D., Sc.D., F.R.S. Sir William Dunn Reader in Biochemistry, University of Cambridge. Scientific Adviser, UNESCO. Foreign Member of the National Academy of China. Terry Lecturer, Yale University. Boyle Lecturer, Oxford University, 1948. Hobhouse Lecturer, London University, 1950. Noguchi Lecturer, Johns Hopkins University, 1950.

BOHUMIL NĚMEC, Ph.D. Professor of Plant Anatomy and Physiology in the University of Prague. President of the National Research Council of Czechoslovakia.

MAX NEUBURGER, M.D. Emeritus Professor of the History of Medicine in the University of Vienna, and formerly member of the scientific staff of the Wellcome Historical Medical Museum, London. Elected in 1913 an Honorary Member of the History of Medicine Section of the Royal Society of Medicine, and in 1939 an Honorary Fellow of the Society.

HUBERT JAMES NORMAN, M.B., Ch.B., D.P.H. Formerly Medical Superintendent, Camberwell House, London. President of the History of Medicine Section, Royal Society of Medicine, 1947–8.†

JAMES MONTROSE DUNCAN OLMSTED, M.A., Ph.D., D.Sc. Professor of Physiology in the University of California. Author of biographies of the French physiologists.

CHARLES DONALD O'MALLEY, M.A. Professor of History in Stanford University, California. Joint-translator of works by Vesalius, and writer on Renaissance medicine.

WALTER TRAUGOTT ULRICH PAGEL, M.D.(Berlin). Pathologist to the Central Middlesex Hospital. Formerly Lecturer on Pathology and on the History of Medicine, University of Heidelberg. Writer on Van Helmont and the seventeenth century.

JAMES RIDDICK PARTINGTON, M.B.E., D.Sc. Emeritus Professor of Chemistry in the University of London. President of the British Society for the History of Science, 1949–51. Author of works on the history of chemistry.

ARTHUR LESLIE PECK, M.A., Ph.D. Fellow of Christ's College, and University Lecturer, Cambridge. Translator of Aristotle.

JEAN PELSENEER, Professor of the History of Scientific Thought in the Université Libre, Brussels. Member of the editorial staff of the *Archives Internationales d'Histoire des Sciences*.

HUMPHREY THOMAS PLEDGE, B.A. Librarian of the Science Museum, South Kensington.

NORMAN JOHN GREVILLE POUNDS, M.A., Ph.D. Professor of Geography, University of Indiana. Formerly Tutor, Fitzwilliam House, University of Cambridge.

FREDERICK NOËL LAWRENCE POYNTER, B.A., F.L.A., F.R.S.L. Deputy Librarian of the Wellcome Historical Medical Library, London.

CHAIM RABIN, M.A., D.Phil. Lecturer in Post-Biblical Hebrew in the University of Oxford. Joint-author with Charles Singer of *A Prelude to Modern Science*.

GEORGE ROSEN, B.S., M.D., Ph.D., M.P.H. Associate Medical Director of Health Insurance Plan of Greater New York, and Professor of Health Education, School of Public Health, Columbia University, New York. Formerly editor of the *Journal of the History of Medicine and Allied Sciences*.

EDWARD STUART RUSSELL, O.B.E., M.A., D.Sc., F.L.A. Formerly Director of Fishery Investigations, Ministry of Agriculture and Fisheries; Honorary Lecturer on Animal Behaviour, University College, London.

REDCLIFFE NATHAN SALAMAN, M.A., M.D., F.L.S., F.R.S. Formerly Director of the Potato Virus Research Station, University of Cambridge, Honorary Fellow, National Institute of Agricultural Botany.

GEORGE ALFRED LEON SARTON, B.Sc., Sc.D., L.H.D., LL.D., Ph.D. Professor of the History of Science in Harvard University. Lowell Lecturer, Boston, 1916. Colver Lecturer, Providence, Rhode Island, 1930. Hitchcock Professor, University of California, 1932. Elihu Root Lecturer, Washington, 1935. Fielding H. Garrison Lecturer, American Association of the History of Medicine, 1941. Special University Lecturer in the History and Philosophy of Science, University of London, 1948. University Lecturer, University College, London, 1949. Honorary President, History of Science Society. Founder and editor of *Isis* and *Osiris*.

JOHN BERTRAND DE CUSANCE MORANT SAUNDERS, M.B., F.R.C.S.(Ed.). Professor of Anatomy, and Lecturer on Medical History and Bibliography in the University of California. Joint-translator of works by Vesalius.

SIR CHARLES SCOTT SHERRINGTON, O.M., G.B.E., M.A., M.D., D.Sc., LL.D., F.R.C.P., F.R.C.S., F.R.S. Formerly Waynflete Professor of Physiology in the University of Oxford. President of the Royal Society, 1920–5. Nobel Laureate for Medicine, 1932. Thomas Vicary Lecturer, Royal College of Surgeons, 1937. Gifford Lecturer, University of Edinburgh, 1936–8. Elected in 1919 an Honorary Fellow of the Royal Society of Medicine.†

HENRY ERNEST SIGERIST, M.D., D.Litt., LL.D. Research Associate, Yale University. Formerly Professor of the History of Medicine, Johns Hopkins University, Baltimore. Terry Lecturer, Yale University, 1938; Messenger Lecturer, Cornell University, 1940. Formerly President of the American Association of the History of Medicine, and of the History of Science Society. Elected in 1940 an Honorary Member of the History of Medicine Section of the Royal Society of Medicine. Editor of the *Bulletin of the History of Medicine*, 1934–47.

ARNOLD SORSBY, M.D., F.R.C.S. Research Professor in Ophthalmology, Royal College of Surgeons and Royal Eye Hospital. Director of the Research Unit, Royal Eye Hospital.

EDWARD CLARK STREETER, A.B., M.D. Formerly Lecturer on the History of Medicine, Harvard Medical School, and Curator of the Museum Collections in the Historical Library, Yale University School of Medicine. Writer on art-anatomy, the history of pharmacy and on metrology.†

FRANK SHERWOOD TAYLOR, M.A., B.Sc., Ph.D. Director of the Science Museum, South Kensington. President of the British Society for the History of Science, 1951–3. Editor of *Ambix* since 1937.

OWSEI TEMKIN, M.D. Associate Professor of the History of Medicine, Johns Hopkins University, Baltimore. Editor of the *Bulletin of the History of Medicine* since 1947. Writer on Graeco-Arabic medicine, and on the history of disease.

SIR HENRY THOMAS, D.Litt., Hon. LL.D., D.Lit., F.S.A., F.B.A. Formerly Principal Keeper of Printed Books, British Museum. President of the Anglo-Spanish Society, 1931–47, and of the Bibliographical Society, 1936–8.†

SIR D'ARCY WENTWORTH THOMPSON, C.B., D.Sc., D.Litt., LL.D., F.R.S. Professor of Natural History in the University of St. Andrews. Herbert Spencer Lecturer, University of Oxford, 1913. Huxley Lecturer, University of Birmingham, 1917. Lowell Lecturer, Harvard University, 1936. President of the Royal Society of Edinburgh, 1934–9. President of the Classical Association, 1929, and of the Scottish Classical Association, 1935.†

LYNN THORNDIKE, M.A., L.H.D., Ph.D. Emeritus Professor of History in Columbia University, New York. Fellow of the Medieval Academy of America. President of the History of Science Society, 1928–9.

Rev. JOHN TODD, M.A., F.S.A. Rector of Waterstock, Oxon. Formerly Lecturer in Divinity, Trinity College, Toronto.

JOSIAH CHARLES TRENT, M.D. Assistant Professor of Surgery (in charge of thoracic surgery), Duke University, Durham, North Carolina. Formerly Instructor in Thoracic Surgery, University of Michigan Hospital.†

JEAN JOSEPH TRICOT-ROYER, M.D. Chevalier de la Légion d'Honneur. Formerly Professor of the History of Medicine in the University of Louvain. Président d'Honneur of the Fédération Médicale Belge, of the Cercle Médicale de la Province d'Anvers, and of the Société Internationale d'Histoire de la Médecine. Founder of the International Congresses of the History of Medicine. Elected in 1940 an Honorary Member of the History of Medicine Section of the Royal Society of Medicine. Founder of *Yperman* (1922), and editor-in-chief of *Le Scalpel* (1942–51).

DOROTHY MABEL TURNER (Mrs. D. M. FEYER), M.A., B.Sc., Ph.D. Senior Lecturer at the Maria Grey Training College, London. Formerly Research Assistant, University College, London. Writer on the history of science and of the teaching of science.

EDGAR ASHWORTH UNDERWOOD, M.A., B.Sc., M.D., D.P.H., F.L.S. Chevalier de la Légion d'Honneur. Director of the Wellcome Historical Medical Museum and of the Wellcome Historical Medical Library, London. Honorary Lecturer, University College, London. Thomas Vicary Lecturer, Royal College of Surgeons, 1946. Fielding H. Garrison Lecturer, American Association of the History of Medicine, 1947. President of the History of Medicine Section, Royal Society of Medicine, 1948–50. General editor of the ' Publications of the Wellcome Historical Medical Museum '.

JOHAN ADRIAAN VOLLGRAFF, Candidat-ingénieur, Matheseos et Physices Doctor. Formerly Privat-docent in the History of Science in the University of Leyden, and Professor of Mathematics in the University of Ghent. President of the Académie Internationale d'Histoire des Sciences, 1950–3. Editor-in-chief of *Janus*, 1938–41.

ERNEST WICKERSHEIMER, M.D. Formerly Administrateur of the Bibliothèque Nationale et Universitaire, Strasbourg. Elected in 1914 an Honorary Member of the Section of the History of Medicine of the Royal Society of Medicine. Author of works on the history of medicine, and especially medieval medicine. Editor of the *Bulletin de la Societé française d'Histoire de la Médecine*, 1910–14.

DOROTHY WRINCH, M.A., M.Sc., D.Sc. Lecturer in the Department of Physics, Smith College, Northampton, Massachusetts. Formerly Member of the Faculty of the Physical Sciences, University of Oxford, and Lecturer in Pure Mathematics, University College, London.

PREFACE

FOR the convenience of the reader it may be well to indicate that this tribute to a great historian is arranged according to the following plan. The text as a whole is divided into eight books, the first seven of which treat the history of science and of medicine as it unfolds itself in chronological periods. The eighth book includes essays which deal with the history of individual subjects over long periods, or with bibliographical and similar matters which find no place in a chronological arrangement. The sequence of the essays in each book is similar, the usual order being :— General problems of science; the physical sciences; the biological sciences; anatomy and physiology; the history of medicine from the scientific aspect; the history of clinical medicine. In the earlier books the arrangement is also based partly on the various civilizations or periods dealt with.

I am much indebted to certain colleagues for the help which they have given me in seeing this work through the press. Mr. W. J. Bishop, Mr. F. N. L. Poynter and Miss S. R. Burstein have on many occasions saved my time by checking various specific points. Miss Jean Hall and Miss Jennifer Willison have assisted with the clerical work. Mr. J. W. Michieli prepared for me a number of excellent photographs. To my former secretary, Miss Peggy Brister (Mrs. Bernard Farrell), and my present secretary, Miss Eileen J. Baker, I am deeply indebted for the great assistance which they have given me in the long process of preparation of the typescript and the checking of proofs. Miss M. E. Rowbottom has throughout given me the most unstinted assistance with the proofs, and my indebtedness to her is difficult to acknowledge. In the preparation of the index of persons I was greatly assisted by the expert advice on many points which was freely given to me by Mr. C. A. Earnshaw. He also undertook to prepare from my rough subject slips the very valuable subject index as it now appears. This heavy task involved the detailed reading of the whole of the text several times.

It is a pleasure to me to express my appreciation of the advice on detailed points given me by various friends; of these I would wish to mention especially Professor K. J. Franklin, Professor Edv. Gotfredsen, Dr. Douglas McKie, and Mr. C. B. Oldman. I am much indebted to Professor Henry E. Sigerist for vital assistance at a time when it seemed possible that the difficulties associated with publication might prove insuperable. It gives me pleasure to express my most sincere gratitude to Sir Arthur Salusbury MacNalty for his constant encouragement, for writing the introduction, and for reading through the whole of the final proofs.

The Nuffield Foundation came to my assistance at a critical period, and it is impossible for me to express adequately my indebtedness to its Trustees for having, out of regard for the recipient's eminence, made an exception to their usual practice and taken a step which enabled the work to be published. To them, and to Mr. L. Farrer-Brown, their Secretary, and Mr. W. A. Sanderson, their Assistant Secretary, I am deeply indebted.

E. A. U.

CONTENTS

VOLUME ONE

BOOK I. THE ANCIENT WORLD

BOOK II. THE MEDIEVAL WORLD

BOOK III. THE RENAISSANCE

BOOK IV. THE NEW PHILOSOPHY

VOLUME TWO

BOOK V. THE INSURGENT CENTURY

BOOK VIII.   CONSPECTUS GENERALES

LIST OF PLATES

VOLUME ONE

VOLUME TWO

ERRATA TO VOLUME ONE

Page 51, line 26 : the Edwin Smith Papyrus is now in the New York Academy of Medicine.

Page 73, note 44, *after* Adams, *op. cit.* (1(a)) *add* vol. iii.

Page 88, note 23, *for* Karsen *read* Karsten.

Page 106, note 25, *for* Spenser *read* Spencer.

Page 127, note 16, *for* Gundev-Shapur *read* Gunder Shapur. (The transliteration Jundi Shapur is now preferred.)

Page 199, line 33, *for* (112) *read* (122).

Page 216, line 42, *for* latter *read* later.

Page 272, lines 17 and 47, *for* Thorndyke *read* Thorndike.

Page 322, legend to Fig. 2, *for cicones read eicones.*

Page 346, line 16, *for* Johnston's *read* Jonston's.

Page 365, line 8, *for* Arantius (d. 1619) *read* Arantius (d. 1589).

Page 555, order : *read* Buragna *before* Burnet.

Page 558, line 40, *for* Giovani *read* Giovan.

INTRODUCTION

by

SIR ARTHUR SALUSBURY MacNALTY, K.C.B., M.A., M.D., F.R.C.P., F.R.C.S., Hon.F.R.S.(Ed.)

AS one who has been a close friend of Charles Singer since the years when we were both young practitioners of the Healing Art, and who, like him, has held the honourable office of President of the History of Medicine Section of the Royal Society of Medicine, it is my high privilege to write an Introduction to this work. It is a mark of the affection and admiration of the contributors for him, our dear colleague and master.

ἡ εὐδαιμονία ἐνέργειά τίς ἐστι.

'Happiness consists in the active employment of the faculties.'

Charles Singer, now advanced in years but ever young in spirit, must indeed be happy when he reflects on the great contributions to knowledge which he has made during his long life. He has founded a School of historical research in Medicine and Science, illuminated it with thought and wisdom, and given forth its teaching with eloquence and literary distinction. Colleagues, pupils and friends, on the invitation of Dr. Ashworth Underwood, have gladly joined in a tribute to the Master of research in the History of Medicine and Science.

The essays in this work—ninety in number—range over a very wide field in the history of Medicine, Science and Learning. They were chosen by the editor to illuminate important and interesting problems in these fields. We contributors put aside our wonted avocations to add our leaves to the chaplet of laurels, which we offer as a tribute to our honoured leader. Charles Singer's fame is world-wide, and the contributions come from Great Britain, the United States of America, and from the leading writers in these fields on the European Continent. Significantly they show the influence and spirit of the master's teaching. To all and each of the writers this self-imposed task has been a labour of love. We are grateful to Dr. Underwood for giving us the opportunity of contributing to this work, and for the care and trouble which he has taken in arranging and editing the material and seeing it through the press.

In reading the essays Charles Singer will recognize the influence which he has exerted by his writings and stimulating conversations on those who have contributed to this work. It is a source of gratification to us all that he continues to give historical Medicine and Science the fruits of his knowledge, and we wish him health and strength for further years to come in which to enrich sound learning. Our good wishes are tendered also to Mrs. Singer, herself an historian of distinction, who has often collaborated in her husband's studies and who shares his triumphs and high ideals.

The contributions in these two volumes, with the illustrations, range from the twilight of history, when early man made his first designs on the rocks of caves and on monoliths, to the nineteenth century and after. The reader from studying the foundations of medicine in the Ancient World in Book I will see continued in Book II its maintenance in the Medieval World, which, at all events by the fifteenth century, was less dark than has been commonly supposed. In Book III the sudden radiance of the Renaissance blazes on mankind, and in the work of Vesalius and others we can mark the beginnings of modern experimental medicine.   Book IV treats comprehensively of the New Philosophy and in Book V the reader is introduced to the Insurgent Century, Charles Singer's own term for the wonderful seventeenth century in which William Harvey discovered the circulation of the blood and the Royal Society was founded. Book VI deals with several medical pioneers of the eighteenth century, so productive in medical discovery and clinical observation.   In Book VII several aspects of medical research in the nineteenth century and after are described, which brings the reader to the threshold of medical history in modern times. Finally in Book VIII, *Conspectus Generales*, he is presented with delightful general essays on various aspects of the history of medicine and science. Among these essays will be found last tributes, *ave atque vale*, from those no longer with us, like Sir Charles Sherrington, Sir D'Arcy Thompson and Major Greenwood.

If any stars in this galaxy shine less brightly in comparison with the greater ones, the recipient of these essays in his charity will not regard them with a too critical eye.   For we may say to Charles Singer, as Sir Thomas Browne said to Nicholas Bacon: " To wish all Readers of your Abilities, were unreasonably to multiply the Number of Scholars beyond the Temper of these Times ... and knowing you a serious Student in the highest *arcanas* of Nature, with much excuse we bring these low Delights and poor Maniples to your Treasure."

April, 1953.   ARTHUR S. MacNALTY.

BOOK I

THE ANCIENT WORLD

THE CONSTITUTION OF ARCHAEOLOGY AS A SCIENCE*

by

V. GORDON CHILDE

AS a humble tribute to a distinguished historian of science and representative of the oldest science, I venture to summarize some of the steps by which the youngest science has developed distinctive methods of its own that justify its pretensions to that status. The purest archaeological methods have been elaborated for, and are best exemplified in, that branch termed prehistoric. But though prehistory will figure prominently in my exposition, the same methods are applicable to all branches. I take archaeology to be the systematic search for, and comparison and classification of, the substantial remains of human handiwork. It originates in two distinct branches of learning—in the humanities on the one hand, in natural science on the other—and must blend both traditions. They could hardly coalesce till Darwin's vindication of Evolution had broken down the barrier between human history and natural history, and Marx's materialist conception of history, announced in the same year, had emphasized the significance of the instruments of production that constitute so large a part of the archaeologist's materials.

The humanistic component begins with the Renaissance; for that meant a revived study not only of classical literature, but also of classical art and architecture. Soon indeed the historians of antiquity themselves turned to coins and inscriptions as supplements to the traditional manuscript sources.[1] Then in the eighteenth century the reaction against classicism, termed the Romantic Movement, and the first stirrings of nationalism turned the attention of some educated Europeans to ancestral monuments not only of the Middle Ages, but of the prehistoric pagan past, termed 'Ancient British', 'Gaulois', 'Germanische', and so on. The same search for local colour penetrated even to classical studies when the first excavations at Herculaneum (1738) and Pompeii (1748) showed how the actual everyday life of an ancient city might be reconstituted.

The scientific survey of Egypt initiated by Napoleon I included a systematic examination and recording of the monuments of the Nile Valley. The consequent decipherment of hieroglyphics by Akerblad and Champollion (1802–32) unlocked a volume of ancient history extending two millennia further back than the oldest Greek texts, but preserved in native sources that had to be recovered and reconstructed by archaeological means rather than by the criticism of literary narratives. A parallel volume came into view when Botta in 1842 dug up the first known monuments of Assyrian art. Its contents were made accessible by Rawlinson, Hincks, Talbot and Oppert between 1837 and 1857, though the first Sumerian chapters were available only at second hand till 1880 when the French started excavations

* This essay was written in 1946. [Editor.]

[1] The title of the French foundation of 1716—Académie des Inscriptions et Belles-Lettres—is symptomatic.

at Tello (Lagash). But classical archaeology, Egyptology and Assyriology
remained engrossed in the discovery and study of inscriptions, objects of
art and monumental architecture till the irruption of the Romantic,
Schliemann, into the Aegean (Troy, 1870), of the prehistorians, Petrie and
de Morgan, into Egypt (1895–6), and of Petrie's disciples, Mackay and
Woolley, into Mesopotamia (Kish, al Ubaid, Ur, 1923–4), compelled the
proper collection and observation of less impressive, but not less significant,
antiquities.

For the romantic gentlemen, who like Stukeley (1724–43) surveyed and
excavated 'Druidic temples', 'Celtic tumuli' and 'Danish camps', had been
obliged by the very poverty of their material to lavish as much care on
unsculptured stones, rude flint implements, sherds of unpainted vases and
scraps of corroded metal as classicists and orientalists bestowed on more
spectacular remains. But though the devotees of prehistory had been
slowly amassing material and were elaborating appropriate methods for its
classification, they received little encouragement from their more fortunate
colleagues. In 1851 Daniel Wilson[2] pleads for an alliance with natural
science; Worsaae[3] in 1869 exults in its establishment. In the interval,
The Origin of Species had appeared.

Ere then the naturalist tradition had substantially enriched the material
and the methodology of archaeology. The prescription of 'powdered
mummy, unicorn's horns and giants' bones' in pharmacopœias as late as the
eighteenth century brought archaeological objects within the ken of medical
science. The antique belief in the curative properties of nephrite was
responsible for the observation and accurate description[4] of a burial in a
megalithic tomb exposed in 1685 at Cocherel near Evreux. Stone axes,
popularly regarded as thunderbolts and learnedly labelled 'keraunia', were
admittedly a proper subject for natural philosophy. Mercati (1541–92),
Curator of the Vatican Botanical Gardens, had correctly interpreted them as
human implements by comparison with the stone hatchets of the newly
discovered aborigines of America, but in 1778 Buffon still had to mention
them as 'les premiers monuments de l'art de l'homme dans l'état de nature
pure' in his *Époques de la Nature*.

The vitrified forts of Scotland attracted the attention of eighteenth-century
geologists under the impression that they were products of volcanic activity.[5]
But the geologists themselves established the existence and status of relics
of pleistocene man. Dean Buckland,[6] indeed, in the interest of Bishop Usher's
chronology, 'rejuvenated by some 20,000 years' what was really the first

[2] Daniel Wilson, *Archaeology and prehistoric annals of Scotland*. Edinburgh, 1851. In
the preface he complains of 'the spirit of Antiquarianism limiting its range within the mediaeval
era and abandoning to isolated labourers that ampler field of research which embraces the
Prehistoric period of nations and belongs, not to literature, but to the science of Nature'.

[3] J. J. A. Worsaae: 'Les érudits classiques de l'école ancienne se moquèrent longtemps de
cette Archéologie nouvelle, qui ne s'occupait que de temps barbares. Mais les naturalistes
vinrent au secours des Archéologues nationaux.' (Presidential address, *Compt. rend. Congrès
internat. d'Arch. et d'Anthrop. préhistoriques, Copenhagen, 1868*. Copenhagen, 1875, p. 4.)

[4] The description of this burial is preserved in Bernard de Montfaucon, *L'antiquité expliquée
et représentée en figures*. Paris, 1719, vol. v, pt. ii, pp. 194–7.

[5] Their artificial character was recognized in 1777 by John Williams. See his *An account
of some remarkable ancient ruins, discovered in the Highlands*. Edinburgh, 1777.

[6] W. Buckland, *Reliquiae diluvianae*. London, 1823, pp. 82–98.

PLATE II

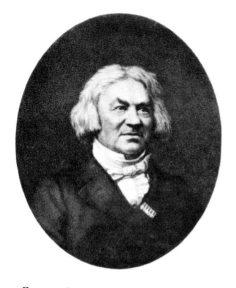

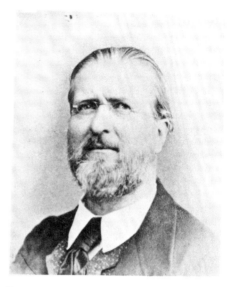

FIG. 1. CHRISTIAN JÜRGENSEN THOMSEN
(1788–1865)

FIG. 2. GABRIEL DE MORTILLET (1821–1898)

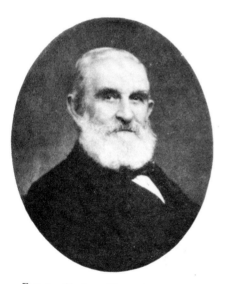

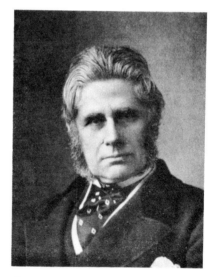

FIG. 3. SIR JOHN EVANS (1828–1903)

FIG. 4. Lieut.-Gen. A. H. LANE FOX
PITT-RIVERS (1827–1900)

recorded Palaeolithic burial that he uncovered in Paviland Cave. Similarly, French savants rejected Boucher de Perthes' copious proofs, set forth in 1847 as a result of long researches in gravel pits on the high terraces of the Somme. But in 1859 John Evans and Prestwich visited his sites and endorsed his implements. Henceforth, the tools of pleistocene man were admitted as objects of study by archaeologists and geologists alike. It remained to blend both the materials and the methods contributed by the two traditions.

By the end of the eighteenth century antiquaries and naturalists had amassed collections of 'curios', and compiled atlases of monuments sufficiently comprehensive to show that even products of human activity could be reduced to a manageable number of abstract types, comparable to the genera and species of animals and plants in the old zoological and botanical gardens. Mercati had at least shown how to discover the use of types if that was not obvious. To become a science archaeology must now produce a distinctive classification for its types.

The decisive step was taken by C. J. Thomsen.[7] Called upon to arrange a large collection of types obtained by systematic excavations in the tumuli and kitchen-middens of Denmark, he decided about 1818 to group together those used at the same time. His principle of classification was thus historical, but, as the relics concerned were uninscribed and undescribed in any contemporary records, Thomsen could not define his period by dynastic labels (like our 'Tudor') nor yet by centuries. He chose instead as the basis of classification the material used for the principal cutting implements and so defined 'the Three Ages' as 'Stone', 'Bronze', and 'Iron' respectively. His successor, Worsaae, by applying the naturalist principle of stratigraphy, borrowed from geology, showed that the assemblages of types thus classified together did in fact follow one another in that order. Indeed, stratigraphical observations have since shown that Stone, Bronze, and Iron Ages in this sense do follow one another in the same order wherever they can be distinguished at all.

Thomsen's principle of classification is both easy to apply and obviously significant. It was accordingly rapidly adopted in other countries besides Denmark. But then the term 'Age', though perfectly legitimate as applied to a homogeneous area like Denmark, was liable to suggest a definite period of sidereal time like the geologists' 'pleistocene'. The danger was aggravated as soon as attempts were made to subdivide the Ages. As early as 1861 Worsaae[8] was calling for a subdivision of the Stone Age into an Older and a Younger even in Denmark. Elsewhere it was perhaps more urgent; the discoveries of Boucher de Perthes, followed by those of Lartet and others, left the relics of pleistocene man to be classified while the exposure of lake-dwellings through the low waters of the Swiss lakes in 1853–4 had brought the late Stone Age to life. The contrast was given terminological expression in the names Palaeolithic and Neolithic proposed by Lubbock[9] in 1865. Unhappily, new bases of division had crept in, and three disparate criteria

[7] G. Daniel in *The Three Ages*. Cambridge, 1943, has given a good account of Thomsen's principles and their subsequent development.

[8] J. J. A. Worsaae, 'Om Tvedelingen af Stenalderen'. *Videnskabs Selskabs Oversigt*, 1861, pp. 273–5.

[9] Sir John Lubbock, *Prehistoric times*. London, 1865, p. 2.

were accepted—technological (the use of simple flaking or polishing in sharpening stone implements), palaeontological (association with extinct or recent fauna), and economic (hunting or farming).

For further subdividing the Ages the typological method, inspired by contemporary biology, had been devised. In its first application in 1841 to trace 'The Evolution of Ancient British Coins from Philippi', John Evans had, as he himself later said, 'attempted to apply the principles of "evolution" and "natural selection" to numismatic enquiries'. The method was subsequently applied to the evolution of bronze axes by Franks in 1863,[10] and then refined and given extended application especially by Montelius, beginning in 1876.[11] Typology does enable the archaeologist to distinguish a sequence of periods, but only within a single province and culture and when the direction of the evolution can be controlled by independent criteria. Failure to observe these reservations was to give rise to absurd confusions.

All these confusions and dangers were exemplified and sanctified in the system devised by Gabriel de Mortillet[12] for the arrangement of the Musée des Antiquités Nationales, founded in 1862 by Napoleon III as an adjunct to the *Histoire de César* he was engaged in writing. The prehistoric collections to be classified were derived from the whole of Roman Gaul, a much more diversified area than Denmark, and few types had as well authenticated contexts as those handled by Thomsen. Yet de Mortillet's system was applied extensively in Europe and even to relics from Asia, Africa and America. The exposure of its inherent contradictions and confusions accordingly involved a re-examination of the Three Age system itself, and ultimately revealed what archaeology ought to classify.

In the division of the Stone Age de Mortillet accepted under protest the technological as well as the palaeontological criterion; he qualified *paléolithique* as '*âge de la pierre simplement taillée*' and *néolithique* as '*âge de la pierre polie*', apparently believing that both criteria led to a concordant result. It was soon shown that polished stone axes did not appear as soon as the pleistocene fauna vanished. In 1874 Torell[13] told the Stockholm Congress: 'Nous aurions dans le Nord les restes d'une étape de civilisation et d'une période, qui paraissent s'intercaler entre la période du renne et l'âge du silex poli. Il faut distinguer dans le vaste âge de la pierre, une subdivision nouvelle, la période mésolithique.' After the stratigraphical observations of Piette at Mas d'Azil (1899) and Capitan's misinterpretation of le Campigny (1898), the Mesolithic (or Epipalaeolithic) was accepted as a major division of the Stone Age to accommodate all pre-neolithic but post-pleistocene assemblages of relics. The 'Three Ages' have thus grown to five and one is equated with a geological period.

---

[10] A. W. Franks, in J. M. Kemble, *Horae ferales; studies in the archaeology of northern nations.* Ed. R. G. Latham and A. W. Franks. London, 1863, p. 143.

[11] Oscar Montelius, 'Sur le premier âge du fer dans les provinces baltiques de la Russie et en Pologne'. *Compt. rend. Congrès internat. d'Arch. et d'Anthrop. préhistoriques, Buda Pest, 1876.* Budapest, 1877, pp. 481–93.

[12] Gabriel de Mortillet's first version was published in *Matériaux pour l'histoire primitive et philosophique de l'homme,* 1868; his first revised version in *ibid.,* 1876, pp. 545 ff.; the last in 1904. The geological qualification 'Quatérnaire' is confined to the first subdivision of the Palaeolithic in 1868.

[13] Otto Torell, *Compt. rend. Congrès internat. d'Arch. et d'Anthrop. préhistoriques, Stockholm, 1874.* Stockholm, 1876, p. 876.

Not content with bisecting the Stone Age, de Mortillet subdivided the Palaeolithic into (Chellean) Acheulian, Mousterian, Solutrean (Aurignacian),[14] and Magdalenian, all named after French sites. These subdivisions are defined by types and techniques of flint-work, but treated as of the same kind as the major division, Palaeolithic itself. In so far as this sequence was based on typology—a supposed evolutionary series of bifacial tools—it simply did not conform to observed stratigraphical facts. Breuil[15] in 1906 just completed the work of d'Acy, Boule, Piette and Rivière when he secured the re-admission of the Aurignacian as a phase between Mousterian and Solutrean.

A much graver defect in de Mortillet's system was that it exalted or degraded types of knife or techniques of flint-work to the role of *Leitfossilen* that could define periods of geological time like fossil elephants and fossil reptiles. Now no serious archaeologist had imagined that the types of bronze and iron artifacts used to define Thomsen's later Ages had anything like this universal significance as indicators of sidereal time. On the contrary, it had always been recognized that these prehistoric Ages in northern and western Europe were partly contemporary with historical periods in Italy, Greece, Egypt and Hither Asia.[16] Indeed, throughout the nineteenth century prehistorians have been trying, by identifying dateable imports from literate civilizations in the graves of illiterate barbarians, to estimate a local 'Age's' duration and determine its position within a universal frame of reference provided independently by the written historical record.[17]

Before 3000 B.C., when the written record fails, an independent chronometer could be sought in the geological-palaeontological record to which appeal had in fact been made in defining the Palaeolithic. The general recognition of several glaciations, foreseen by Morlot as early as 1854, provided an equally independent time scale within the pleistocene into which the subdivisions of the Palaeolithic should be fitted. Since Boule in 1888 published his pioneer *Essai de Paléontologie stratigraphique de l'Homme*, archaeologists were offered the prospect of being able to say whether any two assemblages of types, at least in Europe, belonged to the same glacial or interglacial, i.e., whether they were contemporary in terms of the independent chronometer provided by climatic fluctuations.

[14] Suppressed in 1876.

[15] H. Breuil, 'Les gisements présolutréens du type d'Aurignac'. *Compt. rend. Congrès internat. d'Arch. et d'Anthrop. préhistoriques, Monaco, 1906*. Monaco, 1907, pp. 323–46.

[16] In 1870 indeed L. Lindenschmidt (in the foreword to *Die Alterthümer unserer heidnischen Vorzeit*. Mainz, 1870, vol. ii) abandoned—unnecessarily—the 'System des Stein-, Erz-, und Eisenalters' in the belief that bronze implements found north of the Alps were just Phoenician, Etruscan or Greek imports. Alexandre Bertrand insisted that bronze was not used synchronously even all over Greece (*Archéologie celtique et gauloise*. Paris, 1876, p. 10).

[17] The beginning of the Bronze Age—for example in Central Europe—which is in practice as far as 'historical chronology' is likely to get, can, it was assumed, be dated by local imitations of historical Oriental types. 'About 1000 B.C.' was admitted by Montelius in 1873. After Schliemann's discoveries were better appreciated, Montelius in 1882 raised the limit about five centuries, and then in 1900 to the 'allerersten Jahrhunderten des zweiten Jahrtausends' ('Chronologie der ältesten Bronzezeit in Nord-Deutschland', *Archiv f. Anthrop.*, 1898, xxv, 443–83)—a rise not accepted by Sophus Müller, Naue, Hoernes and others. In 1909 Hubert Schmidt, however, raised Montelius' estimate by half a millenium (*Praehist. Zeitschr.*, 1909, i, 138). In the light of the new evidence accumulated since 1930 and the revision of Oriental chronology, the date must lie between 1600 (when European products appear in dated contexts in the Aegean for the first time) and 2400 (the earliest emergence in Mesopotamia of types copied in barbarian Europe).

The further development of a chronological framework, whether by historical or geological[18] means or by the more recent palaeobotanical[19] or astronomical[20] methods, is no part of the history of archaeology as such. Here then it suffices to point out that the potential existence of such an independent frame of reference renders superfluous the use of archaeological types as indicators of geological age. But this misuse of Palaeolithic types, both by geologists and archaeologists, was in practice only ended by the extension to the whole of the Stone Age of another conception and another classificatory principle, this time again derived from the humanist tradition.

The early antiquaries of the eighteenth century had labelled Roman, Celtic, Gaulois, Germanische the tumuli or camps they dug and the stone or bronze relics they collected, because they assumed them to have been made and used by these 'nations'. That at least implied that the recurrence together of similar types was due not to contemporaneity alone, and that differences between types depended partly on the same factors as those between Roman and Egyptian sculptures or architecture. In the same spirit nineteenth-century prehistorians had 'explained' the changes in the archaeological record, indeed the transition from one Age to the next, by the advent of new peoples; so the Bronze Age north of the Alps would begin with Phoenician colonists (Nilsson) or immigrants from Asia (Worsaae and many others)—often labelled Aryans under the influence of linguistic theory. In the same spirit de Morgan (1897)[21] and Petrie (1896)[22] would attribute the rise of Egyptian civilization to immigrants from a still unknown Asia, like de Rougé in 1894.[23] In default of detailed evidence such identifications and migrations remained just guesses that relieved the prehistorian of the duty of explaining cultural change, till on the one hand prehistoric types could be correlated with historical data, on the other the coexistence, within the same Age or subdivision of an Age, of several distinct recurrent assemblages of types was established.

The excavations at Alesia instigated by Napoleon III from 1862–5 did show what types of weapon the Celts of Gaul had been really using at the time of the Conquest. That enabled Desor and Keller to recognize as Celtic also a great collection of iron weapons and implements just discovered at La Tène on Lake Neuchâtel. By 1871 de Mortillet could identify similar swords from graves in Upper Italy as memorials of the historically-attested Gaulish invasion, and in 1875 on the same principles Pulszky described the 'Denkmäler der Keltenherrschaft in Ungarn'.[24] So a recurrent assemblage

[18] By a study of varved clays, initiated in 1884, de Geer was enabled by 1910 to offer a 'geochronology of the last 10,000 years' in terms of solar years.

[19] Dendrochronology, based on tree-rings, has been successfully applied in America to archaeology. In north-western Europe pollen-analysis (v. infra, note (51)) reveals a succession of climatic phases, presumably contemporary all over the area and capable of being dated by geochronology.

[20] If the fluctuations in solar radiation effectively reaching the Earth explain ice ages, Milankovich's curve reflecting them will date the glaciations and interglacials.

[21] Jacques de Morgan, Recherches sur les origines de l'Égypte : II. Ethnographie préhistorique. Paris, 1897.

[22] W. M. Flinders Petrie and J. E. Quibell, Naqada and Ballas, 1895. London, 1896.

[23] Vicomte J. de Rougé, 'Origine de la race égyptienne'. Mém. de la Soc. nat. des Antiquaires de France, Paris, 1894, liv, 264–87.

[24] I take these points from J. M. de Navarro, A survey of research on an early phase of Celtic culture. Oxford, 1936. (British Academy, Rhys Memorial Lecture.)

of types, first taken to be distinctive of a subdivision of the Iron Age, was recognized as expressive of the common traditions of a people who shared also a common language.

A dramatic demonstration of the coexistence of two distinct assemblages of types repeatedly associated together in the Stone Age of so small and uniform an area as Denmark was given by Sophus Müller[25] in 1898. His excavation of a number of 'separate graves', distinguished as a class from the collective megalithic tombs by Reeh and Smith in 1891, revealed that these normally contained types of weapons, pottery and ornaments quite different from those regularly found in the collective tombs, but were strictly contemporary with the latter, as exceptional types, common to both, proved. Such arbitrary differences in burial customs, armament and fashions could only be due to divergent social traditions; their coherence in recurrent assemblages must reflect the unity of social groups.

About the same time a similar multiplicity of distinct but recurrent assemblages had been recognized in Central Europe by Czech and German investigators, not only in the Stone Age but also in Roman and post-Roman times; some of the latter were more or less successfully identified with the Celtic, Teutonic and Slavic tribes known from literary sources. Such assemblages were termed *Kulturgruppen* or simply *Kulturen* in German, and were most easily distinguished by, and often named after, pottery styles. By the end of the nineteenth century Kossinna, trained originally as a philologist, after plotting the distribution of the relevant types, felt justified in asserting: 'Scharf umgrenzte archäologische Kulturprovinzen decken sich zu allen Zeiten mit ganz bestimmten Völker oder Volkstämmen; Kulturgebiete sind Volksgebiete, Kulturgruppen Völker.' In 1902 he added: 'Wir stehen also vor der altbekannten Tatsache dass die Völker zwar durch Kulturgruppen repräsentiert werden, nicht aber, auch nicht in der neolithischen Zeit, mit bestimmten Rassen zusammenfallen.'[26]

The new refined concept, most unhappily expressed by the overworked word 'culture', won rapid recognition in the twentieth century. It was brilliantly applied in Britain by Abercromby[27] in 1901 in tracing the origin of the Beaker folk. But it was never welcomed by French archaeologists, and was scarcely applied to the Old Stone Age till the middle twenties. The types of de Mortillet were still taken as representing the one culture of each temporal subdivision of that Age.

Admittedly, in 1880 Boyd Dawkins[28] had dared to assert that Mousterian, Solutrean and Magdalenian did not represent a sequence but local differences due to tribal isolation. Moreover, by 1906 it was becoming obvious that the Upper Palaeolithic industries of the Mediterranean area would not fit neatly into de Mortillet's series. Indeed, in 1912 Breuil[29] disengaged from the

[25] Sophus Müller, 'De jydske Enkeltgrave fra Stenalderen'. *Aarböger for Nordisk Oldkyndighed og Historie.* Copenhagen, 1898, xiii, 157–282; cf. *ibid.,* 1891, vi, 329–45.

[26] G. Kossinna, 'Die indogermanische Frage archäologisch beantwortet'. *Zeitschr. f. Ethnol.* 1902, xxxiv, 218.

[27] J. Abercromby, *Journ. Roy. Anthrop. Inst.,* 1902, xxxii, 390 ff.

[28] Boyd Dawkins, in article 'Early Man' in *Encyclop. Britannica,* 9th edition, 1880.

[29] H. Breuil, 'Les subdivisions du Paléolithique supérieur'. *Compt. rend. Congrès internat. d'Arch. et d'Anthrop. préhistoriques, Geneva, 1912.* Geneva, 1913, vol. i, pp. 165–238.

series not only the Mediterranean types but also the Solutrean. But the first systematic exposition of the plurality of cultures coexisting in the last phase of the last Ice Age, corresponding to the Upper Palaeolithic in archaeology, was given by Menghin in 1925 as an appendix to the third edition of Hoernes, *Urgeschichte der bildenden Kunst in Europa*.

To the Lower Palaeolithic the idea was applied in the next year. Obermaier[30] had indeed pointed out in 1919 that the core implements—hand-axes— typical of the Chellean and Acheulian 'periods' were absent from regions where nevertheless flake implements did occur in geologically contemporary strata. Yet such flakes were labelled either 'Chellean-Acheulian' regardless of typology, or Mousterian to the general confusion of chronology. In 1926 Breuil[31] showed in detail that assemblages of flake tools, made by the peculiar Levallois technique, existed throughout the last interglacial, contemporary with Acheulian hand-axes but unmixed with them. In the sequel, by a comparative survey of material gathered from all over the world, he[32] and his school, and Menghin[33] and his disciples, claim to have established the coexistence throughout the pleistocene of at least two distinct traditions of flint-working.

It has thus emerged that the first step in the classification of archaeological types should be to define recurrent assemblages, i.e. 'cultures'. It is only such cultures that are to be classified serially in Ages. But the Ages themselves are not periods of time everywhere contemporary, but technological Stages, universally homotaxial.[31] This interpretation of the Ages as Stages is of course no novelty; it is indeed just the original usage of Lucretius. But its revival has required a reconsideration of the basis of classification. One of the advantages of Thomsen's scheme was that the use of stone, bronze or iron for instruments of production seemed patently to denote progressive steps in Man's control over Nature that might be expected to have far-reaching social consequences. This advantage has been sacrificed in the subdivision of the Stone Age, for which, as we say, three discrepant criteria were once simultaneously invoked.

Of these, the palaeontological introduced an entirely alien principle of division and, though unhappily still retained in the definition of the Palaeolithic, has been abandoned for the Neolithic by all archaeologists.[35] The technological criterion of the latter, the polishing of stone for axe-heads, does not seem likely to have had anything like the same effect on the life and economy of a society as did the substitution of metal for stone as the material for their manufacture. There is no logical reason why polished stone axes should go together with stock-breeding and agriculture, the third criterion, and in fact they do not either in the archaeological or in the

[30] Hugo Obermaier, 'Los derroteros del Paleolítico antiguo en Europa'. *Bol. Real. Acad. Hist.*, Madrid, 1920, lxxvi, 214; also 'Das Paläolithikum u. Epipaläolithikum Spaniens'. *Anthropos*, 1919–20, xiv–xv, 147.

[31] H. Breuil, *Man*, 1926, xxvi, 176.

[32] *idem*, 'Les industries à éclat du Paléolithique ancien'. *Préhistoire*, 1932, i, 125–90.

[33] Oswald Menghin, *Weltgeschichte der Steinzeit*. Vienna, 1931.

[34] This geological term, coined by Huxley, was revived in archaeology by H. Peake in his Huxley Lecture (*Journ. Roy. Anthrop. Inst.*, 1940, lxx, 131).

[35] Some geologists still misuse 'Neolithic' to designate any post-pleistocene 'Stone Stage' assemblage.

ethnographic record. The inhabitants of Esthonia in early post-glacial times and the recent Indians of British Columbia both used polished stone for axe-heads; neither cultivated plants nor bred animals for food.

On the other hand the immense importance of stock-breeding and agriculture was from the first adequately emphasized by Nilsson, Lubbock, de Mortillet and their successors. In the twentieth century Elliot Smith joined de Morgan to insist most eloquently on the revolutionary significance of the contrast between what he termed 'food-gatherers' (hunters, fishers and collectors) and 'food-producers' (cultivators and/or stock-breeders). 'Food production' in this sense has been taken as the criterion of the Neolithic by Childe and Peake, and is now rather widely current. Thus in archaeological classification the Neolithic has recovered the same sort of general significance as the other Ages.

The remaining divisions of the Stone Age need similar revision. In the last thirty years it has become obvious that the cleavage between the cultures designated serially Lower and Middle Palaeolithic on the one hand, and those bracketed together as Upper Palaeolithic on the other, is as great or greater than that between the latter and the Mesolithic. Even in 1909 the veteran French prehistorian and Orientalist, de Morgan,[36] to recognize this real cleavage in the Palaeolithic, proposed to restrict that term to the earlier half, and to label the Upper Palaeolithic 'Archaeolithic'. In view of the circumstance that up to date all the skeletal remains associated with Lower and Middle Palaeolithic cultures, or geologically contemporary therewith, belonged to extinct species, while Upper Palaeolithic industries seemed associated exclusively with men of *Sapiens* type, Elliot Smith[37] proposed the terms Palaeanthropic and Neanthropic respectively. But that would again introduce a palaeontological criterion into archaeological classification and is liable to be upset, since the makers of Lower Palaeolithic hand-axes are too imperfectly known for confident diagnosis. In 1926 Menghin[38] proposed the term 'Protolithic' for the older assemblages and adopted the name 'Miolithic', originally coined by Rellini, to comprise both the Upper Palaeolithic and the Mesolithic. This change would eliminate the double principle of classification and the ambiguous status of the Mesolithic. But Soviet archaeologists[39] have recently drawn attention to aspects of the European Mesolithic—fresh emphasis on collecting and fishing and a consequent increase in the stability of settlement—that might entitle it to a distinct status or even a rank parallel to the Neolithic in an economic hierarchy.

Preoccupation with classification involved the danger of an exclusive concentration on types, obviously useful for the determination of chronology

[36] Jacques de Morgan, *Les premières civilisations*. Paris, 1909. In his classification he admitted an Éolithique before Paléolithique and revived Mésolithique before Néolithique, but insists again that all these terms denote 'États' not 'Ages'.

[37] G. Elliot Smith, 'Primitive man'. *Proc. Brit. Acad.*, 1915–16, p. 475. Since then some antler implements that in Europe would be called 'Mesolithic' have been found in Java, at least in the same geological horizon as, if not associated with, skeletal remains of the distinctly Palaeanthropic *Homo soloensis* (see *L'Anthrop.*, 1936, xlvi, 360).

[38] Oswald Menghin, 'Zur Terminologie des Paläolithikums'. *Wien. prähist. Zeitschr.*, 1926, xiii, 7–13.

[39] For example, V. Krichevskiĭ, 'Mezolit i Neolit Evropy'. *Kratkie Soobshcheniya o dokladakh i polevykh issledovaniyakh*, 1940, iv, 6–12.

or the discrimination of cultures, that might be almost as one-sided as the classical archaeologists' and orientalists' absorption in inscriptions and objects of art. In particular the concept of culture had been used at first mainly for tracing the migrations. Even when not perverted to political ends, as it was by Kossinna, this pursuit was liable to turn prehistory into a pale imitation of old-fashioned politico-military history. Excluded by the nature of a science from observing individuals, some twentieth-century prehistorians have been content with abstract figures—cultures equated with tribes or races—that ape the motions of historical actors. The nineteenth-century pioneers of the science, like Anderson,[40] Montelius[41] and Gross,[42] had tried to reconstitute the life of the prehistoric inhabitants of Scotland, Sweden and Switzerland. In Childe's *Prehistory of Scotland*, Schuchhardt's *Alteuropa* or Reinerth's *Die jüngere Steinzeit der Schweiz*, interest seems to be focused on a succession of invasions or migrations.

Marxist archaeologists[43] in the U.S.S.R. have not altogether unjustly complained that 'bourgeois prehistorians' bring on their stage a succession of societies, generally from some vaguely defined starting-point, but when each has arrived, nothing happens until another society is introduced, equally mysteriously, to be just as passive before the footlights. On the other hand the Marxists, Kruglov and Podgaetskiĭ[44]—to take a single example—did extract a realistic and plausible account of the development of one prehistoric society on the Pontic steppes from the poor material from which Gorodtsov had deduced only a succession of nameless immigrant tribes.

Equally legitimate criticism with the same trend has been levelled by the functionalist school of ethnographers against the Diffusionists. Their concentration on types or traits, supposed to have been diffused, fostered a 'threads and patches conception of culture as a collection of disparate entities—the so-called culture-traits—brought together by pure historical accident and having only accidental relations to one another'.[45] But in fact the old objective, if overshadowed, has never been forgotten. In the thirties the ideal of presenting each culture as an integrated whole, which worked to achieve an adaptation to the environment and make life worth living, was at least revived, clarified by more precise definition and classification, and enriched by new techniques for filling the lamentable gaps in the archaeological record.

The reconstitution of the environment to which each culture was an adaptation was imposed on all students of the Palaeolithic by their dependence

[40] J. Anderson, *Scotland in pagan times: Iron age.* Edinburgh, 1883. *Idem, ibid., Bronze and stone ages.* Edinburgh, 1886.

[41] Oscar Montelius, *Om Lifvet i Sverige under Hednatiden.* Stockholm, 1873.

[42] V. Gross, *Les Protohelvètes ou les premiers colons sur les bords des lacs de Bienne et Neuchatel.* Berlin, 1883.

[43] For example, Bogayevski in a review of V. G. Childe's 'East European relations of Dimini culture'.

[44] Kruglov and Podgaetskiĭ, 'Rodovoe Obshchestvo na Stepeĭ vostochnoĭ Evropy'. *Izvestiya Gos. Akademiya Istoriĭ Materialnoĭ Kultury,* [Leningrad-Moskva] 1935, 119.

[45] Radcliffe Brown, *Amer. Anthrop.,* 1935, xxxvii, 401. His criticism applies both to the English school led by Elliot Smith (*The Ancient Egyptians.* London, 1911), who derive everything from Egypt; and the 'Kultur-historische Schule' of Graebner ('Kulturkreise und Kulturschichten in Ozeanien'. *Zeitschr. f. Ethnol.,* 1905, xxxvii, 28–53); and P. W. Schmidt in ethnography and Menghin in archaeology, who postulate several Kulturkreise spread all over the world apparently by migrations.

PLATE III

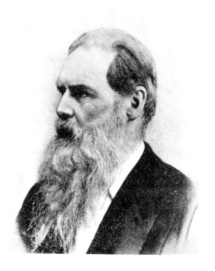

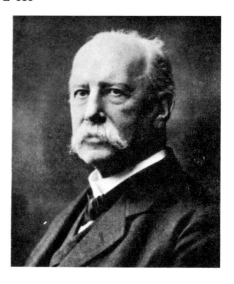

FIG. 5.   Sir EDWARD BURNETT TYLOR
(1832–1917)

FIG. 6.   OSKAR MONTELIUS (1843–1921)

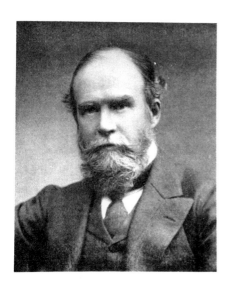

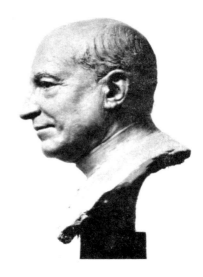

FIG. 7.   Sir JOHN LUBBOCK, Bt., first Baron
Avebury (1834–1913)

FIG. 8.   L'Abbé H. BREUIL (1877–   )
(From the bust by B. Champion, *Musée des
Antiquités nationales*)

on palaeontology for dating and by their geological training. For later periods, too, archaeologists now successfully invoke the aid of geographers, palaeobotanists, and meteorologists. By plotting type distributions on soil maps Schliz (1906)[46] and then Wahle (1920)[47] in Germany, and Crawford (1912)[48], Fleure (1917)[49] and Fox (1923)[50] and their school in Britain, began to work out the relations of prehistoric and later settlements to forests and other natural features. Variations in the composition of the temperate forests and fluctuations in the post-glacial climate have been revealed by the study of peat-bogs, initiated in 1877 and greatly refined by the technique of pollen-analysis since 1905.[51] Reference to these climatological and botanical results has enriched and corrected the archaeologists' pictures of the European environment since 1923.[52]

Organic materials have almost universally disappeared from the archaeo-logical record. But appropriate techniques have been developed to supplement its deficiencies. For instance, while remains of vegetable foods survive only exceptionally, casts of grains can regularly be observed on pottery. This clue, discovered by a Danish school-teacher in 1894, has been systematically followed up by Danish specialists, who extended their investigations successfully to the British Isles in 1939.[53] Dwelling-houses and many other constructions normally made of wood have vanished. They can be reconstructed from the impressions left by supports and founda-tions in the undisturbed subsoil. Pitt-Rivers in 1878[54] was the first to recognize post-holes in the chalk of Sussex. A suitable technique for the detection of such impressions in all soils was worked out by the Römisch-germanische Limeskommission between 1892 and 1902, and was being applied to prehistoric sites on löss soils as early as 1911, on drift hardly before 1923. After Crawford discovered its archaeological use in 1923, air-photography has come to the help of prehistory, since post-holes like any other disturbance in the subsoil show up as crop-marks.

Air-photographs also reveal ancient field boundaries far better than surface observations. With their aid Curwen[55] has shown how largely it is possible to reconstruct the rural economy of southern England in prehistoric, Roman and early medieval times. With the total excavation of a complete

---

[46] A. Schliz, 'Die schnurkeramische Kulturkreis'. *Zeitschr. f. Ethnol.*, 1906, xxxviii, 320 ff.

[47] Ernst Wahle, *Die Besiedelung Südwestdeutschlands in vorrömischer Zeit nach ihren natürlichen Grundlagen. XII Bericht der Römisch-Germanischen Kommission, 1920.* Frankfurt-am-Main, 1921.

[48] O. G. S. Crawford, 'The distribution of early Bronze Age Settlements in Britain'. *Geog. Journ.*, 1912, xl, 184–203, 304–17.

[49] H. J. Fleure, 'Ancient Wales: Anthropological evidences'. *Trans. Hon. Soc. Cymmrodorion, 1915–16.* London, 1917.

[50] Cyril Fox, *The archaeology of the Cambridge region.* Cambridge, 1923.

[51] J. G. D. Clark, in his *Mesolithic Settlement of Northern Europe.* Cambridge, 1936, summarizes the history of these methods.

[52] That is, after the publication of Helmot Gams and Rolf Nordhagen, *Postglaziale Klimaänder-ungen und Erdkrustenbewegung in Mitteleuropa.* Munich, 1923.

[53] Knud Jessen and Hans Helbaek, 'Cereals in Great Britain and Ireland in prehistoric times'. *K. Danske Vidensk. Selskab, Biol. Skrifter,* 1944, iii, No. 2.

[54] A. H. Lane-Fox [Pitt-Rivers], 'Excavations at Mount Caburn Camp'. *Archaeologia*, 1878, xlvi, 423–95.

[55] E. C. Curwen, 'Prehistoric agriculture in Britain'. *Antiquity*, 1927, i, 261–87.

Iron Age farm in 1938–9[56] the further prospect opened up of calculating the yield of a harvest and the area of a holding.

The total excavation of a whole settlement, whether a prehistoric village, an Oriental town or a Roman city, can provide information on population, social organization and economy that is seldom obtainable even from literary sources. It seems to have been the ideal of excavations on classical sites since the first operations at Pompeii. It could seldom be realized there owing to the magnitude of the task, and was only relevant in other domains when the culture sequence had been established by minor operations. Still, it was accomplished for Aegean prehistory in 1899–1901 at Phylakopi on Melos, in Neolithic Europe first at Köln-Lindenthal in 1928–31.[57]

As opposed to means of production, one aspect at least of the relations of production, trade,[58] has always been recognized as falling within the purview of archaeology. In fact the distribution of vases, gems and coins tells us more about Greek trade than the classical authors. The sources of information have been augmented both by the finer definition of 'cultures' and by closer co-operation with natural scientists. Petrographic analysis has shown for instance that the Blue Stones at Stonehenge had been brought to Salisbury Plain from Pembrokeshire, and that quite a number of Neolithic pots, used and broken at Köln-Lindenthal, had been made on the lower Main and transported downstream fifty miles.

The same study of the distribution by human agency of materials and manufactures is an index not only of trade, but of intercourse between the populations of different regions, and so of opportunities for diffusion—the pooling of ideas.

By the application of such techniques it should be possible to clothe dead bones with flesh, to present an archaeological culture as a functioning organism, and to recover not only the technology but also the economy at least of deceased societies. Thus interpreted, archaeological cultures might legitimately be compared with living societies as studied functionally by ethnography. Now archaeologists, particularly prehistorians, since Mercati, have turned to ethnography to supplement the deficiencies in their own sources. At the same time comparative ethnographers of the mid-nineteenth century, like Morgan and Tylor, made use of archaeological results. These were trying by comparative methods to trace the evolution of culture and the prehistory of institutions. In so far as Bachofen, Spencer, Maine and Tylor abstracted elements from their functional context and arranged them in evolutionary series, such could be charged with adopting the unscientific 'threads-and-patches' theory of culture. But Morgan's[59] divisions of savagery, barbarism and civilization did provide a hierarchy of stages into which societies could be classified as wholes. Yet it was rightly objected that the

---

[56] Gerhard Bersu, 'Excavations at Little Woodbury, Wiltshire'. *Proc. Prehist. Soc.*, 1940, n.s., vi, 30–111.

[57] W. Buttler and W. Haberey, *Die bandkeramische Ansiedlung bei Köln-Lindenthal.* (Römisch-Germanische Forschungen, No. 11). Berlin and Leipzig, 1936. Of course the total excavation of the Glastonbury Lake Village by Bulleid and Gray had revealed the value of total excavation on a prehistoric site as early as 1911.

[58] Prehistoric trade in amber between the Baltic and the Mediterranean has been studied in particular detail since the Budapest Congress in 1876.

[59] Lewis Henry Morgan, *Ancient Society.* New York, 1877.

position of societies in the hierarchic series was assigned on *a priori* grounds and subjective criteria.

Archaeology on the contrary can observe cultures that do succeed one another in time and classifies them into Stages precisely because of that succession. If then archaeological cultures be compared with living societies, and if the two classifications be thus correlated, the ethnographers' evolutionary series would become a sequence. There would then be a prospect of realizing the practical expectation expressed by Tylor in 1881:

> The knowledge of man's course of life from the remote past to the present will not only help us to forget the future, but may guide us in our duty of leaving the world better than we found it.[60]

Archaeology is certainly in no position to make any such forecasts. But if the formulation of hypotheses, based on induction and capable of verification by observation, be the mark of a science, archaeologists do already know enough about certain domains of man's past to say where to dig to test a theory, where to look for certain classes of remains, and what is likely to be found in a given area. Since Arthur Evans correctly predicted that the clue to the Mycenaean labyrinth would be found in Crete—and found it, quite a number of modest hypotheses have been 'experimentally' verified.

[60] E. B. Tylor, *Anthropology*. London, 1881. The last sentence in the book.

THE EVOLUTION OF THE KNIFE IN THE OLD STONE AGE

by

A. D. LACAILLE

Introduction

OUR most delicate surgical manipulative instruments are but refinements of ordinary tools. Unquestionably the most important is the knife, whose ancestry lies in dim antiquity. Even variants of its essential feature, the cutting-edge, became standardized countless centuries before metal was used for tools. The back, adapted for the application of finger pressure, and the tang, by which the blade could be fitted into a handle, are glimpsed even among implements made by the forerunners of the first representatives of *Homo sapiens*.

In this paper I shall consider some relics of the principal classic western European cultures which illustrate stages in this development. These cultures belonged to the Old Stone Age which comprised three parts: (*a*) The Lower or early Palaeolithic; (*b*) the Middle Palaeolithic; (*c*) the Upper or late Palaeolithic. The Lower Palaeolithic included the Abbevillian, Clactonian and Acheulian cultures; the Middle Palaeolithic the Mousterian and Levalloisian; and the Upper Palaeolithic the Aurignacian, Solutrean and the Magdalenian. All fell within the Pleistocene period of perhaps just over half a million years, during which the Northern Hemisphere witnessed great climatic changes brought about by the fluctuations of immense ice-sheets. These changes determined man's environment, dictated his habitat, had a bearing on his health, governed his food (plant and animal), influenced his cultures, and were a factor in his social organization.

The Pleistocene consisted of four major glaciations or advances of the ice, named after Alpine valleys: (I) Günz; (II) Mindel; (III) Riss; (IV) Würm.[1] These advances were separated from one another by three retreats, each of which gave rise to a period of interglacial climate. The last extension of the ice was threefold, pauses intervening between its maxima. (For the last important glacial episode in the cycle the term Würm III is now preferred to Bühl.) Man's Palaeolithic cultures and their associations in western Europe have been fitted into this scheme of glacial and interglacial periods. The Lower Palaeolithic cultures ranged possibly from some time before the first glacial episode (Günz) until the third interglacial (Riss–Würm) period. The Middle Palaeolithic cultures had their beginnings before the third (Riss) glaciation. Developing thereafter, they were superseded by the Upper Palaeolithic during the period of climatic improvement between the first and second maxima of the last (Würm) glaciation. The Upper Palaeolithic cultures flourished until, with a changing environment due to the general deglaciation after the last advance of the ice, they came under new influences which varied according to regions.

[1] A. Penck and E. Brückner, *Die Alpen im Eiszeitalter*. Leipzig, 1909.

In the evidence from such regions as the valleys of the Thames and Somme, which provide standards for comparisons and correlations, the Abbé Breuil[2] sees the movements of the Lower Palaeolithic human groups: one, southern manufacturers of core-tools (such as hand-axes made in lumps of stone), associated with warm climatic conditions; the other, manufacturers of flake-tools (made in pieces struck from lumps of stone), associated with cold periods. During overlaps at the end and beginning of each spell the stone industries blended. The alternations generally held good throughout Middle Palaeolithic times until cultural elements fused before the coming of man in the stages of Upper Palaeolithic culture.

Whereas physical anthropologists can say little about the exponents of Lower Palaeolithic culture, they regard the Middle Palaeolithic as that of Neanderthal human types and assign the Upper Palaeolithic cultures to *Homo sapiens*. The Lower and Middle Palaeolithic culture-groups belonged to Palaeanthropic Man, those of the Upper Palaeolithic onwards to Neanthropic Man.[3]

The Earliest Tools

(a) It is probable that man learned to scrape before he discovered how to cut. For scraping he could have used any hard material such as a splintered stone, shell or bone with a convenient edge due to natural conformation or break. Because of its durability he would prefer hard stone for most purposes. In time man learned to adapt and trim edges. When he found how to fracture stones and dress the resulting margins a great landmark in human history was reached. His earliest tools, being but improvised, will never be recognized. And it is unlikely that the simplest edge-retouched forms can ever be distinguished from naturally injured pieces of stone. They belong to the 'Eolithic' Age of man's cultural development.

(b) Man may be supposed to have found how to cut when scraping with an improvised tool whose edge was more than usually sharp. This discovery would lead to his selecting suitable spalls of stone for cutting. Of course the employment of such occasional tools continued throughout the whole of the prehistoric period. (It obtains to-day among peoples living in primitive conditions.) Another step forward was made when man began to prepare stone expressly for the extraction of pieces for manufacturing into implements. This did not happen, however, until the early part of the Palaeolithic Age when he was already a skilled craftsman.

(c) From making shift with improvised tools, man found a way of shaping implements in lumps of selected stone. He favoured flint and kindred rocks, for having observed how they fractured under blows and responded to trimming, he found that he could exercise some control over them. His first standardized tool was the hand-axe,[3, 4] *coup-de-poing* or *biface*, made by flaking over a cobble or piece of stone, by striking upon an anvil-stone, or by hitting the lump of raw material with a hammer-stone. The hand-axe was a tool of all work. With it man could hack, scrape, cut, dig, even stab.

[2] H. Breuil, 'Le Paléolithique Ancien en Europe Occidentale et sa chronologie'. *Bull. Soc. Préhist. Française*, 1932, xxix, 573.

[3] G. Elliot Smith, *Human history*. London, 1930, p. 92.

[4] V. Gordon Childe, *The story of tools*. London, 1944, p. 3.

I   B

Lower Palaeolithic

Abbevillian. The earliest well-defined hand-axes are relics of the Abbevillian culture of the first interglacial period (Günz–Mindel). Characteristic examples are marked by the boldness of their flake-scars and their sinuous long edges. With the development of the culture the scars became shallower and the edges straighter, owing probably to shaping or finishing by softer hammers, possibly of antler, bone or hardwood. Waste flakes from the manufacture of hand-axes were used as scrapers, most of them quite untrimmed but some slightly retouched along the edges. (To these the surgeon's rugine and raspatory trace their ancestry.) Many assuredly served as knives and saws, but this cannot be proved because it is difficult to distinguish edge-wear in Abbevillian artifacts from injuries caused by natural agencies.

The Abbevillian culture was associated with the vegetation of a warm temperate climate and with a fauna having strong Pliocene affinities. Though man of the time would be mainly frugivorous, we may, nevertheless, infer from his use of flake-implements that he prepared the flesh of animals and that meat formed part of his diet. He would thus have evolved beyond his vegetarian ancestors.

Clactonian. During the reign of the Clactonian, which intervened between the Abbevillian and Acheulian core-tool or hand-axe cultures in England and generally in France, virtually all the implements used by man were flake-tools. Great numbers of his large and small plain flakes must have served as knives without any special treatment. For long any such treatment was given mainly to the dressing of an endless variety of scrapers, at their best as products of the evolved Clactonian industries of Suffolk in which Acheulian influences appear. In these advanced industries flakes of pre-determined form were struck from cores to answer specific needs, including a demand for cutting-tools. In this respect the writer considers as knives rather than side-scrapers many of the most developed Clactonian artifacts, particularly those dressed flatly along a long margin to a sharp and straight edge. Such implements usually exhibit some natural feature or accident of fracture (as in Figs. 16 and 17) left untreated, or possibly wrought to serve as a sort of knob or holder.

These masterly products well support the contention that Mousterian industry derives from the Clactonian.[5] Tools of fairly evolved Clactonian facies occur in some deposits in association with Acheulian artifacts and prototypes of Levalloisian forms.[6] It is not surprising, therefore, that resemblances should exist among some of the dressed edge-tools of all these cultures.

Since the main development of the Clactonian flake-industries took place during the cold conditions, which heralded and immediately followed a glaciation (Mindel), man depended more than ever on animals. Groups of Clactonian implements proclaim that he was becoming skilful in the chase,

[5] H. Breuil, *op. cit.* (2), p. 572.
[6] A. D. Lacaille, 'The Palaeoliths from the Gravels of the Lower Boyn Hill Terrace around Maidenhead'. *Ant. Journ.*, 1940, xx, 259–62.

that he possibly prepared skins for clothing and shelter, and that he knew
something of the anatomy of the beasts which he hunted.

Acheulian. Acheulian culture is known principally for the imposing
array of bifacially flaked implements produced by its prolific industries.
Hand-axes, cleavers and ovates speak for the skill of their manufacturers.
Owing to prevailing methods, the waste from the fashioning of these tools
consisted mainly of much thinner flakes than those struck off lumps of stone
in the Abbevillian hand-axe industries. Much of this waste was pressed
into service for scrapers and knives. That many flakes, such as plain
untrimmed occasional tools and a variety of dressed forms, were attractive
without retouch was due partly to their sharpness and partly to their

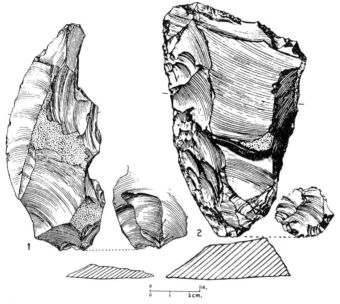

convenient shape. Those found unaltered in containing deposits, and
showing signs of wear from their having been used to cut, are probably the
earliest objects which can confidently be called knives. The specimen
illustrated in Fig. 1 is characteristic.

Besides using convenient flakes struck off hand-axes in the shaping, the
Acheulian knappers detached flakes from nodules and cores expressly for
making into fine hand-axes, stout scrapers and knives. As a specimen of the
last, a heavy implement is shown (Fig. 2). Its carefully dressed straight
working-edge would distinguish this tool from a contemporary true side-
scraper.

Cutting-tools belonging to industries as early as Middle Acheulian were
also made in parallel-sided blades. The preparation and removal of these
from cores marked yet another step forward in man's development. Blades
have since formed part of man's equipment. A slightly dressed and well-worn
Middle Acheulian specimen from the Thames valley is shown in Fig. 3.

Since the Acheulian industries evolved during the second (Mindel–Riss) and the third (Riss–Würm) interglacial periods, it is probable that man lived longer in the Acheulian stage of culture than in any other in the whole of his history. It would be surprising then if industries which endured so long and owed much to contacts during overlap periods had not added considerably to man's equipment. From among a wide range of well-defined forms, illustrating the comprehensiveness of the industries referable to this long-lasting phase of man's cultural development, I have chosen a remarkable

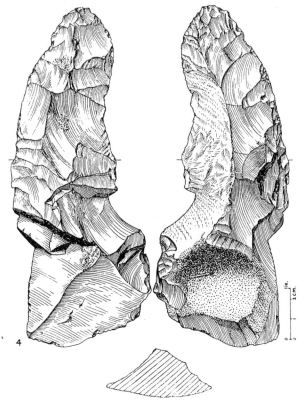

large, flaked Acheulian implement (Fig. 4). This narrow bifacially worked piece may be regarded as a variant of the hand-axe as well as a powerful long-edged cutting-tool. By reason of its flattish faces and convenient untreated basal crust, it fits the grasp perfectly. As held naturally in the right hand, the instrument presents an efficient and somewhat concave cutting-edge suggestive of a flesher's knife.

Middle Palaeolithic

The advance denoted by the deliberate production of blades in Acheulian industries went farther in the succeeding complex of culture, now usually considered as Middle Palaeolithic and attributed to Neanderthal Man.

The most important of the new industries were a locally evolved Clactonian, the Levalloisian of the open periglacial regions in northern France and in England, and the true Mousterian of the rock-shelters, chiefly in the valleys of south-western France. In the Levalloisian and the Mousterian various methods of stone-working were followed in the fashioning of fine hand-axe forms and other implements on flakes and blades. Frequently this basic material was prepared in a highly specialized manner on cores from which

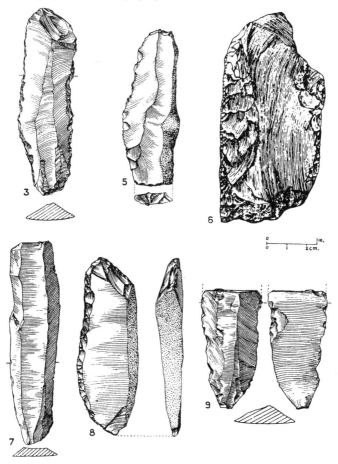

the artisans extracted a great variety of pieces, ranging from short to long and from narrow to wide. So comprehensive an output is not to be wondered at in a complex which grew under the different conditions of a time-span extending from the end of the second interglacial period (Mindel–Riss) until the spell of climatic improvement between the first and second maxima of the Würm or fourth glaciation.

Levalloisian. Apart from bifacial and other finely surface-flaked objects, Levalloisian tools seldom exhibit signs of such careful retouch as appears on

Mousterian, Acheulian and Clactonian implements. This is particularly true of the longer and heavier flakes and blades, the lateral edges of which so often are seen merely to be serrated and worn from use as scrapers and knives. Dressing, if other than just the restricted treatment of a cutting-edge, may sometimes have been meant to facilitate holding.

A small Levalloisian flake, well worn, probably as a knife (Fig. 5), is figured here together with a secondarily retouched tool (Fig. 6), which would have served for scraping and cutting. The scarring on the second shows how Levalloisian flat flaking resembles that expended on well-developed Acheulian and on Mousterian bifacial implements.

Mousterian. The Mousterian industries produced far more definable artifacts than did the Levalloisian. Standardized objects with trimmed straight and convex long margins were now frequently used. Quite a range of true knife shapes appeared, many made in flakes sliced out of nodules. The working-edge of Mousterian scraping- and cutting-tools was fashioned either on the right or the left of the parent flake. That this suggests ambidexterous users is supported by the manner in which the finger adjusts itself to the natural or trimmed back so often present opposite the working-edge. Since Mousterian knives occur in a variety of sizes, with little difference in basic shapes, those shown here (Figs. 18 and 19) may be taken as typologically representative.

Upper Palaeolithic

The process of refrigeration, to which the territory open to man in western Europe had been adapting itself, culminated in the fourth or Würm glaciation. This, with its arctic spells and periods of relaxed severity, was the background of the Upper Palaeolithic cultures. The earliest, the Aurignacian, extinguished the Mousterian and Levalloisian. It throve during the Laufen retreat, or 'Aurignacian oscillation', between the first and second Würm maxima of the Alpine glaciers. In several parts of continental Europe the second Würm onset witnessed its replacement by the Solutrean. By the time of the Achen recession, about twenty-five thousand years ago, both cultures had generally given way before the Magdalenian.

During the predominantly cold conditions, which saw the rise and development of Upper Palaeolithic culture, most of man's implements were related to the chase and made to deal with animal substances. As the Middle Palaeolithic industries of Neanderthal Man gave place to those of modern human types, so blades were increasingly produced in an apparent carrying down of an industrial tradition, which arose in Acheulian culture and was dominant in the Levalloisian.

Aurignacian. Already a well-advanced form by the end of the Middle Palaeolithic Age, the knife reached the peak of its evolution not long after. For it was in the industries of the Aurignacian, the first of the great Upper Palaeolithic cultures, that the principal shapes, the back and the tang, were developed. All these growths from remote forerunners induced the manufacture of most delicate and even sharply pointed stone implements, which must have been employed in such work as piercing and making fine cuts in skins as well as perforating bone and wood. It is easy to see in many of these fine instruments (*v. infra*, pp. 26–30), which developed during the early part of the Upper Palaeolithic Age, the prototypes, if not the very counterparts in stone, of our scalpels and bistouries. The fact that there is no evidence that these Upper Palaeolithic knives were actually used for primitive surgery is beside the point. The only evidence of prehistoric operations which we possess is found in crania on which trephination had been performed, and this operation was not introduced until much later. But bone operations are naturally the only ones which would leave evidence of this type. Palaeolithic man could not have been unaware of the relief obtained on the bursting of a superficial abscess, and by inference it seems probable that he would learn that bursting could be hastened by incision. Some of these stone knives would certainly be satisfactory for this purpose.

As innumerable edge-worn specimens testify, untrimmed flakes and blades (Fig. 7) were freely used as knives at Aurignacian stations. When worn out they could quickly be replaced, especially in localities where tractable raw material abounded. Knives of more permanent character were also fashioned in blades by edge retouch, as in Fig. 8.

In the brilliant array of tools, made in convenient sizes for use unhafted or fixed into handles, we see types which bear comparison with our common domestic knives of to-day. But so many variants and improvements were devised in response to the endless needs of the Aurignacian communities that it is impossible to illustrate more than a few forms. These observations apply equally to the more ordinary types of cutting-tools employed by man living in the succeeding stages of Upper Palaeolithic food-collecting economy.

Solutrean. An innovation in the working of stone appeared in the industries of the Solutrean culture that locally superseded the Aurignacian. This was the application of surface flaking to certain implements made in blades, the principal being tanged points and leaf-shaped artifacts. By analogy with the beautiful North American bifacially flaked leaf-shaped implements,[7] some of them (for example, Fig. 38), besides serving to tip weapons, may well have been used as knives. In the comparable Solutrean forms the Upper Palaeolithic stone-knapper's craft reached its pitch. It was surpassed only by the flint-work of predynastic Egypt, the late Neolithic and early Bronze Age of north-western Europe. While it has always been stressed that the dressing of edges by retouch attained its peak in Solutrean industries, it is sometimes overlooked that man in this stage of culture also used untrimmed flakes (as in Fig. 9) and blades (as in Fig. 10). A bilaterally retouched Solutrean blade (Fig. 11), narrowed by trimming for fitting into a handle, is shown for its delicate workmanship and because its edges are worn from use in cutting.

Magdalenian. Owing probably to their superior equipment the Solutrean invaders became dominant for a while in certain lowland regions. Their influence, however, did not prevail, for the succeeding Upper Palaeolithic culture, the Magdalenian, followed Aurignacian lines. Bone-working became one of its chief crafts, to the detriment of the lithic industries. Still, the Magdalenian kit of stone implements was most comprehensive. It included the principal forms of knives which had been developed or devised in Aurignacian industries (*v. infra*, pp. 26–29). Hence, it is interesting to

[7] Warren K. Moorehead, *The Stone Age in North America*. London, 1911, vol. i, pp. 48–79.

find types recalling the transition from Middle to Upper Palaeolithic, forms of early Aurignacian aspect, and shapes of late Aurignacian facies occurring in Magdalenian levels, of course with great numbers of plain flakes (Fig. 12) and blades (Fig. 13), which show signs of use as cutting-tools. This association epitomizes the development of the blade during the Old Stone Age.

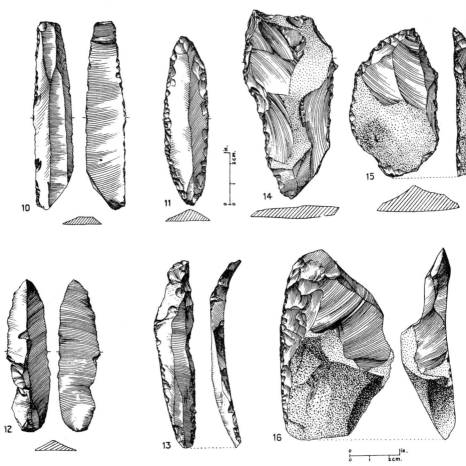

The Back

(a) The thick back, whereby finger pressure can be exerted upon a long cutting-edge without injury to the user's hand, goes back to man's accidental discovery of the usefulness of a convenient flank opposite a working margin. That this discovery was early used in the case of knives appears from Middle Acheulian examples bearing characteristic signs of wear (cf. Fig. 1) and some trimming (Fig. 14). It also occurred to man to *fashion* knife backs in imitation of the fortuitous steep finger-rest, by abruptly retouching or blunting the margin opposite the cutting-edge. An example of this (Fig. 15), assignable to a Middle Acheulian industry of the Thames valley, shows that the prepared knife back would be of far more ancient origin than is generally suspected.

(*b*) The writer can recall no Clactonian knife with a trimmed back. Though as an artificial feature it may be quite absent from many of the industries of the great complex of Lower and Middle Palaeolithic flake-cultures, the knife back is nevertheless present in several as an incorporated natural feature. We find it among corticated surfaces and peculiarities of edges used as finger-rests, stops and grips in the products of the evolved Clactonian (cf. Fig. 16), and the Mousterian of south-western France. Another specimen illustrated here (Fig. 17), a typical late Clactonian leaf-shaped flake from Suffolk, is injured along its left convex edge from long use as a knife. Opposite, at the upper end, the pronounced well-rounded hinge-fracture forms an excellent back.

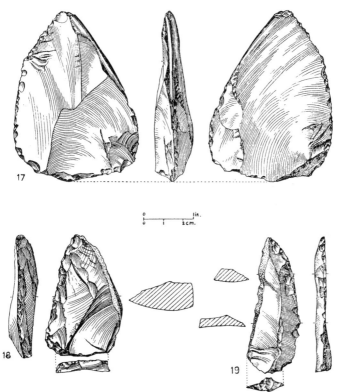

In Mousterian collections from classic rock-shelter stations, including the name-site, wide natural backs are features in many broad and narrow single-edged knives delicately dressed in corticated flakes. These implements have been carefully fashioned so as to leave untreated a long steep surface of crust, (cf. Figs. 18 and 19). This is in keeping with contemporary side-scrapers upon which crust remains opposite the working-edge. Long and short knives with delicately treated curved backs, much after the model of the natural crusted finger-rest, were turned out by early and late Mousterian industries (for example, Fig. 20, Lower Mousterian; and Fig. 22, Upper Mousterian). Experiment shows how well they were made for easy manipulation.

(c) Since implements with prepared backs occur in Acheulian industries in England, referable to the Mindel–Riss interglacial period, and in true Mousterian series from classic sites in the Vézère valley, it is not surprising that in the latter region backed knives (cf. Fig. 21) should be numerous in the relic bed of Würm age between two Mousterian levels. At a number of sites this intermediate layer yields a mixed industry aptly called by Peyrony *Moustérien de tradition acheuléenne*.[8] Though widely separated in space and time, these finds yet point to the prepared knife back as an Acheulian development and feature. That shrewd observer Commont long ago recognized and understood its true purpose in early Palaeolithic artifacts from the Somme valley deposits.[9]

(d) As indicated above, the dressed knife back, foreshadowed in the Acheulian and occurring in later industries, was an important feature of certain tools made during the period of Neanderthal Man's supersession by early representatives of *Homo sapiens*. The typical implements of this phase of transition from Middle to Upper Palaeolithic are characterized by their abruptly dressed backs, which are markedly curved as in earlier industries. The Abri Audi knife, so named from a rock-shelter at Les Eyzies-de-Tayac (Dordogne), is regarded as the standard. Examples for use in the right and left hand are shown (Figs. 23 and 24). Their resemblance to the steeply retouched tools of Acheulio-Mousterian manufacture from Le Moustier (cf. Fig. 21) is manifest.

(e) The able Aurignacian heirs to so many stone-working traditions developed the more advanced knife forms. Their prolific workshops turned out increasing numbers of small delicate backed knives in response to the growing use of animal substances for hunting and domestic gear and for articles of wear.

The trend in Upper Palaeolithic times towards the use of blades rather than flakes is shown by the increasing numbers of fine retouched tools in evolutionary series of Aurignacian artifacts. The backed form, which succeeded the Abri Audi knife of the transition from the final Mousterian, is held to typify early Aurignacian industry. It is the Châtelperron knife, so called after a locality in the Allier *département* where it was first recorded.[10] Whether its working-edge is on the left as in Fig. 25, or on the right as in Fig. 26, its resemblance to the modern knife is striking. This was commented on by Dr. Joseph Bailleau, the finder. Unlike their predecessors trimmed mainly in flakes, backed tools of Châtelperron type are invariably manufactured in blades. Effective as was the knife back of classic Châtelperron form, yet even in early Aurignacian industries it was subjected to such modifications as notching at the upper end for the pressure of the user's finger-tip (cf. Fig. 27).

[8] D. Peyrony, 'Le Moustier, ses gisements, ses industries, ses couches géologiques'. *Rev. Anthrop.*, 1930, xl, 48–76, 155–76.

[9] V. Commont, 'Les Hommes Contemporains du Renne dans la Vallée de la Somme'. *Mém. Soc. des Antiq. de Picardie*, 1913, xxxviii, 285, 327.

[10] J. Bailleau, *L'Homme pendant la Période Quaternaire dans le Bourbonnais*. Moulins, 1872, p. 31.

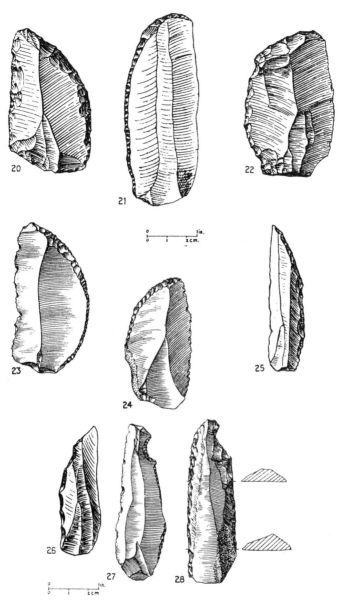

The preparation of this slight hollow was of course quite a natural development from the fortuitous convenient configuration of a piece. A much worn, more advanced Aurignacian knife preserved in the Wellcome Historical Medical Museum is illustrated as a specimen in which advantage has been taken of a fortuitous notch (Fig. 28).

With the growth of Upper Palaeolithic culture thinner and narrower blades were increasingly used.   Retouch on them became finer and the curved back gradually gave place to one which was straight.   This in a small tool may have appeared to present a better surface for the direct application of finger pressure.   It characterizes the graceful La Gravette points and knives of late Aurignacian manufacture (cf. Figs. 35 and 36).

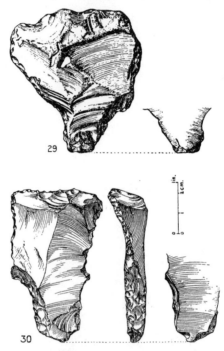

The backed knife was produced by the Solutrean craftsmen, and was also an important item in the equipment of the Magdalenian hunters.   As these late Upper Palaeolithic industries ran to seed with the passing of the Pleistocene into Post-Glacial time, so they tended increasingly to produce small knife forms made in past Aurignacian traditions.[11]

(f) That the knife back became thinner was due partly at least to improving methods of hafting and the devising of composite implements.   The forms of hafts and the later history of the knife do not concern us.   We have, however, briefly to review the tang, which attribute of the knife seems to have developed concurrently with the back.

The Tang

The idea of hafting stone tools assuredly occurred to man long before he had reached an advanced stage of Palaeolithic culture.   The possibility that his earliest and improvised tools were held otherwise than in direct contact

[11] H. Breuil, *Les subdivisions du Paléolithique Supérienr et leur signification.* Second edition, Paris, 1937, p. 72.

with the hand can be ruled out. It may never be known if hand-axes were mounted in some form of handle. The trimming of some Lower Palaeolithic flakes indicates however that these were hafted, as much to protect the user's hand as to impart greater efficiency to the tool.

It seems to the writer that hints of the tang are found in some Abbevillian utilized waste flakes. It is of course impossible to say whether or not the scraper-like object illustrated as an example (Fig. 29) was ever hafted. Such a form, however, might have suggested the working down of the lower and thicker ends of flakes for hafting, say, by inserting the stone in a bone or piece

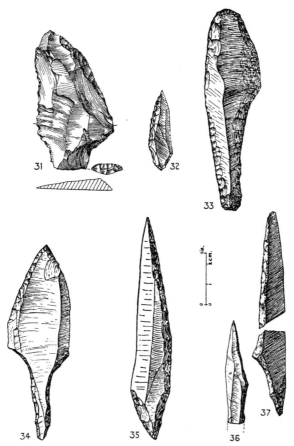

of wood. Continuous study of immense series of Lower Palaeolithic flake-implements later than Abbevillian tempts the writer to suggest that the parentage of the well-made Aurignacian tang is to be found in Acheulian industries. A square-ended scraper (Fig. 30) is illustrated in support of this view. Its lower end has been restricted and shouldered by steep retouch on the left side, while the opposite edge on the nether surface has been flatly dressed. Made in this way, the stem could be fitted into a handle. An

Acheulio-Mousterian specimen (Fig. 31) from the type-station of Le Moustier is particularly significant. Made in a waste flake from the manufacture of a hand-axe, its edges exhibit the wear and retouch of a knife. The dressing on the right of the lower end is particularly good. Together with the fortuitous narrowing opposite, it affords a substantial and fairly symmetrical stem. This piece is also interesting because its butt is finely faceted in the Levalloisian style (cf. Fig. 5).

Not unexpectedly, numbers of Levalloisian and Mousterian flakes and blades have been observed to be narrowed by retouch along the sides of the lower end. Greater interest, however, attaches to the true Châtelperron knives and points in which an incipient tang appears, seemingly for the first time with the curved wide back in the same artifact (cf. Fig. 32).

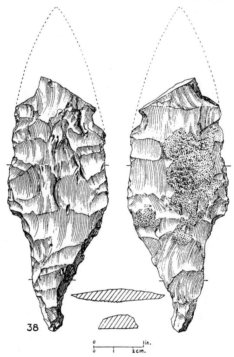

38

Solutrean influences during the final stages of the Aurignacian led to the perfecting of the tang or stem, whereby edged and pointed implements could be firmly fixed into handles or secured to shafts. This development is associated with the steeply trimmed back, and according to Breuil,[11, 22] with the progressive narrowing down of the large Aurignacian *lame-à-coche* or laterally hollowed blade (Fig. 33), the prototypes of which may be found in relics of Acheulian facies (v. pp. 19–20). It eventually culminated in the double-shouldered and centrally-tanged La Font-Robert point (Fig. 34). Stages in the passage from the incipient tang of some Châtelperron knives are illustrated in La Gravette forms (cf. Fig. 35), La Font-Robert ordinary (Fig. 36), and feebly spurred types (Fig. 37).

Attention can be drawn here to an exceptional Solutrean specimen consisting of a bifacially, flatly-flaked *feuille-de-laurier* in the Wellcome Museum (Fig. 38). This is worked bilaterally in the lower part to a tapering tang, the slight recurving of which could allow the user either to manipulate the implement without its being hafted or to fit it into a handle. In this object we see a forerunner of the classic Egyptian tanged surface-flaked knife.

The classic single-shouldered points of the Solutrean industries were further developments of greater importance in the evolution of weapons than domestic implements. They consist of plain and surface-flaked forms. The plain single-shouldered type, and the double-shouldered with central tang, reappeared in the latest Magdalenian industries in south-western France, and spread widely over the continent of Europe as the northern ice-sheets melted away.[12]

APPENDIX

Description of the specimens illustrated (all flint)

Fig. 1. Flake, waste from the manufacture of a Middle Acheulian hand-axe; the sharp convex edge on the left worn; irregular right edge well adapted to finger pressure. Om. 113 by Om. 049. Furze Platt, Maidenhead, Berks. Specimen from author's collection, now in the Wellcome Historical Medical Museum, London.

Fig. 2. Heavy side-scraper knife made in a flake, Middle Acheulian; retouched along left edge and in places along the right edge and top, probably for finger pressure. Om. 118 by Om. 075 by Om. 019. Furze Platt, Maidenhead, Berks. Specimen from author's collection, now in the Wellcome Historical Medical Museum, London.

Fig. 3. Middle Acheulian blade, edges much worn. Om. 093 by Om. 028. Lent Rise, Burnham, Bucks. Specimen from author's collection, now in the Wellcome Historical Medical Museum, London.

Fig. 4. Narrow bifacially flaked knife-like implement, apparently referable to a Middle Acheulian industry; crusted hollow at lower end affords good grip. Om. 17 by Om. 068 by Om. 024. Broomleigh, Kent, now in the Wellcome Historical Medical Museum, London (R 13820/1936).

Fig. 5. Small Levalloisian flake with worn left edge, crusted along the right. Om. 078 by Om. 029. Iver, Bucks. Specimen from author's collection, now in the British Museum, London.

Fig. 6. Side-scraper knife, with carefully retouched working-edge on the left, the product of a well-developed Levalloisian industry. Om. 105 by Om. 052. Saint-Acheul-lès-Amiens (Somme). After Commont.[13]

Fig. 7. Fine Aurignacian blade, edges slightly worn. Om. 102 by Om. 025 by Om. 004. Laussel, Marquay (Dordogne), now in the Wellcome Historical Medical Museum, London, (33093).

Fig. 8. Knife, Aurignacian, dressed along left edge; retouched at top and crust left on the right for finger pressure. Om. 089 by Om. 031 by Om. 013. Beauregard near Nemours (Seine-et-Marne). Specimen from author's collection.

Fig. 9. Broken Solutrean flake, edges worn. Now measuring Om. 059 long, Om. 031 wide and Om. 099 thick. Fourneau du Diable, Bourdeilles (Dordogne). Specimen now in the Wellcome Historical Medical Museum, London (R 1838/1938).

Fig. 10. Fine Solutrean blade, edges much worn. Om. 093 by Om. 019 by Om. 004. Solutré (Saône-et-Loire), now in the Wellcome Historical Medical Museum, London (R 14081/1936, C.Sh.).

[12] J. G. D. Clark, *The Mesolithic Settlement of Northern Europe*. Cambridge, 1936, chap. ii.
[13] V. Commont, *op. cit.* (9), p. 324, Fig. 51 (1).

Fig. 11.   Knife, Solutrean; both edges retouched, the left worn slightly. Om. 085 by Om. 022 by Om. 006.   Grotte du Placard, Vilhonneur (Charente), now in the Wellcome Historical Medical Museum, London (R 14079/1936, C.Sh.).

Fig. 12.   Flake, Magdalenian, edges worn.   Om. 076 by Om. 021 by Om. 005. Grotte des Eyzies, Tayac (Dordogne), now in the Wellcome Historical Medical Museum, London (32502).

Fig. 13.   Blade, Magdalenian, edges much worn; steep right flank suitable for finger pressure.   Om. 093 by Om. 02 by Om. 0085.   Grotte des Eyzies, Tayac (Dordogne), now in the Wellcome Historical Medical Museum, London (32496).

Fig. 14.   Knife; waste flake from the manufacture of a Middle Acheulian hand-axe; the left edge much worn, the right edge and top adapted to the embrace of the index finger of the right hand.   Om. 096 by Om. 047 by Om. 006.   Baker's Farm, Farnham Royal, Bucks.   Specimen from author's collection, now in the Wellcome Historical Medical Museum, London.

Fig. 15.   Knife; flake struck from a pebble and retaining much crust; right edge dressed and worn, the left steeply retouched along the whole length; referable to Middle Acheulian workmanship.   Om. 075 by Om. 048 by Om. 016.   Baker's Farm, Farnham Royal, Bucks.   Specimen from author's collection, now in the Wellcome Historical Medical Museum, London.

Fig. 16.   Side-scraper knife, evolved Clactonian, retaining much crust.   This specimen is illustrated with the dressed cutting-edge on the left and bulbar end at top, since it was probably used in the right hand for which the central ridge, due to the removal of a large plunging flake, would serve conveniently.   Om. 095 long, Om. 059 wide and Om. 023 at thickest.   High Lodge, Mildenhall, Suffolk.   Specimen from author's collection.

Fig. 17.   Leaf-shaped flake, evolved Clactonian; edges much worn.   The well-rounded facet of hinge-fracture on the right would serve as a rest for the user's finger. Om. 084 long, Om. 063 wide and Om. 0295 thick.   High Lodge, Mildenhall, Suffolk. Specimen from author's collection.

Fig. 18.   Knife, of the full typical Mousterian facies; made in flake sliced out of pebble, working-edge on left dressed, crust on left serving as a rest for the finger. Om. 061 by Om. 036 by Om. 014.   Le Moustier, Peyzac (Dordogne), now in the Wellcome Historical Medical Museum, London (R 1216/1938, C.Sh.).

Fig. 19.   Knife, referable to the typical full Mousterian facies; made in a flake; dressed along part of the right edge, crust on the left serving as a rest for the finger. Om. 067 by Om. 022 by Om. 0065.   Le Moustier, Peyzac (Dordogne), now in the Wellcome Historical Medical Museum, London (R 1969/1938, C.Sh.).

Fig. 20.   Lower Mousterian knife, with prepared back on the right and dressed working-edge on the left.   Om. 073 by Om. 04.   Laussel, Marquay (Dordogne). After Lalanne and Bouyssonie.[14]

Fig. 21.   Acheulio-Mousterian knife, the prepared back on the left.   Om. 095 by Om. 037.   Le Moustier, Peyzac (Dordogne).   After D. Peyrony.[15]

Fig. 22.   Upper Mousterian knife; cutting-edge on the right untreated but worn, prepared back opposite.   Om. 072 by Om. 044.   Laussel, Marquay (Dordogne). After G. Lalanne and Bouyssonie.[16]

Fig. 23.   Knife, transitional form from Middle to Upper Palaeolithic (Abri Audi); cutting-edge on left much worn; prepared curved back on right.   Om. 075 by

[14] J. G. Lalanne and J. Bouyssonie, 'Le Gisement Paléolithique de Laussel'. L'Anthropologie, 1946, l, p. 25, Fig. 7 (2).

[15] D. Peyrony, op. cit. (8), p. 25, Fig. 11 (8).

[16] J. G. Lalanne and J. Bouyssonie, op. cit. (14), p. 61, Fig. 37 (5).

Om. 036, Abri Audi, Les Eyzies-de-Tayac (Dordogne), now in Musée Royal d'Histoire Naturelle de Bruxelles. Redrawn from Rutot.[17]

Fig. 24. Knife, transitional form from Middle to Upper Palaeolithic (Abri Audi) cutting-edge on the right, lower part of back formed by untreated crust on the left, the upper retouched to a curve. Om. 064 to Om. 034. Abri Audi, Les Eyzies-de-Tayac (Dordogne), now in Musée Royal d'Histoire Naturelle de Bruxelles. Redrawn from Rutot.[18]

Fig. 25. Knife, early Aurignacian; working-edge on the left, prepared steep curved back opposite. Om. 072 by Om. 018. La Grotte des Fées, Châtelperron (Allier), now in the Wellcome Historical Medical Museum, London. After Breuil.[19]

Fig. 26. Knife, early Aurignacian; working-edge on the right, prepared steep curved back opposite. Om. 064 by Om. 02. La Grotte des Fées, Châtelperron (Allier), now in the Wellcome Historical Medical Museum, London. After Breuil.[20]

Fig. 27. Knife, early Aurignacian; working-edge on right worn, the opposite treated for finger pressure by retouch and a dressed notch. Om. 078 by Om. 025. Gorge d'Enfer, Tayac (Dordogne), now in Musée Royal d'Histoire Naturelle de Bruxelles. Redrawn from Rutot.[21]

Fig. 28. Knife, referable to full Aurignacian industry; trimmed cutting-edge on left and slightly retouched on the right below fortuitous notch. Om. 08 long, Om. 025 wide and Om. 008 at thickest. Le Moustier, Peyzac (Dordogne), now in the Wellcome Historical Medical Museum, London (R 14082/1936, C.Sh.).

Fig. 29. Waste flake from the manufacture of an Abbevillian hand-axe. Om. 072 by Om. 066. Burnham Beeches, Bucks. Specimen from author's collection, now in the Wellcome Historical Medical Museum, London.

Fig. 30. End-scraper, Middle Acheulian; retouched and worn edges, dressed at lower end to a shoulder and asymmetric tang. Om. 076 by Om. 046 by Om. 0021. Furze Platt, Maidenhead, Berks. Specimen from author's collection, now in the Wellcome Historical Medical Museum, London.

Fig. 31. Acheulio-Mousterian tanged implement, retouched along right margin, left edge much worn. Om. 069 by Om. 039 by Om. 006. Le Moustier, Peyzac (Dordogne), now in the Wellcome Historical Medical Museum, London (R 1974/1938, C.Sh.).

Fig. 32. Early Aurignacian pointed knife (Châtelperron form); feebly shouldered and tanged. Om. 04 by Om. 012. Grotte des Fées, Châtelperron (Allier), now in the Wellcome Historical Medical Museum, London. After Breuil.[22]

Fig. 33. Middle Aurignacian *lame-à-coche*. Om. 10 by Om. 0785. Coumba del Bouitou (Corrèze). After Breuil.[23]

Fig. 34. Typical double-shouldered tanged late Aurignacian Font-Robert point. Om. 097 by Om. 031. La Font-Robert (Corrèze). After Breuil.[24]

Fig. 35. Typical late Aurignacian La Gravette knife or point; steeply dressed back and short well-defined tang. Om. 11 by Om. 02. La Gravette (Dordogne). After Breuil.[25]

---

[17] A. Rutot, 'Qu'est-ce que l'Aurignacien?' *Compt. rend. Congrès préhist. de France, 1910.* Tours, 1911, p. 132, Fig. 1 (2).

[18] idem, *ibid.*, p. 132, Fig. 1 (1).

[19] H. Breuil, 'Etudes de Morphologie Paléolithique. II.—L'Industrie de la Grotte de Châtelperron (Allier) et d'autres gisements similaires'. *Rev. Anthrop.*, 1911, xxi, p. 33, Fig. 4 (23).

[20] idem, *ibid.*, p. 33, Fig. 4 (30).

[21] A. Rutot, *op. cit.* (16), p. 135, Fig. 2 (2).

[22] H. Breuil, *op. cit.* (19), p. 33, Fig. 4 (33).

[24] idem, *ibid.*, p. 22, Fig. 12 (4).

[23] idem, *op. cit.* (11), p. 22, Fig. 12 (1).

[25] idem, *ibid.*, p. 6, Fig. 1 (8).

I

Fig. 36. Late Aurignacian knife or point; La Gravette ordinary type with feeble indication of spur in middle of steeply dressed back. Now Om. 051 long and Om. 011. La Font-Robert (Corrèze). After Breuil.[26]

Fig. 37. Late Aurignacian knife or point, La Font-Robert type feebly spurred; broken. La Font-Robert (Corrèze). After Breuil.[27]

Fig. 38. Solutrean leaf-shaped implement (*feuille-de-laurier* type) with tang; upper end wanting. Now measures Om. 127 by Om. 0395 by Om. 006 in middle. In the Wellcome Historical Medical Museum, London (R 1785/1938).

[26] *idem, ibid.*, p. 7, Fig. 2 (2).
[27] *idem, ibid.*, p. 7, Fig. 2 (4).

CHEMISTRY IN THE ANCIENT WORLD

by

J. R. PARTINGTON

IN considering the subject of 'Chemistry in the Ancient World' two questions arise. In the first place it must be stated what is to be understood by 'Chemistry' in such a remote period, and in the second place the parts of the ancient world of particular interest in connection with the development of chemical processes must be defined. Ancient Applied Chemistry included, among other things, the extraction of metals from their ores, the formation of alloys, the production of glazed pottery and other glazed articles, and of glass and coloured pastes, the preparation of pigments, inks and dyes, and salts, the extraction of vegetable oils, the compounding of ointments and perfumes, the production of intoxicating drinks, and the preparation of drugs. All these operations were carried out by the old nations, and what we know of the methods and results shows that the ancient peoples were often very highly skilled in the technical arts, and that they were not at all primitive in this respect.[1] In some cases a high standard of work was reached by mere patience, as when a block of hard stone such as granite or porphyry was shaped into a thin-walled vase by the use of stone grinders and abrasives, and without the assistance of the wheel, but in many other cases the processes were executed in a way which leaves nothing to be supplied in order to make them rank with the best achievements of the modern craftsman. The culture of the Bronze Age was, in fact, on a high level. The manual worker, it is true, was not very highly esteemed, and his hard life is graphically described in some Egyptian papyri, which show that he often wished to become a scribe or clerk, in which capacity he had the opportunity of rising to a higher level of comfort and appreciation. The goldsmiths of Egypt were better thought of than other manual workers, and even the god Ptah was not above assuming the title of 'master of arts and artisans', his priest being called 'foreman of artisans', and 'master of art'. An old Egyptian official is called 'superior of the secrets and chief of the metallurgists of the house of Amen', i.e. of the temple, and another of about 2700 B.C. is styled 'keeper of the king's laboratory and the king's workshops'. It seems as if the finer work was actually carried out in temple workshops, and the Egyptian priests probably busied themselves in producing ornamental materials in much the same way as this was done in the monasteries during the Middle Ages in Europe.

The outstanding achievements in Applied Chemistry in the earliest period were made in some special areas. The principal regions of the ancient world which may engage our attention are Egypt, Mesopotamia and Crete. Although iron was known in Egypt and Mesopotamia before 3000 B.C., and was in quite extensive use from about 1700 B.C., almost the whole period which we shall consider was in the Bronze Age, since the beginning of an Iron Age is properly

---

[1] J. R. Partington, *Origins and development of applied chemistry*. London, 1925, pp. xii+597. References to the sources of information given in the text, and not otherwise indicated, will be found in this book. The stock of the book was destroyed by enemy action during the war, and it is now very scarce.

associated with the use on the large scale of iron weapons. The date 1000 B.C. marks the beginning of an intrusion of an iron-using race or races into Mediterranean sites long previously occupied by peoples of higher culture with a Bronze Age civilization. This immigration, called by the Greeks the Dorian invasion as far as their particular experience was concerned, marked a definite break in the continuity of craftsmanship, and a lowering of standards in many directions. The Classical period, which lies in the Iron Age, is in some respects a period of decadence in the technical arts.

Of the three regions to be considered, Crete was less important. The older Cretan culture was not Greek but Mediterranean, and had greater affinities with Egypt than with later Greece; it was continued in the Mycenaean civilization on the mainland and a similar culture in later Cyprus. As a whole, this region was lacking in originality in the technical arts, most of which were borrowed from Egypt in a period when there was close contact with the Aegean.

The materials and processes known in antiquity are shown in the chart, from which it is clear that an extensive range of metallic and non-metallic products was available. The table gives a view of the occurrence of metals and other materials requiring skill in Applied Chemistry for their preparation. Materials found only very rarely are enclosed in brackets.

B.C.	EGYPT	MESOPOTAMIA	AEGEAN, etc.
	PREDYNASTIC : gold, silver, lead, copper, (iron), glaze, (glass).	SUMER-AKKAD : *Lagash, Kish, Ur:* gold, silver, lead, (iron), copper, tin-bronze, glaze, (glass)	—
3400 3000	I DYNASTY : (tin-bronze)	lead and antimony bronzes, (tin-bronze), metallic antimony	EARLY MINOAN : *Knossos:* copper, gold, silver, lead, tin-bronze
2500			purple dye glaze
2000	XII DYNASTY : (tin), iron tools		*Mycenae:* glass
1700–1500	XVIII DYNASTY : tin-bronze common, tin, glass factories, cobalt glass, indigo, useful iron Ebers Papyrus (medicine)	tin-bronze common, useful iron. Amarna letters, steel weapons, tin oxide glaze, cobalt glass	THE HITTITES : iron working in the Black Sea region ('Chalybes') *Tiryns:* lead-copper glass
1350–1200			*Palestine:* zinc brass
1000	Nubian iron industry, Assyrian iron common in Egypt	Assyrian iron common	THE PHOENICIANS : tin traffic ? IRON AGE : *Classical Greece*
650		Assyrian chemical tablets, imitation gems.	

In considering the materials we may begin with the metals. The earliest discovery of metals is still in many ways mysterious, and has been supposed to go back to 4000 B.C. at least in Egypt. The old authors preserve fragments of legends in which the great inventors are gods and kings.[2]

In ancient Egypt, the god Ptah was regarded as the inventor of metallurgy. In an inscription of Rameses II (1250 B.C.) at Abu-Simbel the god says to the king: 'I have wrought thy body of gold, thy bones of copper, thy vessels of iron'; and this is the first definite reference to iron in a text in Egypt, although the metal was known long before. King Sennacherib, the Assyrian, in 700 B.C. says he made great clay moulds at the command of his god, and cast in them great bronze statues of bulls and lions weighing over 10,000 talents, 'as if making half-shekel pieces'.

The earliest known working in metals appears before 3500 B.C. in Egypt and Mesopotamia, and rather later (2800 B.C.) in Crete and Cyprus. The Egyptians and Sumerians are rivals in the claim for the origin of metallurgy. The earliest known metal was probably gold, which was encountered in alluvial washings and could not escape attention, although mining from the rock was very soon in use. Copper has, however, been found in some of the oldest Egyptian graves without gold. The earliest specimens of gold are unrefined and contain varying amounts of silver, from 3 to 16 per cent, and usually some copper. When the silver reached 20 per cent or more, the resulting pale-yellow natural alloy, now called electrum, which is harder than gold, was given a special name in Egypt, and this name, *asem*, is perhaps the oldest name of a metal to be recorded. It occurs on an ebony tablet of King Menes (about 3400 B.C.). Electrum was a metal of peculiar sanctity in Egypt and was associated with the sun. The kings of the XVIIIth dynasty covered the summit-pyramids of obelisks with sheets of the metal. Queen Hatshepsut built 'two obelisks of electrum, whose points mingled with heaven, their summits being of electrum of the best of every country, which are seen on both sides of the river: their rays flood the Two Lands [Upper and Lower Egypt] when the sun rises between them as he dawns in the horizon of heaven'. One is still standing (without electrum) at Karnak. Asem is also mentioned in the inscription on the obelisk of Thothmes III, now standing on the Thames Embankment and incorrectly called 'Cleopatra's needle', which may at one time have been plated with the metal. This king once received about four tons of electrum as tribute from Asia and Nubia.

Gold seems to have been used in great profusion in Egypt during the XVIIIth dynasty, since a gold coffin in Tutankhamen's tomb was over 6 ft. long and weighed 110·4 kgm., and in the Amarna Letters (1375 B.C.) the King of the Mitanni in the Euphrates region writes to Pharaoh begging him to 'send me so much gold that it cannot be measured, for in my brother's land gold is as common as dust'. He also mentions that: 'thou sentest my father a great deal of gold . . . but the tablet thou sentest me was as if it were alloyed with copper'. The King of Babylon wrote to Ikhnaton (1375–1350 B.C.) saying his gold was not as good as his father's; from 20 minas of this gold put in the furnace only 5 minas of fine gold remained. These letters are interesting, for they show that Egypt was then correctly regarded by other nations as a kind of El Dorado, and also that some kind of refining process was in use in Asia Minor about 1400 B.C., i.e. long before its use in Lydia in 550 B.C., the

[2] *J. R. Partington,* 'The discovery of bronze'. *Scientia,* 1936, lx, 76–83.

traditional date for the introduction of the process of refining gold. Since Pharaoh had sent the base metal in the hope that it would pass as gold, the processes of testing and refining gold were perhaps not well known in Egypt in his time, a deduction which is borne out by the fact that almost pure gold first occurs in Egyptian remains at the beginning of the Persian period, about 525 B.C. It is very probable that this process of purification was that described about 113 B.C. by Agatharchides, extracts from whose lost work are preserved by Diodorus Siculus. Agatharchides also gives a graphic picture of the conditions of slave labour in the mines, and there is no doubt, from incidental allusions in old Egyptian texts, that these conditions were equally severe in the older period, when gold was got from mines in the so-called Arabian Desert, between the Nile and the Red Sea. The appalling conditions of work in the intense heat of this region are more than once mentioned in the chronicles, in which it is said 'the rocks brand the skin'. The method of purification of the gold obtained by stamping the quartz rock and washing is thus described by Agatharchides: 'At last others take it by weight and measure, and putting it with a fixed proportion of lead, salt, a little tin and barley bran into earthen crucibles well closed with clay, they leave it in a furnace for five days and nights together, after which it is allowed to cool. The crucibles are opened and nothing is found in them except the pure gold, a little diminished in quantity'. The utility of tin (which would harden the gold) seems doubtful, but the use of crude vitriols, known at an early period in Egypt, seems possible. The powder used in fairly recent times for the purification of gold, and called the 'royal cement', consisted of brick dust, calcined green vitriol, and common salt.

Silver was of little importance in Egypt, but it occurs in fairly large amounts in early Sumerian remains at Ur. It does occur, however, in small quantities in predynastic remains in Egypt and generally contains appreciable amounts of gold and copper. The silver at Ur is in the form of useful objects such as tumblers, as well as ornamental, so that the metal was probably in fairly extensive use. Probably most of this early silver came from Asia Minor. The Hittites were particularly important in the development of the metallurgy of silver, the ores of which occur in large amounts in Asia Minor, although some of the old mines are now worked out. In the XVIIIth dynasty Egypt received much silver from this source, and so did, probably, the Babylonians and Assyrians. Silver was used fairly early in Crete, and there are interesting finds of artistic silver on the Phoenician coast at Byblos, going back to 2000 B.C. A silver coinage was early in use in Phoenicia and Palestine; the Egyptians used weighed rings of gold, silver and copper, which are shown as tribute.

The metallurgy of copper is very early in Egypt, going back to the early predynastic period. The metal used was probably not native copper but smelted metal from malachite, used as an eye-paint from a very early period. The malachite ore was obtained from the peninsula of Sinai, this ore being readily reduced in charcoal fires, and abundant remains of an early copper industry were found in this region. The wrinkled slag on the surface of molten copper is mentioned in the Edwin Smith Surgical Papyrus, the oldest parts of which go back to 3000 B.C. There is a copper axe-head of $3\frac{1}{2}$ lb. of the middle predynastic period (4000 B.C. ?). In the IInd dynasty the art of working copper had reached a high stage of perfection, as the actual articles show.

Equally remarkable are the highly artistic works in copper from early Sumerian sites, perhaps as early as 3000 B.C. In both regions the copper was obtained in a very pure condition, and very good castings were made, as well as hammered work.

We do not know enough about the actual processes used by the metallurgists, since the reports of excavations are often confused and inaccurate, and many so-called smelting furnaces are probably merely the remains of fire-places or bakers' ovens. We are better informed of the working of metal, as there are good representations of metal-worker's workshops in Egypt, for example one of the Old Kingdom (2980–2475 B.C.) showing the weighing of precious metals and malachite, a furnace with men blowing the fire with a mouth blow-pipe (probably a reed tipped with clay and formerly mistaken for a glass blower's blow-pipe), the cutting and hammering of metal, and the putting together of necklaces and costly ornaments. Blow-pipes were used to a much later period, down to the XVIIIth dynasty, where they are also shown, although bellows were in use in Egypt at least as early as 1580 B.C., and are represented. They were dish bellows, still used in Africa, being wooden or clay dishes covered with leather, the skins being pressed down by stepping on them and raised by pulling strings. There are no valves, the air entering through leaky places. The metal was melted in clay crucibles, actual specimens of which are known, and poured through funnels, probably also of clay, into the moulds. Quite large castings were made, and the drawings seem to indicate that a quantity of metal was poured simultaneously from a number of crucibles.

Really good castings were first possible with the alloy bronze, containing copper and tin, which has a lower melting point than pure copper. Bronze occurs in small amounts in Egyptian remains of the Old Kingdom, but first became abundant in the Middle Kingdom (XIIth dynasty). It seems probable that the two metals, copper and tin, were used separately and melted together to form the bronze, since they are shown brought to the furnaces in blocks of different shapes. The copper was in large hide-shaped blocks, which were traded in the Aegean in the Cretan period, actual specimens being known. The source of the tin for the early bronzes is a matter of speculation. In some Egyptian representations, blocks of a material called *dhty* are shown carried by Cretans. The Cretans (Keftiu) are often shown in the XVIIIth dynasty bringing precious metals made into vases, etc. into Egypt. It is possible that they brought the tin. Later on, the trade in this metal appears to have been in the hands of the Phoenicians, who seem to have been especially important in the later tin traffic. It is known, however, that maritime trade was flourishing before they appeared on the scene, and their importance in the early period has probably been over-estimated.

The source of the tin for all early bronze is a matter of speculation, but it is possible that the tin came at first from some place in Khorassan in Persia, called by the older authors Drangiana. Strabo in A.D.7 says tin was found there and there are later accounts of it, although the mines are now said to be worked out. It is possible[3] that early tin used in Egypt came from the mountains of the Kasrwan district in Syria, not far from the very ancient port of Byblos, which traded with Egypt at least as early as the Ist dynasty. Both tin and

[3] G. A. Wainwright, *Journ. Egyptian Archaeology*, 1934, xx, 29.

copper ores have been found in this locality.   It has also been suggested[4]
that the tin came ultimately from Central Germany, where it is supposed
to have been exploited before 2500 B.C.   This theory may hold for the bronzes
of Troy II, which town was apparently in close relation through the north of
the Balkans with the Danube basin and Hungary.   Bronzes from the Second
Town of Troy (2400–1900 B.C.) contain up to 11 per cent of tin.   British tin
may have been used from about 1500 B.C.   The early Egyptian bronzes are
poor in tin, and normal bronze containing about 10 per cent of tin came into
general use there about 2000 B.C.   Later, there was sometimes a tendency to
replace the tin by lead, a metal known from the predynastic period, and some
early Egyptian bronzes also contain lead.   Later Mesopotamian bronzes
contain lead and antimony in place of tin, and old Chinese bronzes also contain
much lead[5]   Tin itself occurs in Egypt from the XIIth dynasty (2000–1788
B.C.) and was perhaps known earlier, although no actual specimens of still
earlier tin are known.   It is customary among archaeologists to distinguish
between a Copper Age and a Bronze Age, following in this order, but it is
surprising to find that, if the objects are correctly dated, very good normal
tin-bronze occurs in early Sumerian remains at Ur, and is followed, not
preceded, by a Copper period, when the objects are of nearly pure copper.
This is, apparently, peculiar to Ur and Eridu, since on other Sumerian sites
copper is the earliest common metal.   Since the Sumerian culture is closely
related to, if not the same as, that at Mohenjo-daro and Harappā in the Indus
Valley, the possibility of the source of early tin being in Drangiana, which
connects Chaldea and India, seems to be strengthened.

The Sumerian and Egyptian metal workers had different techniques.   This
is especially noteworthy in the axes.   Those of the early Sumerians are cast
in the more fusible bronze, and are socketed, whilst the Egyptians used flat
hammered axes of the more difficultly-fusible copper, not socketed but bound
to the haft by thongs, and such copper axes were also used by the Sumerians.

Copper and bronze also occur in Crete, but later than in Egypt and
Mesopotamia, so that Crete presents nothing very noteworthy in this respect.
Cyprus, which was in relation with the very old site of Râs Shamra on the
mainland, and thus formed a bridge for the transmission of materials and
ideas into Palestine, had a very old copper industry going back at least to
3000 B.C., the ores being smelted on the island, and, somewhat later, bronze
was made there.   Even more important from our point of view was the brass
industry of Cyprus.   Egyptian brass of the predynastic period was found by
Petrie.   There is no definite knowledge of early brass in Mesopotamia, but
some of about 1400–1000 B.C. was found at Gezer in Palestine, containing up
to 23 per cent of zinc.   In the Roman period, the brass industry of Cyprus is
mentioned by Galen and Dioscorides, although they could not obtain any
detailed information about it (the process being, apparently, kept a trade
secret), and the rather extensive use of brass by the Romans, who established
the brass industry at Cologne about the beginning of the Christian era and
made brass known to the rest of Europe, may have been derived from Cyprus.

[4] W. Witter, *Mannus*, 1936, xxviii, 446.

[5] The suggestion by O. Davies, in his admirable book, *Roman Mines in Europe*, Oxford, 1935,
that the presence of lead in a copper alloy indicates the use of a liquation process, seems to me
doubtful; the lead bronzes were probably made by melting together the two metals.

The zinc ore was probably called *cadmia*, a name also given to varieties of zinc oxide produced in the smelting furnaces and used in medicine. The smelting furnace[6] was built into a house of two storeys, the roof being open to the air. In the wall was a charging door and the apertures for the bellows, which were in a separate house. The fuel was put in first and kindled, then the cadmia broken into small pieces, and more fuel. The zinc oxide driven off was collected in the upper storey like fleeces of wool. This process is the one used for making zinc oxide, not brass. The same type of furnace was used for making brass in Rammelsberg in the seventeenth century A.D., and small quantities of metallic zinc were collected there from the cooler walls of the furnace. The same process seems to be mentioned by Strabo. The passage in Strabo (XIII, i, 56; p. 610 C), which seems to be the first account of the production of metallic zinc, is very obscure and is almost certainly corrupt. With two slight emendations, however, it becomes perfectly intelligible. It reads as follows: 'There is an ore ($\lambda i\theta os$) near Andeira [in the Troad] which when roasted produces an ash [reading $\sigma\pi o\delta\delta s$ for the meaningless $\sigma i\delta\eta\rho os$, iron]. Next, being put into a furnace with coal ($\mu\epsilon\tau\grave{a}$ $\gamma\hat{\eta}s$ $\tau\iota\nu os$, 'a certain mineral') it runs into drops ($\grave{a}\pi o\sigma\tau\acute{a}\zeta\epsilon\iota$: Leaf's translation 'distils' is improbable, and the sense is that of running as drops, as water 'distilling' through the roof of a cavern; in medieval chemical works, a liquid is 'distilled' through a filter) of mock-silver ($\psi\epsilon v\delta\acute{a}\rho\gamma v\rho os$) which when alloyed with copper produces brass ($o\rho\epsilon\iota\chi\alpha\lambda\kappa\acute{o}s$)'. Almost the same process is described by Dioscorides (V, 84, 85), who lived about the same time as Strabo, and he supplies the readings $\sigma\pi o\delta\delta s$, and $\ddot{a}\nu\theta\rho a\xi$, coal, adopted above. Writers on the history of Chemistry have been misled by supposing that a process of distillation would be necessary to obtain zinc, whereas the production of the metal by merely heating the ore with coal in a crucible is described as late as 1743 by an English author.[7] A similar process, carried out in crucibles without distillation is described,[8] somewhat obscurely, in the Chinese work *Tien kung k'ai wu* (1637), written by a scholar with an imperfect knowledge of the technical processes he describes. He describes and illustrates the heating of the ore in crucibles, but omits to mention that coal is put in along with it. The early history of zinc is much in need of revision, the modern historians of Chemistry having added to its obscurity by misplaced scepticism and imperfect knowledge of the processes they describe. Finds of objects of metallic zinc of about Strabo's time have been reported, e.g., from the island of Rhodes, and there seems no reason to doubt that the metal was occasionally obtained in the brass furnaces. There seems to have been an early brass industry in Persia, where there are rich deposits of calamine, and brass was also made in China, where there are deposits of zinc ores. The accounts of the industry in both places are, however, quite late.

The working of iron probably originated neither in Egypt nor in the Euphrates valley; old Greek and Jewish legends point to the Chalybes, tribes

---

[6] See Agricola, *De re metallica*, trans. Hoover. London, 1912, p. 395, for a representation of a furnace which is probably identical with a brass furnace as used in the Roman period.

[7] R. James, *Medicinal Dictionary*. London, 1743–5, art. 'Zinc'.

[8] S. Julien and P. Champion, *Industries anciennes et modernes de l'empire Chinois d'après des notices traduites du Chinois*. Paris, 1869, p. 46, Plate II (also reproduced in Partington, *Everyday Chemistry*. London, 1947, p. 73, Fig. 68, and in Li Ch'iao-p'ing, *The Chemical Arts of Old China*. Easton, Pa., 1948, p. 44, Fig. 22).

related to the Hittites and living in the regions between the Caspian and Black
Seas, as the first workers in iron, which they traded with the Egyptians and
Babylonians.

Iron occurs in Egypt in the predynastic period as a valuable metal, and
since the rusted beads found by Petrie are rich in nickel they are probably of
meteoric iron. In the Great Pyramid (about 2900 B.C.) there was found a
wedge of iron, which has lately been shown not to contain nickel, and hence
is probably not meteoric. An early Sumerian iron blade found at Ur in
Mesopotamia contained over 10 per cent of nickel, and was probably of
meteoric metal. Other early iron found at Tall Asmar, however, is free
from nickel, and is probably terrestrial iron.

The process used in making iron is not known, but it probably involved the
reduction of pure oxide ore with charcoal in a shaft furnace provided with
bellows, a spongy mass of metal being obtained which was afterwards
hammered into bars whilst hot. This process is still carried on by African
tribes, no flux being used, the metal being subjected to heat treatment after
forming into small bars. Ancient steel was probably obtained by some kind
of cementation process, the iron being heated in contact with carbonaceous
material. Micrographical examination of Egyptian iron of 1200–800 B.C.
indicates that the metal was carburized and quenched. Although some
supposed early references to cast iron have been discussed, it seems improbable
that the iron could ever have been melted in the furnaces then available, and
it is still disputed when cast iron was first made.

Iron was in use in Egypt from about 2000 B.C. but only sparingly. The
source of this early useful iron was probably the Hittites around the Black
Sea, who were very skilled in the working of iron. A text from Boghazköi
of the fourteenth century B.C. speaks of 'black iron from heaven', and iron
smelting was well known in Syria, Palestine, and Asia Minor in an early period.
Petrie in 1927 found extensive remains of an iron foundry at Gerar, near
Gezer, in Palestine, dating from about 1200 B.C., and also found a steel dagger
of 1350 B.C.

Rameses II obtained presents of iron from Kitzwatna, which is probably
the Pontos region. In a Boghazköi text of about 1250 B.C., Rameses asks the
Hittite king for iron, and receives the reply: 'As for pure iron [steel] about which
you have written, there is no iron in my warehouse at Kitzwatna now, and to
make it would be inconvenient, but I have given written orders that it shall be
made. As soon as it is ready I will send some; at the moment I send only a
dagger'. The Pharaoh had come to know the value of steel weapons in his
wars against the Hittites. There was a well-developed iron industry among
the later Assyrians, and the remains of the palace of Ashurnazirpal at Nimrud
(885–860 B.C.) included large masses of iron. This king also obtained large
amounts of iron as tribute from Hittite kings. The later Assyrians probably
owed their period of military success to their possession of iron weapons.

The prehistoric Egyptian pots of soft body faced with red 'haematite' (the
Egyptologist's name for a clay rich in ferric oxide) were usually baked
upside-down with the brim covered with fuel, the process giving a black rim
and interior, partly due to carbon from smoke and partly to reduction of ferric
oxide to magnetic oxide, Fe_3O_4. It has been said that most pots are blackened

by carbon, but some contain both carbon and magnetic oxide of iron, as I have found by analyses. In some experiments made by Mercer a well-defined red with a sharply defined black top, never achieved except in Egypt and at one period in Cyprus under Egyptian influence, was obtained as follows. The pot, rubbed with haematite and water, was set with the mouth in fine sawdust in the centre of which, just under the vessel, was placed a piece of resin the size of a chestnut. Over the whole was an arch of wire netting, and over this, a fire of dry rye straw, which burned for forty-five minutes. Two kinds of heat, smokeless and smoky, are required, and when the pot becomes red-hot the sawdust, igniting last and smothering its own flame, ends the baking in a smoky heat. It has often happened that primitive industries have proved very difficult to imitate, but this was achieved by Mercer after many others had failed.

The ancient pigments were mostly natural, an exception being the Egyptian blue. This colour was used in the predynastic period, but its preparation is first given by Vitruvius from an Alexandrian source. He says: 'Sand and *natron* (native Egyptian soda) are powdered together as fine as flour, and copper is grated by coarse files over the mixture. This is made into balls by rolling with the hands. The dry balls are put in an earthen jar and this jar put into a furnace. When the copper and sand have coalesced in the intense heat and the separate things have disappeared, the colour *caerulium* is made'.

This colour was carefully examined in specimens from Pompeii by Sir Humphry Davy, who also obtained a similar product by heating sodium carbonate, silica and copper filings. This did not give the true Egyptian blue, which has been shown to contain a definite crystalline compound, $CaO, CuO, 4SiO_2$. This is formed by heating fine sand, calcium carbonate, copper carbonate, and a little alkali carbonate as a flux, for several hours in the temperature range 830–900 deg. C. Below and above this limited range it is not formed, and if too much alkali is used, only a slag results.

There was no glazed pottery in Egypt. Pottery was glazed in Assyria in the 15–12 centuries B.C. in the so-called egg-shell ware, brightly coloured, but later this product died out, only coarse pottery being made. Lead glaze appears both in Egypt and Mesopotamia about 950 B.C. In Assyria also, in the period 900–600 B.C., very artistic glazed bricks were made, the blue colour being copper silicate, the red cuprous oxide, the white a tin oxide enamel (the earliest known example of enamel), and the yellow lead antimoniate ('Naples yellow'). The bright yellow of some Egyptian glass may have been obtained with lead and antimony. Glazed pottery was made in Crete about 2200 B.C., and this is perhaps the earliest known use of the art.

In the case of a powdered quartz body, the glaze was probably first made as a frit, then powdered, mixed with water and painted on the object, which was then dried and fired. This is the process used by modern forgers in Cairo, who carry out the firing in closed boxes of copper or in pots to prevent discoloration by smoke, and their products are the same as the ancient Egyptian, being made by the same process.

Glass itself was known very early in Egypt and Mesopotamia. There are finds of glass in both localities before 3000 B.C. in the form of beads, and a large piece of blue glass of about 2400 B.C. was found at Abu Shahrain (ancient Eridu) in Mesopotamia. The Egyptians were very skilled in the making of glass; the remains of a factory, with a profusion of glass objects, was found at Amarna (1350 B.C.). Apparently quartz sand and alkali were made into a frit in clay pans, some of which were found. The alkali was native soda, found in Egypt. The frit was then melted in small crucibles 2–3 in. deep and wide. Petrie says the glass was never cast in moulds, but was pressed when viscous into the moulds; others say it was pressed over clay forms, or the clay forms dipped into the glass, or glass threads were wound round over the mould, and then 'dragged' while soft so as to give a wavy pattern. The colours are very good. The blue was usually copper, and the red cuprous oxide; the yellow may have been lead antimoniate, lead and antimony being found in XIXth dynasty yellow glass. Cobalt occurs in some Egyptian glasses of the fourteenth century B.C. Colourless glass had been made in Egypt from about 1400 B.C., probably from very pure materials, although some glass found at Amarna contains manganese and had probably been decolorized by pyrolusite.

Glass objects were ground, but the wheel was used in Egypt only in the Roman period. The analyses indicate that the Egyptian glasses are of good quality and of relatively high melting point. Blowing glass was unknown in ancient Egypt, and it seems to have been invented in Sidon about the beginning of the Christian era. Both Seneca and Pliny speak of blown glass as something new in their time.

Assyrian glass is represented in the British Museum by the glass bottle of Sargon II (722–705 B.C.), which was almost certainly of native manufacture, the old idea that it was imported from Egypt being improbable from recent knowledge. Blue glass coloured with cobalt occurs in Mesopotamia. About two-thirds of the so-called lapis lazuli found in Nippur in Mesopotamia, probably of the fourteenth century B.C., was a blue lead glass coloured with copper (1·94 per cent CuO) and cobalt (0·93 per cent CoO). This blue glass imitating lapis lazuli was a speciality in Babylonia, where it was called *uqnu*. A series of Assyrian tablets of the period 668–628 B.C., found in the library of Assurbanipal and now in the British Museum, contains lists of stones, liquids, etc., and although they have long been known their translation is fairly recent.[9] Some of them deal with the production of false gems and coloured glass pastes. They have been rather hastily called 'alchemical' texts, but in reality they are technical treatises. One tablet contains instructions for building the furnace, with an appropriate ritual, and for the production of coloured glasses. It seems as if the traditions preserved in these chemical tablets go back to much earlier times, since a similar tablet of the seventeenth century B.C. was found[10] at Tall Umar on the Tigris. It is written in a difficult style, perhaps intentionally cryptic, and describes the production of a blue glaze containing lead and copper by an unnecessarily complicated process. The Babylonians and Assyrians seem to have been just as expert in Applied Chemistry as the Egyptians, and unlike the latter they have left some of their actual recipes. The collection of Egyptian recipes in the Greek papyri of Leyden and Stockholm, written in Alexandria about 300 B.C., may go back to much earlier, still unknown, originals.

[9] R. C. Thompson, *A dictionary of Assyrian chemistry and geology.* Oxford, 1936; *Ambix*, 1938, ii, 3.

[10] C. J. Gadd and R. C. Thompson, *Iraq*, 1936, ii, (I), 874.

On the side of Organic Chemistry, perhaps the use of dyes is the most interesting. Dyeing was very old in Egypt, where red, yellow, and green clothing is shown in the oldest pictures. Ancient Egyptian dyes definitely established by analysis are indigo and safflower (*Carthamus*). The use of indigo (perhaps obtained from a kind of woad) is especially interesting, since the Romans, who then obtained it from India, were unable to get it into solution and used it only as a pigment (Pliny puts it among the minerals). The Egyptians seem to have been acquainted with the use of mordants, since Pliny mentions that they first impregnated the fabric with chemicals (probably alum[11] and vitriols) which did not give it any colour, but when it was put into a cauldron of boiling dye it was drawn out showing various colours, although there was only one colour in the cauldron. Parti-coloured fabrics, some printed, were found in Egypt at Ikhmim from about Pliny's time, and the process probably went back to an earlier period. The use of the so-called Phoenician purple (a dibromoindigo), obtained from mollusca, appears to have begun in Crete, where large heaps of the murex shells have been found. In later times dyeing in purple was carried out on the large scale in Tyre and Sidon. The process is rather fully described by Pliny and has been successfully imitated in modern times. There were two kinds of mollusc used, the *buccinum* (with trumpet-shaped shells) and the *pelagium*.[12] The juices were combined, mixed with a little salt, and boiled in a lead cauldron. The liquor was tested by putting in a piece of washed wool, and the boiling continued until this came out the required shade, which was a very dark red or crimson rather than what we now call purple. The wool was then put in, left for five hours, taken out, and immersed in a new bath, producing the so-called 'double dyed' purple, which was very expensive. Pliny says 1 lb. of double dyed wool cost £31 5s. It had a rather unpleasant fishy smell.

In Mesopotamia we have the beginnings of the petroleum industry. Bitumen occurs in some of the oldest Sumerian remains, and was obtained from Hît on a river of the same name flowing into the Euphrates about a hundred miles north of Babylon. It was extensively used by the Babylonians for cement, for asphalt drains, floors, etc. Bitumen was also obtained in other places. From these sources was also obtained naphtha (Babylonian *naptu*) or crude petroleum, used for lamps. There were two kinds, a black and white. Strabo says the naphtha of Susiana (which he calls a kind of sulphur) when brought near a fire was ignited and could only be extinguished by a large quantity of water, or by mud, vinegar, alum and glue (an ancient anticipation of the 'foamite' process). Pliny speaks of a white naphtha which Dioscorides calls 'filtered asphalt'. Perhaps it was refined by filtration through kaolin or some kind of absorbent earth, although the possibility of distillation at this time cannot be dismissed.

Taken all in all, the ancient achievements in Applied Chemistry present an impressive picture. They represent far more than is commonly realized or appreciated. It is only by looking at the whole, pieced together from fragments often insignificant, that its magnitude stands revealed for those to see who

[11] Charles Singer, *The Earliest Chemical Industry. An essay in the historical relations of economics and technology illustrated from the alum trade.* London, 1948.

[12] G. Moatsu, *H ΠΟΡΦΥΡΑ*. Alexandria, 1932.

know what effort each part must have cost. The history of Chemistry apart from this neglected part is incomplete, and if the ancient world had little to teach us in theory, its contributions to the practical side of chemical knowledge are worthy of recognition.

EGYPT'S PLACE IN MEDICAL HISTORY

by

WARREN R. DAWSON

I

THE medicine of ancient Egypt undoubtedly occupies an important place in the history of the science, but it has generally been unfortunate in the manner of its treatment by medical historians. In most of the standard medical histories, as well as in innumerable separate pamphlets, lectures and papers, general accounts of Egyptian medicine are to be found, but most of them give a very erroneous notion of the real nature of the medical knowledge and practice of the Egyptians. The reason for this state of affairs is not far to seek : medical historians, not being Egyptologists, have been unable to consult the original documents for themselves, and have been obliged to collect their data at second or third hand from various old and pre-existing published sources, most of them written many years ago when the knowledge of the ancient writing of the hieroglyphs (or in manuscripts, its derivative, hieratic) was in a far less advanced state than it is to-day. Moreover, the nature of Egyptian magic, which is the parent of medicine, was so completely misunderstood as to give a quite false picture of the real state of affairs. Most of the information imparted by medical historians, and the writers upon whom they drew, has been based upon a single document— the Ebers Papyrus—of which, unfortunately for science, a very incorrect and unsatisfactory German 'translation' appeared as long ago as 1890.[1] It is to this well-intended but unfortunate work that most of the errors and misconceptions of later historians can be traced. Even so learned an Egyptologist as Professor Ebers, a former owner of the document (who named it after himself), so entirely mistook its nature and purport as to call it a 'Hermetic Book'.[2] An attempt will be made in the following pages to indicate the true nature of the Ebers and the other so-called Medical Papyri, but in the meantime sufficient has been said to show the unsatisfactory nature of the principal materials hitherto available to historians. For nearly thirty years, I have made a special study of Egyptian medicine directly from the texts themselves, and have endeavoured to form conclusions uninfluenced by the statements of other writers. I am well aware that in order to handle the subject really adequately we must await the advent of a qualified medical man who is also a competent Egyptologist, and whilst this combination of elements has not so far appeared in one individual, medical historians have been obliged to borrow their Egyptological data more or less untested; and conversely, Egyptologists writing on so highly technical a subject must necessarily depend upon borrowed plumes on the purely medical side. If I may lay some claim to Egyptological knowledge, I can certainly lay no claim to medical qualifications; but I have been at pains to acquire some acquaintance with the elements

[1] *Papyros Ebers. Das älteste Buch über Heilkunde* . . . übersetzt von Dr. H. Joachim. Berlin, 1890.

[2] *Papyros Ebers. Das hermetische Buch über die Arzeneimittel der alten Ägypter in hieratischer Schrift.* 2 vols. Leipzig, 1875.

of anatomy and physiology, and hope I may claim, without undue immodesty, to know enough of these subjects to enable me to appreciate the purport, if not the actual words, of the ancient medical writings.   I mention these facts, because it has frequently been assumed, from my previously-published writings on Egyptian medicine, that I am a medical man; but I wish to make it quite clear that I have no academic connection either with Egyptology or with medicine, and am most anxious that I should not be thought to sail under false colours.

The ancient Egyptians have always enjoyed a great reputation for their medical knowledge, especially in classical times.   In the *Odyssey*, for instance, it is stated that the physicians of Egypt were skilled beyond those of all other lands, and Herodotus several times mentions the medical practitioners of Egypt, each of whom, he says, was a specialist, applying himself to the study of a particular branch.   The same writer relates that Cyrus sent to Egypt for an oculist, and that Darius held that the Egyptians enjoyed the highest reputation for their medical skill: elsewhere similar references are to be found.[3] The 'wisdom of the Egyptians' is indeed proverbial, and although they were incapable of that characteristic of the Greek mind—true philosophy and abstract thought—there is no doubt that they were a very highly gifted people, with a great capacity for practical achievement.   There can no longer be any reasonable doubt that the foundations of medical science were laid in Egypt more than fifty centuries ago, and although many modern writers have credited the Egyptians with medical and scientific knowledge of profound extent, others have denied this claim almost to the point of its non-existence,[4] though the writers on both sides of the question usually display a lack of true knowledge of the facts.   The truth, of course, lies between these extremes; and indeed a nation which had acquired sufficient knowledge and skill to plan and carry out feats of engineering and architecture, such as the Pyramids, as early as the fourth millenium before Christ, and whose mathematical knowledge, whilst wholly practical in aim, included highly complex calculations involving the principles of angles, cubic capacity, the square-root and fractional notation was obviously far ahead of its contemporaries in intellectual capacity.   That this real knowledge evolved and developed amidst the meshes of a complex web of magic and super-stition, does not in the least detract from its value, but rather enhances it.   It may appear to be a sweeping generalization, but I believe it is nevertheless quite true, that magic was the basic motive that prompted almost all the practical achievements of the Egyptians.   The real purpose which inspired the erection of the gigantic pyramids and temples, of the preservation of the dead and the vast and valuable equipment with which they were provided, was essentially *magic*, and the impressive and multifarious remains of the ancient civilization which extend from the Delta to the Cataracts and far into Nubia, are but the translation of the magical motive into practical fact.   In medicine, as we shall see, magic played the leading part, and time has spared for us a considerable number of written documents—the so-called Medical Papyri—

[3] In 1924, I published an article on Herodotus as a Medical Writer in the *Annals of Med. History*, vi, 357–60.   I was not then aware that the same subject had been dealt with many years before by Dr. Carl Moeller, in his pamphlet *Die Medizin in Herodot*, Berlin, 1903, which I did not see till more than ten years later.

[4] e.g. T. Wingate Todd, *American Anthropologist*, 1921, xxiii, 460–70.

in which Egyptian ideas on magic and medicine are formulated, and which, as the oldest body of medical literature in the world, are the foundation upon which our knowledge of Egyptian medicine and its derivatives must necessarily be based.   It will be convenient, before proceeding further, to enumerate and comment on these documents.

II

The contents of these papyri fall into two groups: those which may claim to be called medical books, and those which are mainly magical in purport or are collections of popular recipes.   These two groups I will indicate respectively by the letters A and B.   The contents of some of the papyri fall wholly in group A, a few wholly or mainly in group B, and others again contain elements of both groups, more or less indiscriminately combined.

(1) *The Ebers Papyrus.* This document is placed first in the list (although in point of age it deserves no such priority), because it is the longest, most complete, and most famous of all these documents.   It was found, together with the Edwin Smith Papyrus (below, No. 5), in 1862 by Edwin Smith (1822–1906), an American resident in Egypt, who traded in antiquities.[5] Smith sold it a few years later to Professor Georg Ebers of Leipzig, who named it after himself and published a sumptuous facsimile of it.[6]   In this edition, Ebers did not attempt a translation, but he gave an introductory account of the manuscript, the nature of which, as already mentioned, he wholly mis-conceived.   It also contains an Egyptian-Latin Glossary by Ludwig Stern, which is still useful as an index of words, but as a glossary is almost valueless, as it is full of mere guesswork.   A transcript of the hieratic text into hiero-glyphic characters was published without letterpress in 1913 by the late Dr. Walter Wreszinski.[7]   This convenient edition of the text is that most generally used by Egyptologists, although frequent reference must still be made to Ebers's facsimile in order to control Wreszinski's readings.   This editor has conveniently divided the 110 pages of the original manuscript into 877 numbered sections.   A courageous attempt at a full translation into English was made by Dr. B. Ebbell a few years ago, but, whilst this is an immense improvement on Joachim's translation of 1890, it cannot be considered as altogether satisfactory.[8]

Physically, the Ebers Papyrus is in perfect condition and is easily legible from beginning to end.   Its contents, written on the recto, are medical and magical throughout, but on the verso, and quite unrelated to the recto, is written a short calendar which has been of great importance in the study of the difficult problems of Egyptian chronology.   The rest of the verso is uninscribed.   The document was written at the beginning of the XVIIIth dynasty, but there is abundant evidence, based on philological and other grounds, that it was copied from a series of books many centuries older.   It is not a book in the

---

[5] Concerning Edwin Smith and his connection with Egyptology, see my *Life of Charles Wycliffe Goodwin.* Oxford, 1934, pp. 111 ff.

[6] *op. cit.* (2).

[7] *Der Papyrus Ebers. I Teil: Umschrift.* Leipzig, 1913.   No further parts have appeared.

[8] *The Papyrus Ebers: the greatest Egyptian medical document.* Copenhagen and London, 1937.   I have examined this publication in *Journ. Egyptian Archaeology*, xxiv, 250, and have there stated the reasons for my opinion.

proper sense of the word, but a miscellany of extracts, recipes and jottings collected from at least forty different sources, and it is in this respect exactly analogous to the collections of household and medical recipes of Europe in later times. To speak of the Ebers Papyrus, as many writers have done, as an authoritative Egyptian medical treatise from a temple library, is manifestly absurd. The text consists mainly of a large collection of prescriptions for numerous ailments, most of which are named but not diagnosed, specifying the drugs to be used, the measures of each, and the method of preparing and administering them. A few of the sections are extracts from a more serious general medical treatise belonging to the group A, specified above, and of which treatise some portions have come down to us in the Edwin Smith and Kahûn Papyri. The extracts in the Ebers Papyrus just referred to relate to diseases of the stomach, to the action of the heart and its vessels, and to the surgical treatment of cysts, boils, carbuncles and similar conditions. All these excerpts can be readily identified by the fact that in them alone symptoms are described and diagnoses made, and that certain distinctive formulae occur in them which are absent from the rest of the text. Freely interspersed amongst these elements are magical spells and incantations.

(2) *The Ramesseum Papyri.* These two papyri, and that to be next described, are the oldest of the known medical papyri. They belong to the Middle Kingdom, and were written in the XIIth or XIIIth dynasties. The name that has attached itself to them is therefore misleading, for the Ramesseum (the great mortuary temple of the famous Pharaoh Rameses II) dates of course from the XIXth dynasty, some centuries later. Actually they were found, together with many other fragmentary papyri, in a Middle Kingdom tomb beneath the foundations of the Ramesseum, the existence of which was not known to the builders of the latter. The discovery was made in 1896 by the late Mr. J. E. Quibell. Some of the literary papyri from this important find have long since been published, but many of the others (including the medical) are still unpublished. In 1923, Sir Alan H. Gardiner kindly lent me photographs of the two medical papyri from which I made hieroglyphic transcripts. Both are fragmentary and full of lacunae, but sufficient is preserved to establish the nature of the texts. No. 1 is written in vertical columns of hieratic writing, and from the surviving fragments I can distinguish parts of eighteen different recipes for the protection of mothers and their babies.[9] The remedies are sometimes incantations, sometimes prescriptions of drugs. Amongst the recipes may be mentioned one for ascertaining whether a new-born infant will live or die, and one for contraception. Some passages of this text occur also in the Kahûn Papyrus (below, No. 3). The second Ramesseum Papyrus contains a collection of prescriptions for rheumatoid or arthritic complaints, and many of them closely resemble the similar recipes in the Ebers and Hearst Papyri. This document is also written in vertical columns, but in a form of script known as linear hieroglyphic or semi-hieratic. The larger five fragments contain the remains of twenty-six prescriptions. Both papyri belong wholly to group B.

(3) *The Kahûn Papyrus.* This was discovered at Lâhûn in the Faiyûm

---

[9] The text is similar to, but not a duplicate of, a later papyrus (Berlin 3027) published by Erman as *Zauberspruch für Mutter und Kind*. Berlin, 1901,

district of Lower Egypt in 1889. Like those just described, it is of Middle Kingdom date. Although fragmentary, it contains the remains of thirty-four sections, all of which are gynaecological. Most of the sections are extracts from the general medical treatise of which the Edwin Smith and parts of the Ebers Papyri are excerpts (group A), but there are also some medico-magical recipes and incantations of group B, doubtless brought together because of their subject-matter. The prescriptions are for affections of the uterus and vagina, and there are also nostrums for ascertaining pregnancy and the sex of unborn children, these sections occurring in three other papyri (below, Nos. 7, 9, 12). The text was published many years ago with a translation and commentary.[10]

(4) *The Hearst Papyrus* was found at Deir et Ballâs in Upper Egypt in 1899, and is now preserved in the University of California. A photographic facsimile, with an introduction and index of words, but without translation, was published by the late Dr. G. A. Reisner a few years later.[11] The outermost folds of the roll are fragmentary, but otherwise the document is in good condition and consists of fifteen almost undamaged columns, which Dr. Wreszinski, who has published a hieroglyphic transcript, has divided into 250 sections.[12] The papyrus is very similar to the Ebers, of which it contains a number of duplicate passages. It is somewhat later in date than the Ebers, and may be assigned to the time of Tuthmosis III (XVIIIth dynasty).

(5) *The Edwin Smith Papyrus.* This manuscript was found in Egypt, together with the Ebers Papyrus and other documents, in 1862. Edwin Smith did not sell it, and it remained in his possession until his death. His daughter presented it to the New York Historical Society in 1906. In 1930, the late Professor J. H. Breasted of Chicago, having devoted several years to a close study of it, published the papyrus in a sumptuous edition, consisting of a photographic facsimile and transcript in a folio volume, and a stout quarto containing a translation, commentary and glossary.[13] The greater part of this valuable document belongs to our group A, and is devoted to the treatment of wounds and fractures, extracted from the same general medical treatise as the before-mentioned sections of the Ebers Papyrus and the Kahûn Papyrus. It contains forty-eight long sections, each dealing with a particular case, i.e. the affection of a particular organ or region of the body. In addition to these rationally and almost scientifically described cases, the papyrus contains thirteen medico-magical incantations and prescriptions, as well as some explanatory glosses. The medico-magical elements fall into group B.

(6) *The Chester-Beatty Papyri.* Eighteen of this valuable collection of nineteen hieratic papyri of Ramesside period were presented to the British Museum by Mr. and Mrs. A. Chester-Beatty and edited by Sir Alan Gardiner in 1935.[14] The series contains literary and magical documents, two of which

[10] *Hieratic Papyri from Kahûn and Gurob*, by F. Ll. Griffith. London, 1898, 5–11, and Pls. V, VI.

[11] *The Hearst Medical Papyrus.* Leipzig, 1905.

[12] *Der Londoner Medizinische Papyrus und der Papyrus Hearst.* Leipzig, 1912, 1–133 (text, German translation, and commentary).

[13] *The Edwin Smith Surgical Papyrus.* Chicago, Univ. Press, 1930. The late Sir D'Arcy Power published two interesting articles on this papyrus in *Brit. Journ. Surg.*, 1933, xxi, 1–4; 385–7.

[14] *Hieratic Papyri in the British Museum. 3rd series: Chester-Beatty Gift.* 2 vols. London, 1935.

are entirely on medical subjects. The recto of Papyrus No. VI (Brit. Mus. 10686) may be described as a fragment of a treatise on proctology, as it is concerned exclusively with the treatment of affections of the anus and rectum. Although the prescriptions of drugs resemble the familiar pattern of those in the Ebers, Hearst and other papyri, this document differs in an important respect from all the others, and this difference, which will be indicated later in this paper, entitles the papyrus (in my opinion) to be placed in our group A. The verso contains spells and incantations for epilepsy, and these are to be placed in group B. Papyrus No. X (Brit. Mus. 10690) is a book of aphrodisiacs consisting of spells and drugs against impotency, etc. Several of the longer papyri in the Chester-Beatty Collection are filled with magical incantations which are medical in so far as their purport is the cure and prevention of disease.

(7) *The Berlin Medical Papyrus.* This document, of the XIXth dynasty (Berlin Museum 3038), came to Europe early in the nineteenth century with the Passalacqua Collection, and is said to have been found at Sakkara. A lithographic facsimile of it, not very satisfactory, was published many years ago by Brugsch,[15] and more recently a photographic facsimile, with a hieroglyphic transcript, German translation and glossary, appeared under the editorship of Dr. Wreszinski, who divided the text into 204 sections.[16] The contents are very similar to those of the Ebers and Hearst Papyri, of which it contains several duplicate passages. The text is extremely faulty and corrupt, often to the pitch of unintelligibility. On the verso occur the nostrums for the ascertainment of pregnancy, etc., which occur in several other papyri. Nearly all the contents must be relegated to group B, but there is one extract of group A.

(8) *The London Medical Papyrus.* A fragmentary papyrus of the latter part of the XVIIIth dynasty: it is a badly written palimpsest, many traces of an earlier erased text being discernible. It consists entirely of medico-magical recipes and prescriptions, all of group B. A photographic facsimile with a hieroglyphic transcript, German translation and glossary has been published by Dr. Wreszinski.[17] This document was formerly in the library of the Royal Institution, but how it came there is not known. It was presented to the British Museum in 1860 (Brit. Mus. 10059).

(9) *The Carlsberg Papyrus.* The papyrus known as Carlsberg No. VIII is a mere fragment, but it is of considerable interest. The recto contains the remains of prescriptions for the eyes, duplicating a passage of the Ebers Papyrus, and the verso is filled with the birth-prognoses known to us in three other Egyptian papyri (Nos. 3, 7, 12), and is the prototype of many popular birth-prognoses which appear in popular medical (or rather, pseudo-medical) literature over a period of many centuries.[18]

(10) *Magical Papyri.* The museums of London, Paris, Leyden, Turin, Budapest, Rome (Vatican), Berlin, and other cities contain considerable

---

[15] *Recueil de monuments égyptiens.* Ed. by H. Brugsch and J. Dümichen. Leipzig, 1862–85, vol. ii, Pls. 85–107.

[16] *Der grosse Medizinische Papyrus des Berliner Museums.* Leipzig, 1909.

[17] *Der Londoner Medizinische Papyrus und der Papyrus Hearst.* Leipzig, 1912, 137–237.

[18] *Papyrus Carlsberg No. VIII, with some remarks on the Egyptian Origin of some popular Birth Prognoses*, by Erik Iversen. (Kgl. Danske Videnskobernes Selskab, Hist-Filologiske Meddeleser XXVI. 5.) Copenhagen, 1939.

numbers of magical papyri, which, although not generally therapeutic in character, are medical in so far as their purpose is the treatment and cure of disease, injury and the attacks of venomous animals. The Chester-Beatty Collection, as already mentioned, contains several documents of this class, but the richest stores are those of the museums of Leyden and Turin. All these, fantastic as they often are, have a place in the development of medicine, and they well exemplify the *modus operandi* of the magician.[19]

(11) *Ostraca.* All the medical texts described in the foregoing paragraphs are collections of prescriptions, some of which are large and all of which, when complete, were probably extensive. Isolated prescriptions are rare, but a few have been found written on ostraca, i.e. limestone flakes or potsherds. Thus an ostracon in the Louvre (3255) contains two prescriptions for the ear; Milne Ostracon C.I. is a spell for the protection of the limbs on the principle that 'like influences like'; Ramesseum Ostracon 35 is a protection against snake-bite; Medineh Ostracon 1091 is a prescription for a 'cure-all' in any part of the body.

(12) *Later documents.* The texts enumerated above are all of the Pharaonic Period, that is to say of the Middle and New Kingdoms, but in addition to these we have some documents of Ptolemaic and later date. An important magical papyrus,[20] part of which is in the British Museum and part in Leyden, written in the demotic script and of the third century A.D., contains a good deal of medical matter, though all of it belongs to group B. Of Coptic material, the great medical papyrus of Mashâykh, discovered in 1892, is the most important item. This long document contains 237 prescriptions, and is, in the main, very similar to the medical papyri of Pharaonic times. Although it was written as late as the ninth or tenth century A.D. it closely adheres to the traditional forms, albeit some Greek and Arabic elements have obtruded themselves. It was published *in extenso* in a bulky volume in 1921.[21] Other Coptic medical texts, much smaller in extent, exist in the British Museum;[22] the John Rylands Library at Manchester;[23] the Vatican;[24] the Berlin Museum[25] and the University of Michigan,[26] and Paris.[27]

[19] See my Frazer Lecture, *Folk-Lore*, 1936, xlvii, 234–62 on the subject of the magical papyri generally.

[20] *The Demotic Magical Papyrus of London and Leiden*, by F. Ll. Griffith and [Sir] Herbert Thompson. 3 vols. London, 1904–9.

[21] *Un Papyrus Médical Copte*, by Emile Chassinat. Cairo, 1921. See also my paper in *Proc. Roy. Soc. Med.*, 1924, xvii (Sect. Hist. Med.), 51–7.

[22] MS. Or. 4920(3), W. E. Crum, *Cat. Coptic MSS. Brit. Mus.* No. 527, p. 255; an ointment for the eyes, Ostr. 27422, H. R. Hall, *Coptic and Greek Texts*, 1905, p. 64.

[23] W. E. Crum, *Cat. Coptic MSS. John Rylands Library*, Nos. 102, 104, 106–10.

[24] G. Zoëga, *Catalogus Codicum Copticorum*. Rome, 1810, pp. 626–30. (Contains 45 prescriptions, written on leaves of a vellum book, numbered ⲤⲙⲆ to ⲤⲙⲆ (i.e. 241–244).) This book, when complete, must have contained nearly 2000 prescriptions up to p. 244 if the average number per page revealed by the surviving fragment held good throughout. This assumes, of course, that the whole of its contents consisted of prescriptions, but the earlier leaves may have contained other matter.

[25] Ostracon 2173, *Zeitschr. f. äg. Sprache*, 1878, xvi, Taf. i (prescription for spitting blood); Ostr. P. 4984, *Koptische Urkunden*, No. 27 (preparation of a drug); Ostr. P. 8109, *op. cit.*, i. p. 24 (prescriptions for insomnia, palpitation, menstruation, etc.).

[26] Coptic MSS. 593–603. W. H. Worrell, 'A Coptic wizard's hoard.' *Amer. Journ. Semitic Languages*, 1930, xlvi, 239–62.

[27] Urbain Bouriant, 'Fragment d'un Livre de Médecine en Copte.' *Compt. rend. de l'Acad. des Inscr. et Belles-Lettres*, 1887, xv, 374. A single leaf from a vellum book containing eleven prescriptions for the breasts. The pages are numbered ⲤⲓⲆ and Ⲥⲓⲉ (214, 215).

From various sites in Egypt, chiefly in the Faiyûm, has come to light a series of medical papyri wholly Egyptian in character, though written in Greek. These are now dispersed in various museums. Most of them follow the ancient pattern and are obviously of native origin. Thus we find in one fragment eleven prescriptions for the ear,[28] in a second, five prescriptions for the eyes,[29] and in a third, fourteen prescriptions for a variety of ailments.[30] Three fragments deal with the making of lozenges (τροχίσκοι) and tooth-powder (ὀδοντότριμμα).[31] But in addition to these collections of popular recipes, medical papyri not only written in Greek, but also of Greek origin, have been found in Egypt. Thus the Golenischef Papyrus, a Greek medical fragment of the third century A.D., although too fragmentary to be translated as it stands, contains a text closely resembling a passage from the Gynaecology of Soranus of Ephesus.[32] Another document, the Cattaui Papyrus, contains 2 columns of 27 lines each, a fragment of a surgical treatise of the third century A.D.[33] A papyrus in the John Rylands Library describes the omens and significance of the quivering or twitching of every part of the body. It begins with the abdomen and enumerates 41 organs or parts of the body from that point to the soles of the feet. Presumably, when complete, it began at the top of the head.[34] A Greek medical papyrus from Egypt of late first or early second century A.D. deals with luxation of the jaw.[35]

Such, in outline, is the documentary material available for the study of Egyptian medicine, and it is at the same time voluminous and fragmentary. Tradition ascribed to various gods, to certain early kings, and to sages such as Imhotep (the Imouthes of the Greeks) the authorship of medical treatises. Whilst we have no indication of the authenticity of such attributions, we do know that one or two general treatises did exist, by whomsoever they were compiled, and that fragments of them have come down to us in several papyri.

III

As already mentioned, magic played a very prominent part in the social and religious life of the Egyptians: it affected not only the relations of men with their living fellows, but also with the dead and with the gods.[36] By the Egyptian, magic was believed to be a sure means of accomplishing all his necessities and desires, and of performing indeed everything which the common procedure of daily life was inadequate to bring about. It was, theoretically at least, the private faith of the magician in his own omnipotence, his *credo quia*

[28] Grenfell and Hunt, *Oxyrhynchus Papyri*, 1899, ii, 134, No. 234 (2–3 century A.D.).

[29] *Tebtunis Papyri*, 1907, ii, 22, No. 273 (late second or early third century A.D.).

[30] *Oxyrhynchus Papyri*, 1911, viii, 110, No. 1088 (early first century A.D.).

[31] A. S. Hunt, *Cat. Greek Papyri, John Rylands Library*, 65–9, Nos. 29, 29A, 29B.

[32] A. Bäckström, *Archiv für Papyrusforschung*, 1906, iii, 157–62. The passage from Soranus is in ed. Huber, Munich, 1894, 148 ff.; ed. Rose, ii, 31, 85.

[33] Jules Nicole, *Archiv für Papyrusforschung*, 1908, iv, 269–71, with commentary by Johannes Ilberg, *ibid.*, 271–83; E. Chassinat, *Bull. de l'Inst. Franç. d'Arch. Orientale*, 1910, viii, 111–12 and 1 Pl.

[34] Rylands Greek Papyrus, No. 28. A. S. Hunt, *Cat. Greek Papyri, John Rylands Library*, i, 56–65.

[35] Brit. Mus. Pap. Gr. 155, purchased from the Rev. Greville Chester, who obtained it in Egypt. F. G. Kenyon, *Cat. Greek Papyri*, 1898, ii, xiv, 144.

On Egyptian Magic generally, see my paper in *Folk-Lore*, 1936, xlvii, 234–62.

impossibile. The Egyptians, naturally a gifted and practical people, were incapable of abstract thought, yet in very early times they so far recognized the existence and importance of the mystical power of magic upon which they placed so much reliance, as to conceive it as an entity and to name it. In very early texts we meet with the word *hike*, 'magic', a mystic power that was soon personified as a god, and it was by virtue of this *hike* that they carried out throughout their long history the complex series of rites, customs and beliefs which we to-day describe as magical. The power of magic was coextensive with the whole range of human activity and desire, and it was employed explicitly or implicity for almost every conceivable purpose.

The magic art was most often exercised for defensive, protective, preventive, productive and prognostic purposes. The services of the magician are most commonly met with in the prevention and cure of sickness, injury, the bites or stings of noxious animals and other similar calamities befalling the individual. These medical applications of the magic art, besides being the most numerous, well exemplify the method of procedure of the practitioner, and enable us to discern the steps by which the germs of rational scientific ideas grew out of mere magical jargon.

In the numerous medico-magical texts which have come down to us, the leading idea is possession, for diseases are treated as if personified and are harangued and addressed by the magician. It is generally stated or implied that disease or suffering is due to the actual presence in the patient's body of the demon itself, but frequently it is implied that the suffering is due to some poison or other evil emanation that the demon has projected into the body of his victim. The possessing spirit is usually conceived as a god or a goddess, a dead man or a dead woman, an enemy male or female, or a pain male or female. This collocation of words with endless variations is an oft-recurring formula in the magical spells.

Once installed, the demon made the patient ill and the business of the magician was primarily to eject the intruder. The simplest method of procedure was the recitation of a spell in which the demon was summarily ordered to quit, or the poison to flow forth from the infected body. These spells, of varying length and elaboration, are full of references to the gods and are often of the highest mythological interest. Some of the more elaborate spells embody threats and exorcisms of the most daring character. In these simplest cases, the magician operated by word of mouth only, but in most spells the spoken words are accompanied by a ritual—by gestures or by the use of amulets or other objects. These two essential parts of the magician's art have been very aptly termed by Sir Alan Gardiner the *oral rite* and the *manual rite* respectively. It is usual in the magico-medical texts to find a rubric at the end of the spoken formula (or oral rite) giving directions as to the performance of an accompanying manual rite. The manual rite often took the form of reciting the spell over an image, a string of beads, a knotted cord, a strip of inscribed linen, an amulet, a stone, or some other object. These articles, thus magically charged, the magician is directed to lay upon or attach to some part of the patient's body. In cases of illness or injury, the manual rite often takes the form of repeating the formula over a mixture of substances which were then given to the patient to swallow, or were applied to his body externally as ointments or poultices, the medicine so given being thus rendered efficacious by the recitation of the oral rite.   The medical papyri, which consist for the most part of prescriptions of drugs, are interspersed with magical spells, the object of which was to impart efficacy to the prescriptions which follow them.   Such spells are the oral rites belonging to each group of prescriptions, the preparation and administration of each of which constitute the corresponding manual rite.   Many of the doses contain noxious or offensive ingredients (coprotherapy being especially frequent), and their object is manifestly to make them as unpalatable as possible to the possessing spirit so as to give it no inducement to linger in the patient's body.

It is characteristic of the magician at all times that he should have more than one string to his bow, for if one remedy fails, another may succeed, and at all costs his prestige must be maintained.   Thus it is that we find in the medical papyri numerous alternative prescriptions for each complaint, and in the magical texts alternative spells to be recited with the same object.   Some of the remedies contain drugs that are really appropriate and beneficial, and such prescriptions, actually accomplishing their purpose, would tend to survive their more fantastic fellows.   By such means, more and more reliance would come to be placed on the drugs themselves (i.e. upon the manual rite) and less and less upon the recited spells (i.e. the oral rite).   The magicians, therefore, who would be most in request in case of sickness would be those who were skilled in the knowledge of the preparation of drugs and manipulative treatment. Such men were no longer mere magicians, but were becoming physicians—and thus out of magic grew medicine.   But the evolution of the physician did not extinguish magic.   It is rare in human experience for any new order to supersede the old completely.   The first physicians kept magic as a stand-by: magical methods continued to be employed side by side with the more rational procedure, as the medical papyri of Pharaonic times clearly show.   Moreover, the existence of many magical papyri dating from Ptolemaic times and later, written in demotic Egyptian, Coptic and Greek, reveal unmistakably that magical practices for the cure of disease were in active operation long after the influence of scientific medicine, which was mainly due to the Greeks, had made itself felt.   Magic maintained powerful sway throughout the early centuries of the Christian Era and throughout the Middle Ages: it persisted into the sixteenth, seventeenth and eighteenth centuries, and is by no means extinct to-day, even among highly civilized nations.   The magician has survived: he has merely changed his role from time to time, becoming successively the palmer, the quack and the advertiser of medicines.   The ancient magician, when, *malgré lui*, he had become physician, refused to part with the mysticism of his craft, and he often disguised his more rational treatment under a veneer of mystery, a method which has been followed throughout the ages by his successors.

The very multiplicity of the prescriptions in the medical papyri is of itself a confession of their purely arbitrary and unscientific character: the very fact that numerous alternative remedies are provided for one and the same complaint implies that if one fails, another should be tried until, perchance, an effective one was found.   The procedure according to most of the medical papyri really amounts to this—Try X, *or* Y, *or* Z, and so on.   A definite advance on this haphazard method is manifested by the Chester-Beatty Papyrus VI, where the plan is: Do X, *then* Y, *then* Z, etc. That is to say the prescriptions for each case were to be *all* employed successively, and not merely selected at will from many alternatives. It is for this reason that I would place the papyrus in question in the group A, as defined above.

IV

Had the Egyptians any knowledge of anatomy and physiology, or was their medical lore confined to therapeutic treatment? There cannot be any doubt that they did indeed possess such knowledge in a far greater measure than any of their contemporaries. They had opportunities for acquiring such knowledge which elsewhere were entirely lacking, for the custom of embalming the dead, involving as it did the removal and handling of the viscera, had a profound influence upon the growth of medicine, although it was not carried out by physicians but was a religious observance. Not only did the custom of mummification familiarize the Egyptians with the appearance, nature and mutual positions of the internal organs of the body—opportunities that were denied to all people who interred or cremated their dead—but it also made them acquainted with the preservative properties of the salts and resins they employed in the process. Mummification thus provided also for the first time in human history opportunities for observations in comparative anatomy, for it enabled its practitioners to perceive the analogies between the human viscera and those of animals, the latter long familiar from the time-honoured custom of cutting up beasts for food or sacrifice. It is worthy of note that the various hieroglyphic signs representing parts of the body, and especially the internal organs, are pictures of the organs of mammals and not of human beings. This proves that the Egyptians' knowledge of mammalian anatomy is older than their knowledge of that of man, and that they recognized the essential identity of the two by devising signs based on the organs of mammals, and using them unaltered when referring to the corresponding organs of the human body.

It is significant that the knowledge of a people in respect of any technical subject can be gauged by the richness or paucity of its terminology. In the ancient Egyptian language there are considerably over one hundred anatomical terms, and this fact of itself proves that the Egyptians were able to differentiate and name a great many organs and organic structures, that a less enlightened people would have grouped together or would have failed to perceive. For instance, every part of the alimentary canal had its separate name. Whilst, however, their terminology for the gross anatomy of the body is accurate, they entirely failed to understand the nerves, muscles, arteries and veins. They had but one word to denote all these structures, and appear to have regarded them all as parts of a single system of branching and radiating cables forming a network over all parts of the body. The word used for the blood-vessels communicating with the heart is the same as that employed for the muscles and nerves in the prescriptions for stiff joints and rheumatoid complaints.

I need not recapitulate the well-known passage in the Ebers Papyrus which describes the heart and its 'vessels', a passage which is duplicated in the Berlin Medical Papyrus, and triplicated by a fragmentary copy in the Edwin Smith Papyrus. Nothing like a system of physiology can be reconstructed from this corrupt and garbled text, but one fact clearly emerges—the appreciation that the heart was the centre of the vascular system and that all the vessels were dependent upon it.   The Egyptians certainly regarded the heart as the most important organ of the body, and they attached no importance at all to the brain.   The heart was held to be the seat of intelligence and of all emotions, and its presence in the body was so important that it was not ablated during mummification, but was carefully left, together with its great vessels, in its place in the thorax, although all the other viscera were removed.   The 'vessels' were believed to be the vehicles, not only of blood, but also of air, water, mucus, semen, and other secretions.   This erroneous conclusion doubtless arose from the post-mortem manipulations of the embalmers, and could not have been derived from the functional vessels of a living body.   The exposure of organs by wounds and fractures also afforded opportunites for observation. It was observed, for instance (as we learn from the Edwin Smith Papyrus), that the brain is enclosed in a membrane and that its hemispheres are patterned with convolutions; that injury to the spinal column may cause priapism, and that such an injury may also cause meteorism.   A passage in the Ebers Papyrus dealing with affections of the stomach, and another in the Kahûn Papyrus dealing with uterine and other female disorders, introduce a novel feature in that they describe symptoms and give a diagnosis.   In nearly all the other medical texts the diagnosis is assumed and only treatment is provided.   These passages, together with the greater part of the Edwin Smith Papyrus, and the concluding part of the Ebers Papyrus, are evidently drawn from one source, quite different from that of the bulk of the medical papyri, and belong to the type which has been designated above as Group A.

V

Space compels me to pass over in silence the subjects of pathology, therapeutics and materia medica, and indeed all these have been fully dealt with elsewhere, but it is necessary to recur again to the 'scientific' texts of Group A. These are clearly extracts from one and the same book, and their form and arrangement is far in advance of those of the greater part of the medical papyri, which consist merely of prescriptions.   These surgical and physiological texts are drawn up with definite formulae in a fivefold form: (i) title, (ii) examination (symptoms), (iii) diagnosis, (iv) opinion (i.e. whether curable or not) and (v) treatment.   In many cases glosses are added which help us to understand the obscurities and idioms of the text.   From the rational and almost methodical manner in which these texts are presented, the late Professor Breasted claimed that the former belief in the magical origin of medicine is no longer tenable, that there is now evidence that anatomy was studied for its own sake, and that the Edwin Smith Papyrus is in the true sense a scientific book.   He failed to recognize, however, that this particular papyrus is only a part of a larger body of texts into which magic enters to no small extent, as it does, indeed, into that very papyrus itself.   It does not in the least detract from the interest and importance of this text to prefer the opinion that, whilst it undoubtedly affords evidence that an attempt was being made to understand the structure of the body, yet it must be remembered that it deals only with wounds and fractures— injuries of palpable and intelligible origin—and not with diseases, the causes of which, to the ancients, were impalpable, invisible and unknown. A wound or injury caused by a fall, or by a weapon or tool, was well understood and generally treated by rational means; but the causes of headache and fever, of skin eruptions and swellings, and of countless other maladies, were wholly mysterious and attributed to possession. In the collections of remedies, in the papyri of Group B, each prescription is headed by a title in which, instead of the simple phrase 'prescription for curing' such and such a disease, we have 'prescription for banishing', 'driving-out', 'terrifying' or 'killing' such disease. In such phraseology the idea of possession is manifest, and when in the Edwin Smith Papyrus, in cases where the physician's opinion is favourable as to the possibility of a cure, the formula used is 'it is a malady that I will contend with', or 'wrestle with', words which clearly imply the ancient belief in magic, it is evident that the physician was still a magician at heart. As has already been indicated, even after rationalism began to pervade Egyptian medicine, the magical and the medical elements marched side by side, and the same age produced both the Edwin Smith and Ebers Papyri with their widely differing contents. Indeed, in the Edwin Smith Papyrus there is a magical incantation in the body of the surgical text itself, and on the back of it there is written a collection of charms and prescriptions of the familiar type that fills page after page of the once so-called medical papyri. The ancient owner of the Edwin Smith Papyrus saw no incongruity in copying into the same note-book elements that appear to us to-day as absolutely antagonistic in nature and content.

VI

Finally, having considered the foregoing statements, we may ask—what is the place in Medical History that Egypt may justly claim? I think the answer must be: a place of high priority. From Egypt we have the earliest medical books, the first observations in human and comparative anatomy, the first experiments in surgery and pharmacy, the first use of splints, bandages, compresses and other appliances, and the first anatomical and medical vocabulary, and that an extensive one. In general terms it may be said that the popular medicine of almost every country of Europe and the Near East largely owes its origin to Egypt, and in its various migrations it has preserved its ancestral form and its very words and phrases almost intact throughout the ages. Not only were many well-known drugs of universal vogue first used by the Egyptians, but in addition to the more obvious examples, many of the drugs, as well as the properties and traditions ascribed to them by the Egyptians, that occur in the works of Pliny, Dioscorides, Galen, and even in the Hippocratic Collection itself, are clearly borrowed from Egypt. These later writers, and others who followed them, are the sources from which the compilers of herbals and books of popular medicine mainly drew for their materials, and the works of classical writers are often merely the stepping-stones by which much of the ancient medical lore of Egypt reached Europe, apart from direct borrowings. Early medical books in Arabic, Hebrew and other Semitic languages have also drawn largely from the same stock. When a drug really possesses the virtues attributed to it and is an effective remedy, its survival into modern times is natural enough, but the fact that many quite fantastic and arbitrary remedies have been carried on almost to our own times is definite proof of the slavish copying from the works of one writer to the works of another, in a continuous line that originated many centuries ago on the banks of the Nile.[37] The use of certain arbitrary preparations, the use of the same formulae, idioms and colophons in the popular medical literature of many countries through many centuries, are all indications with an unmistakable interpretation.

In two other ways, most important of all, Egypt has served the history of medical science. First, through the distinctive custom of mummification, aided by favourable climatic conditions, hundreds of actual bodies, many of them accurately dateable, have carried down to us the earliest actual cases of the effects of disease. The history of the incidence of many diseases and morbid conditions can be thrust farther and farther back into antiquity from the evidence provided by Egyptian mummies and skeletons: of calculi, bilharzia, arterial diseases, tuberculosis, arthritis and other bone diseases, as well as many inflammatory and other conditions. Nor is the evidence confined to that afforded by the bones, for many affections of the soft parts and viscera are likewise recognizable, such as pleural and appendicular adhesions, tumours, cysts, eruptive conditions of the skin, and other manifestations of disease. And secondly, and most important of all, the Egyptians, by that same custom of mummification, had the greatest of all influences on the history of medicine—for that practice had reconciled the popular mind for more than twenty centuries to the idea of cutting open the dead human body. It was in Egypt that it became possible for the Greek physicians and anatomists of the Ptolemaic age to practise for the first time openly and unhampered the systematic dissection of the human body, which religious and popular odium and prejudice forbade in their own country and in all other parts of the world. To this one fact above all others the true science of medicine ultimately owes its origin, and the possibility of its development through the sister-science of anatomy. Making every allowance for the magical and more fantastic elements in Egyptian medicine, which were the necessary forerunners of more rational methods, it can be justly claimed that the earliest dawn of medical science broke over the Valley of the Nile.

[37] Many instances might be quoted, but one may here suffice. "The milk of a woman who has borne a male child" occurs as a drug twelve times in the Ebers Papyrus, three times in the London Medical Papyrus, twice in the Berlin Medical Papyrus, and once each in four other papyri. It occurs in Coptic, in the Hippocratic Collection, in Dioscorides, in Pliny and in other classical writers, as well as in countless European medical works, both MS. and printed, from the Middle Ages until the eighteenth century. See my *Leechbook* (1934), p. 14.

THE MANAGEMENT OF FRACTURES ACCORDING TO THE HEARST MEDICAL PAPYRUS

by

CHAUNCEY D. LEAKE, SANFORD V. LARKEY *and* HENRY F. LUTZ

ABOUT twenty years ago a notable attempt was made at the University of California to establish the history of science as an independent academic discipline. William Henry Welch was a stimulating visitor, and George Sarton, the distinguished historian of science, now at Harvard, was a special lecturer. The most significant inspiration, however, came from Dr. and Mrs. Charles Singer of London, who spent two separate years at Berkeley. Their lectures and seminars were enthusiastically received, and fortunately have been preserved in part in a well-illustrated volume.

In connection with this effort, Dr. Herbert M. Evans, Professor of Anatomy and Director of the Institute of Experimental Biology, undertook the collection of significant classics in the history of science. These were exhibited in 1934 when the American Association for the Advancement of Science met on the West Coast. A feature of the exhibit was the eighteen brown crumbly sheets of the Hearst Medical Papyrus. The excitement over the history of science suggested the propriety of undertaking an English translation of the Hearst Medical Papyrus. The authors of this tribute to Dr. Singer herewith acknowledge their debt to him, and in this small way hope to indicate to him their gratitude for his ever-helpful encouragement and interest.[1]

The Hearst Medical Papyrus

In 1901 the late distinguished Egyptologist, Dr. George A. Reisner, was in charge of an Egyptian expedition sent by Mrs. Phoebe Apperson Hearst, a Regent of the University of California, to study Egyptian antiquities. A peasant brought him a roll of eighteen rumpled sheets of papyrus as a thank-offering. These eighteen sheets, which are mutilated at the beginning and end, were printed in facsimile by Dr. Reisner in 1905, with a rough outline of their contents.[2] Under the direction of Professor Edward W. Gifford, Curator of the Anthropological Museum at the University of California, the sheets were mounted for preservation, and were formerly displayed in the

---

[1] The following works may be helpful in reading the texts:—
  (a) Adams, F. *The seven books of Paulus Aegineta.* Translated with commentary by Francis Adams. (Sydenham Society.) 3 vols. London, 1844–7.
  (b) Dioscorides. *The Greek Herbal of Dioscorides.* Edited by R. T. Gunther. Oxford, 1934.
  (c) Ebbell, B. *The Papyrus Ebers, the greatest Egyptian medical document.* Copenhagen, 1937.
  (d) Leake, C. D. 'Ancient Egyptian therapeutics.' *Ciba Symposia,* 1940, i, No. 10.
  (e) *National Standard Dispensatory.* Edited by H. A. Hare, C. Caspari, and H. H. Rusby. Third edition. Philadelphia, 1916.
  (f) Ranke, H. 'Medicine and Surgery in Ancient Egypt.' *Bull. Inst. Hist. Med.,* 1933, i, 237–57.
  (g) Reisner, G. A. *The Hearst Medical Papyrus.* University of California Publications, Egyptian Archaeology, vol. i. Leipzig, 1905.
  (h) Temkin, O. 'Recent publications on Egyptian and Babylonian medicine.' *Bull. Inst. Hist. Med.,* 1936, iv, 247–56.
  (i) Wreszinski, W. 'Der Londoner medizinische Papyrus und der Papyrus Hearst in Transkription, Übersetzung und Kommentar.' *Die Medizin der Alten Ägypter.* Vol. ii. Leipzig, 1912.

[2] Reisner, *op. cit.* (1 (g)).

Egyptian Antiquities Room of the Anthropological Museum on Parnassus Heights in San Francisco. Since 1933 they have been in storage in Berkeley.

In 1912 Walter Wreszinski[3] published a scholarly and accurate hieroglyphic transcription and partial translation of the Hearst Medical Papyrus in German. The contributions of Reisner and Wreszinski were used in connexion with the preparation of the present translation into English. The numbering of prescriptions follows Wreszinski in our text.

The Management of Fractures in the Hearst Medical Papyrus

Prescriptions 10 to 14 in the Hearst Medical Papyrus are recommended for 'causing broken bones to knit'. They are similar to the terminal group of remedies recommended in the Hearst Medical Papyrus, all of which deal with orthopædic conditions such as fractures, injured muscles, or lacerated wounds caused by the bites of large animals. Hearst prescriptions 10–14 and 217–25 form a series designed for the purpose of providing a sort of cast for the immobilization of a fractured bone.

Both Hearst 10 and Hearst 217 seem to have the same heading: 'A Prescription To Knit a Broken Bone on the First Day'. The phrase 'on the first day' suggests that the flour or honey casts of the prescription were to be applied only on the first day of the fracture, while the terminal directions in each prescription seem to imply that the bandaging was to continue on subsequent days.

There seems to be some correlation between the two series of similar prescriptions. Hearst 217 is similar to Hearst 10, but Hearst 10 includes $^cm^c$ flour. Hearst 218 is similar to Hearst 12, but Hearst 12 lacks the parts of the drugs.

Hearst 219 is similar to Hearst 11, but the different arrangements of the drugs suggest different sources. Hearst 220 is questionably related to Hearst 13. The two prescriptions have dough and honey in common. Hearst 221 is similar to Hearst 14 although the latter is incomplete. Hearst 222–5 are not duplicated by similar prescriptions elsewhere.

These prescriptions, for the purpose of 'causing broken bones to knit', are essentially starch pastes made of various kinds of flours from glutinous sources mixed with cream or honey. On slow drying in contact with the skin, such pastes would become quite hard, and the effect would be similar to that obtained by modern plaster casts. Particularly is this the case when such pastes are incorporated with cloth in bandaging. This explanation of the rationale of these prescriptions becomes more probably correct when one considers that the 'builder's lime', added to the mucilaginous plant, gum, and honey mixture of Hearst 14, must have been a cement.

Classical surgeons (Graeco-Roman, Arabic, and Renaissance) followed the admirable system of treating fractures outlined in the Hippocratic writings, *Fractures*, *Joints*, and *Mochlicon*.[4] The significant features of these writings are the emphasis on anatomical details in the reduction of dislocations,

---

[3] Wreszinski, *op. cit.* (1 (i)).

[4] The most recent and authoritative English translation of these Hippocratic works is by E. T. Withington in *Hippocrates*, vol. iii, Loeb Classical Library. London and New York, 1927.

on the care necessary in bandaging to avoid too great pressure, and on the necessity of proper extension to avoid shortening. Adams[5] gives a very full account of the classical writings on the treatment of fractures. The bandages used were ordinarily impregnated with 'cerate', which was also applied directly to the skin. This was a waxy preparation which may have hardened on drying. It is noteworthy that Adams closes his commentary on the Hippocratic section relating to the treatment of fractures of the upper arm with these words: 'We are certain it will be generally admitted that the waxed apparatus of the ancients in the case of fractures was probably quite as efficacious as the starched bandages which have been introduced of late years with so much advantage.'[6] In speaking of fractures of the nose it is interesting that the Hippocratic writer says, 'After all, the best treatment is to use a little fresh flour, worked and kneaded into a glutinous mass, as a plaster for such lesions'.[7]

Dr. John B. de C. M. Saunders, Professor of Anatomy in the University of California Medical School, who has kindly assisted us in preparing this commentary, called our attention to two recent historical studies by Monro and Bacon on the development of casts in the treatment of fractures. Monro[8] suggests that the ancient Egyptians used plaster bandages. Bacon[9] credits Rhazes (Al-Razi, A.D. 860–923) with discovering in treating fractures that 'an apparatus with lime and white of egg . . . will become hard as stone and need not be removed until the healing is complete'. That the 'apparatus' of Rhazes may have persisted in Arabia is apparent from the reference given by Eton[10] to the Arab method of using gypsum ('plaster-of-Paris') in making casts for fractured bones. Sir George Ballingall[11] tells of the natives of India treating fractures with moulds of clay. William Cheselden, describing the method of Mr. Cowper, a bone-setter, wrote: 'His way was after putting the limb in a proper posture, to wrap it up in rags dip'd in the whites of eggs, and a little wheat flour mixed . . . I think there is no way better than this in fractures, for it preserves the position of the limb without strict bandage'.[12] The use of gums and pastes was brought to its greatest perfection by Sentin[13] in the Belgian Army. He probably inspired the modern development of the plaster-of-Paris cast by Antonius Mathijsen[14] and by van de Loo.[15] A full description of the modern technique may be found in such a standard text as Pye's *Surgical Handicraft*, which states, 'Starch is the least efficient material for making a supporting case . . . It is applied like gum and chalk, by rubbing starch-paste into the interstices of ordinary bandages'.[16]

[5] Adams, *op. cit.* (1 (a)), vol. ii, pp. 427–511.

[6] *ibid.*, vol. ii, p. 464.

[7] Hippocrates, *Joints*, ch. xxxvi, *op. cit.* (4), p. 267.

[8] J. K. Monro, *Brit. Journ. Surg.*, 1935, xxiii, 257.

[9] L. W. Bacon, *Bull. Soc. Med. Hist.*, Chicago, 1923, ii, 122.

[10] W. Eton, *Survey of the Turkish Empire.* London, 1798, p. 218.

[11] Sir George Ballingall, *Outlines of military surgery.* Fourth edition. Edinburgh, 1852, p. 358.

[12] W. Cheselden, *Anatomy of the human body.* Fifth edition. London, 1740, p. 38.

[13] Sentin, *Traité de la méthode amovo-inamovible.* Brussels, 1849.

[14] A. Mathijsen, *Nieuwe wijze van aanwending van het gips-verband bij beenbreuken.* Haarlem, 1852. A much-extended second edition appeared as *Du bandage plâtré et de son application dans le traitement des fractures.* Liége, 1854.

[15] J. H. P. van de Loo, *Der amovo-inamovible Gypsverband.* Venlo [1862].

[16] Pye's *Surgical Handicraft.* Ninth edition. Bristol, 1924, pp. 102–6,

At the present time, plaster casts for broken bones are made by soaking gauze bandages in a mixture of 'plaster-of-Paris' (gypsum, or desiccated calcium sulphate) with half its weight of water, and 'bandaging therewith'. From Hearst 10–14 to modern times, then, one may trace a fairly continuous method of treating fractures by bandaging with cloth impregnated with soft gelatinous materials, which on drying become hard casts which immobilize the part, thus promoting bone healing without pressure sufficient to block blood flow or to cause skin irritation. In these Hearst prescriptions, therefore, ingredients, which superficially may seem nonsensical, become rationally understandable, and empirically sound when the probable manner of their use is considered. Further, they were probably the best available for the purpose at that time.

The Prescriptions

There follow the Hearst Prescriptions 10–14 and 217–25, in transliteration and translation, together with notes. These will afford some idea of the manner in which we are attempting to treat the whole of the Hearst Medical Papyrus.

HEARST PRESCRIPTION 10

(I: 9) [ph̬r·t nt tsw ḳś śḏ (?)] -f hrw tpj
ḏ'r·t 'wrj·t r-20 ḳ'w ʿmʿ nḏ·w 'mj·w (I: 10) [ḥr mś]t' n
ḥdw wt ḥr-ś r hrw 4

[A prescription to knit a broken (1) bone] on the first day:
gourds (2), beans 20 ro (3), flour of ʿmʿ (4), ground up, mixed with a
mśt (5) of ḥdw liquid (6), bandage therewith for 4 days (7).

Notes

1. Read śḏ or one of the numerous synonyms of 'to break'. This has been restored from comparison with Hearst 26.

2. The number of ro is omitted. It should probably read 5 ro, as in Hearst 217. For discussion of gourds, see Hearst 6, note 1.

3. The text apparently reads the fractional number $\frac{2}{3}$. Wreszinski wishes to emend it to read 20 ro. Since the amount of beans is given in Hearst 217 as 5 ro, the 20 ro seem altogether too large here; nevertheless the reading adopted is one-sixteenth ḥḳ' ·t which equals 20 ro.

The Egyptian bean (Nelumbium speciosium) is specifically described by Dioscorides (ii, 128) under the name Faba Egyptica, to distinguish it from the Faba Graeca. Preparations of beans were used externally in the classical period as astringent poultices.[17] This is the general use for which they are advised in Hearst, as, for broken bones (10, 217); for skin afflictions (71); and to expel swellings (137).

4. Variations of ʿmʿ, which is probably a grain, are recommended in Hearst for external application, as here; to knit a bone (12); to remove sickness from the stomach (48); for skin afflictions (72); and to soothe mt·w (249). In these it seems to be used to obtain a soothing mucilaginous effect. In Hearst 48 it enters into a demulcent mucilaginous mixture again to

[17] Adams, op. cit. (1 (a)), vol. iii, p. 199.

be taken internally for 'sickness of the stomach'. It seems to refer to a part of wheat (*Triticum aestivum*) or barley (*Hordeum vulgare*). Wheat and barley preparations were used in Graeco-Roman times in the same way medically as used by the earlier Egyptians.[18]

5. The *mst'* is apparently not a certain liquid, as the dictionary gives, but may be a measure. The word *mst'* with the second form *mstj* may be related, apart from its meaning as a basket. The latter is a dry measure. In *mst'nj*, the ending *nj* implies 'belonging to', which favours the meaning of a measure rather than the name of a specific liquid. In Ebers 181 occurs '*šfšf·t* kernels ground to the amount of a *mst'*'. Literally it means '*šfšf·t* kernels to be ground—stopping at (an amount equal to) a *mst'*'. Ebbell tentatively renders *mst'* as 'paste', which would make the text understandable here, as well as in Hearst 247. The 'water' must have been drawn off from some sediment or immiscible layer.

6. This is the only place this occurs. We have no idea of its identity.

7. The question may be brought up here regarding the significance of the final instruction to 'bandage therewith for 4 days'. Was it meant to let the bandage remain in place merely for four days? This would not give time to permit healing to occur satisfactorily. Was it meant to increase the cast by building up the layers of the bandage? This method would permit gradual tightening as the initial swelling accompanying the fracture subsided. The Hippocratic writings on *Fractures* caution against too tight bandaging at first.

HEARST PRESCRIPTION 11

pḥr·t śn·tj

k'w n it w'd śmj (I: 11) '[*mj·w ḥr bj·t wt ḥ*] *r-ś r hrw* 4

A second prescription:

flour of fresh barley (1) (and) cream (2) mi[xed with honey (3); bandage] therewith for 4 days

Notes

1. Barley (*Hordeum vulgare* of *H. sativum*) contains about 65 per cent starch, 15 per cent albumin and gluten, 12 per cent cellulose, and fat, sugar, ash and moisture. It has long been used as an ingredient of poultices for ulcers,[17] for which its high starch content would make it well suited. It is a constituent of several Hearst prescriptions for external applications, as here and in 219 for broken bones; for scabs (17); toe-nails (191); and illness in members (33).

In Graeco-Roman times decoctions of barley had a reputation as a cooling and diuretic agent when used internally. Barley decoctions are still recommended as a nutrient demulcent diuretic in inflammatory conditions of the urinary tract.[19] Barley is recommended for oral administration to 'kill pains in limbs' (46) and for 'heat from bladder' (70).

For an interesting discussion of the medicinal and folk-lore uses of barley

---

[18] Dioscorides, *op. cit.* (1 (*b*)), II, 107, 108; Adams, *op. cit.* (1 (*a*)), vol. iii, pp. 195, 314.

[19] *Nat. Stand. Disp.*, *op. cit.* (1 (*e*)), p. 796.

I   E

water or 'ptisan', see John F. Fulton's note on the 1669 *Bromographia* of Richard Lower.[20]

2. Cream occurs only for external application in Hearst. It is used in three prescriptions (11, 15, and 219) for knitting broken bones and once to expel *mssw·t* (167). In the classical period, milk or cream was applied locally to ulcers and in ointments for gout.[21] Milk is a bland alkaline material whose detergent and soothing properties may have suggested these uses.

3. Honey is recommended for external use in Hearst in many prescriptions apparently concerned with bone or skin lesions or ulcers (11, 13, 14, 74, 98, 99, 103, 104, 108, 115, 117, 132, 135, 141, 220–2, 233, 248, 260). It is also used in fracture cases 36, 37, and 38 in the Edwin Smith Surgical Papyrus (J. H. Breasted, Chicago, 1930). In the case of fractures, the honey may simply be added to help form the stiff cartonnage moulded to the broken limb, as suggested by Breasted. Perhaps the Egyptians made no distinction between simple fractures, where the skin is not broken, and what we call compound fractures, where the skin is broken and infection is possible. Even in the case of compound fractures, the honey dressing might have been found by experience to be useful. It is interesting that Lücke[22] reports that honey aids in cleaning wounds and is useful as a surgical dressing. Crude honey contains about 0·1 per cent formic acid, which is antiseptic and locally irritating, thus promoting increased blood circulation.

HEARST PRESCRIPTION 12

$\overline{\underline{p}\underline{h}r·t\ \underline{h}mtnw·t}$
$d'r·t\ r$-20 $^{r}m^{r}\ n\ bd·t\ n\underline{d}·w\ \underline{h}r\ \underline{h}s'w$ (I: 12) [. . .] $n\underline{d}m\ r$
hrw 4

A third prescription:

gourds 20 *ro* (1), $^{r}m^{r}$ of spelt (2), ground up with dough [of *psn* bread] (3) . . . sweet, for 4 days (4).

Notes

1. The text reads $\frac{2}{3}$, which has been changed in accordance with the discussion in note 3 of Hearst 10.

The plant name, *d'r·t*, has been equated with 'gourd' by comparison with the Coptic *GLO*. It seems that *d'r·t*, 'gourd' was subjected to a development similar to that of the word *d'r·t*, 'scorpion', which passed into the Coptic *GLE*. This identification is compatible with the substitute determinative and also with the medicinal use of the seeds of the *d'r·t* plant.

Preparations of gourds and other members of the gourd family, such as cucumber, melon, and pumpkin, occur frequently in Hearst prescriptions. Gourd meal, seeds, and other preparations are recommended externally for bone and joint conditions, for burns, and for healing of contusions. Gourd seeds are suggested internally for expelling 'sickness'. Dioscorides[23] recommends raw gourd as a cooling application for various swellings. See

[20] J. F. Fulton, *A bibliography of two Oxford physiologists: Richard Lower (1631–1691); John Mayow (1643–1679)*. Oxford, 1935, pp. 25–6.

[21] Dioscorides, *op. cit.* (1 (*b*)), II, 75–8.

[22] H. Lücke, *Deut. Med. Wchnschr.*, 1935, lxi, 1638.

[23] Dioscorides, *op. cit.* (1 (*b*)), II, 162–3.

Adams[27] for a general commentary on the use of the gourd (*Cucumis sativus*, cucumber, or *Cucurbita*, gourd) in classical medicine. Various members of the gourd family have been used internally since Graeco-Roman times for gastro-enteric and bladder conditions. Laxative and diuretic properties are still ascribed to all members of the gourd family by the *National Standard Dispensatory* (pp. 551–3).

2. The text seems not to be in order. Spelt (*Triticum spelta*) is a variety of Greek wheat, Zeia.[25] Zeia was employed externally by classic physicians as a desiccative emplastic agent.[26] Variations of spelt are recommended externally here, to grow hair (145), and to expel *tmj·t* (168). Black spelt is suggested internally for curing the heart. *ᶜmᶜ* seems to refer to a grain, from which a mucilaginous mass may have been easily prepared. This would conform to the purpose of this prescription. For discussion of *ᶜmᶜ*, see Hearst 10, note 4.

3. 'Of *psn* bread' is supplied from Hearst 218, which is very similar to this prescription. *psn* probably formed a floury bread, or a sticky dough. The dough of *psn* bread was used externally for broken bones (12, 13, 218, 220). The crumbs of *psn* bread are used the first day (89); to give relief to the interior of a *mt* (100); to drive away swellings in any member (128); and to expel *tmj·t* (168).

4. 'For 4 days' appears to be a senseless addition unless 'bandage therewith' is assumed. The scribe probably omitted it accidentally, but it might have been assumed from the previous prescription.

HEARST PRESCRIPTION 13

snᶜᶜ ḳš šḏ (?)*-f m ᶜ·wt nb·t nt s s·t r'-pw* (1)

ḥš'w n (I: 13) [. . .] . . . *pr·t nš' irj·w m iḥ·t wᶜ·t 'mj·w ḥr bj·t wt ḥr-š*

To cause a broken bone to knit (2) in any limb of a male or female: dough of [*psn* bread] (3) ... fruit kernels of the *nš'* plant (4) mixed together, stirred with honey (5); bandage therewith (6).

Notes

1. Text omits the vertical stroke after *r*.

2. The verb, *šnᶜᶜ*, used here, really means 'to make smooth, to polish'. Wreszinski thinks that as a medical technical term, it signifies 'das richtige Zusammenlagern der Stücke des gebrochenen Knochens, sodass er glatt zusammenwachst'. In Hearst 217 the verb employed is *ts* 'to set'.

3. Restored according to Hearst 218 and 220. For discussion of dough of *psn* bread, see Hearst 12, note 3.

4. Erman[27] tentatively equates this with the pondweed (*Potamogeton lucens*) which was used by the classical medical writers as a cooling astringent agent for external application.[28] It occurs for external application here and

[24] Adams, *op. cit.* (1 (*a*)), vol. iii, p. 182.

[25] *ibid.*, p. 123.

[26] *idem.*, *op. cit.* (1 (*a*)), vol. i, p. 123; vol. iii, p. 123. Dioscorides, *op. cit.* (1 (*b*)), II, iii.

[27] A. Erman, *Wörterbuch der Ägyptischen Sprache*. Edited by A. Erman and H. Grapow. 5 vols. Leipzig, 1925–31. Vol. ii, p. 338.

[28] Adams, *op. cit.* (1 (*a*)), vol. iii, p. 309; Dioscorides, *op. cit.* (1 (*b*)), IV, 101.

for a stiff *mt* (110), to expel *tmj·t* (169). In all of these a cooling astringent seems indicated. There are many varieties of pondweeds of which the water lily, belonging to the family *Nymphoeaceae*, is most common. All contain resins and tannin.[29]

5. In the two sets of prescriptions in Hearst referring to casts for the treatment of fractures, namely 10–14 and 217–25, honey occurs in sequence in 13 and 14, and in 221 and 222. In view of the possible external use of honey in Hearst for cleansing foul wounds (see Hearst 6), it may be that these four prescriptions were originally devised for 'compound fractures' where the skin is broken and infection may set in. On the basis of the recent report of H. Lücke[22] such an ancient empirical use of honey would be justified on modern evidence.

6. Has the omission of the usual 'four days' any significance? Probably the scribe assumed it. But it may indicate that this particular type of cast was not to be built up in layers, as the others may have been. See Hearst 10, note 6.

HEARST PRESCRIPTION 14

sn^{rr} (I: 14) . . .

[. . .] *r-5 ḳmj·t r-5 išd·t nt nḥ·t r-5 išd·t nt nbś r-5 išd·t nt im'* (I: 15) [*r-5*] [. . . *'i*] *wḥ ḏb' ḥmt r-s m bj·t wt ḥr-ś r hrw* 4

To cause to knit . . . :

[builder's lime] (1) 5 *ro*, gum 5 *ro* (2), fruit bunches (3) of the fig-mulberry 5 *ro* (4), fruit bunches of thistle 5 *ro* (5), fruit bunches of the *im'* tree [5 *ro*] (6) . . . stir into it three finger-fulls of honey (7); bandage therewith for 4 days.

Notes

1. *bśn n 'iḳdw*, restored according to Hearst 89 and 221, on the basis of the determinative preserved in Hearst 14. This is probably a cement which when added to the mucilaginous plant and honey mixture of the rest of the prescription, would form a serviceable 'plaster cast' as it dries in the cloth bandage.

2. *ḳmj·t* is identified with *p'j·t* (gum), by comparison between Hearst 40 and Ebers 538, Hearst 63 and Ebers 277, Hearst 65 and Ebers 280, Hearst 66 and Ebers 278. Gum is recommended in Hearst to knit bones, for burns, to expel sores, to remove hair, and for sore fingers and toes. Taken internally, it is suggested for excessive urine and to expel fluid accumulations. The ancient gums are well described in Pliny.[30] Gum acacia from the Egyptian thorn (*Acacia vera*) seems generally to have been used. It was employed in classical medicine as a soothing demulcent agent externally, and internally against coughs and as a stomachic.[31]

3. The Egyptian word *išd·t* is specified in Hearst 14 as 'fruit bunches' of the fig-mulberry, the thistle, and the *im'* tree, respectively. In passages of the text when *išd·t* stands alone it is doubtful what 'clusters' or 'fruit

[29] *Nat. Stand. Disp.*, *op. cit.* (1 (*e*)), pp. 1056–7; *United States Dispensatory*, p. 1492.

[30] Pliny, *Hist. Nat.*, xiii. 20.

[31] Adams, *op. cit.* (1 (*a*)), vol. iii, p. 184; Dioscorides, *op. cit.* (1 (*b*)), I, 133.

bunches' may be meant. However, the Egyptian *išd·t* or *išd* (Hearst 28) is very much like the Arabic ʿ*unqūd* (pl. ʿ*anāqīd*), which may refer to 'grape clusters' when it stands alone, or to the clusters of other fruits such as, for instance, the 'clusters' or 'fruit bunches' of the pepper tree. Thus, whenever *išd·t* is not especially designated as the cluster of a particular fruit, it has been translated as 'grape clusters', and whenever determined with the sign for seeds, as 'grape seeds' or merely 'grapes'.

4. *nkʿw·t* refers to the red berries of the fig-mulberry, the Arabic *ǧummaiz*. A current Arabic description of the sycamore or fig-mulberry (*Ficus morus* or *Morus nigra?*) is to be found in *Maǧānī-el-adab fī ḥadaiḳ el-ʿarab* (Beirut, 2; 270, No. 407, 1882). While it was used as a purge internally, it was recommended for external application as an astringent agent. The buds are advised in Hearst for knitting and cooling a bone (221, 226, 234). Graeco-Roman writers credited the fig-mulberry with the power to reduce swellings. The uses made of it by Egyptian physicians were followed by classical authorities.[32]

5. Regarding the *Zizyphus spina Christi* (thistle or white thorn, see Erman) as being still used in Egypt, as a drug, see Ahmed Bey Kemal.[33] On the basis of Adams's discussion[34] this may be *Cirsium acarna*, or *Onopordon acanthium*. These are said to be astringent and drying, whether used internally or for local application. Dioscorides recommends them as diuretics and to stop bleeding and toothache.[35] The plant here mentioned is more likely, however, to be of the genera *Zizyphus* of the *Rhamnaceae*, the buckthorn family. To this large group belong many plants with laxative, demulcent, or astringent properties.[36] The plant occurs in Hearst chiefly for external use. This is the only place the fruit bunches of the thistle occurs. The buds of the thistle are recommended externally to cool *mt·w* (95, 238), for fingers and toes (173-*b*, 191), to knit a broken bone (221) and for 'cooling' the bone after it is set (226). The bread of thistle kernels occurs once for internal use to expel fluid accumulations (84), and once for local application to expel sores of any member (134).

6. Fruit bunches, fruit, and buds of the *im'* tree occur in Hearst only for external application. The fruit is recommended to expel ills in the head (76), and for a *mt* which throbs in any limb (99). The *ḫs*-fruit is used to prevent white hair (147) and the buds to knit a broken bone (221). Hearst 14 is very similar in purpose and ingredients to Hearst 221. The *im'* tree may be the male date palm.[37]

7. For discussion of the external use of honey, see Hearst 11, note 3. The construction of *iwḥ ḏbʿ ḥmt r-s m bj·t* is very awkward.

HEARST PRESCRIPTION 217

pḥr·t nt ts ḳš šḏ-f hrw tpj

ḳʾ·w n ḏ'r·t r-5 (XIV: 14) *ḳʾ·w n iwrj·t r-5 mw n*
mštj r-5 'irj·w m iḫ·t wʿ·t wt·w ḥr-š r hrw 4

[32] Adams, *op. cit.* (1 (*a*)), vol. iii, p. 256 ; Dioscorides, *op. cit.* (1 (*b*)), I, 180.

[33] Ahmed Bey Kemal, 'Le pain de Nebaq des Anciens Égyptiens'. *Ann. du Service d. Antiquités*, 1912, xii, 240.

[34] Adams, *op. cit.* (1 (*a*)), vol. iii, p. 28.

[35] Dioscorides, *op. cit.* (1 (*b*)), III, 14, 15.

[36] *Nat. Stand. Disp.*, *op. cit.* (1 (*e*)), p. 414; *United States Dispensatory*, p. 1646.

[37] Erman, *op. cit.* (27), vol. i, 79.

A prescription to knit a broken bone, on the first day:

Gourd meal 5 *ro* (1), meal of beans 5 *ro* (2), water to the amount of *mśtj*
5 *ro* (3); to be mixed together (and) bandaged therewith for 4 days.

Notes

1. For discussion of gourds, see Hearst 12, note 1.
2. For discussion of beans, see Hearst 10, note 3.
3. For discussion of *mśtj*, see Hearst 10, note 5.

HEARST PRESCRIPTION 218

pḫr·t śn-nw·t

$\overline{k'·w \ n \ ḏ'r·t \quad r\text{-}5 \ k'·w \ n}$ (XIV: 15) *ꜥꜥm   r-5 ḥs'w n psn*
r-5 fśj m iḥ·t wꜥ·t wt·w ḥr-ś

A second prescription:

Gourd meal 5 *ro* (1) meal of the *ꜥꜥm* plant 5 *ro* (2), (and) dough of *psn*
bread 5 *ro* (3); to be cooked together (and) bandaged therewith.

Notes

1. For discussion of gourds, see Hearst 12, note 1.
2. The *ꜥꜥm* plant occurs only here in Hearst. There is no clue to its identity
except that it has the designation for a plant.
3. For discussion of *psn* bread, see Hearst 12, note 3. In the present
prescription dough is specified, probably for the purpose of providing a
mucilaginous paste with the other ingredients so that it might gradually
harden as a sort of cast.

HEARST PRESCRIPTION 219

pḫr·t ḫmt-nw·t

$\overline{śmj \ n \ iḥ \ [·t] \ r\text{-}5 \ k'·w \ nw \ it \ w'ḏ \ r\text{-}5 \ irj·w \ m}$ (XIV: 16)
iḥ·t wꜥ·t wt·w ḥr-ś r hrw 4

A third prescription:

cow's cream 5 *ro* (1), (and) fresh barley meal 5 *ro* (2); to be mixed
together (and) bandaged therewith for 4 days.

Notes

1. For discussion of cream, see Hearst 11, note 2.
2. For discussion of barley, see Hearst 11, note 1.

HEARST PRESCRIPTION 220

ktj pḫr·t .

$\overline{pr·t \ ś'w \ r\text{-}5 \ pr·t \ twn \ r\text{-}5 \ bj·t \ r\text{-}5 \ ḥs'w \ n \ psn \ r\text{-}5}$
(XIV: 17) *irj·w m iḥ·t wꜥ·t wt ḥr-ś r hrw* (!) 4

Another prescription:

fruit of coriander 5 *ro* (1), fruit of the *twn* plant 5 *ro* (2), honey
5 *ro* (3), (and) dough of *psn* bread 5 *ro* (4); to be mixed together
(and) bandaged therewith for 4 days.

Notes

1. Coriander (*Coriandrum sativum*) occurs in Hearst usually in remedies for external use against skin afflictions (71, 75, 77, 161), to soothe *mt·w* (97, 101, 107, 119, 228, 250), and to knit broken bones, as here. It appears in three prescriptions for internal use to expel fluid accumulations (84, 86 and 87). Among the Graeco-Roman physicians it had a reputation as a cooling agent and astringent, and was recommended for applications to ulcers and carbuncles.[38] Coriander is now used chiefly as a condiment.[39]

2. The *twn* plant occurs in Hearst only for external applications for sores, broken bones, or to cool (99, 116, 181, 200, 201, 220, 251). Ebbell translates *twn* as acacia, but this is improbable since acacia is a tree and would require a tree determinative, while *twn* always has plant determinatives. These indicate that *twn* was a meadow plant used as cattle food. *snd* with a tree determinative is usually identified with acacia.

3. For discussion of the use of honey, see Hearst 11, note 3.

4. For discussion of *psn* bread, see Hearst 12, note 3.

HEARST PRESCRIPTION 221

ktj pḥr·t

bśn n ỉḳdw r-5 drd n nḥ·t r-5 drd n nbś r-5 drd n
ỉm' r-5 (XV: 1) *drd n śnd·t r-5 bj·t r-5 ḳmj·t śnd·t*
ỉrj·w m iḥ·t wˁ·t wt·w ḥr-ś

Another prescription:

lime of the potter 5 *ro* (1), buds of the fig-mulberry 5 *ro* (2), buds of the thistle 5 *ro* (3), buds of the *ỉm'* tree 5 *ro* (4), acacia buds 5 *ro* (5), honey 5 *ro* (6), (and) acacia gum ? parts (7); to be mixed together (and) bandaged therewith.

Notes

1. Or alkali, lye? The text is in disorder, with the reading taken as *bśn*. This prescription would seem to be well devised for making a cast to immobilize the part to permit the broken bone to knit.

2. For discussion of fig-mulberry, see Hearst 14, note 4.

3. For discussion of thistle (zizyphus), see Hearst 14, note 6.

4. For discussion of *ỉm'* tree, see Hearst 14, note 7.

5. *śnd* is generally identified with *Acacia vera*, a thorny tree indigenous to Egypt. *drd*, actually written to be 'bud' or 'leaf', is erroneously translated by Ebbell in Ebers 616 as 'juice'. *drd* is rendered here as 'buds'. Acacia buds are consistently recommended in Hearst for external application for burns, skin conditions and broken bones. They are also suggested internally for purgation. Acacia preparations were used by the classical medical writers for cooling and astringent external applications to sores and ulcers.[40] At present acacia is described in all pharmacopoeias, and almost the entire source is from Egypt. Gum acacia consists of various mixtures of calcium, potassium, and magnesium salts of arabic acid, which form mucilages with water. It

---

[38] Adams, *op. cit.* (1 (a)), vol. iii, p. 189; Dioscorides, *op. cit.* (1 (b)), III, 71.

[39] *Nat. Stand. Disp.*, *op. cit.* (1 (e)), p. 532.

[40] Adams, *op. cit.* (1 (a)), vol. iii, pp. 26–7; Dioscorides, *op. cit.* (1 (b)), I, 133.

would seem to be well suited for incorporation into a mixture which on drying would form a cast for a broken bone. Acacia is still advised medicinally for soothing application in water solution to irritated skin areas. It has a mild detergent and astringent effect, reducing inflammation and relieving pain due to surface drying. Acacia helps to emulsify materials not easily soluble in water. A full description is given in the *National Standard Dispensatory* (pp. 5–8).

6. For discussion of the external use of honey, see Hearst 12, note 2.

7. The number of parts was omitted in the text. This is the only place the phrase 'acacia gum' is used.

HEARST PRESCRIPTION 222

ktj phr·t

$\overline{bj·t\ r}$-5 $š^ʿm\ r$-5 $pr·t\ šnj\ r$-5 (XV: 2) *fšj m iḫ·t wʿ·t wt·w ḫr-š r hrw* 4

Another prescription:

honey 5 *ro* (1), *š^ʿm* plant 5 *ro* (2), (and) juniper berries 5 *ro* (3); to be cooked together (and) bandaged therewith for 4 days.

Notes

1. For discussion of the external use of honey, see Hearst 12, note 2.

2. *š^ʿm* is apparently only a variant spelling for *š^ʿm*. *š^ʿm* has only the plant determinative, while *š^ʿm* has both plant and tree determinatives. *š^ʿm* plant is mentioned in Hearst 8 for external application to a tooth 'about to fall out'. It is probably mentioned in Dioscorides[41] under the name *sum*, which is said was the Egyptian name for the chaste tree (*Vitex Agnus-castus*), so-called because chaste matrons slept on branches of it in rites to Ceres in ancient Greece. Dioscorides recommends it externally as a 'counter-irritant' and internally as a purgative. It has locally irritating and astringent properties from the acrid oils and bitter compounds in it. It was used by classical authorities as an emmenagogue.[42]

3. Juniper berries are often mentioned in Hearst for external use in reducing swellings, and internally for diuretic effect. *Juniperus communis* is a large spreading shrub widely distributed in Europe and Northern Africa. Its berries contain much resin and volatile oil. They have been used medicinally since classical times for diuretic action and for local astringent effects.[43]

HEARST PRESCRIPTION 223

ktj phr·t

ḏrḏ n šnḏ·t r-5 *kmj·t r*-5 *mw r*-5 *irj·w m iḫ·t wʿ·t wt·w ḫr-š r hrw* 4

Another prescription:

acacia buds 5 *ro* (1), gum lotion 5 *ro* (2), (and) water 5 *ro*; to be mixed together (and) bandaged therewith for 4 days.

[41] Dioscorides, *op. cit.* (1 (*b*)), I, 135.

[42] Adams, *op. cit.* (1 (*a*)), vol. iii, p. 20.

[43] *ibid.*, pp. 50, 164; Dioscorides, *op. cit.* (1 (*b*)), I, 103.

Notes

1. For a discussion of acacia, see Hearst 221, note 5.

2. 'Lotion' is suggested since *kmj·t* is determined by a vase. In the following prescription we read *mw nw kmj·t*, 'gum-water'. For discussion of gum, see Hearst 14, note 2. 'Gum lotion' was probably some sort of mucilage kept in a covered vase.

HEARST PRESCRIPTION 224

(XV: 3) *ktj phr·t*

mw nw kmj·t r-5 mrh·t ś r-5 mnhj r-5 fśj m ih·t wʿ·t
wt·w hr-ś r hrw 4

Another prescription:

gum lotion 5 *ro* (1), goose fat 5 *ro* (2), (and) wax 5 *ro* (3); to be cooked together (and) bandaged therewith for 4 days.

Notes

1. For discussion of gum lotion, probably a sort of mucilage, see Hearst 14, note 2.

2. Goose-fat is quite often recommended for internal use in Hearst prescriptions, but only thrice for external application. In these instances it may have contributed to a soothing effect, or as here, to assist in 'working' stiffer material, such as wax, to the shape desired.

3. Wax occurs often in Hearst for external use in skin or muscle ailments, for bone injuries, and to promote healing of wounds. Among classical physicians wax was used for cooling and detergent purposes externally on wounds, or in liniments.[44] Wax (*Cera*) is ordinarily obtained from the honeycomb of the bee, and is a mixture of complex organic acids. Vegetable waxes were probably unknown to the ancient Egyptians. Wax is still used in preparing surgical dressings, and as a protective and soothing agent on wounds or burns.[45]

HEARST PRESCRIPTION 225

ktj phr·t

pkrw n mrh·t śdr (XV: 4) *n iʾd·t wt·w hr-ś*

Another prescription:

the *pkrw* worm that occurs in oil (1), exposed to the dew over night (and) bandaged therewith.

Notes

1. The *pkrm* worm occurs only here in Hearst. It is not known what kind of a worm was meant, nor is it known what kind occurs in oil.

Summary

Examples are offered in transliteration and translation of the ancient Egyptian method of immobilizing fractured bones by means of starch paste

[44] Adams, *op. cit.* (1 (*a*)), p. 169; Dioscorides, *op. cit.* (1 (*b*)), II, 205.
[45] *Nat. Stand. Disp.*, *op. cit.* (1 (*e*)), pp. 428–30.

casts.   These illustrations are taken from the Hearst Medical Papyrus, which was probably a practising physician's formulary, copied from various sources sometime about 1500 B.C.   Fom this ancient time to the present, one may trace a continuous method of treating fractures by bandaging with cloths impregnated with soft gelatinous materials which on drying become hard casts immobilizing the bone, thus promoting healing without pressure sufficient to block blood flow or to cause skin irritation.   While the ancient Egyptian physicians made no attempt to analyse the advantageous mechanism of their procedures derived from experience, their practical recommendations were apparently followed by the Greeks, who began the inquiry into the problem of why these procedures 'worked'.   This inquiry still continues!

THE APOTHEOSIS OF ASTRONOMY*

by

Sir RICHARD GREGORY

AT all stages of civilization, men have observed the movements of the Sun, Moon and the starry sky, and have arrived at explanations of them in relation to the Earth which satisfied the state of knowledge at the time. To a child, as to primitive people, the Earth seems to be generally flat, even though hills or mountains occur here and there upon it. The Sun rises on the eastern horizon and gives the light and warmth required by all living things; and people in very early times began to wonder what became of it at night. The ancient Egyptians taught that a new sun was created every day, reached the prime of life at noon, and died at sunset. In an early papyrus the Earth is represented as a reclining figure covered with leaves and the heavens as a star-spangled body of a sky-goddess stretching over it, with two boats over her, one carrying the rising, and the other the setting, Sun. In the centre of this allegorical picture was another god which represented divine intelligence.

Representations of the Earth as a wide expanse upon which rested the vault or canopy of heaven appear in the histories of the Hindus, Greeks, and many other peoples. Between the heavens above and the Earth beneath was the region of the clouds and of the brightness which gave dawn and twilight when the Sun was not visible. This conception of a flat Earth with the heavens above it was believed in for many centuries, in spite of the fact that, in the sixth century before the Christian era, a Greek philosopher, Pythagoras, held that the Earth was spherical in shape. The view generally accepted in his time and much later was that the human race lived on a wide expanse which was surrounded by mountains or a sea. The whole Earth itself was regarded as having the shape of a short cylinder, or a cube, and people were living on one of the flat faces of it.

Ancient Hindus conceived the Earth as a hemisphere supported by four elephants standing upon an immense tortoise which floated on the face of a universal ocean. This recognition of the curved character of the Earth's surface was an advance upon the flat-Earth theory, and it provided an imaginary support for the Earth as well as a course for the Sun under the Earth between sunset and sunrise. Whatever shape the Earth was supposed to be, early people thought that it needed a support or foundation of some kind. One view was that it floated on water; another was that it had roots; but neither of these ideas could explain what happened to the Sun when it disappeared below the horizon at sunset. To get over this difficulty, it was suggested by Vedic priests that the Earth was supported by twelve pillars, and that it was only through sacrifices to gods that the pillars were kept upright. The Sun travelled between the pillars from sunset to sunrise. These ideas are less

* Certain portions of this essay have been published in the author's *Gods and Men*, London, 1949, and are reproduced by permission. [Editor.]

fantastic than those held by the Christian Fathers so late as the eighth century. The Venerable Bede, and others who followed him, believed that the Earth had the shape of an egg which floated in water and was surrounded by fire.

Such primitive conceptions as these of a flat or curved Earth fixed in space, with or without foundations supporting it, and of the Sun and other celestial bodies moving around it, had to be abandoned when it was explained by Copernicus, and proved by Galileo, that the Earth was a globe which turned daily on its axis and travelled around the Sun in a year. As there is endless space in all directions, there is no reason why the Earth should need support of any kind, except when it is pulled by other bodies. 'Up' and 'down' have no meaning in infinite space.

Whatever shape the Earth was supposed to be in early times, the Sun, Moon, and stars appeared to travel around it as a centre and were used to mark the day, the month and the year. Five thousand years ago the Sun as the source of all heat, light and life on the Earth was the central object of religious belief in ancient Egypt and was personified and worshipped under the name of Ra, or Amon-Ra. At Karnak, near Luxor, there are still impressive remains of a great temple with its open end pointing to where the Sun set on the longest day of the year when it was built. When the Sun sank to the horizon, its rays would shine right along the main aisle to the Sanctuary at the far end and be reflected by jewels on the altar.

Our own great historic monument, Stonehenge, seems originally to have been constructed to mark the position of the Sun at sunrise on the longest day; and every year people still go there on that day to watch for the Sun rising in the direction of a particular stone as seen from the altar-stone. Primitive people in various parts of the world still mark the beginning of their year by noticing when the Sun rises in a certain direction on the horizon.

In the latitude of Egypt, the duration of dawn and twilight is very short, and bright stars are therefore visible near the Sun at sunrise and sunset. The star Sirius is the brightest in the sky, and it was observed by the Egyptians to appear above the eastern horizon, just before the rising of the Sun, each year towards the end of July, which was very near the time of the annual inundation of the Nile. From such observations the astronomer-priests of Egypt were able to predict when the Nile could be expected to rise.

They and other ancient watchers of the skies noticed also that different groups of stars were near the Sun at sunrise and sunset at different times of the year. A group near the Sun at sunrise in any month would be above it at sunrise in the following month, and would not be with the Sun again until a year had passed. A certain group of stars, or constellation, is thus associated with each month, and twelve such groups make up the constellations of the Zodiac. Several representations of these stellar configurations have been found in Egyptian temples, and one of them from a ceiling of the temple at Denderah is now in a museum in Paris.

The groups of stars just above the Sun at dawn and twilight were thus used as figures on a celestial dial, and the Sun took a year to pass round the complete circle of the heavens upon which they were fixed. The division of the circuit into twelve parts, or signs, made up the Zodiac, as recognized and used for religious and seasonal observances by the Chaldeans, the Chinese, the Egyptians, Hindus, Persians, Greeks, Romans, and other peoples. The order of the constellations of the Zodiac is given in rhyme as

The Ram, the Bull, the Heavenly Twins,
And next the Crab, the Lion shines,
The Virgin and the Scales,
The Scorpion, Archer, and He-goat,
The Man that bears the watering-pot,
And Fishes with glittering tails.

The constellations of the Zodiac begin with that of the Ram, and this was the group in which at one time the Sun appeared at sunrise at the spring equinox, 20 March, when days and nights are equal in length. On account, however, of a change in the position of the Earth's axis, the positions of stars in relation to that of the Sun vary in a cycle of about twenty-six thousand years, with the result that the constellations of the Zodiac move backwards in this period through the so-called signs of the Zodiac, which are geometrical divisions of the Zodiac from the point of the spring equinox. In consequence of this movement, the star-group in which the Sun is now at the spring equinox is not the Ram but the Fishes, though the first sign of the Zodiac still starts with Aries.

The constellations of the Zodiac were known a thousand years or more before the days of Joseph, and were no doubt referred to in his second dream when he said: 'Behold I have dreamed a dream more; and, behold, the sun and the moon and the eleven stars made obeisance to me.' The sun signified his father; the moon, his mother; and the eleven stars, or constellations, his eleven brethren. Hence the rebuke of Jacob: 'What is this dream that thou hast dreamed? Shall I and thy mother and thy brethren indeed come to bow down ourselves to thee to the earth?'

There is a certain amount of evidence to associate all the twelve tribes of Israel with constellations of the Zodiac; and the description given to each son in the blessing of Jacob affords support for this view. Judah was referred to as 'a lion's whelp'; Reuben 'unstable as water'; and Dan as 'a serpent by the way'. Moreover, the traditional devices upon the sacred standards of the four chief tribes were for Judah a lion, for Reuben a river, for Ephraim a bull, and for Dan an eagle or serpent—all of which are identified with constellations of the Zodiac. These tribes always pitched their tents around the tabernacle in the four corners of the camp, representing the four quarters of the heavens.

In addition to the twelve constellations of the Zodiac, thirty-two other well-marked groups of stars were described in verse by a Greek poet, Aratus, in the third century before our era. These, with four additions, are still used by astronomers, with few changes, to mark the grouping of stars in the sky. When the Apostle Paul spoke to the Athenians on Mars' Hill about the Altar to the Unknown God, he used the words 'as certain also of your own poets have said, For we are also his offspring'. The particular poet to whom Saint Paul referred was Aratus, who, like the Apostle, was a native of Cilicia, though he lived three centuries earlier.

Aratus was esteemed by both pagan and Christian philosophers, and in a beautiful dedication of his poem to Zeus or Jove he used the actual words mentioned by Saint Paul, 'And we his offspring are'. The poem was translated into Latin by Cicero and other authors, and was quoted largely by several Latin poets, especially Virgil. Though it is purely a didactic picture of the division of the heavens into regions represented in stories of Greek mythology, yet for half a dozen centuries its influence upon writers who followed Aratus was immense from the point of view of both astronomy and theology.

Aratus could scarcely be called an astronomer, but what he did was to bring together in a remarkable poem the traditional knowledge of the constellations and certain stars in them. The heavens as described by him were as they were known long before his time and as seen in latitude forty degrees or so north. There is, indeed, evidence that the celestial phenomena as described by Aratus did not actually represent conditions in his time but about a couple of thousand years earlier.

The star-list of Hipparchus and Ptolemy agrees with that of Aratus with a few exceptions. Hipparchus, 'who had ventured to count the stars, a work arduous even for the Deity' (Pliny, *Hist. Nat.*, ii. 26), made a catalogue of 1,680 stars. Ptolemy's catalogue included 1,022 stars, of which 914 form constellation figures. He placed two additional constellations among the unformed stars, while recognizing the ancient groups. The constellations of the Greeks were adopted by the Romans and other peoples, and are still used to designate divisions of the celestial sphere.

From whatever source the Greeks derived their knowledge of the heavens and particular groupings of stars upon them, the actual origin of the association of constellation figures with characters in Greek mythology has been the subject of much discussion. As several of the constellations represent characters in the voyage of the Argonauts, and none is named after the heroes of Troy, the grouping must have been settled after the expedition of the Argonauts and before the destruction of Troy.

Whatever the origin of the names, all the characters in a particular drama or legend are represented together in the heavens. Thus, Cepheus and his wife Cassiopeia, Andromeda, their daughter, waiting to be devoured by Cetus, but rescued by Perseus, who was flying through the air after slaying the Gorgon, the sea-monster turned into stone by being shown the head of Medusa. The apotheosis of all these figures is easy to understand if the myth was the origin of the constellations bearing names imposed upon them by imaginative observers, but the history of many such star-groups goes back much beyond Greek times; and it is closely connected with astronomical relationships.

From this point of view, the story of Hercules, which was derived from a group of cosmic myths going back to the very remote times in Mesopotamia and western Asia, originated in the sky, the giant being a solar hero, and his twelve labours, representing the Sun's course along the Zodiac, quenching the star light of the twelve signs one after another, and renewing every year his round of labours. A brilliant presidential address by Sir D'Arcy Thompson, delivered to the Scottish Classical Association in 1936, contains many similar explanations of early astronomical origins of constellations independent of Greek mythology.

In addition to his renowned poem, *Phainomena*, on astronomy, Aratus described weather portents and signs in another poem, *Diosemeia*. In his great didactic poem, the *Georgics*, Virgil uses the two works with stimulative imagination to bring man into intimate contact with Nature.

Agriculture and its relation to the seasons and deities associated with them is the theme of the first book of this poem. To know the proper times of sowing and other operations on the land, the stars must be watched as closely by the farmer as by the navigator. At the autumnal equinox, when days and nights are equal in length, the Sun is in the constellation of the Balance. The constellation of the Scorpion was regarded at one time as occupying two-twelfths of the Zodiac, but later the Balance was introduced between Scorpion and the Virgin. When the Sun enters the constellation of the Bull on 17 April, certain seeds may be sown, but the sowing of some other seeds should be postponed until the setting of Maia (one of the Pleiades) and of Boötes in November. The movement of the Sun through the twelve signs of the Zodiac guides the husbandman in his annual tasks. The changes of the seasons are thus connected with celestial signs and reveal orderly design and purpose.

Virgil's five zones of the sky and the Earth are derived from a work by Eratosthenes (276–196 B.C.), and the description is not altogether clear. The Earth is regarded as flat, with the celestial sphere revolving around it on an axis, one end of which rises towards the north (Scythia), while the other pole is in the gloomy Styx of the underworld. Arctos, the constellation of the Bear, or, in plural, the Great and Little Bears, is so close to the pole that, unlike some other groups of stars, it does not sink into the ocean which surrounds the world.

Comparable with Virgil, the next great poetic genius was Dante (1265–1321), a typical university scholar of the period, and a poet who made accurate use of existing scientific knowledge, as well as a politician and a patriot. He was steeped in the learning of his times, and he combined this knowledge with mysticism and Christian faith in his immortal poem *Commedia*, which after his death was given the title *The Divine Comedy*. He was the first to give a complete picture of the Christian European Cosmos. The theme of the poem opens with Dante being met in a gloomy forest by the poet Virgil, who promises to show him the punishments of Hell, and afterwards of Purgatory, after which he is conducted into Paradise. The three stages of his journey are represented in the *Inferno*, the *Purgatorio*, and the *Paradiso*.

When Virgil leaves Dante on the summit of the Earthly Paradise, Beatrice guides him through the celestial spheres, which are described according to the astronomy and theology of the time. The outermost of ten heavens is the Empyrean, the heaven of pure light and the seat of the Godhead. Within it are nine celestial spheres, the first in order below the Empyrean being the *Primum Mobile*, which bounds the material universe. Then come the heaven of the fixed stars and the seven lower heavens of Saturn, Jupiter, Mars, the Sun, Venus, Mercury, and the Moon, which are kept in motion 'by blessed movers', or angels. Dante is finally taken to the heaven of the fixed stars and apostrophizes the constellations, stating that the Sun was in the constellation of the Twins when he was born and thus fixing the date of his birth. In 1265 the Sun entered this constellation on 18 May and left it on 17 June.

Dante's ideas of the Celestial Universe were derived from the work of Aristotle, known to the Middle Ages in Arabic and Latin translation under the title *De Caelo et Mundo*, by which Dante refers to it; although on occasion it may be that he is to be taken to refer rather to the work with the same title by Albertus Magnus (1193–1280). Albertus was a voluminous writer and the first Schoolman and great Aristotelian scholar. He was the teacher of Thomas Aquinas; and to these two scientists and theologians belong the credit of being the first to reconcile the Christian and Aristotelian philosophies.

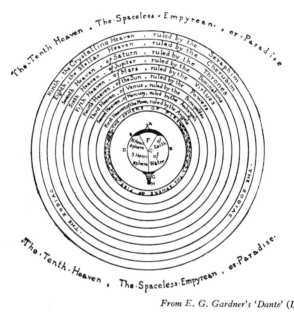

From E. G. Gardner's 'Dante' (Dent, 1900).

The Universe, as represented in Dante's *Divine Comedy*. A, Jerusalem ; B, Italy; C, Centre of Earth; D, Spain; E, the Ganges; G, Purgatory; H, Eden.

Dante obtained the data for his knowledge of the planets from Alfraganus' *De Orbibus Planetarum*. Alfraganus was a celebrated Arab astronomer who flourished at the beginning of the ninth century of our era. He wrote in Arabic on sundials, the astrolabe, and the elements of astronomy, the last a work in thirty chapters based on the principles of Ptolemy and first translated into Latin in the twelfth century. Dante himself calculated the periods for Saturn, Jupiter, Mars, the Sun, Venus, Mercury, and the Moon. The working of the system is explained to Beatrice (*Par.*, xxvii. 78–120).

In Dante's time, the study of any branch of science other than astronomy, especially of experimental natural philosophy, was regarded as belonging to the 'black arts' and any who practised it as magicians. It was believed that they could see into the future by supernatural means obtained by selling their souls to Satan. One of the foremost wizards of the Middle Ages was the Scotch astrologer and alchemist, Michael Scot, who died about 1235, and with another astrologer, Guido Bonatti of Forli, and Asdente of Parma, a shoemaker who became a diviner, is placed in Hell by Dante, together with witches:

> That other, round the loins
> So slender of his shape, was Michael Scot,
> Practised in every slight of magic wile.
> Guido Bonatti see: Asdente mark,
> Who now were willing he had tended still
> The thread and cordwain, and too late repents.
> See next the wretches, who the needle left
> The shuttle and the spindle, and became
> Diviners: baneful witcheries they wrought
> With images and herbs.
>
> (*Inferno*, xx. 113–122.)

Though Michael Scot was an intellectual giant in his day, his name is associated in the popular mind with legends relating to his magical powers. He translated into Latin several of Aristotle's works, and also Arabic works on astronomy; and he was the author of treatises on astrology, alchemy and physiology. Sir Walter Scott's *Lay of the Last Minstrel* refers particularly to Michael Scot.

After the discovery of America and the voyage of Vasco da Gama around the Cape of Good Hope, Dante was credited with the gift of prophecy. In *Purgatorio* Dante wrote: 'Io mi volsi a man destra, e posi mente all altro polo, e vide quattro stelle, non vista mai, fuor ch'alla prima genta.' (I turned on my right hand, and I looked upon the other pole, and there I saw four stars, which had never been seen since the days of earliest men.)

As Dante had written nearly a hundred years before the voyage of da Gama, this was considered to be a prevision of the constellation of the Southern Cross. Voltaire refers to both prophecies in his treatise on the voyages of the Portuguese sailors. With reference to the passage in Dante, he says that, like so much else that Dante wrote, it must be taken symbolically.

It has, however, been pointed out that Marco Polo, who returned to Italy from the East in Dante's time, might well have seen the Southern Cross on his voyages in Asia, while Pietro d'Abano, Dante's contemporary, mentions that Marco Polo had delineated to him a star, which might have been one of the four to which Dante refers.

Chaucer (1340–1400) was another astronomer-poet who was indebted to Arabian science for much of the astronomical knowledge revealed in his works. The poems of this first great master of English verse contain many references to celestial objects and movements, chiefly from the point of view of their relationships to human life and events. The planet Saturn is thus associated with a malign influence; the Sun's position in the Zodiac at different times of the year is mentioned; the *Primum Mobile*, or motive power of the system of the universe described by Ptolemy, to whom Chaucer refers; and within it are the celestial spheres carrying the fixed stars, the six planets, the Sun, and the Moon. In the Franklin story in the *Canterbury Tales*, the Zodiac is placed in the outermost of the nine spheres or circles, and the astrologer is represented as calculating the precession of the equinoxes by the

I F

distance between the true equinoctial point in Aries and the bright star
Alnath. His words were:

> For his equacions in every thyng;
> And by his eighte speere in his wirkyng
> He knew ful wel how fer Alnath was shove
> Fro the heed of thilke fixe Aries above,
> That in the nynte speere considered is.

In his poem *The Complente of Mars* Chaucer refers to the planet Venus being
in conjunction with the planet Mars in the zodiacal sign of Taurus, and to
the sign of Gemini.

Chaucer's prose writings included a *Treatise on the Astrolabe*, written for
the instruction of 'Lytel Lowys my son'. This is a simple and clear description
of the parts of the oldest form of astronomical instrument and their uses in
measuring altitudes of stars and other celestial objects for the determination
of latitude and time. The treatise was based upon a Latin translation of a
work by a ninth-century Arabian astronomer, Messahalla, entitled *De
Compositione et Utilitate Astrolabii*, supplemented by extracts from a treatise
written in the thirteenth century by an English mathematician and astronomer,
John of Halifax or Joannes de Sacrobosco. This work was entitled *Tractus
de Sphaera*, and the astronomy in it was derived from Alfraganus' work on
astronomy already mentioned.

DEMOCRITUS' THEORY OF VISION

by

KURT von FRITZ

OUR knowledge of Democritus' theory of vision is mainly and, in many very important respects, even exclusively, derived from the report given by Aristotle's disciple Theophrastus in his treatise *On sense perception*.[1] This report is critical and historical. It is historical in the sense that Theophrastus does not only present the theories of pre-Aristotelian philosophers, including Plato, in chronological sequence, but is also careful to point out the agreements and disagreements between a philosopher and some of his predecessors. Like his master Aristotle,[2] Theophrastus is also specifically interested in the answers given by each philosopher to specific stereotyped questions, as, for instance, the question whether like is perceived by like or rather opposites by opposites. Theophrastus' report is critical inasmuch as he tries to prove the insufficiency of all pre-Aristotelian theories of perception by pointing out what he considers their self-contradictions and their discrepancies when compared with observable facts.

All this would not necessarily impair the value of Theophrastus' report. But in his desire to elicit from every individual philosopher an answer to the same recurring question, he very often fails to see that, within the framework of a different philosophical system, the nature of the question itself has changed, and that this may be the reason why seemingly no clear answer can be found, or why the answers actually given appear contradictory. An example of the unjust criticism to which this may lead is the following. One of the stereotyped questions which recur again and again is whether the world which we perceive is the real world or whether there is a real world different from the world which we perceive with our senses. In section 60/61 of his treatise Theophrastus accuses Democritus of self-contradiction because, on the one hand, he considers what we perceive is a mere effect in our sensory organs, yet on the other hand tries to determine the real nature of the objects perceived. In this case we can see very clearly from literal fragments of Democritus' work preserved by other authors[3] that he was very well aware of the problem, and tried to solve it by the assumption that we cannot have any knowledge of the real world except through our senses, but that the picture of the world which the senses give us directly is blurred and incorrect, and that we can acquire a knowledge of the world as it really is only by analysing the testimony of our senses critically with our intellect or νοῦς.[4]

In this case it would perhaps not be entirely impossible to criticize

---

[1] Theophrastus, *De sensu*, 49–54 and 73–82; cf. also H. Diels, *Die Fragmente der Vorsokratiker* (4th edition by W. Kranz. Berlin, 1922), Democritus, fragm. A 135.

[2] For Aristotle's method see H. Cherniss, *Aristotle's Criticism of Presocratic Philosophy*. Baltimore (The Johns Hopkins Press), 1935.

[3] Democritus, fragm. B 9, B 10, B 11, and B 125; cf. also K. von Fritz, '*NOYΣ, NOEIN* and their Derivatives in Presocratic Philosophy. Part II, The Postparmenidean Period'. *Classical Philology*, 1946, xli, 28 ff.

[4] For Democritus' concept of νοῦς and its relation to the senses, see *op. cit.* (3), pp. 24–30.

Theophrastus' criticism on the basis of his own preceding and following report on Democritus' theory of the various senses. But it would certainly be extremely difficult if we did not have the direct testimony preserved by other authors. One of the main reasons for this difficulty is that Theophrastus very often mingles his report with his criticism in such a way that important details of Democritus' theory are revealed only implicitly through his criticism, a procedure which does not make for clarity. Furthermore, Theophrastus never quotes a whole sentence of Democritus' works literally, but reports everything in his own language; though it seems reasonably certain that he does use not infrequently individual Democritean terms in his report, since many of the words occurring in it show the characteristics of Democritus' terminology[5] and are not characteristic of peripatetic philosophy. Finally there is the additional difficulty that the text of Theophrastus' work, as preserved in the extant manuscripts, is in a great many places undoubtedly corrupt.

In order to overcome these difficulties it is not sufficient to interpret the text of Theophrastus' report as carefully as possible, by itself or with the help of other ancient testimonies concerning Democritus' theory of vision or of sense perception in general. It is necessary to relate everything that Theophrastus says to Democritus' whole system and, above all, to the main questions which he has everywhere in mind and to the characteristic methods which he everywhere applies to their solution. In order to overcome the difficulties resulting from the deficiencies of Theophrastus' historical method, it is further necessary to distinguish from the beginning Democritus' main problems and methods as clearly as possible from those characteristic of his predecessors and successors, including Theophrastus himself. Even if this is done, there will still remain some questions concerning which it is impossible to give an absolutely conclusive answer. But a good many obscure points can perhaps be clarified in this way.[6]

[5] Concerning the characteristics of Democritus' terminology see K. von Fritz, *Philosophie und sprachlicher Ausdruck bei Demokrit, Platon, und Aristoteles.* New York (G. E. Stechert), 1938, pp. 1–38.

[6] Of books and articles dealing with important aspects of the problem and published within the last few decades the following have come to my notice: A. Brieger, 'Demokrits Leugnung der Sinneswahrheit'. *Hermes,* 1902, xxxvii, 56–83; I. Beare, *Greek theories of elementary cognition from Alcmaeon to Aristotle.* Oxford, 1906; A. E. Haas, 'Antike Lichttheorien'. *Archiv für Geschichte der Philosophie,* 1907, xx, 370 ff.; Ingeborg Hammer-Jensen, 'Demokrit und Platon'. *ibid.,* 1909, xxiii, 101 ff.; W. Kranz, 'Die ältesten Farbenlehren der Griechen'. *Hermes,* 1912, xlvii, 126 ff.; G. M. Stratton, *Theophrastus and the Greek physiological psychology before Aristotle* (including the Greek text of Theophrastus, *De sensu,* with English translation and commentary). London and New York, 1917; Cyril Bailey, *The Greek Atomists and Epicurus.* Oxford, 1928, pp. 162 ff.; W. Jablonski, 'Die Theorie des Sehens im Griechischen Altertum bis auf Aristoteles'. *Sudhoffs Archiv für Geschichte der Medizin,* 1930, xxiii, 306–31; H. Langerbeck, *ΔΟΞΙΣ ΕΠΙΡΥΣΜΙΗ* in *Neue philologische Untersuchungen,* 1935, x, 75–118; together with the two interesting reviews of this book by E. Kapp in *Gnomon,* 1936, xii, 65–77 and 158–169, and by V. E. Alfieri in *Giornale Critico della Filosofia Italiana,* 1936, xvii, 66–78 and 264–277. Because of the conditions created by the war and certain other factors I am not certain whether I have not missed some more recent publications.
Of the books and articles quoted, the work by G. M. Stratton, who availed himself of the help and advice of such outstanding classisists as A. E. Taylor and I. Linforth, seems by far the best so far as the interpretation of Theophrastus' work is concerned. This seems all the more worthy of mention since apparently none of the authors who wrote later about Democritus' theory of perception has taken cognizance of Stratton's work. Since Stratton's main interest, however, is in Theophrastus and not in Democritus' system as a whole, he did not deal with some rather important aspects of Democritus' theory of vision, though he made some very important contributions to its better understanding.

It is Democritus' most fundamental belief that there is an absolute truth, to some extent accessible to us, but hidden (ἄδηλον) or, in other words, that the real world is different from the world which we perceive, but that within certain limits it is nevertheless possible for us to acquire a correct knowledge of the world as it really is. The real world consists of nothing but the atoms and the void or empty space. The void is nothing but extension. It is a real nothing which nevertheless exists. The atoms are filled space. Their qualities are the following: (1) Impenetrability. This means essentially that the space occupied by one atom cannot at the same time be occupied by another atom. But it is also considered to imply absolute rigidity and hence indivisibility, since nothing can penetrate into the atom so as to separate its parts from one another. In regard to these interrelated qualities all atoms are absolutely alike. From their indivisibility they have received their name. Their other qualities are: (2) Size. (3) Shape (ῥυσμός). (4) Position in space (τροπή). (5) Position in relation to other atoms (διαθιγή). (6) Motion in space (κίνησις or σοῦς).[7] In regard to the qualities (2) to (6) the atoms differ from one another. For though all the atoms are very small they are of different size, shape, position, etc.

All other things are nothing but compounds of atoms plus the void separating the individual atoms from one another. Their primary qualities, size, shape, weight, relative rigidity, etc., are direct consequences of the size, shape, position, arrangement, motion, etc., of the atoms of which they are composed. Their secondary qualities, on the other hand, that is, their tastes, smells, colours, etc., are not in fact qualities of the real things in themselves but merely the effects produced by them in our sensory organs. It is however possible within certain limits to draw conclusions from the effect to the cause, and hence to acquire a certain knowledge of the structure of those real things which are the ultimate causes of our sensations. The limitations of this possibility are determined by the following considerations. Democritus believes that the same sensations must essentially always have the same cause, that is, they must be caused by atoms of essentially the same size, shape, motion, and arrangement. In this respect there is no uncertainty. But the principle is not entirely reversible. For whether certain atoms can cause a sensation depends also on the state of the sensory organs.[8] Where the sensory

---

[7] For a more detailed analysis of this part of Democritus' theory and of its provenance, see *op. cit.* (5), pp. 15 ff.

[8] See Democritus, fragm. A 112, A 113, B 9 (Sext., *Adv. math.* vii. 136), and B 11. The information given by ancient authors on this part of Democritus' theory is very unsatisfactory. But, on the one hand, Theophrastus' whole report on Democritus' theory of sense perception and most of the evidence found in other authors do not leave the slightest doubt that Democritus believed that, generally speaking, certain sensations were always caused by definite types of atoms. On the other hand, we are also told that Democritus believed that our sensations depended on the condition (διαθήκη) of our body, and that hence we could never have a certain knowledge of anything. The only plausible solution of this seeming contradiction seems to be the one given above, which may perhaps be further elucidated as follows, though no direct confirmation of this elucidation can be found in the extant fragments of Democritus' works. If, for instance, the tongue of a person is affected in such a way that certain types of atoms, contained in the food juices, cannot reach the sensory parts of the taste organ because of their size or shape, while other atoms can, only the latter type of atoms will be sensed or tasted, though they may be in the minority. Hence for a person so affected, the food will have a different taste from that which it would have for a normal person, and if the first person is not helped by his other senses, he will come to wrong conclusions concerning the nature of the food which he is tasting. Nevertheless, the same taste is still caused by the same kind of atoms.

organ is defective or differently constructed, the sensation may therefore also be defective or altered, and hence the conclusions drawn from it would be partly erroneous. Further limitations have to be acknowledged where distant objects are under ordinary circumstances the ultimate cause of certain sensations. For since, according to Democritus' belief, all sensations are caused by direct contact with the sensory organs, the perception of distant objects must be caused by effluences from these objects which come in contact with our body.[9] These effluences, like everything else, are of course combinations of atoms. But such combinations of atoms can also be formed both inside and outside our body without having emanated from distant objects.[10] Hence the conclusion from the sensation to the existence of such distant objects is not absolutely conclusive in the individual case unless it can be confirmed by further evidence. But this uncertainty in the individual case does by no means preclude the possibility of determining accurately in what way generally certain sensations are caused, and to what sorts of reality they, generally speaking, correspond.

It is then perfectly clear what the main aims of Democritus' theory of sense perception must have been: (1) To determine as far as possible the real, and therefore purely atomistic, structure of the objects causing certain sensations; and (2) to determine and analyse the atomistic mechanism by which the actual sensation is finally produced. Democritus' passionate interest in this causal analysis is beautifully illustrated by his famous exclamation that he 'would rather wish to discover one causal relation than to become king of the Persian realm'. It is true that Democritus' theory has one great defect in common with all purely materialistic systems. He does not recognize anything as really existing except filled space and empty space. But there is no bridge from atomistic kinetics to sensation. It is, however, very interesting to see how he tries to overcome this fundamental difficulty.[11] Apart from this, all the remainder of the different parts of his system, to some extent even of his ethics,[12] show how much the two main questions formulated above were always foremost in his mind.

The idea that the real world is different from the world which we perceive is by no means foreign to Democritus' predecessors and contemporaries in Greek philosophy. In a way it is anticipated in the belief of both Heraclitus and Parmenides that reality is quite different from what people in general believe it to be. But it was Parmenides who first raised the problems with which most of the Greek philosophers of the fifth century, including Democritus and his master Leucippus, are struggling.

[9] There is, of course, the opposite possibility that something reaches out from our eyes and establishes contact with distant objects. This theory seems to have been adopted by some Pythagoreans and by most representatives of scientific optics in antiquity, beginning with Euclid, if Theon (*Euclidis opticorum recensio*, ed. Heiberg, pp. 148–50) is to be trusted. But no trace of this theory can be found in the fragments of Democritus' works.

[10] Cf. fragm. A 77 Diels.

[11] See *infra*, pp. 95 ff.

[12] The ethical fragments of Democritus can be roughly divided into two groups. The fragments of one group show little relation to Democritus' atomistic system, but rather contain the observations of a man who has seen much and has made his reflections on what he has seen. The other group seems to belong to a more systematic work, and here the connexion with Democritus' atomistic philosophy is very marked. Cf. *op. cit.* (5), pp. 34 ff. and the excellent article by G. Vlastos, 'Ethics and physics in Democritus' in *The Philosophical Review*, 1945, liv, 578–92, and 1946, lv, 53–64.

Parmenides is not primarily concerned with sense perception. It is to the νοῦς or intellect[13] that he attributes the fundamental error which makes men split up the world into types or forms,[14] one positive, the other negative, while in reality there can be nothing but solid positive *being*. Yet in a way even he seems to find the ultimate origin of the error in our senses, when he says[15] that our νοῦς depends on 'the mixture of our much-erring limbs (or body)'. This statement meant, according to Theophrastus,[16] that we feel warmth, light, and sound, as *being*, because they are prevalent in us, while for the dead cold, darkness, and silence would be positive, because they are prevalent in them; and because, as a general principle, like is recognized only by like.[17] At any rate, if Parmenides does not mention the senses expressly in the extant fragments of his works, but speaks only of our 'limbs' or body, his disciples Zenon and Melissus did attribute the origin of the error to seeing and hearing, etc., that is, to sense perception.[18]

While in this respect there may seem to be a certain similarity between the philosophy of Parmenides and his disciples on the one hand, and that of Democritus on the other, Parmenides is certainly very far from a materialistic concept of the world. It is very difficult to define clearly what those fundamental contrasts of warmth, light, sound and cold, darkness, silence are, which our 'limbs' reveal to us correctly or incorrectly. They can hardly be called qualities since they are not qualities of something else, but rather the stuff of which the world fundamentally consists. From a modern point of view one might be tempted to call them energies. But they are not purely physical energies; they have also an emotional character. This explains the adoption of the principle that only like can be perceived by like. For it is in the emotional sphere that a cold heart, for instance, cannot feel the warmth of love. In a philosophy like this Democritus' problem of explaining the sense qualities of colour, sound, smell, etc. in terms of shapes, motions, etc. of merely space-filling atoms obviously did not exist.

In this respect the philosophy of Empedocles forms an interesting link between Parmenides and Democritus. He has two groups of first principles, the 'material' elements of fire, air, water, and earth, and the two 'immaterial' driving forces Love and Hate. It is characteristic that the latter still belong to both the physical and the emotional world. As in Parmenides' philosophy, the perception of these forces is not connected with any specific sensory organ,[19] and the way in which they are perceived does not seem to require any specific explanation. It is in regard to the 'material' elements that a specific theory of perception becomes necessary.

The 'physico-emotional energies' of warmth, light, love, hate, etc. are not in the same sense definitely here or there as material objects are. Hence, as long as the problem of perception was mainly conceived in connexion with these

---

[13] For Parmenides' concept of νοῦς see K. von Fritz, 'ΝΟΥΣ, ΝΟΕΙΝ and their Derivatives in Presocratic Philosophy. Part I, From the Beginnings to Parmenides'. *Classical Philology*, 1945, xl, 236 ff.

[14] Parmenides, fragm. B 8, 11 ff. Diels.   [15] Parmenides, fragm. B 16 Diels.

[16] *De sensu*, 3; cf. Parmenides, fragm. A 46 Diels.

[17] Concerning the origin of this principle see *infra*, and for a more detailed discussion the article quoted in *op. cit.* (3), pp. 19 ff.

[18] See *ibid.*, p. 12.   [19] See *op. cit.* (13), p. 239.

energies,[20] the question of how knowledge of distant things could come to us did not arise. On the other hand, together with Empedocles' material elements, there appears at once the principle that matter can affect something only by direct contact. The perception of distant objects becomes then immediately a special problem, and Empedocles has tried to solve this problem by the assumption that there are constant effluences (ἀπορροιαί) from all things which come to our sensory organs. But the old Parmenidean and probably pre-Parmenidean principle, that like is perceived only by like, has still an important function in Empedocles' philosophy,[21] and in regard to the material elements —but not in regard to Love and Hate—it now receives a partly materialistic interpretation.

According to Theophrastus' report,[22] Empedocles assumed that the eye contains the four elements fire, air, water, and earth. In the human eye the fire is inside, while air and earth (and water?)[23] form the external part. There are alternate pores or passages of fire and water in the eye. By the fire pores we perceive white, by the water pores black. In the eyes of some animals the fire part is more external. This and the difference in the quantitative relation of fire and water in the eyes of various animals is the reason why some animals see better by day, others better by night. Finally, in order to be perceived, the particles must 'fit' into the corresponding pores or passages.[24]

It seems obvious that Theophrastus' report is not quite complete. Something must certainly have been said about the function of air and earth in the eye. But what Theophrastus says is sufficient to draw some conclusions which are essential for the interpretation of Democritus' theory in its relation to Empedocles. The principle that like is perceived by like is now partly used to explain the fact that different animals may have different perceptions, though the external conditions are the same. How this principle itself functions in regard to the 'material' elements is now partly explained in purely materialistic terms, that is, in terms of purely spatial arrangements: in order to be perceived the particles must fit into the corresponding passageways of the sensory organs. Yet no such 'materialistic' explanation seems to have been applied to the perception of Love and Hate. What is more, Empedocles' material elements are distinguished from one another not merely by size, shape, motion, and other spatial relations, like Democritus' atoms, but have other inherent qualities also, of which colour seems to be one.[25] Therefore, though it is true that

---

[20] The earliest Greek philosophers who, in a way, seem to have started with the assumption of material first principles, in so far as this latter concept can be attributed to them, seem not to have had any theory of perception.

[21] See *infra*. [22] *De sensu*, 7 ff. and 12 ff.

[23] Water is not mentioned in this connexion in the Theophrastus text as preserved in our manuscripts. Yet the remainder of the report leaves no doubt that water is part of the eye. Hence it seems that it must have been mentioned somewhere in the enumeration of the elements constituting the eye, and that ὕδωρ should be inserted in the text, following the suggestion of Karsen, accepted by Diels, in spite of the objections raised by Stratton, *op. cit.* (6), p. 163.

[24] This theory is stressed again and again in Theophrastus' report, and in such a way that one can hardly doubt that the word *to fit in* was actually used by Empedocles.

[25] W. Kranz's theory (*op. cit.* (6), p. 126) that, according to Empedocles, the colours exist merely in our sensory organs and are not properties of the elements and their mixtures in themselves, seems to have no foundation in the evidence and is directly contradicted by Emped. fragm. A 92 from Aëtius. The passages which he quotes in support of his assumption merely say that in order to be perceived the effluences must fit into the sensory passages, but not that colour is merely subjective.

black, which is the colour of water, cannot be perceived unless it can penetrate into the water pores of the eye, the real and fundamental reason for its perception is still the affinity of water to water. In spite of the 'materialistic' additions the original meaning of the principle that like is perceived by like is still essentially preserved in Empedocles' theory.

In peripatetic philosophy the physical contrasts of warmth and cold, light and dark, etc. are no longer identified with or even closely related to emotional qualities. But they are still, at least δυνάμει, qualities of the objects belonging to the real world, not merely effects produced in our sensory organs. Aristotle, furthermore, has a very elaborate answer to the question of how far or in what respect qualities must be alike, and how far they must be different or even contrasts in order to affect one another.[26]   Both from the point of view of the development of the theory of sense perception before Democritus and from the point of view of peripatetic philosophy, therefore, Theophrastus must have been keenly interested in eliciting from Democritus an answer to the question of whether like is perceived by like or opposites by opposites.   Yet in regard to this problem the position of a philosopher who did not recognize the real existence of anything except atoms and the empty space must have been fundamentally different from that of either Empedocles or Theophrastus. It seems important to keep this in mind when analysing Theophrastus' report on Democritus' solution of the problem.

Theophrastus begins his report with the statement[27] that Democritus did not indicate whether in his opinion sense perception was perception of like by like or of opposites by opposites.   By inference, however, Theophrastus says, one can arrive at opposite conclusions.   For if, according to Democritus' own theory, sense perception is the result of a 'change' or 'alteration' (ἀλλοιοῦσθαι) produced in our sensory organs, one has to conclude that perception is produced by opposites.   If, on the other hand, 'to be changed' (ἀλλοιοῦσθαι) means 'to be affected' (πάσχειν), and if one accepts Democritus' theory that only like can be affected by like, then it follows that perception must be of like by like.

This whole argument is very characteristic of Theophrastus' method. The principle that ἀλλοιοῦσθαι is effected by opposites is an Aristotelian— and to some extent a pre-Democritean—principle,[28] but there is no evidence of its having been accepted by Democritus. On the other hand, there cannot be the slightest doubt that ἀλλοιοῦσθαι, or rather μεταρυσμεῖσθαι—for this seems to have been the term used by Democritus—by external objects, as is the case with sense perception, implies πάσχειν. Hence only the second inference drawn by Theophrastus applies really to Democritus in terms of his own philosophy.

It would, however, be much more interesting to know what Democritus had in mind when he said that only like could be affected by like, and whether in stating this principle he merely adopted in a slightly different form the old principle that like is perceived by like.   Obviously Theophrastus' statement that Democritus did not say whether perception was of like by like does not favour the latter interpretation.   But there are more cogent reasons for its rejection.   In pre-Democritean philosophy (Anaximander, Anaximenes,

---

[26] See the second book of Aristotle, *De generatione et corruptione*.
[27] *De sensu*, 49.   [28] See *infra*.

Heraclitus, and even Parmenides, as far as the realm of δόξα is concerned), and in early Greek medicine the theory is quite prevalent that in the physical world the opposites struggle with one another and 'affect' one another. So, in Anaximander's theory, when the hot fire meets the cold water, part of the latter is evaporated into air while part of it is dried and becomes solid.[29]   But when fire meets fire or water water, nothing happens, since, being alike, they do not affect one another.   The rules therefore in pre-Democritean philosophy for causation of change in the physical world, which is effected by opposites, and for perception, which is of like by like, are the not same but opposite.   It follows that Democritus' doctrine that only like can be affected by like can hardly be an adaptation of the early theory that like is perceived by like.   It obviously belongs from the outset to the theory of physical causation and was formulated in opposition to earlier doctrines.   This is confirmed by an Aristotelian passage where Aristotle says[30] that Democritus, in contrast to earlier philosophers, contended that only like can act on like, and that even where qualitatively different things act upon one another, this can happen only in so far as there is nevertheless something identical in them.

Aristotle does not explain the meaning of Democritus' doctrine any further. But he does say somewhat later that in his opinion the whole controversy is due to the fact that the early philosophers did not distinguish clearly between the different ways in which the term 'like' is used.   For, he says, it is obvious that interaction can exist only between what belongs to the same field, as, for instance, colour and colour, taste and taste, but not between colour and taste, which belong to entirely different fields.   But within each field it is the opposites which affect one another, that is, white affects black but not black black.

This is, of course, an Aristotelian, not a Democritean theory, but, together with the quotation from Democritus to the effect that 'even where qualitatively different things act upon one another there must be something identical in them', it shows clearly that Democritus does not speak of things which are qualitatively absolutely alike, as his predecessors did in their theory of sense perception.   Considering the fundamental differences between Democritus' system and the systems of his most famous contemporaries, it seems then most likely that Democritus' doctrine was directed against theories like those of Anaximander, who made an immaterial νοῦς move material particles, or of Empedocles, who made immaterial forces like Love and Hate act upon the material elements, and that it meant simply that only a body can act upon a body.[31]   At any rate it appears certain that Democritus' doctrine that only like can act upon like has nothing to do with the earlier doctrine that like is perceived by like, and that it was only Theophrastus' eagerness to elicit from

---

[29] Anaximander, fragm. A 27 Diels.   [30] *De generatione et corruptione*, i. 7; 323[b] 10 ff.

[31] In view of Democritus' theory of the soul, which has been very well analysed by G. Vlastos in the article quoted in note 12, p. 578 ff., one is even tempted to assume that Democritus pointed out explicitly that it is quite true that the (human or animal) body is moved by the soul, but that in order to be able to move the body the soul itself must be matter.   This would fit exactly the Democritean principle mentioned by Aristotle, to the effect that what acts upon something else may be qualitatively different from it, but that there must be something identical in them if one is to act upon the other.

It will hardly be necessary to mention that since perception, according to Democritus, is an action of atoms on atoms, the principle mentioned applies also to perception, but that the principle in this form is very different in its origin and implications from the earlier principle that like is perceived by like.

every philosopher an answer to the same stereotyped question which seemed to establish a historical relation which in reality does not exist.[32] To make this quite clear seems rather important in view of the ever-repeated assumption that a good many of Democritus' doctrines are taken over from his predecessors, and do not really fit in with his system.

Against the interpretation given, it may be said that a little later Theophrastus does attribute to Democritus the theory that like is perceived by like, when he credits him with the statement that 'everyone perceives best what is akin or homogeneous' (τὸ ὁμόφυλον). In fact it has been held[33] that here Theophrastus openly contradicts his earlier statement to the effect that Democritus did not say whether like is perceived by like or opposites by opposites. The very fact, however, that Theophrastus appears to contradict himself so flagrantly should prevent us from drawing rash conclusions. For while Theophrastus is apt to see the opinions of earlier philosophers in a wrong perspective, because he often looks at them from the peripatetic viewpoint rather than from the point of view of their own fundamental philosophy, he is, as his works show everywhere, always extremely careful in marshalling his evidence when he wishes to make a point. It is therefore not quite believable that, when he tried to find out what Democritus thought about the old problem of whether like was perceived by like, he failed to see that Democritus had expressed himself on this problem in very clear terms, and that in fact he quoted Democritus' clearly formulated answer after having stated only a few sentences earlier that Democritus did not give any explicit answer at all. It seems much more likely that in Theophrastus' opinion the sentence quoted was not an answer to the traditional problem. An analysis of the context in which it occurs will show us that he was probably right.

Before entering upon the interpretation of the difficult chapter on ἔμφασις in which Democritus' statement about perception of ὁμόφυλα occurs, it will be useful to discuss briefly another theory concerning the relation of like to like which is attributed to Democritus. Sextus Empiricus quotes[34] a fragment from a work of Democritus in which Democritus says that everywhere like associates with like. This law can be observed in the animal kingdom, where doves associate with doves and cranes with cranes, and also in the inanimate world. For when the pebbles are beaten by the waves on the beach of the sea, the round pebbles become separated from the oblong, and likewise if one shakes lentils, barley, and wheat in a sieve the lentils will be lined up together, and the barley and wheat will be separated from them and from one another. Sextus connects this observation of Democritus with the traditional theory that like is perceived by like, and in fact, a passage in a work of Aëtius,[35] which ultimately seems to go back to Posidonius, confirms that it must have had something to do with Democritus' theory of perception. Again, however, the evidence must be analysed carefully in order to avoid rash conclusions.

The observation that like associates with like is, of course, very old.[36]

---

[32] *De sensu*, 50. The expression is repeated in 54.

[33] See, for instance, J. I. Beare, *op. cit.* (6), p. 24, note 1.

[34] Sext. Emp., *Adv. math.* vii. 116/17; cf. also Democritus, fragm. B 164.

[35] Aëtius, iv. 19, 3: cf. Democritus, fragm. A 128 Diels.

[36] Cf. Homer, *Odyssey*, xvii. 218 and the proverb 'a crow sits always with a crow', which seems to have been quoted by Democritus.

But the available evidence does not favour the assumption that it was in any way brought into connexion with the doctrine that like is perceived by like in early Greek philosophy. In Empedocles' philosophy certainly they are completely dissociated from one another. For, while the principle that like is perceived by like, according to Empedocles, is true of all things and at all times, it is his doctrine that under the influence and the rule of Love the opposites mix and associate with one another, while Hate makes the opposites separate from one another and brings like together with like. If therefore Democritus used the observation that like associates with like in this theory of perception, this was not a continuation of the theories of Parmenides and Empedocles but something essentially new. What is more, the way in which the observation that like associates with like is elaborated by Democritus reveals also an interesting new approach. In its application to human beings and animals the observation was old. Democritus not only extended it to the inanimate world but, at least in this field, expressed it in terms of size and shape, that is, in terms of purely spatial properties. In those parts of his work which have come down to us he did not try to reduce the phenomenon to the first principles of atomistic mechanics. But the tendency in this direction is very marked. Nothing of this kind can be found in earlier formulations or applications of the observation.

It remains to find out how Democritus used the observation that like associates with like in his theory of vision. Aëtius (or probably rather Posidonius) speaks of it[37] not in connexion with Democritus' theory of vision but with his theory of sound and hearing. He says that, according to Democritus, the air is broken into little bodies or pieces of like shape under the influence of the beatings of the voice, and so is rolled along with the beatings. But it is clear that here Democritus does not speak of a likeness of the pieces, into which the air is broken, with anything in our sensory organs or in our soul, but of a likeness of these pieces among themselves, or, if one pays attention to the explanation which follows, rather of an arrangement of the particles of the air in homogeneous patterns like those created by the waves of the sea among the pebbles on the beach.[38]

The interpretation of the Theophrastus passage in which the term ὁμόφυλα occurs is somewhat more difficult. But the general idea cannot be completely different from that found in the theory of sound which is discussed by Aëtius. Theophrastus explains[39] that vision is caused by a 'reflection'[40] in the eye. This 'reflection' is first produced in the air. Then it penetrates into the eyes, which are moist. For what is dense does not admit it, but what is moist (or rather liquid) lets it pass. Therefore moist eyes have a better vision than hard eyes, especially if the outer coat is extremely thin,[41] and the inner part

---

[37] Aëtius, *Placita*, iv. 19, 3; cf. Democritus, fragm. A 128 Diels.

[38] For the function of this observation in Democritus' theory of hearing see *infra*, p. 94 and note 48.   [39] *De sensu*, 50.

[40] For the real meaning of the Greek word ἔμφασις which is usually translated by *reflection*, see *infra*, pp. 94–5.

[41] The Greek text says 'very thin and very dense'. But since Democritus insists that all other parts of the eye must *not* be dense so that the ἔμφασις can easily penetrate into it, the statement that the outer coat must be very dense is difficult to understand. Perhaps Democritus made such a statement and explained it in some way. But since the manuscript tradition is rather bad, there is also the possibility that the text is corrupt.

is extremely spongy and free from dense and strong flesh and also free from thick and oily moisture,[42] and if the ducts in the eye are straight and dry so as to correspond perfectly to the imprints (which enter the eye). This explanation is directly followed by the sentence: 'For everyone [or everything][43] perceives best what is akin [or homogeneous]'. Obviously this last sentence, beginning with 'for' and in the connexion in which it stands, is a complete *non sequitur* if it is to be interpreted in the sense of the old principle that like is perceived by like. For with Democritus' predecessors to be like meant to be of the same, irreducible quality which was partly of an emotional character, while in the context of Theophrastus' report likeness, if it is to make any sense at all, can only mean likeness of pattern, and this not even in the sense that the shape of the atoms or their combinations in the perceived imprint and the perceiving sensory organ are exactly alike, but merely in the sense that they are sufficiently alike to fit into each other.[44] Again, therefore, in perfect agreement with the fundamental concepts of the Democritean system, the explanation is given in terms of purely spatial relations.

If this interpretation is correct—and it does not seem that any other interpretation agrees with the context in which Theophrastus' statement concerning the ὁμόφυλα in Democritus is found—it explains easily the seeming or real contradictions in the tradition concerning Democritus' attitude towards the old principle that like is perceived by like. It is no longer surprising that Theophrastus, when discussing this problem, considered first Democritus' theory that only like acts upon like and not the statement that ὁμόφυλα are always best perceived, though, if one considers merely the wording, the second statement seems to come so much nearer to the old principle that like is perceived by like than the first one. For, if one is not deceived by words but considers the realities to which they refer, the doctrine that only bodies can act upon bodies is at least somewhat more closely related to the doctrine that only like qualities can affect one another so as to be perceived, than the theory that perception depends on homogeneous spatial arrangements. It is not surprising either that Sextus, who always explains everything in terms of a few traditional concepts,[45] missed the fundamental difference between Democritus and his predecessors and contemporaries altogether.

In his report on Democritus' discussion of the structure of the eye Theophrastus had spoken of the ἔμφασις which is first produced in the air but then penetrates into the eye and there produces vision. Ἔμφασις is usually translated by 'reflection'. But this word suggests a throwing back or reflecting of the rays, while ἔμφασις suggests merely that something appears in something. The theory of ἔμφασις seems to have originated from the observation that we can see in the eyes of a person a small picture of the objects that he faces. If this picture is identified with the combination of particles which causes his vision the question can, of course, be asked how we can see this picture, since the particles, in order to be seen by the person, should penetrate into his eye and

---

[42] Here I follow (like Stratton, *op. cit.* (6), p. 111 and note 133) the reading of the manuscripts against Diels' conjecture μεστά.

[43] Since ἕκαστον is used in the accusative it is not possible to tell whether the masculine or the neuter is meant.

[44] See also *infra*, note 47.

[45] For a striking example, see *op. cit.* (13), pp. 234 ff.

not be thrown back or reflected so as to be seen by us.   But apart from this difficulty the idea seems natural enough.

There is, however, another element in Democritus' ἔμφασις-theory which has puzzled both ancient and modern commentators and critics.   This is the assumption that the ἔμφασις is first produced in the air and at some distance from the eye, namely, it seems, in the place where the effluences from the object which is seen and from the body or the eye of the person seeing it come together.   According to Theophrastus, Democritus believed that in this spot the air was compressed so that an imprint was formed in it.   It is, then, this imprint which penetrates into the eye and appears in it.

Theophrastus himself points out that it would have been so much simpler to assume that the effluences penetrate directly into the eye than to assume that there is first an imprint in the air, an assumption which leads to all sorts of difficulties.   Some modern commentators[46] have pointed to a fragment in which Democritus says that, if the space between object and eye were pure void, an ant could be clearly seen in the sky, and have drawn from it the conclusion that the imprint in the air serves merely to explain why we do not see very distant objects as clearly as near ones.   This explanation, however, seems hardly sufficient.   That the effluences from the visible objects are disturbed and blurred by the air through which they have to pass is perfectly understandable, without the assumption of a special imprint produced in the air at the place where the effluences from opposite directions meet.   What is more, while their passing through the air over a great distance may blur the effluences, the imprint itself, according to Theophrastus' report, seems rather to consolidate the image.   For the ἔμφασις produced in this way is said to be hard.[47]

The matter can perhaps be further elucidated by referring again to Democritus' theory of hearing.   The theory that the beating of the air by the voice makes the particles of air fall into homogeneous patterns seems to have served to explain the articulation of sound.[48]   On the other hand, Theophrastus[49] says that, according to Democritus, the sound-producing particles enter the body through the ear, which of all the parts of the body contains the most empty space, and then scatter.   One may then perhaps conjecture that the ἔμφασις-theory

[46] For instance J. I. Beare, *op. cit.* (6), p. 27.

[47] Theophrastus, *De sensu*, 50.   This statement shows also how different Democritus' theory concerning the perception of ὁμόφυλα is from the old doctrine that like is perceived by like. For the ἔμφασις must be hard in order to be seen as a definite shape, while the eye must be moist and soft in order to receive it.   In this respect, therefore, there is certainly no likeness between the ἔμφασις which produces the vision and the sensory organ.   Also water, according to Democritus, must be in the eye, so that the ἔμφασις does not find resistance, and has not, as in Empedocles' theory, the function of perceiving water or the colour black which is inherent in it, while the fiery parts perceive fire and white.

[48] This seems to follow from Aëtius' report on Epicurus' theory of hearing which precedes his report on Democritus' theory (cf. H. Diels, *Doxographi Graeci*, p. 408).   This report on Epicurus contains also another detail which illustrates the close relation between the theory of hearing and the theory of vision within the atomistic system.   According to Aëtius, Epicurus illustrated the formation of fields of similarly shaped particles in the air under the impact of voice-beats, by a phenomenon which can be observed 'when fullers blow on clothes'.   What this means is explained by Seneca (*Qaest. Nat.* i. 3, 2), who says that, when a fuller sprays clothes with water, the water in the air separates into the various colours of the rainbow.   Obviously, then, the assumption is made that the same phenomenon which produces the articulation of sound, namely, that under an impact similarly shaped particles come together, can also be observed by the eye as the regular arrangement of the rainbow colours.   It should, however, be noticed that the illustration by reference to the fuller does not come from Democritus, but from Epicurus.

[49] *De sensu*, 55.

serves to explain how it comes about that the vision-producing effluences retain a definite shape, so that we are enabled to know the shape of the external objects from which they have come,[50] while sound, though it has a certain pattern and is articulated, does not reveal the shape of the object by which it was produced. It would then seem that Democritus found the reason for this phenomenon, on the one hand, in the fact that all things are constantly vision-producing during day-time, and that hence the vision-producing effluences from opposite directions can be assumed to meet and to produce a consolidated imprint in the air; and, on the other hand, in the structure of the eye, which, in contrast to the ear, is such as to hold the ἔμφασις together, while sound scatters after having penetrated into the ear. It is true that Theophrastus' criticism is justified to some extent when he finds it difficult to explain how a substance as volatile as air could be compressed into a hard image by an impact of two different images from opposite sides. But even so, an analysis of the theory shows how much attention Democritus paid to the atomistic mechanism of sense perception.

Another and most interesting problem is presented by Democritus' theory of colour. Theophrastus reports[51] that Democritus reduced all colours to mixtures of four primary colours, white (λευκόν), black (μέλαν), red (ἐρυθρόν), and green (χλωρόν).[52] Only these four colours therefore have to be explained directly in terms of atomistic mechanics.

Aristotle declares[53] that Democritus reduces all sense perception to sensations of touch. That this is actually so is most conspicuous in regard to Democritus' theory of taste sensations, though one may say that Democritus' actual procedure is a little more complicated. His ultimate aim is of course to find out the atomic pattern of the objects creating certain sensations. Now one cannot say that the touch sensations of rough, smooth, sticky, etc. give us a knowledge of this structure directly. But the transition from these touch sensations to a visualization of the surface structure of the objects causing it seems easier and more direct than in the case of taste, smell, or colour sensations.[54] Hence Democritus tries to reduce taste and smell sensations to what seem to him related touch sensations, and so to arrive at a conclusion concerning their atomic pattern or structure.

No such complicated procedure is of course necessary to explain the perception of the shape of objects by the sense of vision. For shape is a quality of

---

[50] What Democritus means by ἔμφασις is obviously not merely a negative imprint on the air, which, as Theophrastus points out, would mean that we get a negative picture of the real things, but which would also mean that the effluences themselves do not penetrate into the eye at all, which is contrary to Democritus' statement. It is rather a consolidated image formed both by the effluences and by the air compressed by them.
In this form the theory is not irreconcilable with the assumption that the effluences are blurred to some extent by a long passage through the air before the imprint is formed, though it is difficult to understand how there could be an ἔμφασις or imprint of the ant in the sky (see above p. 94) at all, if there was only empty space between it and the eye of the person seeing it. But this is an inconsistency which cannot be explained away by any possible interpretation, and which, after all, is not too difficult to understand.

[51] De sensu, 73 ff.

[52] χλωρόν means the yellowish green of young leaves or dark honey, and is different from πράσινον (blue-green), which Democritus probably considered a mixed colour, though Aristotle contends (Meteor. iii. 2; 372ᵃ 8) that it cannot be produced by mixture.

[53] De sensu, 4; 442ᵃ 29; cf. Democritus, fragm. A 119 Diels.

[54] For a more detailed analysis see the article quoted in note 3, p. 29.

the real things themselves and directly given in perception through the sense of vision. But colour, which is not a quality of the things as they really are, has to be explained. Here then we may expect Democritus to have followed the same procedure as in the case of taste and smell, and Aristotle, when he says that Democritus reduced all sensations to sensations of touch, seems to imply that he did. In this case, however, Theophrastus' report, if one follows the generally accepted interpretation, presents serious difficulties.

Concerning Democritus' explanation of white and black, Theophrastus has this to say. White is what is smooth. For what is neither rough nor shadow-making nor difficult to penetrate, that is bright.[55] What is bright must also have straight pores and be transparent. Now things which are both hard and white consist of such shapes (or patterns) as the inner surface of a cockle shell. For in this way they will be shadowless, bright, and with straight pores. But white things which are friable and crumbling consist of round shapes obliquely arranged in their position and their combination by pairs, but in their whole arrangement as uniform as possible. If this is their arrangement, they will be friable because they touch one another only a little; they will have straight pores because uniformly arranged,[56] and shadowless because smooth and with an even surface.

The black will consist of the opposite shapes or patterns, namely, such as are rough, irregular, and differing from one another. For these will make shadows and will have pores that are not straight and are difficult to pass. Furthermore, their effluences will be sluggish and disturbed. For the effluence makes a difference in regard to what appears (to the perception), and it is also affected by aggregating with air.

It is generally assumed that the shapes, figures, or patterns ($\sigma\chi\dot{\eta}\mu\alpha\tau\alpha$)[57] of which Theophrastus (or Democritus) speaks here are the shapes of the atoms of which the white or black objects consist, and hence also the shapes of the atoms which constitute the effluences from them. But this assumption can hardly be correct. The straight pores of white objects and the irregular pores of dark objects can hardly be in the atoms but must be between them. In the analysis of the black colour the effluences are clearly distinguished from the figures or patterns and they are characterized by their motion, while the figures are characterized by the position of particles to one another. Aristotle, furthermore, when speaking of Democritus' theory of colour,[58] says that colour is produced by the *position* ($\tau\rho\sigma\pi\dot{\eta}$) of atoms, which is in clear contrast to

[55] For the ancient Greeks the notions of white and of bright, shining, brilliant were always very closely connected and appear often as interchangeable (see, for instance, Callimachus, *Hymn* vi. 120 ff.).

[56] The manuscripts have here the word $\epsilon\ddot{v}\theta\rho\upsilon\pi\tau\alpha$, which means friable or crumbling. But this word is almost synonymous with the preceding $\psi\alpha\theta\upsilon\rho\dot{\alpha}$, so that one does not see why another explanation should be needed. It is also difficult to see why an object should be friable if its particles are uniformly arranged, since they can nevertheless be interlaced. One misses an explanation that the body in this way will have straight pores, which previously was mentioned as a most essential property. If the particles are uniformly arranged the pores obviously will be straight. Hence it seems very likely that $\epsilon\ddot{v}\theta\rho\upsilon\pi\tau\alpha$ is corrupted from $\epsilon\dot{v}\theta\dot{v}\pi\sigma\rho\alpha$, a very similar word.

[57] $\Sigma\chi\hat{\eta}\mu\alpha$ can have all three meanings. It very ofte nmeans, for instance, the figures or configurations in a dance. Hence the special meaning of the word in a given instance depends on the context.

[58] *De generatione et corruptione*, i. 2; 316ᵃ 1. Cf. Democritus, fragm. A 123 Diels. See also Theophrastus, *De sensu*, 75; $\tau\hat{\eta}\ \theta\dot{\epsilon}\sigma\epsilon\iota\ \kappa\alpha\dot{\iota}\ \tau\dot{\alpha}\xi\epsilon\iota\ \delta\iota\alpha\lambda\lambda\dot{\alpha}\tau\epsilon\iota\nu\ \tau\dot{\eta}\nu\ \chi\rho\dot{\sigma}\alpha\nu$.

Democritus' theory of taste, which explains the different tastes by the difference in the *shapes* of the atoms affecting the sensory organ.[59]

All this seems to indicate that what Democritus had in mind in his analysis of the colours of white and black was the structural arrangement of the atoms in white and black objects rather than the shapes of the individual atoms themselves. This is further confirmed by his distinction of hard and friable white objects. Hard bodies, according to Democritus,[60] consist of atoms which are strongly interlaced so that they do not easily change their relative position; while friable bodies consist of atoms which are not interlaced, though otherwise they may be more densely arranged, which will be the case if a heavy body is soft or friable, while a light but hard body will have large empty spaces of void within a tightly interlaced structure. Since round or spherical atoms can hardly be interlaced, it would naturally follow that a hard object will not consist of spherical atoms but of atoms with hooks, while a friable object will not consist of hooked but of more rounded atoms. On the basis of these considerations one can easily understand why Democritus felt compelled to explain how hard and friable objects, in spite of their different internal structure, nevertheless can have the same colour. He points out that, in spite of their structural differences, in both of them the particles can be so arranged as to form straight pores in regular patterns and with a comparatively smooth surface.[61]

This alone, it would seem, proves conclusively that the σχήματα of which Democritus spoke cannot possibly have meant the shapes of the atoms but must have referred to their configurations. It is then also easy to explain Democritus' statement that the pores of white objects are 'shadowless' while those of black objects produce shade. Theophrastus[62] found this statement difficult to understand, and W. Kranz[63] goes so far as to contend that by introducing shade Democritus brings in colour as an objective quality by the backdoor. These objections, however, are entirely unjustified. Shade is produced where an object obstructs the path of light rays, or, in Democritean terms, of vision-producing effluences, and prevents them either wholly or partly from proceeding in a straight line. Obviously this is the case where the pores through which the effluences emanate from a body are not straight and regular. Everything, therefore, in this explanation is explained in terms of matter particles, their shape and arrangement. No 'objective' colour is brought in at all. This becomes even clearer through another passage in which Theophrastus describes how it is possible that a white object, in spite of the earlier statement that the configuration of a white body must be smooth, can have a rough surface. Such objects, he says, consist of big particles and their junctures are not rounded but protruding, and the shapes of the configurations[64]

[59] See Theophrastus, *De sensu*, 65 ff.   [60] Cf. Democritus, fragm. A 60.

[61] There seems to be a certain inconsistency inasmuch as Democritus later (*v. infra*) tries to explain that white objects can also have a rough surface. But his σχήματα are neither the atoms nor the shape of the surface as a whole, but rather the small-scale or finer structure of the latter. What is necessary for the production of the white-effect is obviously that there be no rough protrusions which would hamper the outflow of the effluences. Hence the requirement of (small-scale) smoothness. But since it is obvious that white objects can have rough surfaces, Democritus tries to show how this kind of roughness is reconcilable with the absence of protrusions which would obstruct the effluences.

[62] *De sensu*, 81.   [63] *op. cit.* (6), p. 131.

[64] In this passage where Theophrastus speaks of μορφαὶ σχημάτων it seems crystal clear that σχήματα cannot mean the shapes of the atoms as has always been assumed, quite apart from the absurdity that atoms should have the shape of the zigzag walls on the approaches of a fortress.

are broken or zigzag-shaped like the earthworks in the approach to a city wall. For if arranged in this way they will still throw no shadow and will not hinder the brightness.

The evidence collected leaves hardly any doubt that Democritus' σχήματα designate the small-scale structures of the bodies which to human vision appear as white or black. The fundamental principle is extremely simple. If an object has straight pores which do not obstruct the emanation of the effluences it will appear white; if its pores are not straight, so that they hinder and disturb the effluences, it will appear black. But the straightness of the pores will be a product of different configurations in a hard and in a friable object, or in objects with a rough or a smooth surface.

The connexion between the nature of the pores and the colour-effect in the sensory organ is perhaps not too difficult to explain, though Theophrastus says hardly anything about it. He does say that coming from black objects the effluences are sluggish and confused. This is natural enough if their motion is obstructed and disturbed while they flow out of the pores. By contrast, then, the effluences from white objects with straight, regular, and uniform pores must be quick and regular. It follows, further, that the white-effect in the eye is produced by quick and regular, the black-effect by slow and irregular effluences. This theory is not difficult to understand if one takes into consideration that, especially in the clear and limpid air of Greece, a shining white hits the eye, so to speak, with great intensity, and that white objects stand out with bright clear contours, while the opposite is true in both respects of the black colour.

It remains to show very briefly that Democritus' theory of red and yellow-green agrees with the explanation given. It is obvious that it must have been difficult to explain the nature of any other colour except black and white in terms of the motion of the effluences producing them. This difficulty is clearly illustrated by Democritus' theory of red and green. Of green he says nothing but that it is an effect of a combination of the solid and the void.[65] This means that he despaired of a detailed scientific explanation. But that he mentions the void is again a clear proof of the fact that he has in mind the structure of the object from which the effluences come, but not of the effluences themselves. For the void is a real nothing. It exists inasmuch as it is between the solid atoms. But it cannot act on anything. Hence its presence in the effluences which act on the sensory organs is not of essential importance. Its presence in the seen object, on the other hand, is most essential, since without it the effluences cannot emanate from it and hence not reach the eye.

In his theory of the red colour Democritus has tried to overcome the difficulty by connecting it with the phenomenon of heat, explaining that red objects have the same configurations as hot ones, only larger. In another passage[66] we learn that a body is heated by producing empty space in it. So there is another explanation in terms of empty space. In still another passage[67] we are informed that Democritus believed that fire atoms are of spherical shape. The seeming contradiction disappears if one assumes that the empty space in a heated body

---

[65] Theophrastus affirms positively that Democritus did not give any further explanation of the yellow-green colour.

[66] Theophrastus, De sensu, 65.   [67] Democritus, fragm. A 74.

lets the fire atoms pass easily and without obstruction. The theory of the red colour then agrees perfectly with the interpretation given above, especially since red, like white, is an intense colour, which, so to speak, hits the eye.[68]

If the interpretation of his theory of colours given here is correct, one must admire the energy with which Democritus, not content to find out something about the nature of the effluences which produce a certain colour sensation in our eye, pursued the question further and asked what the structure of an object must be, if it is to give off effluences producing a white-sensation and at the same time is hard and smooth or friable and rough.

Much more important, however, is another conclusion that can be drawn from the interpretation of all the various phases of Democritus' theory of vision. For if these interpretations are accepted, it follows that Democritus was much more consistent in reducing everything to purely spatial properties, relations, and motions, and that the difference between him and his predecessors and contemporaries (with the exception, of course, of his teacher Leucippus), all of whom believe in objective non-spatial properties, is much greater than is generally believed. In fact, one may say that down to the present day nobody has ever surpassed, or perhaps even reached, the degree of consistency with which he carried out a purely materialistic and mechanistic explanation of all phenomena. This is perhaps all the more interesting because both the provenance of Democritus' philosophy through Leucippus from Parmenides, and the elaboration of his system in detail, show very clearly that materialism has anything but a purely empirical basis, as so many moderns seem to believe.

[68] There is one very important problem which cannot be dealt with here because of its difficulty and the limited space available. This is the question of whether the effluences themselves were supposed to consist of particles of the objects from which they emanate or of light, fire, air, or still something else. Theophrastus criticizes Democritus first on the assumption that the effluences are particles of the objects from which they emanate. But then (*De sensu*, 82) he becomes doubtful, and mentions the possibility that they might consist of light. Obviously he did not find Democritus very explicit on this point. The problem, if it can be solved at all, would have to be attacked together with a new discussion of the question whether and how far Plato has made use of Democritus' theory of vision in his *Timaeus*.

ANCIENT DOCUMENTS AND CONTEMPORARY LIFE, WITH SPECIAL REFERENCE TO THE HIPPOCRATIC *CORPUS*, CELSUS AND PLINY *

by

W. H. S. JONES

FOR a long time classical scholars have been much interested in the search for sources. Since F. A. Wolf in 1795 published his *Prolegomena* the importance attached to this branch of scholarship has perhaps epualled that attached to textual criticism. Accordingly, while creative literature, such as drama and lyric poetry, has attracted, as it always will attract, the attention of all kinds of interpreters, the significance of less artistic material, derived from compilations and text-books, has tended to be passed over in the eagerness to look for origins.

This *Quellenkritik* has a very necessary function to perform. Without critical examination the *Lives* of Plutarch cannot be used as evidence for events which took place perhaps hundreds of years before he wrote. The credibility of Plutarch's statements is weighed by considering the credibility of the writers from whom Plutarch derived his information, from their opportunities, ability and honesty, as well as by a reasoned judgement of his own abilities and character. There is, however, another side to the question. Whoever were Plutarch's authorities, whatever his merits or demerits, the testimony given by him has a value independent of its value for the history of the lives and events with which he deals.

Such a differentiation does not arise when historians deal with an original writer, one who puts on record his own experiences and convictions without conscious borrowing from the past. Of such a nature for instance are the *Letters* of Cicero. These may be used as first-hand evidence, subject only to such precautions as are taken when any direct witness, however capable and honest, is under examination. Books, however, dependent upon the testimony of others, are perhaps equally valuable as authorities for contemporary history. For this purpose what is required is not the source but the date, and if possible the provenance. The problem is roughly this: at such a date, a work of such a character was written containing such information. What can be justly inferred from these data about the knowledge, culture and taste of the author and his contemporaries? The *Meditations*, for instance, of Marcus Aurelius may be studied either as a late source for Stoic ethics, or as the self-revelation of

---

* The following are the chief works dealing with the questions raised in this essay :—

Allbutt, T. C., *Greek Medicine in Rome*. London, 1921.
Ilberg, J., *A. Cornelius Celsus und die Medizin in Rom*. Leipzig, 1907.
Jones, W. H. S., *Dea Febris*. Liverpool, 1909.
idem, Malaria and Greek History. Manchester, 1909.
idem, Hippocrates. London and Camb. (Mass.) (Loeb Library), vol. iv, 1931.
Marx, F., *A. Cornelii Celsi quae supersunt*. Leipzig (*Corp. Med. Lat.*), 1915. (Especially the Prolegomena.)
Münzer, F., *Beiträge zur Quellenkritik der Naturgeschichte des Plinius*. Berlin, 1897.
Spencer, W. G., *Celsus de Medicina*. London and Camb. (Mass.) (Loeb). 3 vols., 1935–8.
Wellman, M., *A. Cornelius Celsus, eine Quellenuntersuchung*. Berlin, 1913.

an educated Roman of high position in the latter half of the second century A.D. Again, the *Medicina* of Gargilius, a compilation chiefly from the *Natural History* of Pliny, is not only valuable to the textual critic of that work, but also illustrative of the medical needs of a traveller at the period when Gargilius lived.

There are three classical works on medical subjects which afford some illustration of these remarks—*Regimen* in the Hippocratic *Corpus*, the treatise of Celsus, and Pliny's *Natural History*. The text of all three has been critically examined many times; the sources have attracted the attention of generations of scholars, the first being peculiarly valuable for the reconstruction of Heraclitean philosophy.[1] Little, however, has been done to estimate the light they throw on contemporary culture and ideals. The subject is a vast one, and a short essay can but touch the fringe of it. The chief question to be considered here is this: had the ancients a science of health as distinct from a science of healing? If so, why did it decline?

Regimen

Professor Farrington[2] has discussed *Regimen* with the purpose recommended in this essay as likely to lead to useful results. He argues that the teaching of *Regimen* explains and justifies the bitter attack of Plato[3] on Herodicus and his followers. 'Under these circumstances alone is it conceivable how an eminent scientist like the author of *Regimen* could consider the problem of health on the assumption that the patient had nothing to do but to eat, drink and amuse himself. [He does not assume this. See below.] Only because the narrow basis of this type of medical science has not been clear to medical historians has it been possible to describe the author of *Regimen* as the Father of Preventive Medicine. He in no way deserves such a title. Much more fittingly could he be described, in the spirit of the Platonic attack, as the Father of Valetudinarianism'.[4]

It is true that Plato does attack Herodicus, an invalid who sought to prolong his own and other unhealthy lives by elaborate regimen. But Plato thought that chronic invalids, if their incapacity interfered with the performance of their duties, had much better be left to die, just as he would have exposed all unhealthy or deformed babies. Healthy children in the *Republic* go through a strict if simple course of training and regimen to keep them in health all their lives.

The author of *Regimen*, however, although like Plato and all true Greeks he worshipped physical beauty, and health as the only means of securing it, was more humane than Plato in his views. He took men as he found them, and aimed at keeping them at their maximum efficiency by diet, exercise and nipping all disease in the bud.[5] His thesis in brief is this: 'Health results from a harmony between food and exercise. All must eat and take exercise. Let us

---

[1] Bywater, Diels and A. L. Peck have all used *Regimen* for this purpose.

[2] *The Hand in Healing*, lecture to the Royal Institution, 4 Dec. 1941.

[3] *Republic*, 406 A–408 B.

[4] *op. cit.* (2), p. 17.

[5] He uses such phrases as οὐ χρὴ προέσθαι, ἀλλὰ χρὴ προμηθεῖσθαι, προκαταλαμβάνειν τὴν ὑγείην.

do so in accordance with the laws of health, to which I have discovered the key. To obey them requires no other apparatus than that used every day in our normal lives. Let us use it scientifically'. He does not ask for special equipment, foods, or even drugs, only the usual purges and emetics. In many ways he leans towards asceticism rather than towards self-indulgence. He often recommends, for instance, the habit of taking only one full meal every day. This habit (μονοσιτία) was not an invention or fad of the author. It is mentioned as a common custom, adopted continuously by many because it suited their constitutions, in *Ancient Medicine* and *Regimen in Acute Diseases*, and hundreds of years later in Celsus.

In chapter lxix the author states that he has been writing for the great mass of mankind, who of necessity live a haphazard life (εἰκῆ), with no chance of concentrating on the care of their health; he then goes on to give rules for those who are fortunate enough to be able to do this.

The work begins with a criticism of previous writers (πολλοὶ ἤδη συνέγραψαν), so that the culture of health was popular, and had been so for some time. Besides text-books the author found ready to his hand much elaborate equipment—gymnasia, palaestrae, racing tracks, baths, vapour baths, punch-balls and material for ball games, to say nothing of instructors, attendants and masseurs. There is not the slightest hint that any of these would be costly or difficult to find; if the manifold detail of *Regimen* and its long list, with their qualities, of foods and drinks are proof of valetudinarianism, then the author of *Regimen* was assuredly not the Father of it. The Greeks really seem to have succeeded in devoting a great part of their lives to physical culture without showing any signs of becoming valetudinarians or faddists.[6] They kept healthy and free from morbid preoccupations their ideal, manifest in literature as early as Pindar and implied in the continued popularity of their athletic 'gatherings', of a sound mind in a beautiful body. That there were some unwholesome exceptions was inevitable; the wonder is that literature presents us with so few. Plato's criticisms in the *Republic* may have had some justification, but they are obviously exaggerated, and biassed by his ruthless conception of the function of medicine. Professional athleticism too began in the fifth century B.C., damaging the reputation of the great games and bringing in methods of diet and training which, frowned on by the best medical authorities,[7] were fortunately regarded as a joke by popular opinion. In the first century A.D. appears, as we shall see, considerable evidence of wide-spread valetudinarianism, due to the increase of malaria, but in the great age of Greece there is manifest a spontaneous, natural and almost unconscious desire for physical perfection that fully accounts for the assumption made by the author of *Regimen*[8] that equipment, text-books on dietetics, and personnel were readily accessible to all. Nothing new was required for putting into practice his 'discovery' (εὕρημα) of προδιάγνωσις.

---

[6] The Pythagoreans were very interested in diet as an aid to 'positive' health. See L. Edelstein, *Hippocratic Oath*, p. 50. In the *Corpus*, besides *Regimen* there are *Ancient Medicine*, *Regimen in Acute Diseases*, and *Regimen in Health*. Interest in diet and cooking was wide-spread. See Mahaffy, *Social Life in Greece*, pp. 299 ff.

[7] *Aphorisms* I, iii: ἐν τοῖσι γυμναστικοῖσιν αἱ ἐπ' ἄκρον εὐεξίαι σφαλεραί.

[8] He thinks far more about health than he does about disease. Catarrhs are mentioned (lxx) and pneumonia (lxx), but his chief anxiety is lest strain should lead to fever (lxvi, lxx, lxxi, lxxii, lxxxiii). Twice these fevers are called φρικώδεες, i.e. probably ague (lxx, lxxxiii).

Much of the information given in *Regimen* is of interest only to antiquarians, but some of it, such as the accounts of 'physical jerks', massage and vapour baths, throw light on Greek customs and habits. Of special importance is μονοσιτία, that striking indication of abstemiousness so strangely neglected by writers on Greek life and thought.

The fourth book of *Regimen*, sometimes styled *Dreams*, is the earliest extant attempt to account for unusual appearances in sleep as symptoms of physical disorders. The divine origin of certain dreams is apparently admitted,[9] but is dismissed in a few words : for most dreams 'prayer indeed is good, but while calling on the gods a man should also himself co-operate with them'. The discussion shows no definitely Freudian characteristics, anticipating however the modern view that dreams are sometimes a psychic satisfaction of desires thwarted or inhibited in the waking life.[10] A great number of the dreams mentioned are concerned with the sun, moon, stars and celestial phenomena. Such dreams were apparently common then, though perhaps rare to-day. The reason for the difference is curious. Ordinary men rarely look for long at the sky now-a-days; but a people without clocks, calendars or compasses would be compelled to contemplate the heavens continually. An important interest of their waking life would be certain to affect the content of their dreams.

Stress should be laid on the author's preoccupation with health rather than with diseases, and on his preference for diet and exercise rather than drugs. It is implied throughout the work that, if a normal person pays attention to regimen, disease will be avoided and medicines will rarely be required. There is in fact some similarity between the author's plan for keeping well and the treatment adopted in modern hydropathic establishments.

Celsus

There is a thorny *Celsusproblem*. Who were his authorities? Was he a mere translator? Wellmann[11] thinks that he translated a Greek treatise written by his friend Cassius; Marx[12] holds that the Greek original was the work of Titus Aufidius Siculus, a pupil of Asclepiades. Was he a mere 'general editor' of an encyclopaedia, with assistant editors looking after its different sections? Was Celsus a practising physician or a layman?

These questions are interesting but well-nigh insoluble. Even scholarly writers like Sir Clifford Allbutt[13] and Mr. W. G. Spencer[14] came to contrary conclusions about the status of Celsus, although the balance of evidence is perhaps in favour of his being a layman. Any inquiry, therefore, into the work of Celsus should as far as possible be based, not on uncertainties and speculation, but on a sound foundation of indisputable facts. This foundation can be found in the nature of the contents of the *De medicina*, the first systematic treatise on medicine to come down to us. It was one section of an encyclopaedia,

[9] Chap. lxxxvii.   [10] Chap. xciii.

[11] Max Wellmann, *A. Cornelius Celsus, eine Quellenuntersuchung*, p. 4: 'Er ist gar nicht Verfasser des Werkes, sondern nur Übersetzer.'

[12] See the Prolegomena to F. Marx, *A. Cornelii Celsi quae supersunt.*

[13] *Greek Medicine in Rome*, p. 204.   See also p. 205: 'A not impossible alternative is that Celsus translated or incorporated a Greek treatise, now lost; and invested it with his own qualities of sound judgement and beautiful Latin.'

[14] See Loeb edition, vol. i, pp. xi and xii.

the other sections being on agriculture, warfare, rhetoric, philosophy and law. If the lost books were as good as the one still extant, their loss is deeply to be deplored, for the *De medicina* is a model of orderly arrangement, accurate information, sober judgment and beautiful Latin.   Published about the time of Tiberius, this encyclopaedia met a demand, which had been growing ever since the establishment of the first universities and of the great public libraries, for accurate summaries of scientific knowledge in all its chief departments.   Celsus therefore had an educated public for whom to write, and whose needs he was admirably fitted to supply.   We cannot be certain whether he was an original author, or a compiler, or a translator, but in any case he knew his subject thoroughly, and could expound all its branches in a masterly manner.   It is also certain that he confined his attention to practical information, such as was daily needed by his readers, who may have been medical students, or the heads of big establishments with the 'large hospitals' he speaks of in his 'Introduction'.[15] In fact it would be wrong to limit his public to one class only.   There was in Rome, as elsewhere, no sharp line between professional and amateur; but the paid practitioners—usually Greeks or freedmen—held a far lower position in Roman society than had been held in Greece by the medical 'graduates' (if they may be called such) from the schools of Cos, Cnidos and Alexandria. Much medical supervision, though not all actual carrying out of treatment, must have been undertaken by amateurs for the benefit of their families and dependents.   With no hospitals except 'sick-bays' for slaves, no nursing homes, no trained nurses, with only a few specialists (like Asclepiades) and the lower-grade *medici*, often of dubious ability, the care of the sick must have been a serious question, not only in Rome, but everywhere in Italy and throughout the Empire, especially at the malarial season of the year.   The difficulty of providing skilled attention for the sick helps us to understand why so much care was taken to keep fit and avoid illness, and should be remembered by all who lightly accuse the ancients, whether Greeks or Romans, of valetudinarianism.

Celsus, then, like all writers of all ages, cannot be appreciated when his work is divorced from the context of contemporary life.   The discovery of his sources is important; equally so is it to treat the *De medicina* as a living document as well as a preservative of fossils.   What then are its actual contents? After a short but able survey of medical theories in an historical introduction, Celsus goes on to discuss health, how to keep well and to maintain the maximum of physical efficiency.   Elaborate instructions are given, strikingly similar to those in *Regimen* and implying similar facilities for putting them into practice, but foods and drinks are, naturally enough, not discussed in such great detail. The custom of μονοσιτία[16] is still kept up, τρῖψις appears as *frictio*,[17] voice exercises (φωνῆς πόνοι) as *clara lectio*, and some stress is laid on rocking (*gestatio*)[18] for those without the strength required for ordinary exercises. If the author of *Regimen* encouraged valetudinarianism, so equally did Celsus.

But in spite of these similarities, the reader is conscious of a marked change when he passes from the earlier work to the later.   There is in Celsus an increased anxiety to avoid 'exciting' causes of illness, and certain kinds of illness are

---

[15] See *Procemium*, 65: *ampla valetudinaria*.
[16] *Procemium*, 72; i. 3. 16, 30.
[17] ii, 14.   [18] ii, 15.

much more prominent than others. These diseases are those of the eyes,[19] skin[20] and chest, together with the various forms of malaria.[21] The notice taken of splenic affections, which usually are *sequelae* of malaria, is very significant.

These diseases afflicted the ancient world from the time of Hippocrates, as the *Corpus* proves; the zymotic diseases so common to-day are, with the possible exception of typhoid, nowhere referred to, much less described.[22] Consumption, and affections of the eyes and skin, were certain to be common in countries where dust was all-prevalent but ignored, and hygienic rules for keeping it uncontaminated were unthought of. They appear to have become more common as time went on, if we may judge from the greater attention paid to them in medical writings, but confirmatory evidence is lacking. Such evidence, however, exists for an increase of malaria, although it comes from a Greek source, and from a writer who lived in a very unhealthy region.

The little work in Plutarch's *Moralia* called *De tuenda sanitate* strongly confirms the view that it was malaria that in the course of time changed a devotion to physical culture into an over-anxious fear of falling ill. The writer says that those desirous of being students or politicians, must, if they would be well, follow certain rules.

It is necessary to keep the hands warm, as chill in the extremities invites fever (123 A). Even though fevers are caused by exertion, the liability is increased by over-indulgence (127 B–D). The forewarnings given by fevers must not be neglected (127 D–128 E). Without being over-strict in diet, everybody should moderate appetite before those pains come on which are the forerunners of fever. It is wise to be on the look-out for bad dreams, crossness of temper and melancholy (128 E–129 C). When visiting a sick friend one should inquire whether it was surfeit, heat, lack of sleep, or faulty diet that caused his fever (129 D–130 C). Food should be light; emetics and purges are to be avoided (131 D–134 A). While it is absurd to neglect the duties of life in order to keep healthy, a man should learn all he can about his own constitution, taking care not to tax it at the change of seasons (135 A–137 B). Students should not put a severe strain on their bodies by too much application to study, or they will be forced to lay aside their books owing to fever (137 C–E). The exciting causes of fever are thus said to be fatigue, extremes of temperature, over-indulgence, and an insufficiency of rest or sleep—just the things that residents in malarious countries are warned to avoid. The logical conclusion is that malaria was a controlling factor in the daily lives of those for whom the author wrote. The people of Plutarch's time may possibly have degenerated into valetudinarianism, but it was the valetudinarianism of a race that had set a great value on efficiency, physical and mental, and found this efficiency threatened by an insidious endemic disease.

A great change from Hippocratic therapeutics is manifest in *De medicina*. The Coan physician distrusted the use of medicines, placing his trust in

---

[19] *De medicina* vi. 6.   [20] vi. 1–5.   [21] ii. 1 and iii. 3–20.

[22] For this very difficult question see W. H. S. Jones, *Malaria and Greek History*, pp. 127–9 and *Hippocrates* (Loeb), vol. i, pp. lv, lix. In *Epidemics*, I, 1, there is a description, beautifully clear, of mumps, an epidemic of which is said to have occurred in Thasos. The symptoms are accurately given, but no name is assigned to the disease, nor are there any later allusions, unless it is included under the vague 'parotid swellings' (παρώτιδες) of later writers.

modification of regimen, which he adapted to the constitution of the individual patient, so that the *vis naturae medicatrix* might be impeded as little as possible in its beneficent work; Celsus bases his treatment largely on medicines and drugs. But Celsus did not introduce the change; he only followed a tendency that had been growing for a very long time. He gives numerous prescriptions throughout the treatise, often prefixing the name of the discoverer, but the largest number are to be found in v. 1–25. The use of various drugs, indeed, preceded scientific medicine; Aeschylus attributed medicines and salves to the φιλανθρωπία of Prometheus,[23] calling them his greatest gift to man, but at the same time significantly associating them with seer-craft and the interpretation of dreams. The remarkable thing, however, is that in the interval between Hippocrates and Celsus, popular medicine, with its errors and superstitions, had been adopted by physicians and surgeons of the highest rank, who, though they purged away many of its grossest blunders, left several minor ones behind.[24] Celsus mentions well over two hundred ingredients, and they include, besides vegetable substances, chemicals such as copper, lead, iron, mercury, soda and sulphur.[25] It was doubtless a sign of progress for medicine to recognize the value of simples and drugs, especially for external use, but the recognition involved at least one danger. The preparation and sale of *medicamenta* were encouraged, especially among the poorer and more ignorant classes, who found it easier to prescribe for themselves than to procure the best medical advice. Modern parallels readily suggest themselves. Perhaps Celsus himself had this danger in his mind when he wrote, *optimum medicamentum quies est.*[26]

Pliny

A generation after Celsus Pliny the Elder published his *Natural History*, dedicating it to Titus, son of the reigning Emperor Vespasian. In the dedicatory preface Pliny invites serious criticism for his encyclopaedia, of which is extant the whole, and not merely a section, as is the *De medicina*, of a much longer work. A glance at a few pages, however, shows that it would appeal to a more *dilettante* circle of readers than that catered for by Celsus, who wrote for specialists, while Pliny put together a mass of general information. In Pliny's eyes all information seems to have been of equal value; Sir Clifford Allbutt rather unkindly compares his work to the scrap heap collected by a jackdaw. He was, however, an educated, intelligent man, who wrote for readers at much the same cultural level. His book met the need that is met to-day by popular encyclopaedias, general-science periodicals, and even such papers as *Titbits*, but while satisfying curiosity it also gave useful knowledge of the kind to be found in *Mrs. Beeton's Cookery Book*. Every section of it provides a multitude of details which, if carefully put together, enable the historian to reconstruct many features of the social and family life of the first century A.D. Only the medical section can be discussed here, very briefly and from one aspect.

In the first book Pliny gives a list of the authorities he used, so that the

---

[23] *Prometheus Vinctus*, ll. 478–99.
[24] Galen even used amulets. E. T. Withington in Jones, *Malaria and Greek History*, p. 153.
[25] W. G. Spenser, *Celsus* (Loeb), vol. ii, pp. xv–lx.   [26] v. 26, 28 c.

Quellenkritik[27] is somewhat narrower than usual in scope. Strangely enough he makes no mention of Dioscorides, who according to Wellmann[28] was his contemporary. Yet the parallel passages are very numerous indeed, with frequent mistakes in Pliny's version. That Dioscorides used Pliny as an authority is thus most unlikely; possibly they both drew from the same source, now lost.

The complaints most often mentioned by Pliny include all those that have been shown to be prevalent in the ancient world, together with one or two others presenting some features of interest.

Eye diseases. Jan's *Index*, under *oculi* has: 'Vid. *adustiones, aegilopia, albugines, angulus, argema, caligines, cicatrices, claritas, collyria, epinyctides, epiphorae, excrescentia, fluctiones, frigus, glaucomata, gremiae, hypochyses, impetus, inflammatio, lacrimatio, lacunae, lippitudo, lusciosi, nubeculae, nyctalopes, palpebrae, palpitatio, pili, plumbum, procidentes, prurigines, psilotrum, pterygia, pupilla, pusulae, scabritia, scintillationes, squamae, subfusiones, suggillatio, tumor.'*

Most of these refer to definite ailments, and we are reminded, among other things, that the Romans had no spectacles or eye-glasses.

Skin diseases. (1) Alopecia, a kind of mange, mentioned 30 times; (2) impetigo, mentioned 7 times; (3) lepra, including many skin diseases, 46 times; (4) lichen, 46 times; (5) phthiriasis, caused by lice, of which Sulla died, 18 times; (6) porrigo, 14 times; (7) psora, 24 times.

There are also many references to rashes and to such diseases as erysipelas, which is referred to 54 times.

Malaria. (1) Quotidians, 2; (2) tertians, 22 ; (3) quartans, 39; (4) lethargus, comatose pernicious malaria, 22; (5) phrenitis, pernicious malaria marked by severe delirium, 12.

There are several references to the shivering and hot fits that are so typical of ague. As for splenic complaints, there are about 80 allusions, most of which occur in books XX, XXI and XXII. Malaria tends to cause a swollen spleen, but in a non-malarious country nobody has to worry very much about the spleen and its affections. Its connection with the psychological effects of malaria is preserved in the words 'splenetic' and 'spleenful'.

Cures for the bites and stings of noxious animals are mentioned by Celsus, but Pliny gives nearly 180 prescriptions for keeping snakes away or for neutralizing their poison, and over 100 cures for scorpion stings. Poisonous spiders are referred to in at least 30 passages. Perhaps many harmless creatures were thought to be poisonous. If so, a natural fear might easily grow into over-nervousness.

Pliny, however, does not concern himself with diseases. He is far more interested in the remedies adopted to cure them. The number of such that he describes or mentions is amazingly large.[29] From the summaries given

---

[27] F. Münzer published *Beiträge* on this in 1897.

[28] See Pauly *s. v.* Dioskurides, p. 1131a: 'Demnach lebte er unter Nero, also etwa gleichzeitig mit dem älteren Plinius.'

[29] Pliny apparently wished everybody to doctor himself and to do without physicians (xxii. 14, 15). He complains that his contemporaries laughed at his study of herbs and drugs, thinking it a waste of time, and rejoins by attacking the carelessness and luxury of the day. *Nunquam fuit vitae cupido maior nec minor cura.*

in the first book may be taken a few informative details. Of *medicinae*, with *historiae* and *observationes*, there are: In xx, 1606; in xxi, 730; in xxii, 406; in xxiii, 1418; in xxiv, 1116; in xxv, 1292; in xxvi, 1019; in xxvii, 602; in xxviii, 1682; in xxix, 621; in xxx, 854; in xxxi, 924; in xxxii, 990; in xxxiii, 288; while in xxxiv there are 257 *medicinae*.

There is scarcely a vegetable or herb known to the botanists of the time that Pliny does not use for draught, ointment or plaster, and besides vegetable drugs he gives prescriptions containing copper, iron, lead and various metallic compounds. It should be remembered that these *medicinae* are taken from what may be called the general pharmacopœia of the first century A.D. Pliny makes no claim to be himself a druggist.

As to their character, some, but only a few, might be useful; by far the greater number would be quite useless or even positively harmful. It is therefore remarkable that many of them ever came to be recognized as remedies, having nothing whatever, not even a pleasant taste or smell, to recommend them. In modern times a useless prescription has often enjoyed a long vogue through clever advertising. These ancient medicines, however, were not advertised,[30] and their composition was no secret. Anybody could prepare them for himself or buy them from a herbalist. So far as we know, nobody tried to make a fortune out of the superstitious credulity of the many who were, or thought that they were, suffering from some ailment. The age of the profiteer was not yet.[31] How valueless are most of the prescriptions given by Pliny can be seen by a glance at one of the more modern commentaries. Again and again the commentator remarks that Pliny is mistaken, that certain information is incorrect, or that such and such treatment would be positively injurious. It would be easy but tiresome to quote a score of the most absurd statements. Two must suffice. If a radish be placed upon a scorpion it will kill him.[32] The root of hipposelinon (horse parsley) boiled in wine is a cure for the bite of a mad dog.[33] Even charms, amulets and superstitious remedies find a place. 'The root of the wild mallow, pulled up before sunrise, and wrapped in wool of the colour known as native, taken from a sheep which has just dropped a ewe lamb, is employed as a bandage for scrofulous swellings, even after they have suppurated. Some persons are of opinion that for this purpose the root should be dug up with an implement of gold, and that care should be taken not to let it touch the ground.'[34] It may be remarked in passing that much of the efficacy of such remedies as were not quite useless was due to two of their basic constituents, wine and honey The universal use of the latter, which had in antiquity to do duty for all sweetening substances, must have had a beneficial effect upon the public health.

---

[30] That is, in the ordinary modern sense of advertisement. In another sense Pliny and Dioscorides 'advertised' these remedies by collecting them and giving them wider publicity.

[31] Possibly this statement should be qualified, as there were certainly quacks in Pliny's day, and a quack is very like a profiteer. In the preface to pseudo-Pliny and Gargilius, p. 7 of V. Rose's edition, the compiler remarks that in his time travellers who fell sick suffered because 'some charge top prices for the most worthless medicines, and others through greed undertake to treat ailments they do not understand'. A most informative remark, but unfortunately we cannot date the document with any certainty.

[32] xx. xiii.   [33] xx. xlvi.   [34] xx. xiv.

Summary and Conclusion

Certain books in the Hippocratic *Corpus*, in particular the four books of *Regimen*, by implying a fully developed system and technique of physical training, throw light upon the Greek cult of health and love of a beautiful body. The cure of disease was looked upon as a branch of dietetics, and the maintenance of maximum efficiency another branch. Drugs were very sparingly used, especially by the most enlightened practitioners. The chief diseases with which therapeutics concerned itself were chest diseases and remittent malaria.[35] Other diseases are discussed in the *Corpus*, but these, together with pulmonary consumption (φθίσις), are the physician's chief concern. All this was sensible, hygienic, and as scientific as the science of the day allowed.[36]

Unfortunately there is an interval of 400 years before the appearance of the next extant treatise on medicine, and the home of its public is Italy, not Greece. Probably, however, close intercommunication between the various parts of the Roman Empire resulted in a certain amount of uniformity everywhere in the medical 'field'. In Celsus the preservation of health is treated almost as fully as in *Regimen*, and the means employed are practically the same. But there is now far more attention paid to drugs; in fact the department of pharmacology is on its way to full development. Although chest diseases and malaria occupy a prominent position, eye and skin diseases run them very close, and treatment of minor ailments, with prescriptions for them, take up a great part of the treatise. There is a tendency in therapeutics to subordinate the slow-healing *vis naturae medicatrix*, upon which Hippocratic therapeutics relied, to the use of quick cures.

In Pliny pharmacology has swamped everything else. He catered for a public that was ready to try anything, however silly, a simple or even magic, for complaints of the eyes or of the skin, for wounds inflicted by poisonous creatures, for scrofula, dropsy and affections of the spleen. Acute diseases like phrenitis and pneumonia are sometimes mentioned, but not so often; Pliny possibly thought that they were better left to the skilled practitioner. He does not reject, or at least mentions without condemnation, charms and amulets, which are actually recommended by Dioscorides and Galen.

There were always among the common people much credulity and superstition about the utility of drugs and of magic in the treatment of disease. Especially important evidence is afforded by the famous forty-two inscriptions at Epidaurus, and those on many hundreds of Greek votive offerings. But by Pliny's time the taint had infected all the lower, and had begun to infect the higher strata of the medical profession. The author of *Regimen*, on much the same cultural level as Pliny and Galen, never sinks to the level of many Plinian remedies. This degeneration from rational dietetics to the quick-cure methods of popular pharmacology raises a perplexing problem. Dr. E. T. Withington[37] has a passage which presents this difference

---

[35] In *Regimen in Acute Diseases*, v, it is said that most deaths are caused by πλευρῖτις, περιπνευμονίη, φρενῖτις and καῦσος. The MS.M, adds λήθαργος.

[36] It would be hard to find a better description of the object of Greek dietetics than a phrase from *Regimen*, lxvii: προκαταλαμβάνειν ὑγείην, ὥστε τὰς νούσους μὴ προσπελάζειν.

[37] In Jones, *Malaria and Greek History*, pp. 145, 146, 154.

between the two ages very graphically. 'Cinquefoil, which Hippocrates administered in tertians, is still a popular remedy for ague throughout Europe. But in its next extant recommendation we find a significant change. Cinquefoil, according to Dioscorides, is a valuable remedy for tertians and quartans, but it is important to take three leaves in the former, and four in the latter disease, while the addition of an amulet consisting of three crushed spiders in a bag adds greatly to the efficacy of the remedy.' 'In short, therapeutics tend to revert to the ancient mixture of religion, magic and empiricism.'

If Plutarch's little treatise *De tuenda sanitate* be rightly interpreted as a series of instructions how to keep away the ever-present danger of malaria, and if this danger greatly increased, as it appears to have done,[38] in the interval between Hippocrates and Plutarch, then circumstances encouraged an apprehensive attitude to the risks of life that might easily lead to :

(*a*) valetudinarianism in place of an elaborate cult of health, efficiency and physical beauty;

(*b*) a marked tendency to trust in drugs, and even in magic charms, instead of the slower but surer processes of regimen and dietetics.

Whether these conclusions are correct or not, our documents ought to be studied in relation to contemporary life, and not only in order to throw light upon their sources and authorities.

[38] See Jones *Malaria and Greek History* and *Dea Febris*.

THE CONNATE *PNEUMA*

AN ESSENTIAL FACTOR IN ARISTOTLE'S SOLUTIONS TO THE PROBLEMS OF REPRODUCTION AND SENSATION

by

ARTHUR L. PECK

IN this essay I wish to deal with the solutions offered by Aristotle to a number of fundamental problems which are of primary interest at the present day, including those of animal reproduction, sensation, and animal movement, as I think that, although the details of these solutions are not those arrived at by contemporary science, there may be some who will welcome a reasonably brief account of Aristotle's theories as affording a convenient means of appraising the general framework of the solutions he gives and his method of approach. For this reason I have refrained from any attempt to modernize Aristotle's terminology, and have endeavoured to present these theories as exactly as can be done in another language.

I have chosen as the subject of the essay those problems, in Aristotle's solution of which an essential factor is the concept of what he calls 'connate *pneuma*'. I do not intend to deal with the earlier or later history of this concept, but only with Aristotle's use of it, as my purpose is to show how Aristotle dealt with these problems. The term *pneuma* I have deliberately left untranslated, because there is no satisfactory term to represent it in English. Of the two obvious possibilities, 'breath' would suggest air breathed in by an animal from without, and 'spirit' has come to acquire an almost exclusively non-corporeal connotation. The meaning of *pneuma* will, I hope, become clearer in the course of the essay. All I need emphasize here is that *pneuma* is certainly corporeal; it is, as we should say, a kind of matter; and it is connate, congenital, present in an animal from the moment of conception and so long as the animal remains alive. It is, in fact, the primary vehicle of life and of the processes peculiar to living organisms, and occupies a key position in Aristotle's interpretation of these processes.

On the whole, it is true to say that in modern times the interest in Aristotle of philosophers has been directed chiefly to his non-biological works, and that of scientists to those parts of his biological works in which he has either recorded some notable observation or has indicated some general line of classification or investigation which has proved of permanent interest or value. For example, that he observed the viviparous dogfish (*Mustelus laevis*) is generally known, largely because after an interval of 2,000 years such observations were again recorded by Nicolaus Steno in the seventeenth century, and more fully by Johannes Müller in his classic monograph of 1842.[1] So too is Aristotle's championship of epigenesis as against preformationism, a point on which he was vindicated in the time of C. F. Wolff and K. E. von Baer, at the end of the eighteenth and the beginning of the nineteenth centuries.

---

[1] Johannes Müller, *Ueber den glatten Hai des Aristoteles.* Berlin, 1842. The paper was read in April, 1839 and continued in August, 1840. See *Bericht über die zur Bekanntmachung geeigneten Verhandlungen der Königl. Preuss. Akademie der Wissenschaften zu Berlin*, 1839, 11 April, 49–52; 1840, 6 August, 171–5.

Even his erroneous theory that in reproduction the male contributes the 'form' and the female the 'matter' (the menstrual blood) is not unfamiliar,[2] partly owing to the fact that it was left for Harvey[3] to demonstrate its falsity by his famous experiments on does in the forests of King Charles I. Similarly, to philosophers his doctrines of the four Causes and of moral goodness as a 'mean' are commonplaces. But it is less generally recognized that Aristotle was not content to record observations, or to propound theories in general terms, without at the same time accepting the obligation to offer a detailed account of the mechanism by which he thought the observed phenomena came about. For instance, he did not consider it sufficient to say that an individual is the result of a particular 'form' having become embodied in a particular quantity of 'matter'; he accepted the obligation to explain precisely how he thought this embodiment was effected. In biology, of course, this problem is of crucial importance, and it is with a factor which is an essential part of his answer to this and to other fundamental problems that I wish to deal in this essay. First, then, how is the 'form' of the parent transmitted to its offspring; how is the 'form' reproduced in another individual?

As is well known, Aristotle's philosophy is permeated by his conception of the 'actual' and the 'potential' and by his doctrine of the four Causes.[4] As a translation of Aristotle's own term, 'cause' is open to certain objections, for in modern usage 'cause' has come to be applied almost exclusively to one only out of the four Aristotelian types of cause, viz. the 'efficient' cause, while at the same time the notion of 'cause' in this sense has been extended to include some types of causation which Aristotle would not have regarded as normal causes in his own sense at all, but would have described in an entirely different way. The reason for this discrepancy is that for Aristotle all processes normally proceed to an 'end' or goal (telos) which controls their course; and only exceptionally do results occur which lack this control, in which case they may be ascribed either to 'chance' or to 'necessity'; and if such results coincide with those which are produced by the normal methods of operation, then the processes which produce them can be said to simulate those set up by the 'efficient' causes found either in art or in the world of nature. Indeed, for Aristotle, 'necessity' is regarded as something other than, and often opposed to, the teleological operations of art and nature, and is not a term descriptive of those operations. Thus, Aristotle can say that, if a craftsman wishes to make an axe, he must of necessity use this or that material; so must nature, if her aim is to produce this or that living creature; but these 'necessary' materials may also have certain properties which are irrelevant to the purpose in hand, and may entail certain results or by-products which are similarly irrelevant. Such results are described as occurring 'of necessity'; they are beside the purpose. We must not, therefore, expect to find in Aristotle the conception of a 'necessary' chain of cause and effect as a normal occurrence, but rather the view that art and nature can sometimes be obstructed by 'necessity'. We shall thus not be surprised to find that for

[2] But see below, pp. 114–5.

[3] William Harvey, *Exercitationes de generatione animalium*. London, 1651.

[4] For a fuller account of these and of other Aristotelian doctrines, I may be allowed to refer the reader to the introductions and appendices to my editions of the *Parts of Animals* and *Generation of Animals* (Loeb Classical Library).

Aristotle the 'efficient' cause is normally an individual living being, just as the 'end' to which a process advances, the 'final cause', is normally an individual living being, or an individual object or action. These two 'causes', however, are not sufficient to account completely for the individual which is produced, and in addition to them Aristotle posits a 'formal' cause, or 'form', which expresses the plan or essential character of the thing; and a 'material' cause, the 'matter' in which the 'form' is realized by means of the process originated by the 'efficient' cause or agent. We have then four 'causes', which between them are responsible for the existence of an individual or for the performance of an action:

(1) the 'final' cause, the end or object towards which a process advances;
(2) the 'efficient' cause, the agent responsible for having set the process going;
(3) the 'formal' cause, which is responsible for the character of the course which the process follows; and
(4) the 'material' cause, that out of which the thing is made, or the medium in which the action is performed.

We can therefore say that certain 'matter' is potentially x: it is capable of receiving from an agent the 'form' of x and of becoming an actual x itself. Thus, a piece of wood (a 'material' cause) is potentially a chair: it is capable of receiving from a carpenter (an 'efficient' cause) the 'form' or essential plan of chair (a 'formal' cause), and so becoming a chair itself, thus realizing the 'final' cause. But how precisely is all this brought about? Aristotle's answer is that the 'form' of chair is in the mind of the carpenter; the carpenter moves his hands and instruments with the 'movements' appropriate to that 'form'; and the instruments, being charged with these 'movements', 'move' the material so as to produce a chair. No material part passes from the agent to the material on which he is working: he transmits the 'form' to the material by means of the 'movements' which he sets up in his instruments.

This example of the craftsman shows the pattern of the process in its simplest terms. We have:

(1) the 'end' or final purpose, which is the chair that is to be produced;
(2) the agent, who is the originator of the 'movements' which lead to the realization of that purpose;
(3) his instruments, which he charges with those 'movements'; and
(4) the material upon which those 'movements' operate until they have realized the 'form' in it.

Aristotle follows the same general pattern in his explanations (a) of the way in which the limbs of an animal are moved and (b) of the reproduction of animals. An example of (a) would be the earlier stages of the making of a chair just described, viz. the stages up to and including the moving of the craftsman's hands. I will defer consideration of this for the present and go on at once to consider (b), the reproduction of animals. The main difference to be noted in this process, as compared with the process of making a chair, is that here the 'form' to be realized is not one which is of a different order from the agent (as chair is of a different order from man), but one which is itself the agent's own essential 'form'. In reproduction, it is, as will be shown in more detail presently, 'soul' which has to be transmitted, and according to Aristotle 'soul' is the 'form' of the living body. The agent in this process of transmission is the soul of the male parent; the 'material' is the menstrual blood of the female; and in order to transmit the proper 'movements' to that material the agent employs an instrument, viz. the 'connate *pneuma*' which is contained in the semen. This *pneuma* is charged with the 'movements' proper to the species of animal concerned, and it sets up these same 'movements' in the material. The pattern then is:

(1) the 'end' or final purpose, viz. the new individual to be produced;
(2) the agent, the 'soul' of the male parent;
(3) the instrument employed by the agent, viz. the connate *pneuma*; and
(4) the material in which the 'form' is to be realized, viz. the menstrual blood.

Before examining the character of the connate *pneuma* it is necessary to say a little more about what Aristotle meant by 'soul'. Like all other 'forms', soul is something non-material, non-corporeal. (The term 'soul', which in some ways is unsatisfactory as a translation of the Greek term used by Aristotle, is from this point of view a useful one, since its associations in our language are very definitely non-corporeal. It has also the advantage of being less misleading than some other possible translations.) So far I have spoken of soul both (*a*) as the 'form' to be transmitted in reproduction and (*b*) as the agent concerned in the process of transmission; but in the case of animals at any rate this is not a sufficiently exact statement of the position. As is well known, Aristotle recognizes several 'parts' or levels of soul. The lowest of these is common to all living things, plants and animals alike, and it is the principle which enables them to grow and to maintain themselves, and also to reproduce themselves. This he calls 'nutritive and generative' soul. Beyond this faculty, animals have also the faculty of sensation, which, Aristotle claims, is the distinguishing mark of an animal: this is 'sentient ' soul, and together with it are usually found 'appetitive' soul and 'locomotive' soul. Beyond this again, in man alone, is found 'rational' soul, but this is something outside the scope of biology, since its activity is in no sense physical.

Now, as its name implies, it is nutritive and generative soul which is the agent, the 'efficient' cause, in reproduction; but this, at any rate in animals, is not coextensive with the 'form' which has to be transmitted, for an animal must possess not merely nutritive and generative soul, but also sentient soul; and therefore the 'form' to be transmitted must include sentient soul (and appetitive soul and locomotive soul too, if the animal is one which naturally has these faculties). In animal reproduction, then, the soul to be transmitted is of wider extent than the soul which is the agent of its transmission; and indeed it is the essential function of the male to supply the 'movements' of sentient soul to the female's material. And in this connexion we should note that, although in a way it is true, as mentioned already, to say—as Aristotle himself sometimes does—that in reproduction the male supplies the 'form' and the female the 'matter', such a statement can be misleading unless we are careful to remember that for Aristotle there is not one level but many levels of 'matter'. (Indeed, Aristotelian 'matter' need not necessarily be what we call 'matter' at all; but that does not concern us here.) 'Matter' can be successively 'informed' by various 'forms', beginning from the lowest stage of 'informed' matter, the four elements Fire, Air, Water, Earth; and at each stage the stuff which has been 'informed' can serve as 'matter' for a further stage of 'information'. Thus, the carpenter cannot make a chair out of Fire, Air, Water, and Earth; he needs wood, which is 'matter' that has been much further 'informed'; and similarly in the process of reproduction, the 'matter' concerned, viz. the menstrual blood, must have reached a very high degree of 'information'. This is shown, for instance, in the case of female birds, which are able to produce full-sized eggs without fertilization. These eggs, having reached so advanced a stage of growth, must obviously possess the 'movements' of nutritive soul; but in order to advance further and develop into a chick, an egg also requires the 'movements' of sentient soul, and these only the male can provide. The menstrual fluid, then, is 'matter' possessing 'form' to a high degree already; indeed, it lacks only the 'movements' proper to sentient soul. But why is the female unable to supply these 'movements' to the menstrual fluid?

To understand this difference between the male and the female, we must take into account Aristotle's theory of the function of the heart and the process of nutrition. For him, the central seat of life and of soul is the heart, and the essential characteristic of the heart is that it possesses vital heat. Other parts of the body too possess vital heat, derived from that of the heart. Briefly, the process of nutrition is this. After mastication, food passes into the stomach, where it undergoes some preliminary 'concoction' by the vital heat resident there, and then passes on to the heart, where it undergoes the main stage of its concoction whereby it is turned into blood, which is the 'ultimate nourishment' of the whole body. It is most probable that in Aristotle's view an important part of this process of concoction was the 'pneumatization' of the blood as evidenced by the pulsatory action, that is, the charging of the blood with 'connate *pneuma*' and with the special 'movements' requisite to enable the blood (*a*) to maintain the animal in being ('nutritive and seminal nourishment'), and (*b*) to supply the animal's growth ('growth-promoting nourishment'). Normally, more blood is produced than is required for these two basic purposes, and this surplus blood gives rise, when further concocted in the appropriate parts of the body, to 'residues' (*perittōmata*, superfluities) of various kinds, for example, hair, nails, horn, milk, and (most important of all) the 'generative residues'. Now the difference of sex is due to a difference of vital heat in the heart. The female is less 'hot' than the male, and from this fundamental inferiority all the physical sex-differences derive, including the inability of the female to 'concoct' its generative residue as completely as the male: the female cannot do more than concoct it to the stage of possessing the 'movements' of nutritive soul. But throughout, in the blood wherever in the body it may be, and of course in the concocted blood which forms the generative residues, it is the connate *pneuma* that is the vehicle of 'soul' and of those 'movements' by which soul performs its operations. Thus the function of the male generative residue is to supply to the residue of the female those 'movements' which can constitute a new individual; in other words, which can bring about the formation of a heart with its power to develop an embryo of exactly the same 'form' as its parents. And the instrument which soul uses to do this is, as has been said, the connate *pneuma*.

In view of the fact that the generative secretions are 'residues' of the blood which supplies the whole body, they are, as Aristotle is careful to point out, more correctly described as 'that which is distributed to the whole body' rather than 'that which is drawn from the whole body'—a point against the preformationists, who held that there was a tiny bit of every part of the body already present in the semen. Aristotle's view is that these parts are not present in the semen, but that they are fashioned by the 'movements' with which the *pneuma* contained in it is charged.

Something more must now be said about the nature of this connate *pneuma*. First, it is not the breath which the animal inhales; it is not acquired from outside, but is *connate*. Although it is a sort of air, and although it is 'hot', it is in a class apart from the four regular sublunary elements Fire, Air, Water, and Earth, and Aristotle describes it as being the 'counterpart' (analogue) of the fifth element, *aither*, the substance out of which the celestial spheres and the heavenly bodies are made. The *aither* too, says Aristotle, is generative, for it takes a man *and the Sun* (which is made of *aither*) to generate a man.[5] *Pneuma*, then the vehicle of soul, is a physical substance 'more divine' than the four so-called elements; just as the *aither*, of which it is the counterpart, is ungenerated, indestructible and 'divine'.

This is not the place to describe or to comment on the remarkable observations in embryology which Aristotle made and recorded. His work was not resumed until the time of Hieronymus Fabricius ab Aquapendente (1537–1619) and his successor, our own William Harvey (1578–1657), both of whom were careful students of Aristotle. Harvey, indeed, was the first to make any substantial advance in embryology since Aristotle himself. We must however notice some explanations of the recorded observations which Aristotle gives, which are relevant to our subject. First, with regard to the initial act of 'setting' the embryo. He writes as follows: 'The action of the semen of the male in "setting" the female's secretion in the uterus is similar to the action of rennet upon milk. Rennet is milk which contains vital heat, as semen does, and this integrates the homogeneous substance and makes it "set". As the nature of milk and the menstrual fluid is one and the same [they are both "residues" of the blood, as we have seen], the action of the semen upon the substance of the menstrual fluid is the same as that of rennet upon milk. Thus when the "setting" is effected, that is, when the bulky portion "sets", the fluid portion comes away; and as the earthy portion solidifies, membranes form all round its outer surface'.[6] This reference to 'vital heat' in the semen shows that Aristotle has in mind the connate *pneuma*; and in another passage he says: ' The parts of animals [that is, of embryos] are differentiated by means of *pneuma*; but this is not the *pneuma* [breath] of the mother nor that of the creature itself, as some of the writers on natural philosophy allege [he is probably thinking of the treatise *Of the Nature of the Child* in the Hippocratic *Corpus*, according to which the embryo both received nourishment and breathed through the umbilicus].

⁵ *Physics*, ii. 2.
⁶ *Generation of Animals*, ii. 4.

This point is clear in the case of birds, fishes and insects; thus, some of these [viz. birds] are formed out of an egg, after separation from the mother, and it is in the egg that they get their articulation; and some animals [viz. fishes and insects] do not breathe at all, but are produced as larvae or as eggs; others [viz. the Vivipara], which both breathe and get their articulation within the uterus, do not, however, breathe until their lungs have reached completion: with them, both the lungs and the preceding parts become articulated before they breathe. Further, the polydactylous quadrupeds, such as the dog, the lion, the wolf, the fox and the jackal, all bring forth their young blind, and the eyelid does not separate until some time after birth'.[7] Aristotle is here at pains to make two points clear: (1) It is *pneuma* which is concerned in the development of the embryo, and this *pneuma* is *connate*: it is not breath inhaled from without, either by the mother or by the embryo itself; (2) this connate *pneuma* is responsible for the whole process of development of the embryo, just as it is responsible for the initial 'setting' or constituting of it.

In another passage Aristotle speaks of the growth of the 'imperfect' (i.e. non-cleidoic) eggs of fishes.[8] Again he makes the point that these eggs 'grow of their own means and not in virtue of being attached to something else'. Their increase in size after deposition he compares to the behaviour of yeast, 'which is small in bulk to begin with, and gets larger: this growth is due to its more solid portion turning fluid, and the fluid being pneumatized. This is the handiwork of the substance of the soul-heat in the case of the animals, and of the heat of the humour blent with it in the case of the yeast'. Here again the 'substance of the soul-heat' is the connate *pneuma*, which acts upon the fluid contained in the egg.

Aristotle, however, is not content to offer explanations only for these phenomena already mentioned. He extends his theory to give an account of heredity. The fundamental factor in this explanation is the 'movements' already described, which are contributed to the formation of the embryo by the two parents. If the 'movement' from the male is deficient in any 'power' (*dynamis*), the offspring will be correspondingly deficient, and will 'depart from type' and pass over into the opposite state, for example, into the female state, or even into a monstrosity (the female, according to Aristotle, is a 'natural deformity'). Or the 'movement' may 'relapse', and then the offspring takes after its grandfather or great-grandfather. And similarly if there is any deficiency in the female's 'movement'. The same principle applies to the resemblance of the various parts of the body (other than those already involved in the difference of sex) as well as to the appearance of the body as a whole. 'Departure from type' is due to deficient potency in the 'movement' from the male or to excessive bulk and coldness in the matter provided by the female. The cause of 'relapses' is more obscure: it seems to lie in some reaction or resistance offered by the material to the agent acting upon it.

Reproduction is only one of the operations in which connate *pneuma* is an essential factor. Another has already been mentioned—the movement of the limbs of the body. Here again it is the instrument employed by soul, in this case 'appetitive' soul. All the various stimuli which excite animals can, says Aristotle, be classified ultimately under two headings, objects of thought and

[7] *ibid.*, ii. 6.   [8] *ibid.*, iii. 4.

objects of desire, and these act upon the appetition or appetitive soul in a way which will be described presently. The 'movement' produced in the appetitive soul is communicated by the heart to the connate *pneuma*, and the *pneuma*, in virtue of its ability to expand and contract, can (although not itself subject to qualitative change) bring about qualitative change in the various parts of the body which control the limbs and so cause the limbs to move.

The manner in which the objects of thought and desire exert their influence upon appetitive soul is compared by Aristotle to the way in which the 'unmoved mover' ('God') exerts his influence upon the outermost shell or sphere of the universe, the *primum mobile*, and through it and the other spheres upon the whole sublunary world. In the famous phrase, the unmoved mover causes the *primum mobile* to rotate by being to it as an object of its love (κινεῖ ὡς ἐρώμενον), though not himself in motion. Similarly, the objects of thought and appetition, though not themselves in motion, cause 'movement' in the appetitive soul.

Aristotle's statement that connate *pneuma* is 'analogous' in its nature to the celestial element *aither* has already been referred to. In the present instance we have two further points in which it resembles the *aither*, although these are not remarked upon by Aristotle himself. (1) *Pneuma* is an intermediary between an immaterial originator of movement (the soul) and material objects. *Aither* also is such an intermediary: the unmoved mover moves the outermost sphere of the heavens, which communicates this movement to the inner spheres and the heavenly bodies which they carry, all of which spheres and bodies are made of *aither*, and these heavenly bodies in turn cause movement in the sublunary world, bringing about the transformations of the elements and the whole cyclic process of the seasons and of the succession of generations of living things. (2) *Pneuma* causes the limbs to move without itself undergoing qualitative change. *Aither* also causes the movements just mentioned without being itself subject to any kind of qualitative change.

It may be worth remarking in this connexion that the comparison of *pneuma* and *aither* is not an isolated instance in Aristotle of 'counterparts' or 'analogues'. It is a notion found over and over again in his works. A biological illustration of this will be appropriate. Aristotle recognizes two chief modes of 'difference', (*a*) that of degree, or, as he calls it, 'of excess and deficiency', and (*b*) a wider divergence, where the difference is 'by analogy'. Examples of (*a*) are the minor differences which are found as between different species of one and the same genus, or between different genera, or even between individuals of different sexes. Thus, some birds have long legs or feathers, others have short ones; the male of a species may have the same offensive or defensive organ as the female, but 'to a greater degree'. This same mode of difference applies to skin, membrane, sinew, etc., and again to bone, fish-spine, cartilage, etc.; these are sets of substances which between themselves differ 'by the more and the less'. It is interesting to notice that in the Greek of Aristotle's time the phrase 'excess and deficiency' had a mathematical connexion if not a mathematical origin, and as Sir D'Arcy Thompson has shown, differences of the type which Aristotle characterized by this phrase can be reduced to the terminology of mathematics; thus, for example, the cannon-bones of the ox, the sheep, and the giraffe can be shown as strictly proportionate and successive deformations of one and the same form.[9]

Examples of (*b*), difference 'by analogy', are the feathers of birds, the scales of fishes, and the scales of reptiles: these are the 'counterparts' of each other, as indeed the large groups of animals or of living things themselves may be. Thus, Testacea and plants are 'analogous', and their relationship corresponds to the relationship which subsists between water and fluid matter on the one hand and earth and solid matter on the other: plants, says Aristotle, are a sort of land-shellfish, and shellfish are a sort of water-plant. Water and fluids are better able to support life than earth and solids; and air is better still; it is the 'more perfect' animals which have lungs and breathe. In his treatise on the *Generation of Animals* the most frequent references to 'analogy' are the counterparts of the heart and of the blood in what he calls the bloodless animals; but he also refers to 'analogues' of the menstrual fluid (in bloodless animals), of teeth, of flesh, of fat, of hair, and of sinew. Also, the menstrual fluid in females is 'analogous' to the semen in males: this difference we might have expected to be one merely 'of excess and deficiency', but no doubt the reason why he treats it as being a wider divergence is that the menstrual fluid lacks sentient soul, as we have already noted.

So far we have been considering connate *pneuma* as the vehicle by which 'movements' originated by the soul, which has its seat in the heart, are transmitted and propagated outwards from the heart, or from the semen which contains the *pneuma* and the 'movements' with which the heart has charged it. But the *pneuma* is capable also of being charged with certain other 'movements' derived from outside the body and of transmitting them inwards to the heart from the sense-organs, and it is thus an essential factor in all processes of sensation. It is the instrument by which the 'movements' set up in the sense-organs by external stimuli are conveyed to their destination in the heart, the seat of sentient soul. It is clear that Aristotle considered that these 'movements' were conveyed to the heart through the blood in the blood-vessels, this blood being, as we have seen, instinct with connate *pneuma*. In the case of some senses, the first stage of the journey was covered, not by vessels containing blood, but by 'passages' containing connate *pneuma* only. Thus, we read that from the eyes 'passages' run to the blood-vessels around the brain, and similarly from the ears a 'passage' connects to the back of the head.[10] This is amplified by another statement in the *Generation of Animals*[11] where smell and hearing are said to be 'passages' full of connate *pneuma*, connecting with the external air, and terminating at the small vessels which come from the heart and extend around the brain. Hence there is continuity of connate *pneuma* from the sense-organ, through the 'passages' and then the vessels, right up to the heart. In addition to its own proper 'movements', the connate *pneuma* picks up these 'movements'

---

[9] D'A. W. Thompson, *On Growth and Form*; cf. also *idem*, 'Excess and defect'. *Mind*, 1929, xxxviii, 43 ff.

[10] Aristotle, *Parts of Animals*, ii. 10.

[11] ii. 6.

which are derived from external stimuli and transmits them to the heart, where they are interpreted by the soul as sensations.

It is interesting to note that Aristotle had a parallel theory to account for the transmission of colour from a visible object to the sense-organ. According to this theory, 'colour' means 'that which has the power to set in movement that which is actually transparent', and the latter acts as the medium. The medium must extend continuously from the object to the sense-organ, and in its turn it sets the sense-organ in movement. The medium is indispensable, because colour cannot set the sense-organ in movement direct. Examples of transparent media are air, water, and certain solids. Their transparency is due not to themselves, but to the fact that they contain a certain substance which is also found in the 'eternal substance of the upper cosmos', that is, in the *aither*. This substance, then, is the vehicle by which colour is transmitted to the eye; it conveys the 'movements' set up in itself by the colour of an object, and sets up these same 'movements' in the sense-organ, where they are picked up by the connate *pneuma*, which conveys them in the same manner from the eye to the heart and the sentient soul. Aristotle's theory of sound is similar to his theory of colour-transmission. True, he does not mention *aither* or any substance 'found in *aither*', but the medium here is air, which obviously has certain properties in common with *pneuma*. Again there are three main factors, the sounding object, the air, and the sense-organ. 'A sounding object' means 'an object which can set in movement a continuous volume of air as far as the organ of hearing', and the movement of the air constitutes sound only when the air is thus set in movement as one continuous entity. The 'movement' set up in the air is of course transmitted to the connate air or *pneuma* in the ear, and the rest of the process follows as before.

This brief and condensed account of Aristotle's theories will, I hope, be sufficient to indicate his method of approach to the problems of reproduction and sensation, and to show the essential position in these theories of his concept of connate *pneuma* and other similar substances. It would have been possible to enlarge upon his theory of connate *pneuma* by showing how he applies it to explain the supposed phenomenon of spontaneous generation, but as this is not a problem of interest at the present day no useful purpose would be served. It may, however, be of interest to remark, in conclusion, that in Aristotle's view the continuous succession of generations of plants and animals was an essential feature of the universe, and that this may perhaps account for his willingness to allow the introduction into the sublunary world of *pneuma* and substances comparable to the *aither* of the celestial regions, substances which are really of a different order from the four sublunary elements Fire, Air, Water, and Earth. The regular, continuous rotation of the *primum mobile* and of the other celestial spheres is their way of representing the unmoved eternity of the prime mover; and the cyclic succession of transformation of the elements and the generations of living things in the sublunary world is their way of doing the same thing. If he could have done so, says Aristotle, God would have filled the whole universe through and through with being which was eternal and immutable, such as that possessed by the celestial spheres, but since for some reason this was impossible, he provided for the continuous succession of generation and decay, decay and generation, which is exhibited by the four elements and by plants and animals. And in this process of nature it is *pneuma* which is the indispensable instrument: 'Just as certain things serve many uses in the arts and crafts, for instance the hammer and anvil of the smith, so does *pneuma* in the objects that are constructed by nature. . . . In fact, it is probable that nature makes the majority of her productions by means of *pneuma* used as an instrument'.[12]

[12] *Generation of Animals*, v. 8.

THE ORIGIN OF HOSPITALS

by

GEORGE E. GASK and JOHN TODD

IT is often said that the earliest reference to hospitals is to be found in India in the time of the great Emperor Asoka (264–228 B.C.), but the reference is by no means free from ambiguity. The word in the second Edict of Asoka which is translated 'hospitals' may mean nothing more than 'medical remedies', and is so translated by some scholars. If that is so, the claim that Asoka founded hospitals has no support. Even if this enlightened emperor did actually found hospitals, his foundations had no influence on the development of these institutions, and for the origin of hospitals we must look elsewhere.

It is to Greece, the birthplace of rational medicine, that we naturally turn to find the beginnings of hospitals, and some have found those beginnings in the temples of Aesculapius. It was the custom of sick people to resort to the temples of Aesculapius, or Asclepios as the Greeks called him, but there is no evidence that the sick received in those temples anything that could be called regular medical treatment. They came, indeed, primarily not for medical treatment but for dreams, and believed that in their dreams Aesculapius himself appeared and revealed to them the particular treatment which they ought to follow. The dreams which they received during their 'temple-sleep', or incubation, were told to the priests who interpreted them, but such records as have come down to us of the cures wrought at Epidauros, the site of the chief temple of Aesculapius in Greece, are such as to suggest self-deception and sometimes even trickery, rather than serious medical treatment. The practice in these temples of Aesculapius and its relation to serious Hippocratic medicine has been discussed at length by one of us in a previous communication,[1] and the conclusion seems inevitable that although pleasant places in which to sojourn for a time and doubtless affording welcome refreshment to body and mind, they cannot be regarded as hospitals but may be classed with the watering-places and hydropathic establishments of our own day.

The iatreia of the Greek and Roman physicians. Every Greek physician had his *iatreion*, literally 'healing-place', and to the *iatreion* patients came to consult the doctor and to be treated by him. Had these *iatreia* beds attached to them? Had they provision for nursing the sick? There is no evidence that they had either. True, there must have been occasions when a sick man had to stay in the *iatreion*, occasions when it was too dangerous to move him once he was there. But although such exceptional circumstances might possibly arise, there is not the slightest evidence, literary or archaeological, that such was the common practice.

An attempt was made to introduce the *iatreion* into Rome when the Greek physician, Archagathus, came from the Peloponnesus to that city *c.* 220 B.C.

[1] G. E. Gask, 'Early medical schools. The cult of Aesculapius and the origin of Hippocratic medicine'. *Ann. Med. Hist.*, 1939, 3s., i, 128–57.

He was given Roman citizenship and presented by the city with a *taberna* where he might carry on his work. At first he met with great success and received the honourable name of *Vulnerarius*, 'Wound doctor', but later his drastic methods in surgery earned for him the uncomplimentary title of *Carnifex*, 'Butcher', and he had to leave the city. But there is nothing to imply that his *taberna* was anything more than a house where he saw his patients. In fact, we gather from Plautus (254–184 B.C.), the Roman comic poet and contemporary of Archagathus, that the *tabernae* did not enjoy a high reputation, for he classes them with *tonstrinae*, barbers' shops. A passage from Plautus has been quoted to prove that patients did, indeed, stay in the doctor's *taberna*. In the *Menaechmi* a madman is handed over to the care of the doctor, and the doctor says to the man's friends: 'The best thing for you to do is to have him taken to my house. There, at my discretion, I shall be able to treat the man. . . . I'll make him drink hellebore some twenty days. . . . I shall go home that the things may be got ready which are necessary to be prepared. Bid your servants carry him to my house.' But those words furnished no evidence that the doctor had a hospital attached to his house. On the contrary, do they not suggest that there was no place ready for the sick man, and that the doctor had to go on ahead to make arrangements for his patient's reception? All that can be said of these *iatreia* or *tabernae* is that they were something in the nature of the dispensaries of the modern general practitioner. They cannot, in any sense, be regarded as hospitals.

Valetudinaria. Not the least important part of a wealthy Roman's possessions were his slaves, and, if any were ill, it was to the owner's interest to look after this valuable property. Consequently the wealthy slave-owners arranged for the medical care of their sick slaves, and the place where these slaves received treatment was called a *valetudinarium*. Columella,[2] a native of Spain who lived in Rome in the days of Saint Paul, wrote a treatise on agriculture and in it he points out the need of providing such *valetudinaria* for slaves. These buildings, he says, must be kept clean and aired, and slaves who are ill ought to be allowed to rest there. But these *valetudinaria* were private institutions, part of the organization of large houses or of big estates which depended on slave labour, and their existence was due to the enlightened self-interest of the slave-owners. There is no evidence that they were used by the general public, nor, in the circumstances, would we expect the general public to be admitted to them; and although they possessed beds and medical attendants, they cannot rightly be described as hospitals.

Military Valetudinaria. Much the same may be said of the Roman military hospitals. The Romans were a practical people, and the experience of many wars soon taught them the necessity of looking after their sick and wounded soldiers. Consequently *valetudinaria* were established especially near the frontiers, and remains of such military hospitals have been excavated at Carnuntum on the Danube, about six miles south-west of Bratislava and fifteen miles east of Vienna, and at Novaesium, the modern Neuss, near Düsseldorf. The Roman camp at Carnuntum, headquarters of the 14th Legion, was built *c.* A.D. 73, and lasted for more than 300 years. Here

[2] Columella, XI. i. 18; XII. i. 6; XII. iii. 7–8.

in the second century A.D. were the headquarters of the Emperor Marcus Aurelius, and here that philosopher wrote part of his *Meditations*. It would appear that the hospital belonged to the earliest days of the Roman camp, and may well be assigned to the first century A.D. In that case, it is the earliest Roman military hospital of which we have any trace. The hospital at Novaesium, too, may be dated *c.* A.D. 100, and of this hospital Professor Singer writes: 'It is built on the corridor system. Entering from the north between the administrative offices we come on a large hall on which succeeds a long narrow room placed along the axis of the building. This room was probably used as a refectory. It is surrounded on three sides by a corridor out of which open chambers for the sick. Around this series of chambers runs another corridor also along three sides of the building, and around this outer corridor again is another series of chambers. These outer chambers are peculiarly arranged so that they do not open directly into the corridor but each pair is reached through a small vestibule. The arrangement must be related to sanitation, and traces of the drainage system have been uncovered. The general scheme is much in advance of any military hospital until quite modern times.'[3]   Inscriptions, too, refer to medical attendants, *optiones valetudinarii*, and there is, therefore, no doubt whatever that the Roman army, on the frontier at least, possessed a regular system of military hospitals. But although this is true of the Roman army, there is no evidence that such institutions existed for civilians. Indeed, we may go further and say that there is positive evidence which suggests the absence of civilian hospitals. Tacitus relates that in the year A.D. 27 a terrible disaster took place at Fidena, a town about five miles from Rome, when the amphitheatre collapsed and fifty thousand people were killed and injured. He tells us that the injured were taken to *private houses*, for, after the ancient custom, the nobles 'threw open their doors, they ordered medicines to be distributed and physicians attended with assiduity in every quarter'.[4] Surely if hospitals had existed for civilians it would have been to those institutions, and not to private houses, that the injured would have been taken.

There is no reason to think that these military *valetudinaria* played any part in the evolution of the hospital. Like the slave *valetudinaria*, they existed for a particular purpose and for a particular class, and when that purpose (military necessity) and that class (Roman soldiers) ceased, the military valetudinaria ceased also. So negligible, indeed, was the influence of the *valetudinarium* on the evolution of the hospital that not even its name survived, for when hospitals did arise they were known not by the Latin name *valetudinaria* but by the Greek name *xenodochia*.

The more one searches for traces of hospitals in pre-Christian days, the more one is impressed by the absence of any allusion to them in places where we might well expect to find them. If they had existed in pre-Christian days, surely the city of Alexandria would have possessed them. For three centuries before Christ this city was the chief centre of all medical learning, and students flocked to it from all parts. Celsus, 'the custodian of Alexandrine medicine', discusses Ammonius Lithotomos who flourished in Alexandria in the third

[3] C. Singer, in *The Legacy of Rome*. Ed. C. Bailey. Oxford, 1940, p. 294.
[4] Tacitus, *Annals*, iv. 63.

century B.C., and was renowned for his operation for crushing stone in the bladder. He praises Gorgias who also lived in Alexandria in the third century, and discusses his work on operative treatment of hernia. In neither case does he give any hint of the existence of a hospital. Galen visited Alexandria in the second century A.D. and studied there, but, although he was a most voluminous writer, he does not say one word which would lead us to suppose that there was a hospital in that city. In the early days of the Empire wealthy Romans lavished gifts on the cities. Aqueducts, baths, pavements, libraries, amphitheatres were built by private munificence, and many donors must have well-nigh beggared themselves with the prodigality of their gifts. But for our purpose the remarkable fact is that, amongst all these gifts, there is not a single case of the gift of a hospital. 'I may be permitted to assume,' writes Sir Clifford Allbutt, 'from what we know of the temper of a century or two before Christ, that, partly politically or socially, partly sympathetically, the provision of hospitals, or of institutions virtually hospitals, for the relief of the poor, or the advantage of the affluent, would be not incredible.'[5] We can only reply that, incredible or not, there is no evidence that such institutions existed.

For the movement which ultimately produced the hospitals we must turn to Christianity. The early Christians, remembering the words of their Master, 'I was sick and ye visited me',[6] regarded the care of the sick as a duty specially laid upon them; and the earliest account of a Christian service outside the pages of the New Testament, i.e., c. A.D. 150, shows that it was the custom to make a collection every Sunday for 'orphans, widows, those who are in want owing to sickness or any other cause, those who are in prison and strangers who are on a journey'.[7] With the care of the sick went the duty of hospitality, and twice in the New Testament a bishop is described as one who must be 'given to hospitality'.[8] There was much correspondence between bishops and their clergy in distant parts of their dioceses, and accommodation had to be provided for messengers bringing such correspondence, for fellow-Christians on a journey, for pilgrims who had fallen sick, and, indeed, for all who needed it. It is easy to realize that accommodation in the bishop's house must soon have been inadequate, and so a separate house for strangers would soon be set aside. Such a house, called a *xenodochium*, literally 'house for strangers', is the germ from which the hospital system developed. In addition to the xenodochium arose the *nosocomium* or 'house for the sick', the *ptochotrophium* or 'house for the poor', and the *orphanotrophium* or 'house for orphans'; but, in the earliest days, these names seem to have been interchangeable and xenodochium was used as a general name for the abode of the sick.

Although it is impossible to say when these xenodochia began, it is certain that they were in existence in the first half of the fourth century; for, although Eusebius, who finished his *Ecclesiastical History* in A.D. 342, appears to know nothing of xenodochia, the Emperor Julian the Apostate (A.D. 361–3) is well acquainted with them. When Julian renounced Christianity and

[5] Sir T. Clifford Allbutt, *Greek Medicine in Rome*. London, 1921, p. 461.
[6] Matt. xxv. 36.
[7] Justin Martyr, *First Apology*, i. 67.
[8] 1 Tim. iii. 2; Titus i. 8.

attempted to revive paganism, he tried to attract converts to his revived paganism by establishing xenodochia such as the Christians had.   In a letter to Arsacius, his pagan high priest in Galatia, he wrote: 'In every city establish frequent xenodochia in order that strangers may profit by our benevolence. . . . For it is disgraceful where no Jew has to beg, and the impious Galileans support not only their own poor but ours as well, all men see that our people lack aid from us.'[9]   Julian adds that he has given orders that 30,000 modii of corn shall be assigned every year for the whole of Galatia and 60,000 sexarii of wine, and four-fifths of this are to be distributed to strangers and beggars. Sozomen, the Greek ecclesiastical historian of the fifth century, relates the same story, and there is no doubt that Julian founded his xenodochia in imitation of the Christain xenodochia.   Consequently, by A.D. 362 xenodochia were well-known institutions of the Church.   An early tradition assigns the first xenodochium to Zoticus, and says that he founded it in Constantinople shortly after A.D. 330, for a law of the Emperors Leo and Anthemius in A.D. 470 orders xenodochia to be founded 'after the fashion of Zoticus of blessed memory who is said to have been the first to introduce the duty of compassion of this sort' ('ad similitutindem Zotici beatissimae memoriae, qui primus hujusmodi pietatis officium invenisse dicitur').[10]

Xenodochia spread rapidly in the East.   Eustathius, Bishop of Sebaste in the extreme south of Pontus, founded one there c. 350,[11] and Chrysostom mentions a large xenodochium in Antioch, and when he became Patriarch of Constantinople in 397, he founded two xenodochia in that city.[12]   Not the least famous xenodochium in Constantinople was that of Saint Sampson which stood between Saint Sophia and Saint Irene, and was restored by the Emperor Justinian after it had been destroyed in the Nika Riots in 532.[13]   Constantinople, indeed, appears to have been well provided with institutions for the sick, for records have survived of no less than thirty-five xenodochia or similar establishments in the city.[14]   Ephesus, too, had its xenodochium founded by Bishop Bassianus c. 440, and provided with seventy beds.[15]

Sometimes an emergency led to an improvisation, as when a famine at Edessa was followed by wide-spread sickness, and arrangements, whether temporary or permanent, had to be made for the sick.   In 378 this city was suffering from a dreadful famine, and Saint Ephraim, then living a hermit life in a rocky cavern near the city, having heard of the distress which had befallen the city, quitted his solitary cell and came to Edessa. Gathering the citizens together, he blamed the rich for allowing the poor to die around them. The rich citizens replied that they were willing to contribute money, but they did not know any man sufficiently honest to administer the funds.   ' "We are not intent on hoarding our wealth, but we know of no one to whom we can confide the distribution of our goods, for all are prone to seek after lucre and to betray the trust placed in them." "What think ye of me?" asked Ephraim.

[9] Julian, *Epist.*, 49 (Loeb Class. Lib., *Julian*, vol. iii. p. 69).

[10] *Code of Justinian*, I. i. tit. 3.

[11] Eustathius, *Epiphanes, Adv. Haeres*, I. iii. 4.

[12] Chrysostom, *Hom.* 66 *in Matt.*; *Consol. ad Stagyrum*, I. iii. 13.   Palladius, *Vita Chrys.*, 5.

[13] Procopius, *De aedif.*, I. iii; Du Cange, *Constantinoplis Christiana*, p. 164.

[14] Du Cange, *op. cit.* (13), IV, p. 163.

[15] *Acts of the Council*, 11th Session, Hefele, vol. ii, p. 471.

On their admitting that they considered him an excellent and just man and worthy of confidence, he offered to undertake the distribution of their alms. As soon as he received the money he caused about three hundred beds to be fitted up in the public galleries, and here he tended those who were ill and suffering from the effects of the famine, whether they were foreigners or natives of the surrounding country. On the cessation of the famine he returned to the cell in which he had previously dwelt, and after the lapse of five days he expired.'[16]

By far the most famous hospital in the ancient world was that founded by Saint Basil at Caesarea in Cappadocia. Basil, Bishop of Caesarea, was one of the outstanding men of his age, pre-eminent as a theologian and an administrator, but also mindful of the needs of the sick and poor amongst his people. In 372 he founded a hospital which, in many of its features, is surprisingly modern. Fortunately we are acquainted with many details about this hospital, for when his friend Gregory of Nazianus preached his funeral sermon, he dwelt upon the bishop's work for the sick at Caesarea. 'Go forth', says Gregory, 'a little from the city and behold the new city, the treasure house of godliness . . . in which the superfluities of wealth . . . nay even things not superfluous, have been laid up at his exhortation.'[17] From these words we gather that Basil's hospital was some little way outside the city of Caesarea. It was not a building which had been merely improvised from already existing buildings in a crowded part of the city, but was actually designed and built for its purpose, affording plenty of space for expansion. In this respect Basil's hospital reminds us of the new medical city which has recently been built in the outskirts of Birmingham, where the hospitals and the medical schools have been grouped together in a suburb not too far removed from the centre of the city, but at the same time allowing room for expansion.

The success of Basil's new hospital seems to have excited a certain amount of envy, and some of his critics accused him of aiming at undue power and infringing the rights of the civil authority. Basil met this criticism by writing to Elias, the governor of the province, and fortunately Basil's letter has been preserved, for it contains a description of the most remarkable feature of his hospital, his scheme for the training and rehabilitation of the inmates. After some tactful references to overburdening a man already busy with so many responsibilities, Basil writes:

'Now I should like those who are besieging your impartial ears to be asked what harm the government suffers from me? What depreciation is suffered by any public interests, be they great or small, by my administration of the churches? Still, possibly, it might be urged that I have done damage to the government by erecting a magnificently appointed church to God, and around it a dwelling house, one liberally assigned to the bishop, and others underneath, allotted to the officers of the church in order, the use of both

---

[16] Sozomen, *Ecclesiastical History*, iii, 16. This 'Emergency Medical Service' is not without interest in view of the fact that Edessa later became a famous medical centre with two large hospitals, and when the Nestorians, who taught medicine there, were expelled in 489, they carried the medical tradition to Gundev-Shapur in western Persia which later became the centre from which Arabian medicine spread.

[17] Gregory's Oration, xliii in Migne, *Patrologia Graeca*, vol. xxxvi, col. 578–9.

being open to you of the magistracy and your escort. But to whom do we do any harm by building a place for entertainment of strangers, both for those who are on a journey and for those who require medical treatment on account of sickness, and so establishing a means of giving these men the comfort they want, nurses, physicians (τοὺς νοσοκομοῦντας, τοὺς ἰατρεύοντας) means of conveyance and escort? All these men must learn such occupations as are necessary to life and have been found essential to a respectable career; they must also have buildings suitable for their employment, all of which are an honour to the place, and, as their reputation is credited to our governor, confer glory on him. . . .'[18]

This letter, so simple and direct, shows that Basil realized that the responsibility of the hospital does not cease with the cure of the patient. The patient must be rehabilitated and enabled to earn his livelihood. Hence Basil's insistence on the need for workshops where men could 'learn such occupations as are necessary to life', and it may be noted that in this respect modern hospitals are tending to carry out the ideas which Basil practised nearly sixteen hundred years ago. Very little is known about Basil's hospital, but the memory of this early 'hospital town' long survived in the name Basiliad, or Basil's Town, and if Medicine, like the Church, had any way of canonizing its most worthy sons, it would surely number Basil amongst its elect.

We know little about the medical staff of the xenodochia, but as there are frequent references, both literary and epigraphical, to Christian physicians in the third, fourth and fifth centuries, we may presume that xenodochia were not without skilled medical assistants. Bishops, indeed, seemed to have taken pains to obtain the services of physicians, for in A.D. 450 Theodoret, Bishop of Cyrrhus in northern Syria, writes in commendatory terms of a priest named Peter who formerly practised medicine in Alexandria and was now practising in Cyrrhus; and in another letter (cxv) the Bishop tells how he procured skilful physicians to live in Cyrrhus. It is possible, too, that in their earlier days, the xenodochia were partly staffed by 'parabolani'. The word means 'those who take a risk', and was applied to the Christians who risked their lives in attending to the plague-stricken. But this self-sacrificing body of nurses, who began so nobly, deteriorated rapidly. Organized to attend the sick, they became a body organized for violence, a sort of ruffianly body-guard of Cyril, the factious Patriarch of Alexandria; and in A.D. 416, in consequence of the disturbances in Alexandria in the course of which Hypatia was murdered, Theodosius II reduced their number to 500, took them away from the Patriarch and placed them under Orestes, the Prefect of the city. Two years later the Emperor rescinded the order, raised their number to 600, and restored them to the Patriarch's authority. Their violent behaviour at the *Latrocinium*, or Council of Brigands, as the Second Church Council at Ephesus in 449 was not inappropriately called, so terrorized their opponents that the brutal Abbot Barsumas, who relied upon these ruffians, was able to get his own way. They continued to be a menace to the peace of both Church and State, and it is evident that by A.D. 400, if not earlier, they had out-lived their usefulness, and their history

[18] Basil, letter to Elias (No. xciv).

belongs not to the development of hospitals, but to the bitter ecclesiastical controversies of the fifth century.

Towards the end of the fourth century the xenodochia spread from the east to the west, and it is important to notice that the terms used for the institution in the west are Greek and not Latin, that is, they were not called *valetudinaria* but *nosocomia* or *xenodochia*. The use of these Greek names shows that the hospital was so great a novelty in Rome in the fourth century that there was no Latin word for it, and hence the names already in use for hospitals in the east were adopted in the west. If the hospital had been the product of Rome, as is sometimes asserted, it is difficult to understand why they were not called by Latin names.

The first public hospital in the west was founded by Fabiola *c.* A.D. 390. This Roman lady, a wealthy widow, was a friend of Jerome, and the latter tells us how she founded a νοσοκομεῖον (Jerome calls it by this Greek name) 'into which she gathered the sick from the streets', and he expressly states that Fabiola was the first (evidently meaning the first in Rome) to found such 'a place for the sick'.[19] A few years later, in 398, Fabiola, together with Pammachius, a Roman noble, founded a xenodochium at Ostia, the port of Rome, and so great was the fame of that institution that Jerome, with pardonable exaggeration, declares that the whole world has heard of it ('Xenodochium in portu Romano situm totus pariter mundus audivit').[20] During the excavations at Ostia about eighty years ago, the foundations of this xenodochium were discovered with many of the bases of the columns still in situ, and fragments of columns and capitals lying around. The main building was surrounded by corridors which opened into long rooms, presumably wards, and the total length of the building appears to have been 186 feet.

Only slowly did hospitals spread in the west, and it is remarkable that even so large and important a city as Milan, in the days when Saint Ambrose was bishop (374–397), apparently did not possess a xenodochium; whilst Saint Augustine, the great Bishop of Hippo (d. A.D. 431), appears to have regarded them as a novelty, and he induced Leporius, a priest of Hippo (modern Bone), to found one, which he did, partly at his own expense and partly out of funds contributed by the Christians of Hippo in A.D. 425.[21] The popes, too, were active in this work, and Symmachus is recorded as having founded three hospitals in Rome about A.D. 500,[22] and a hundred years later Pelagius II turned his house into a hospital for old men, *xenodochium pauperum senum*. No pope concerned himself more with hospitals than did Gregory the Great, and his administrative ability was constantly employed to secure the efficiency of the xenodochia. When Isidorus, for example, left a sum of money to found a xenodochium at Palermo, and his heirs were negligent in carrying out the terms of the will, Gregory gave instructions that the bequest, if insufficient for the purpose, was to be used for the support of the xenodochium of Saint Theodorus, which had been founded earlier by a certain

---

[19] Jerome, letter to Oceanus (*Epist.* 77).
[20] *idem, Epist.* 66.
[21] St. Augustine, *Sermons*, 356, 10.
[22] Ado's Chron., Migne, *Patrologia Latina*, vol. cxxiii, p. 106 B.

Peter.   Indeed, the letters of Pope Gregory imply the existence of a large number of xenodochia in Italy, for there are references to them in Naples, in Sicily, in Sardinia, even in the unimportant see of Cagliari.[23]

It is evident that by the middle of the sixth century hosptials were securely established, their rights fully recognized and their property duly safe-guarded, for a Church Council, which met at Orleans in 549 and was presided over by Sacerdos, Bishop of Lyons, regards the property of the xenodochium as inviolable as that of a church or a monastery, and decrees in particular that the property of the hospital founded at Lyons by King Childebert must not be alienated to the Bishop of Lyons or to his church.   This mention of Childebert's hospital at Lyons may fittingly close our enquiry into the origin of hospitals, for that hospital, the oldest in Europe, founded in A.D. 542, still carries on its work, and so provides the living link between the early xenodochia and the modern hospitals.[24]

[23] Gregory the Great, *Letters* iii, viii, x; John the Deacon, *Vita Gregorii*, ii. 51; F. H. Dudden, *Gregory the Great*. London, 1905, vol. i, p. 147.

[24] About A.D. 800 the term xenodochium began to give place to the term hospital.   In A.D. 796 Alcuin wrote to his old pupil Eanbald II, Archbishop of York, urging him to found in his diocese 'xenodochia, id est, hospitalia'.   Alcuin, *Letter* 56, *Ad Eanbaldum*.

SAINT AUGUSTINE AND MAGIC

by

CLAUDE JENKINS

THE student has missed one of the more subtle pleasures of life who has never adventured himself into the pages of *St. Avgvstine, of the Citie of God: with the Learned Comments of Io. Lod. Vives. Englished by J. H. Printed by George Eld, 1610.*[1] And this is true, however well he may know his Augustine in the solemn tomes of a Benedictine edition or the even more austere, if handier, volumes of some modern critical recension. John Healey's version no doubt needs to be checked, though there is certainly no warrant for a later description of it by a rival translator as 'exceptionally bad'; but there is a charm about its Elizabethan prose which leads the reader on, as he becomes accustomed to it, into the heart and even to a complete anatomy of one of the great books of the ancient world, while its verse translations and its renderings of Vives' notes are in many cases an unforgettable delight. Like the printer's elaborate device, on the title-page, of the sun breaking through the clouds with ten-pointed rays upon the rolling earth, it does something at least to justify its motto *Dissipabit sic Avgvstinvs*.

We will venture to quote a few examples from that storehouse of marvels, the twenty-first book of the *De Civitate Dei*, to illustrate a point of view in regard to which a modern scientific student would find much to say by way of criticism. In the first Augustine is calling in the aid of natural history to support a theological conclusion which, in any case, he regards as beyond dispute.

> If therefore the Salamander liue in the fire (as the most exact naturalists record) and if there bee certaine famous hills in Sicily that haue beene on fire continually, from beyond the memory of man, and yet remaine whole & vnconsumed, then are these sufficient proofes to shew that all doth not consume that burneth, as the soule prooueth that all that feeleth paine, doth not perish. Why then should we stand vpon any more examples to prooue the perpetuity of mans soule and body, without death, or dissolution in euerlasting fire and torment? That G O D that endowed nature with so many seuerall and admirable qualities, shall as then giue the flesh a quality whereby it shall endure paine and burning for euer. Who was it but hee, that hath made the flesh of a dead Peacock to remaine alwaies sweete, and without all putrefaction? I thought this vnpossible at first, and by chance being at meate in Carthage, a boyled Peacock was serued in, and I to try the conclusion, tooke of some of the Lyre of the breast and caused it to be layd vp. After a certaine space (sufficient for the putrefaction of any ordinary flesh) I called for it, and smelling to it, found no ill taste in it at all. Layd it vp againe, and thirty daies after, I lookt

[1] Juan Luis Vives (1492–1540), Spanish humanist, educationist and philosopher. Born at Valencia, he studied at Bruges and at Louvain, where he became friendly with Erasmus and received a teaching post (1519). In 1523 he was invited by Henry VIII to come to England as tutor to his daughter the Princess Mary. In 1528 he supported Catharine of Aragon in the case of her divorce and was imprisoned for six weeks by Henry. Vives then returned to Bruges, where he spent the rest of his life. His annotated edition of the *De Civitate Dei* was first published at Basle in 1522. It was translated into French as well as into English. It was criticized by the theologians of Louvain, and as a result Vives was placed on the *Index*. In the following notes this English edition of 1610 is referred to as *Citie of God*. [Editor.]

againe, it was the same I left it. The like I did an whole yeare after, and found no change, onely it was somewhat more drie and solide?...[2]

*   *   *   *   *   *

Wee know that the loade-stone draweth Iron strangely: and surely when I obserued it at the first, it made mee much agast. For I beheld the stone draw vppe an Iron ringe and then as if it had giuen the owne power to the ring, the ring drew vppe an other and made it hang fast by it, as it hung by the stone. So did a third by that, and a fourth by the third, and so vntill there was hung as it were a chaine of rings onelie by touch of one another, without any inter-linking. Who would not admire the power in this stone, not onely inherent in it, but also extending it selfe through so many circles, and such a distance? Yet stranger was that experiment of this stone which my brother and fellow Bishoppe *Seuerus*, Bishoppe of Mileuita shewed me.

Hee told mee that hee had seene *Bathanarius* (some-times a Count of Affrica) when hee feasted him once at his owne house, take the sayd stone and hold it vnder a siluer plate vpon which hee layd a peece of Iron: and still as hee mooued the stone vnder the plate, so did the Iron mooue aboue, the plate not moouing at all, and iust in the same motion that his hand mooued the stone, did the stone mooue the Iron. This I saw, and this did I heare him report, whom I will beleeue as well as if I had seene it my selfe. I haue read further-more of this stone, that lay but a diamond neare it, and it will not draw Iron at all, but putteth it from it as soone as euer the diamond comes to touch it. These stones are to bee found in India. But if the strangenesse of them bee now no more admired of vs, how much lesse doe they admire them where they are as common as our lyme, whose strange burning in water (which vseth to quensh the fire,) and not in oyle (which feedeth it) wee doe now cease to wonder at because it is so frequent.[3]

The engaging picture of these eminent persons solemnly practising scientific experiments is noteworthy whatever we may think of them. Vives' comment on the dead peacock is: 'Many of these examples here are beyond reason, and at the most but explanable by weake coniectures, which wee will omit, least wee should seeme rather to oppose Saint *Augustine* then expound him.'[4] To us the observation may suggest the reflexion that the lapse of more than eleven hundred years between author and commentator had not inspired any great confidence of assertion in the latter where matters of scientific knowledge were concerned. And when in the following chapter,[5] headed by Healey 'Of such things as cannot bee assuredly knowne to bee such, and yet are not to be doubted of', Augustine goes on to confute the scepticism of Infidels in regard to Miracles 'and such things as wee cannot make apparant to their sence' by examples to 'try their cunning in things which are extant for any to see, that will take the paines',[6] Vives contents himself not with criticism or explanation, but with the enumeration of the authors from whom as he supposes Augustine derived his information, such as Pomponius Mela, Pliny, Solinus 'Plinies Ape', and many others of repute. So we learn of the salt of Agrigentum in Sicily which 'beeing put in fire melteth into water, and

---

[2] *Citie of God*, xxi. 4; p. 840.
[3] *ibid.*, p. 841–2.
[4] *ibid.*, p. 842.
[5] Chap. 5.
[6] *Citie of God*, xxi. 4; p. 842.

in water, it crackleth like the fire'[7]; of the fountain of the Garamantes 'so cold in the day that it cannot bee drunke oft: so hot in the night that it cannot bee toucht'[8]; of another in Epirus 'wherein if you quensh a toarch, you may light it againe thereat'; and of the Arcadian Asbest which 'beeing once enflamed, will neuer bee quenshed', and other like marvels including the mode of conception of the mares of Cappadocia—as to which Vives, not to be outdone, observes that 'it is commonly held that the Mares of Andaluzia doe conceiue by the south-west winde'.[9]

In the following chapter,[10] to which Healey gives this title, 'All strange effects are not natures: some are mans deuises: some the deuills', Augustine represents his infidel opponents as endeavouring to evade the force of his instances:

> Perhaps they will answere, Oh, these are lies, wee beleeue them not, they are false relations, if these be credible, then beleeue you also if you list, (for one man hath related both this and those) that there was a temple of *Venus* wherein there burned a lampe which no winde nor water could euer quensh, so that it was called the inextinguible lampe. This they may obiect, to put vs to our plunges, for if wee say it is false, wee detract from the truth of our former examples, and if wee say it is true wee shall seeme to avouch a Pagan deity. But as I sayd in the eighteenth booke, we need not beleeue all that Paganisme hath historically published, their histories (as *Varro* witnesseth) seeming to conspire in voluntary contention one against another: but wee may, if we will, beleeue such of their relations as doe not contradict those bookes which wee are bound to beleeue.[11]

'Ea, si volumus credimus, quae non adversantur libris, quibus non dubitamus oportere nos credere.' A hubristic junior fellow of a college is credited with having distinguished the several grades of the ministry by characteristic modes of verbal expression: the deacon 'One does feel'; the priest 'One learns, does one not?'; the bishop 'I am profoundly convinced'. And here at any rate this utterance of Augustine the bishop tells us much as to the attitude with which, after a somewhat discursively speculative youth, he will find himself approaching natural phenomena and the questions which they raise for the scientific man. To the historian of science, viewing the slowness of its progress through the centuries, such a standpoint with its consequent limitations of outlook will explain much. But lest it be supposed that what would now be deemed 'obscurantism' is the peculiar possession of ecclesiastics, we may venture to add an illustration from a much later age. When Henry Acland in 1853 succeeded John Kidd as Lee's Reader in Anatomy at Oxford (appointed 1816) his methods of teaching, including microscopical illustrations, were regarded as curious and not a little disconcerting. 'A few senior men came from time to time, but could not force their minds into the new groove. . . Dr. Kidd, after examining some delicate morphological preparation, while his young colleague explained the meaning, made answer first, that he did not believe in it, and, secondly that

---

[7] *ibid.*

[8] *ibid.*, p. 843.

[9] *ibid.*, p. 844.

[10] Chap. 6.

[11] *Citie of God*, p. 844. Cf. *De Civ. Dei*, xxi. 6: 'non habemus necesse omnia credere quae continet historia gentium . . . sed ea, si uolumus, credimus, quae non aduersantur libris, quibus non dubitamus oportere nos credere.'

if it were true, he did not think God meant us to know it.'[12]   Yet Kidd was a
man whom Acland in his history of *Oxford and Modern Medicine* described
as 'an admirable man gifted with a real scientific insight'.

In the case of Augustine the consequence of his presuppositions is seen in
his treatment of the example which has just been quoted.

> Experience [he says], and sufficient testimony shall afford vs wonders enow of
> nature, to conuince the possibility of what we intend, against those Infidells.[13]
> As for that lampe of *Venus* it rather giueth our argument more scope then any way
> suppresseth it.   For vnto that, wee can adde a thousand strange things effected both
> by humane inuention and Magicall operation.   Which if wee would deny, we should
> contradict those very bookes wherein wee beleeue.[14]   Wherefore that lampe either
> burned by the artificiall placing of some Asbest in it, or it was effected by art
> magike, to procure a religious wonder, or else some deuill hauing honour there
> vnder the name of *Venus*, continued in this apparition for the preseruation of mens
> misbeleefe.[15]

Vives commenting in 1522 is content to add on 'Asbest'—'Or of a kinde
of flaxe that will neuer bee consumed, for such there is.   *Plin. lib.* 19.   *Piedro
Garsia* and I saw many lampes of it at Paris, where wee saw also a napkin of
it throwne into the middest of a fire, and taken out againe after a while more
white and cleane then all the sope in Europe would haue made it.   Such did
Pliny see also, as hee saith himselfe'.[16]   And on 'art magique': 'In my fathers
time there was a tombe found, wherein there burned a lampe which by the
inscription of the tombe, had beene lighted therein, the space of one thousand
fiue hundred yeares and more.   Beeing touched, it fell all to dust.'[17]   Beside
this the much loved and as often challenged story of the supposed germination
of wheat from Egyptian tombs is a marvel of quite minor interest as a strain
on credulity.

Postulating the reality of 'Art magike' on the warrant of holy scripture
Augustine goes on to enlarge on the activities of devils 'inspiring' man

> . . . with the secrets thereof, or teaching him the order in a false and flattering
> apparition, making some few, schollers to them, and teachers to a many more. . . .
> Nay what cannot that G O D doe, who hath giuen such power to the most hated
> creatures?   So then, if humane arte can effect such rare conclusions, that such as
> know them not would thinke them diuine effects: (as there was an Iron Image
> hung in a certaine temple, so strangely that the ignorant would haue verely beleeued
> they had seene a worke of G O D S immediate power, it hung so iust betweene
> two loade-stones, (whereof one was placed in the roofe of the temple, and the other
> in the floore) without touching of any thing at all,) and as there might be such a
> tricke of mans art, in that inextinguible lampe of *Venus*, if Magicians, (which the
> scriptures call sorcerers and enchanters[18]) can doe such are exploytes by the

[12] J. B. Atlay, *Sir Henry Wentworth Acland, Bart., K.C.B., F.R.S. A Memoir.* London, 1903,
p. 142, where he quotes W. Tuckwell, *Reminiscences*, p. 45.

[13] *De Civ. Dei*, xxi. 6: 'De his autem miraculorum locis, nobis ad ea, quae futura persuadere
incredulis uolumus, satis illa sufficiunt, quae nos quoque possumus experiri, et eorum testes
idoneos non difficile est inuenire.'

[14] *ibid.*   'quae si negare uoluerimus, eidem ipsi cui credimus sacrarum litterarum aduersabimur
ueritati.'

[15] *Citie of God*, p. 844.

[16] *ibid.*, p. 845.

[17] *ibid.*

[18] *De Civ. Dei*, xxi. 6: 'quos nostra scriptura ueneficos et incantatores uocat.'

deuills meanes as *Virgil* that famous poet relateth of an Enchantresse, in these words . . . .

> 'She said her charmes could ease ones heart in paine,
> Euen when she list, and make him greeue againe,
> Stop flouds, bring back the stars, and with her breath,
> Rouse the black fiends, vntill the earth beneath
> Groan'd, and the trees came marching from the hills &c.'[19]

Vives finds the authority for the Iron Image in the temple of Serapis at Alexandria in Ruffinus, *Ecclesiastical History*, lib. xxi and the testimony of the 'nobilis poeta' in the fourth *Aeneid*, and even if we feel that we are being introduced into a queer world of ideas as well as of phenomena, we are at least gaining some further means of understanding this habit of Augustine's mind. In one of his sermons on the martyrdom of Stephen we are suddenly given a vignette of a fifth-century sickroom: 'One of the faithful is sick and the tempter is at hand (in the person no doubt of a pagan friend). The sick man is promised for his recovery an unlawful sacrifice, a baleful and sacrilegious binding, a profane incantation, a magical consecration, and he is told So and so and So and so were in much greater danger than you, and they came through: do it, if you want to live; you will die if you dont. Consider if it does not mean You will die if you dont deny Christ.'[20] But as another sermon shows the tempter need not necessarily be a pagan: 'A man has a pain in the head. A neighbour male or female will say to you, There is an enchanter here, there is a healer here, and a wizard somewhere.[21] You say, I am a Christian, it is not lawful for me. And if he says to you, Why? Am I not a Christian? You should say, But I am one of the faithful. And he will answer, I too have been baptized. The devils become angels, members of Christ. Because the Enemy possesses himself, he is trying to draw in another also.' And we are told elsewhere that on occasion these illegitimate practitioners 'who lead astray by bindings, by precantations, by devices of the Enemy,[22] mix with their precantations the Name of Christ; because they are not now able to lead Christians astray so as to give them poison, they add a little honey, so that that which is bitter may be hidden by the sweet and the draught may be drunk to their destruction'. The illustration may provoke a self-conscious smile in the reader, but Augustine cites from his own knowledge a case in which the 'Pilleati sacerdos' was wont to say 'Et ipse Pilleatus Christianus est '.[23] One thing so far at any rate seems clear, such practices are not rejected as being mere quackery, but as being wicked and for a Christian sacrilegious. In an elaborate answer to the question why Pharoah's magicians did some of the miracles which Moses, God's servant, did, Augustine not only postulates (without references) on the authority of Scripture a remarkable scheme of the ministry and superintendence of

---

[19] Virgil, *Aeneid*, iv. 487–91. The passage quoted is from *Citie of God*, p. 845.

[20] Augustine, *Sermo* cccxviii, 3 (Paris, 1683, v.1273B): 'Illicitum sacrificium, noxia et sacrilega ligatura, nefanda incantatio, magica consecratio promittitur.'

[21] *idem, Sermo* ccclxxvi (*op. cit.* (20), v.1470): 'Est hic incantator, est hic remediator, et nescio ubi mathematicus.'

[22] *idem, In Ioh. Evang.* cap. i, tract. vii (*op. cit.* (20), ii. 344B): 'qui seducunt per ligaturas. per praecantationes, per machinamenta inimici.'

[23] *ibid.*

angels[24] and observes that the faculty of perpetrating some sins is the penalty of others that preceded them, but evolves a theory of operation from which we are to infer that there are some 'miracula' which wicked (*scelerati*) men are able to perform but holy (*sancti*) men cannot. It is of course safeguarded by the assumption of Divine permission justified by the dictum of Saint Paul (Rom. i. 26: 'tradidit illos Deus in desideria cordis eorum') curiously removed from its context and original intention.

We have not, however, as yet even summarily arrived at the whole of what Augustine is prepared to maintain with the subject of Pharaoh's magicians as a theme. He says that he is aware that unrobust thinking (*infirma cogitatio*) may raise the question why those miracles are performed by magic arts as well; for Pharaoh's magicians also likewise made serpents and other like things. But, he adds, it is even more astonishing how that power of the magicians, which was able to make serpents, when it came to the smallest of flies (*ad muscas minutissimas*), wholly failed . . . so that they said This thing is the finger of God (Exod. viii. 19). From this we are given to understand that not even the transgressor angels and the powers of the air, thrust down from the habitation of that ethereal purity on high into that lowest darkness as to an appropriate prison, those powers through which magic arts have any power that they possess, have any avail unless it has been given to them from above. And it is given to them either to deceive deceivers, as it was in respect of the Egyptians and of the magicians themselves, in order that by the seduction of these spirits they should seem marvellous in action but damnable by God's Truth, or for the admonition of the faithful not to account any such thing great—for which reason also they have been handed down to us by the authority of Scripture or for the exercise, proving and manifestation of the patience of the righteous. Job is adduced as an example, and we are warned against regarding such magicians as creators when they made frogs and serpents, since God is the only creator and they produce only what they are allowed to produce. The argument wanders off into a consideration of problems of generation illustrated by a strange, though not of course an original, disquisition on the natural history of bees.[25] Nor are there wanting elsewhere other examples of the limitation of the power of the magician in other directions. In a well-known letter to Marcellinus, Augustine is at pains to point out that, while 'David noster' without any such arts rose from shepherd to king, Apuleius Afer, though of distinguished birth and liberal education and endowed with great eloquence, with all his magical arts was unable to attain not to a kingdom but even to any judicial office in the state.[26] It is noted however that in spite of the exaggerated claims made for his magical skill by his admirers, he himself provided them with a problem by a most eloquent defence against the charge of being a magician. But in any case we are warned against allowing the marvels of the magicians to be compared with the holy prophets pre-eminent by the distinction of great miracles, still less to Christ whose coming those prophets foretold.

[24] Augustine, *Lib. de diversis quaestionibus*, lxxix (*op. cit.* (20), vi. 69–72): 'unaquaeque res visibilis in hoc mundo habit potestatem angelicam sibi praepositam.'

[25] *idem, De Trin.* iii. 13 (*op. cit.* (20), viii. 800B): 'Et certe apes semina filiorum non coeundo concipiunt, sed tamquam sparsa per terras ore colligunt.'

[26] *idem, Epist.* cxxxviii. 19 (*op. cit.* (20), ii. 418).

The intervention of demonic powers in the performance of magical arts is a not unnatural assumption for a man like Augustine, who held at the same time that, while there are some pains which have a purgatorial character in such as take them for correction, 'all other pains, whether temporal or eternal are laid upon everyone as God pleases by men or angels good or bad, either for sins whether past or wherein the person afflicted is now living or else for the exercise or declaration of Virtues'.[27] It can hardly be expected that in Augustine's treatment such consideration will foster a cheerful outlook upon life and, if we may quote Healey's version of the *De Civitate Dei* again: 'Who would not tremble and rather choose to die then to be an infant againe, if he were put to such a choyce? We begin it with teares, and therein presage our future miseries. Onely *Zoroastres* smiled (they say) when hee was borne: but his prodigyous mirth [*monstrosus risus*] boded him no good: for hee was, by report, the first inuentor of Magike, which notwithstanding stood him not in a pins stead in his misfortunes, for *Ninus* King of Assiria ouer came him in battel and tooke his Kingdome of Bactria from him.'[28] On this Vives notes: 'hee smiled at his birth, and his braine beate so that it would lift vp the hand; a presage of his future knowledge. *Plin.* He liued twenty yeares in a desert vpon cheese, which hee had so mixed, that it neuer grew mouldy nor decayed.'[28]

No one who has ever made any extended study of the works of Augustine could justly accuse him of being hostile to advance in knowledge. And when he shows himself distrustful or cautious in regard to the way in which it is used, we must take into account both his own varied experience in early life, the circumstances of his life as a diocesan bishop, and the conventional ideas of the world around him. He can speak of the advantage of knowledge of precious stones and indicate the possibility that ignorance in this respect may on occasion close doors of understanding.[29] But that is quite a different thing from applying them as remedies or devices (*machinamenta*) of some superstition. He gives an example, not from stones but from plants, which may well interest the modern student.

It is one thing [he remarks] to say If you drink that herb pounded, your stomach will not hurt; and another to say If you hang that herb on your neck, your stomach will not hurt. For in the one case a wholesome 'contemporatio' is approved, in the other a superstitious interpretation is condemned. Although where there are not precantations and invocations and signs (*characteres*) there is frequently a doubt whether the thing which is bound on or joined in some way to the body to be healed avails by force of nature—in which case it may freely be used; or proceeds by some significative obligation—in which case it behoves the Christian to beware of it with the greater caution in proportion as it shall seem more efficaciously profitable. But where the cause of anything's power is unknown, it makes a difference in what spirit anyone uses it, especially in healing or tempering bodies whether in medicine or in agriculture.[30]

---

[27] *De Civ. Dei*, xxi. 14 (*op cit.* (20), vii. 634).   [28] *Citie of God*, p. 855.

[29] Augustine, *De doctrina Christiana*, ii. 24 (*op. cit.* (20), iii. 29b): 'ignorantia berilli vel adamantis claudit plerumque intelligentiae fores.'

[30] *idem, ibid.*, ii. 45 (*op. cit.* (20), iii. 37): 'ubi latet qua causa quid valeat, quo animo quisque utatur interest, dumtaxat in sanandis vel temporandis corporibus, sive in medicina, sive in agricultura.'

That is a sentiment to which it is unlikely that any modern scientist would at its face value seriously object. But it must frankly be admitted also in this connexion that Augustine expresses himself elsewhere in terms which call for more jealous scrutiny. The most significant passage is contained in a chapter towards the end of the tenth book of his *Confessions*, part of which we will venture to quote in another seventeenth-century version—that of William Watts. He is discoursing on the evils attendant on 'curiositas', and distinguishes between the pleasure which is derived from the sensible perception of pleasant things, and the unpleasant consequences following from yielding to the instinct which he regards with disapproval.

> Curiosity for trial's sake pries into objects clean contrary to the former, not to engage itself in the trouble they bring, but merely out of an itch of gaining the knowledge and experience of them. For what pleasure hath it, to see that in a torn carcass, which would strike horror into a man? And yet, if any such be near lying, they all flock to it, even of purpose to be made sad and to grow pale at it: they are afraid also to see it in their sleep; as if some one had forced them to go and see it while they were awake. . . . And out of this disease of curiosity (*morbus cupiditatis*) are all those strange sights (*miracula*) presented unto us in the theatre.

So far as concerns what may be called the 'cultus of the horrible' probably many, and even the majority of modern intelligent observers would share the Bishop's disapproval, at any rate in cases where there was no overriding consideration recognized as justification. But he is prepared to carry his argument further, and continues:

> Hence also men proceed to investigate some concealed powers of that nature which is not beyond our ken, which it does them no good to know, and yet men desire to know for the sake of knowing. Hence proceeds it also, if with that same end of perverted learning, the magical arts be made use of to enquire by. Upon this curiosity also even in religion itself, is God tempted; when namely, certain signs and wonders from heaven are demanded of him: not desired for any saving end, but merely for an experience.[31]

Probably if the passage be read as a whole Augustine may be admitted in his reference to 'ad perscrutanda naturae, quae praeter nos non est, operata' to be dissuading, not from the scientific investigation of the secrets of nature such as lie within the possible scope of human knowledge, but from the use of illegitimate means of doing so 'per artes magicas', which most scientific men would regard with contempt—even if for different reasons. It has been said by a modern writer that 'indifference to natural knowledge was the most palpable intellectual defect of Ambrose and Augustine, and the most portentous '.[32] It is a hard saying, and it is only partly true. Considering the natural beauty of the surroundings in which the greater part of Augustine's life was spent, one might indeed have expected a larger number of illustrations taken from natural phenomena to be found in the voluminous writings, especially of a writer so luxuriant in rhetoric. There are enough to discharge him from the imputation of indifference; but it must be remembered also that his whole intellectual history, as well as the bent of his mind, inclined him to view everything at the earliest opportunity from the standpoint of

[31] *idem, Conf.* x. 35.
[32] H. O. Taylor, *The Medieval Mind*. London, 1911, vol. i, p. 300.

metaphysical rather than of natural philosophy; and in later life the permeation of the whole by theological concepts tended to the sublimation of everything patient of such treatment to the sphere of things seen *sub specie aeternitatis*—a sphere in respect of which he would have claimed the authority of Scripture for regarding natural objects as of merely transitory interest and importance. Moreover, the experience of his early philosophical and religious adventures in quest of Truth, whether through Neoplatonism, Manichæanism or in other directions, left a series of marks on the Christian bishop which lasted to the end. It is not an accident that if he refers to plants it is to tell us of what the Manichæans, 'nonnulli nimis errantes haeretici', thought as to their possession not only of sense-perception but intelligence and the power of reasoning.[33] We may wonder what he would have thought of the *Plant Autographs and their Revelations* by Sir Jagadis Chunder Bose,[34] and its correlation of 'transient and persistent spontaneity' with 'a certain phenomenon known among literary and artistic people as inspiration'. If he speaks of trees the thought of the 'arbor scientiae boni et mali' of the Old Testament or of the 'arbor bona' and 'arbor mala' of the New is seldom far away. We know from the record of one of the scapegrace exploits of his adolescence that his home had pear trees as well as a vineyard, but it is on the authority of Ezekiel[35] rather than on his own account that he prefers to tell us that the wood of the vine separated from the tree is useless for any purpose except to be burnt, though there may be personal observation in his expansion into 'useless for farmers' purposes or the making of tools'.[36] The scriptural examples of which he makes such frequent use determine at any rate to a large extent his attitude towards magic arts and the application of natural forces which they seem to imply. They may be the wrong kind of 'miracles', but we recall that for him in any case 'portentum fit, non contra naturam, sed contra quam est nota natura'.[37] The testimony of Scripture guarantees for him the fact that they were wrought, and the unfavourable judgement which he is bound to take of temerarious experiments of this kind, however successful, rests on the same ground.[38] But we cannot doubt that pronouncements against practices condemned alike by civil and divine law were influenced also by secular conditions around him. The proximity of Tagaste, where Augustine was born in 354, to Madaura, where Augustine went to school and where Lucius Appuleius Afer, the 'evening star of the Platonic and the morning star of the Neoplatonic philosophy', as he has been called, had been born in the second quarter of the second century, would not necessarily imply that the fame of its most illustrious name would impress itself on a boyish imagination. But Appuleius was not only the author of *The Golden Ass* but of an oration or Apology *De Magia*, and Augustine's writings show that the marvels associated with his name were still so far current

---

[33] Augustine, *De genesi ad litteram*, 24 (*op. cit.* (20), iii. 101B).

[34] Longmans, 1927. [35] Ezek. xv. 5.

[36] Augustine, *In Ioh. Evang.*, cap. 15, tract. lxxxi (*op. cit.* (20), iii. 704 B).

[37] *De Civ. Dei*, xxi. 8.

[38] This is true even though he speaks in a rhetorical passage as doing 'nonnulla sanctis Angelis similia, non veritate, sed specie, non sapientia, sed plane fallacia' and enquires what view would be taken had the story of Jonah been related of Apollonius of Tyana or Appuleius of Madaura. (*op. cit.*, *Epist.* cii, *Liber ad Deogratias* ii. 285).

as to seem to demand serious notice in answer to a request from so important a person as Marcellinus, delegate of the Emperor Honorius in Africa in 411. He notes it as ridiculous that people should endeavour to compare Apollonius and Appuleius and other masters of magical arts with Christ, and even to prefer them to Him.[39]

Probably of even greater importance in Augustine's intellectural history, considering the number of references that he makes to him, was another, a third-century writer, Porphyry 'nobilissimus philosophus paganorum',[40] wavering between the confession of the true God and the cultus of demons, perchance through fear of offending the 'theurgi', from whom being deceived by 'curiositas' he has learnt these pernicious and insane things as a great benefit,[41] and as Augustine says in the following chapter far exceeding Appuleius in impiety. It is for the most part in connexion with Porphyry that Augustine indulges in the tenth book of the *De Civitate Dei* in so many contemptuous strictures on that 'magia' which in more detestable guise is styled 'goetia', or more honorifically 'theurgy'. An account is given[42] of Porphyry's letter to Anebo the Egyptian, to ask questions and obtain instructions as to different kinds of demons and the methods and results of invoking such powers. The use of herbs and stones, processes of divination, bindings, the opening of closed doors, use of odours, commerce with the spirits of the dead all seem to be involved, and not unnatural surprise is expressed that so great a philosopher should concern himself with things that any old Christian crone (*quaelibet anicula Christiana*) would regard with contempt. And there perhaps we may leave the matter, not certainly for lack of more material but of space, with the reflexion that to the men of his own age at any rate Augustine would have needed no apology for the attitude which he adopted, still less for the vigour of the language which he uses, and that in our day the examination and discussion of such subjects even by scientific men has not always been pursued in the atmosphere of the island-valley of Avilion, still less of a laboratory.

[39] Augustine, *Epist.* cxxxviii. 18 *Ad Marcellinum* (*op. cit.* (20), ii. 417).
[40] *De Civ. Dei*, xxii. 3 (*op. cit.* (20), vii. 657 F).
[41] *ibid.*, x. 26 (*op. cit.* vii. 260–1).
[42] *ibid.* x. 11.

BOOK II

THE MEDIEVAL WORLD

REMARKS ON THE EARLIEST MEDICAL CONDITIONS IN NORWAY AND ICELAND WITH SPECIAL REFERENCE TO BRITISH INFLUENCE

by

FREDRIK GRÖN

SEVERAL Norwegian authors have written essays on this subject, mostly in Norwegian and German,[1] but one particular aspect has been dealt with in English.[2] In 1936 Reichborn-Kjennerud, Grön and Kobro published a complete review of the history of medicine in Norway up to our time.[3] In effect a considerable amount of work has been carried out in this field generally, but it must be admitted that our neighbours, Sweden and Denmark, are a little ahead of us. This present contribution deals with the early period of our medical history. Though no fundamentally new point of view emerges, I will attempt to show that the terminology of diseases indicates influences which are noticeably British in origin. It is well known that the relations between Norway and Great Britain, including Eire and the Isle of Man, were quite close in the age of the Vikings. Norwegian archaeologists, historians and students of topographical nomenclature like A. W. Brögger, Haakon Shetelig, Alexander Bugge, Magnus Olsen and several others, have pointed out the multiple fields of reciprocal interchange, both material and cultural, between the Norwegians on the one hand and the Anglo-Saxons and Celts on the other in the older history.[4] The relations were particularly active in the age of the Vikings. We must of course admit that our ancestors, the Vikings, did not go as friends to the western countries, and indeed they mostly went as warriors and marauders. Our early history gives many details on that subject. When we regard the spiritual relations between the two peoples, it must be admitted that our culture was considerably influenced by the British Isles. It is hardly possible to elucidate direct medical influence, particularly with regard to new medicines and methods of treatment. On the other hand, there are instances of diseases of a kind previously unknown in Norway having been introduced from Great Britain. This is especially true of leprosy, a disease to which I shall refer later. General mention must also be made of the influence exerted by the Anglo-Saxon and Celtic languages. It should be remembered that long ago definite evidence was obtained that the origin of our oldest medical practice, that of the monks, could be traced to southern Europe. It may be mentioned also that the ancient Norwegian folk-medicine, as found in the poems and tales of the Edda, is also of foreign origin.

In Norway the subject of trephination is of great and continued interest.

[1] F. Grön, 'Altnordische Heilkunde'. *Janus*, 1908, xiii, 73, 138, 206 258, 313, 369, 433, 486, 569, 631. (This article contains extensive references to previous papers. There are also many articles of a later date.)

[2] I. Reichborn-Kjennerud, 'The School of Salerno and Surgery in the North during the Saga Age'. *Ann. Med. Hist.*, 1937, n.s. ix, 321–37.

[3] I. Reichborn-Kjennerud, F. Grön, and F. Kobro, *Medisinens historie i Norge*. Oslo, 1936.

[4] A. Bugge, *Vesterlandenes indflydelse paa Nordboernes og særlig Nordmændenes ydre Kultur, Levesaet og Samfundsforhold i Vikingetiden*. Kristiania, 1905.

Up to a few years ago no trephined skull had been found in this country. In 1939 Anders Nummedal, the Norwegian archaeologist, found such a skull in old graves dating from the Neolithic Age, and the discovery shows several points of interest. The skull was found in the most northern part of Norway in the district of Finnmark. The actual place was Nyelv in the parish of Nesseby near Vadsö. The skull was examined and described in detail by K. E. Schreiner, a professor at the University of Oslo.[5]

It is well known that over a period of many years numerous prehistoric trephined crania were unearthed in Sweden and Denmark as well as in Spain, Germany, Austria and Scotland. What is of particular interest is the site at which the Norwegian skull was found, when compared with similar Swedish and Danish finds. The Swedish sites are in south Sweden or in the southern part of the area of mid-Sweden. According to Professor V. Fürst of Lund, in every trephined skull which was examined the operation was done for a therapeutic purpose. In Sweden only one or perhaps two skulls date from the Stone Age, while in Denmark as many as six belong to that period. From the Bronze and Iron Ages only a few cases are known in these countries. The single case from Norway dates from about 2000 B.C. The craniometric measurements of this skull show, according to K. E. Schreiner, Nordic racial characteristics, and the technique of the operation is exactly the same as that used in the Neolithic Age in Sweden and Denmark. Schreiner therefore concludes that either the skull was trephined in Finnmark, or the subject of the operation had it performed in southern Scandinavia and later finished his days travelling in Finnmark. Schreiner finds the second alternative almost unacceptable, and he concludes that the subject belonged to a Nordic Stone Age community in Finnmark. In confirmation he adduces several other archaeological discoveries in northern Norway and especially in Finnmark. Other workers have expressed different opinions on this point, but details need not be mentioned here. Relying on the discovery of the Norwegian cranium which we owe principally to Nummedal, Schreiner insists that towards the end of the Stone Age an aboriginal Nordic settlement existed in Finnmark. In further support of this argument he points out that the climate of northern Norway in the Neolithic Age was more favourable than in any later period, and living conditions were then far easier than at the present day.

It is hardly necessary to emphasize the fact that all medicine has its origin in folk-medicine. As an example we will take knowledge obtained from the effects of certain medicinal herbs, especially when it is combined with much superstitition and is based on a belief in demons and the influence of certain spirits on health and disease. It was this primitive philosophy of nature— under the name of Animism—which Edward Tylor dealt with in his *Primitive Culture.*

We must not forget that primitive people in their simple mode of thought depended largely on different types of superstition, and that while educated people of to-day look with scepticism on their 'medical art' and its childish

---

[5] K. E. Schreiner, 'Om en trepaneret Finnmarkskalle fra Steinalderen'. *Institutt for sammen-lignende Kulturforskning*, Oslo, 1940, civ, 3 ff. (Contains a survey of Swedish and Danish literature on trephination, p. 18.)

conceptions, the medicine of the present day owes some of its more valuable therapeutic agents to primitive peoples. Quinine and cocaine may be taken as examples. In particular, even from the earliest stages of man's evolution, the surgical operations which are known from prehistoric skeletons show surprising ability on the part of the operators. Trephination is probably the best example. Our conclusions on the performance of this operation by prehistoric man are influenced by reports of explorers on its performance by the least-developed of the surviving primitive races. On the other hand, in historic times we can point out influences originating from other more advanced nations, and so far as the Norwegian people are concerned, an effort to do so will be made in this essay. It should, however, be recalled that Oswald Cockayne, in his great work *Leechdoms, Wortcunning and Starcraft of Early England*, which was published as early as 1864–6, repeatedly points out the influence of Anglo-Saxons on old Norwegian folk-medicine, and a partial influence also in the opposite direction. Not only does he quote several of the Elder Edda poems, especially *Hávamál*, *Sigrdrifumál* and others, but also *Njáls Saga*, *Heimskringla*, *Harald Hårfagres Saga*, and *Olav Tryggvasons Saga*. In one passage he says that 'The triumphant barbarians'—as he calls the Vikings—'must have employed herbs before their pouring down over the south seems indisputable, and leeches are not only Teutonic in the form of their name, but are mentioned as driving a profession in the rudest ages' (i, preface, p. xxvii). In this connexion he quotes the famous verse in *Sigrdrifumál*: 'Branch-runes you must know if you want to be a leech and understand healing of wounds. On bark you shall draw them and in the wood on the branches leaning towards East.' Thus he is referring to the 'magic of runes'. Cockayne also quotes extensively (i, preface, p. xxxvi) the tale of the *Ynglinge Saga* about King Vanlande who dies from nightmare. Our word 'mara' is derived from Anglo-Saxon 'mare' (English, 'nightmare'), and it is found in Old Norse also in *Kormaks Saga* (p. 63). But the scald Kormak who died about A.D. 970 had been to Britain and to Ireland.

In the following discussion of some phases from our ancient folk-medicine, it should first be stated that the oldest Old Norse word for physician, 'læknir', is derived from the verb 'lækna' taken from the Anglo-Saxon 'læcnian'; while the later Old Norse word for physician, 'læknari', originated from the Middle High German 'lachenære', 'one who blesses'.[6]

As is well known, Iceland was peopled and colonized from Norway, especially western Norway. The old Norwegian and Icelandic cultures were therefore in general the same. It was the descendants of the old settlers who created the Saga literature, even if some natives of Norway also wrote Sagas. Thus the famous Leiv Erikson, author of *Eirik Raude Saga* and discoverer of 'Vinland' (America) about A.D. 1000, was the son of a native Norwegian, Eirik Raude Torvaldsson, discoverer of Greenland, who was born in Jaederen, Norway. During the reign of King Harald Hårfagre towards the end of the ninth century, there was an invasion of early settlers and Irish monks then living in Iceland. They fled from the Norwegians. Some of the latter had come via Britain and Ireland and brought with them

[6] Reichborn-Kjennerud *et al.*, *op. cit.* (3), p. 3.

Irish thralls to Iceland. Some Celtic words from this period are still preserved in the Norwegian language to-day; for example, 'skjaðak', a poisonous herb, which is the so-called 'svimling' (*Lolium temulentum*), the English bearded darnel. It is pointed out by the Norwegian professor Carl Marstrander that this word came to Norway from Ireland in olden times.[7] The word is the Irish adjective 'scethach', meaning 'which causes to vomit'. A peculiar fact is that this Irish word is found as early as in the original *Kongespeilet* (*Speculum regale*) and in the Old Icelandic Bishop's Saga, which indicates that the bishops used to consecrate the ale to make it potable. It should be noted that the bearded darnel is poisonous. Much later in Norwegian literature we hear of poisoning by 'skjæks' ale, and even as late as 1858 a serious case of poisoning by bearded darnel was known in Norway. This plant was considered to be harmful by the Greeks and the Romans and is repeatedly referred to by Pliny, Virgil and Ovid. Hence, even if the word for *Lolium temulentum* in our language is derived from an old Irish word, it is not certain that the knowledge of the poisonous properties of the plant came to Norway from Ireland in past ages, though this is a possibility. In Old Norse, as we have said, the plant is called 'skjaðak', and it is found in our grain fields as a weed. It has been supposed that the phrase 'klinte in the wheat' (English, cockle) in the Bible refers to this plant. In our language the name of this plant is also used for *Agrostemma githago*, another weed. While the name of a plant like 'skjaðak' only signifies an injurious herb, we find in our oldest literature, the Elder Edda poems, healing herbs jointly called 'urt alls viþar', the leaves of all kinds of trees in *Guðrúnarkviða*.

In the following we shall proceed to quote some extracts from the Elder Edda poems—in all there are about forty of them—and it is well to bear in mind that they are partly mythical and partly heroic. They were written in the Viking Age (*c.* A.D. 800–1050) either in Norway, in Iceland, or even in the British Isles. The old literary dispute between men of letters, represented on one side by the Norwegian professor Sophus Bugge and on the other by the Icelandic professor Finnur Jónsson, is now almost over. Jónsson asserted that the poems originated in heathen times, probably about the tenth century.[8] The poems convey much of the manner of thought and attitude to life which were found in the Viking Age. The most remarkable poem in its field is the *Hávamál*[9] which reflects the growth of religious conceptions, and this work is of particular interest in connexion with the subject of this article, as the medical views of our ancestors are expressed in short and pertinent verses. The most famous stanza (No. 137) reads in prose translation as follows: 'I advise you, Loddfafne, but you follow the advice. It will do you good if you remember it. Wherever you drink ale, choose the power of the earth. Because earth is a remedy against the drunkenness of ale, but fire against disease, oak against "blod-sótt" [tenesmus], corn-ear against witchcraft, helder against grudge, invoke the moon; use earthworm against "bitsótt" [sickness from bite]; against misfortunes use

[7] Reichborn-Kjennerud, *Vår gamle trolldomsmedisin*. Oslo, 1940, vol. iii, p. 153.

[8] Finnur Jónsson, *Den oldnorske og oldislandske Litteraturs Historie*. Copenhagen, 1894, vol. i, p. 230 ff.

[9] *Die Lieder der älteren Edda, herausgeben von Karl Hildebrand*. Second edition, by G. Gering. Paderborn, 1904, p. 53.

runes. The earth will absorb the moist.' Let us comment on these methods of treatment.

It should be said that this part of the *Hávamál* probably dates from the latter part of the ninth century and has its origin in Norway. It is difficult to give a linguistic interpretation of the stanza as a whole, but the attempt of Reichborn-Kjennerud to interpret it from the medico-historical aspect is of interest.[10] The present author has also tried to interpret it from this angle.[11] It may be supposed that the lines 'Wherever you drink ale, choose the power of the earth' are logically related to the last line 'The earth shall absorb the moist'. Beyond doubt reference is made to ale of bearded darnel, as previously mentioned. In other words, the remedy for ale mixed with 'skjaðak' is to take 'earth' acting as an emetic; that which is vomited, 'the moist, is absorbed by the earth'. We may also recall the use of terra sigillata in ancient medicine. We have references to this in an Icelandic medical book dating from the thirteenth century.[12] There it says: 'The earth on which is impressed a seal and on which there is an image of man, is good against worm-bite. . . And if you have taken a poisonous drink, you shall drink of the earth. It expells the poison.' In this connexion we may refer to the therapeutic use of substances such as salt, saltpetre and clay by primitive peoples. Dioscorides in his materia medica refers to 'earth from Samos'.

Still another prescription in the *Hávamál* (stanza 137) merits special mention, namely, the words 'beiti við bitsóttum', which have been variously translated and interpreted. The most probable interpretation is that of Reichborn-Kjennerud: 'earthworm against sickness from bite.' The ordinary earthworm (*Lumbricus terrestris*) was supposed to be used against a disease caused by 'bites', whether of real or hypothetical animals, 'because', says Reichborn-Kjennerud, 'ancient peoples thought that wounds and pains of unknown cause, as well as exanthema and boils, were due to the bites of animals'. This cure originated in classical times (Dioscorides, Pliny and later Marcellus Empiricus). However, it is of interest to note that in one of the Anglo-Saxon medical books referred to by Cockayne, crushed earthworm is recommended in a rather peculiar manner.[13] 'If sinews are cut through, take worms, pound them well, lay on till the sinews be restored.' The use of the earthworm, especially as earthworm oil, has been continuous even up to our own time.

We may deal more briefly with the other medical recommendations mentioned in stanza 137, even though they may point to foreign influence. The fourth line ('Fire against disease') unquestionably reminds one of the wide use of the cautery for various diseases in classical medicine. We may also mention the method called 'Nothfeuer' by the Teutons, that is, the use of smoke for expelling the demons of diseases. Bartels comprehensibly refers to this as something well known to primitive peoples.[14] Grimm in his

---

[10] Reichborn-Kjennerud *et al.*, *op. cit.* (3), pp. 14 ff.

[11] F. Grön, 'Bidrag til den norröne lægekunsts historie'. *Tidsskrift for Den norske Lægeforening*, 1907, særtrykk (reprint), pp. 10 ff.

[12] K. Gislason, 44 *Prövir af oldnordisk Sprog og Literatur*. Copenhagen, 1860, p. 472.

[13] O. Cockayne, *Leechdoms*, etc. London, 1864–6, vol. iii, p. 329.

[14] M. C. A. Bartels, *Die Medizin der Naturvölker*. Leipzig, 1893, p. 191.

Deutsche Mythologie also mentions that the smoke from Nothfeuer was considered as curative.[15] By 'oak' must be meant the bark of the oak or perhaps the fruit. If we assume that 'abbindi' means dysentery—a point which we will discuss later—we cannot be surprised that oak is recommended because of its astringent qualities. Further, Dragendorff states:[16] 'Schon im Altertum sind Eichen und ihre Teile sonst häufig in der Medizin benutzt worden.' Eventually we learn from another Edda poem, *Guðrunarkviða* (II, stanza 22),[17] that 'burnt oak nut' is used as a drink to produce oblivion; the acorn is described as being harmful, together with various particular substances such as 'hearth's dew' (that is, soot), intestines of animals offered in sacrifice, and boiled hog's liver—in other words substances whose effects are based merely on superstition.

As might be expected, several of the methods of treatment mentioned in the Edda poems are purely magical. It is also easy to understand that the Old Norse language has a special word for disease caused by witchcraft. The word is 'gerningasótt', derived directly from 'gerningar' (or 'gjörningar'), performance of witchcraft, and 'sótt', disease. This word is found repeatedly in the Old Norse-Icelandic literature, both in legal phraseology, as for example Borgarthings and in Viken's *Christian Court* (*Kristenrett*, I, 16), and also in the language of the Sagas. Thus the word is found in Saint Olav's Saga (*Fornmanna sögur*, V, p. 326), where one of the men of the king, Egil Halisson, is stated to have contracted 'sótt' by witchcraft. It is there even called by name, 'hjartverkr', which is a disease of the heart ('cardialgia'), and the duration of the illness is given as half-a-day to two days. King Olav, however, cures his men. Of course, he possessed healing power. Also, we get some partial knowledge of the nature of the magical practices. 'Runes' were the oldest form of writing in the north—'galdrar', that is, witchcraft, and songs or formulae of exorcism, also called 'seiðr' (equally one of the forms of witchcraft). These forms of witchcraft may be applied to cause as well as to cure disease. It may further be noted that, in the many rune writings which were preserved and interpreted by Sophus Bugge and Magnus Olsen, there is no word for 'physician'. This in spite of the fact that several titles of social positions are on record, such as 'gode' (priest), 'styresmann' (county sheriff) and 'bryde' (administrator of property). It may be a pure accident that no special word for a 'physician' was used in the runes, but it is more probable that at that time the spoken language did not include such a word. Further, in two places in the Elder Edda the word 'læknir' is found. One is in *Hávamál* (stanza 148) where Oden talks about himself: 'That I know, for the second, as sons of Man need, those who want to live as a leech.' In this verse, the second half-stanza is lost, and Sophus Bugge explains that it is by the laying on of hands that Oden cures.[18] The other place in the Elder Edda where the word is found is in *Sigrdrifumál* (stanza 10), where the word is found in connexion with rune magic. This passage emphasizes the necessity of treating wounds.

---

[15] J. L. C. Grimm, *Deutsche Mythologie*. Göttingen, 1843–4, p. 574.
[16] G. L. N. Dragendorff, *Die Heilpflanzen*. Stuttgart, 1898, pp. 560 ff.
[17] *op. cit.* (9), p. 376.
[18] S. Bugge, *Studier over de nordiske Gude—og Heltesagns Oprindelse*. Christiania, 1881–9.

From this we may probably conclude that the original meaning of the word 'læknir' is equivalent to what we might call a 'wound-healer'. This in itself is reasonable and comprehensible when we recall the warlike life of the Vikings. Further, we must remember that the primitive art of medicine probably began with the art of a 'wound-healer'. This is confirmed by the early appearance of trephination in the Neolithic Age. This does not mean that treatment by wild herbs and parts of animals may not be very old. If we may be permitted to draw conclusions from the apes closely related to man, we may instance a kind of 'wound-healer' among them. From this again, we may venture to conclude that the earliest prehistoric men tried at first by mere instinct to heal wounds by sucking them, and by pressing the edges together to stop the bleeding.

The rune magic, as seen for example in the *Sigrdrifumål* (stanzas 8 and 10), is worthy of note. Here more specific directions are given, both on the manner of writing the runes, and on their use in certain diseases. They are said to be useful both in obstetrics and for the treatment of wounds. Stanza 8 says: 'Aiding-runes you shall know, if you wish to help in delivering women [Old Norse, 'leysa kind frá konum']. They shall be drawn on the palm of the hand and the helper shall tighten around the wrist.' In stanza 10 already quoted, it is said: 'Branch-runes you must know if you want to be a leech and understand the healing of wounds. On bark you shall draw them, on branches leaning towards the East.' On the other hand we also learn that runes are believed to be harmful to a high degree, as in one place in the *Grettis Saga*.[19] The witch Turid, whose thigh bone Grettir has broken with a blow from a stone, takes revenge on Grettir in the following way: 'She took her knife and drew runes on the tree and tinted it red with her blood and said magic words.' Here her revenge is to be effected by a combination of runes and tinting with blood. And so it happens; Grettir injures his foot on the root of the tree and the wound provokes a disease which later causes his death. We would now say that he contracted an infection from which he died.

The expression 'oak against "blod-sótt"' in stanza 137 of the *Håvamål* reads in the Old Norse 'eik vid abbindi'. It is the last word which is peculiar. Lexicographers like Fritzner and Egilsson in his *Lexicon poeticum*, and Cleasby and Vigfusson in their *Icelandic-English Dictionary*, have translated this word by 'stoltvang or tenesmus'. The late Professor Alf Torp, the Norwegian classical scholar and etymologist, said that the word 'abbindi' was the same as 'af-bindi', from a verb 'binda af', signifying hindrance, abstention. In an article on the Icelandic names of diseases Svein Pálsson, however, defines the meaning thus: 'Afbendi (Tenesmus) er, þegar manni finnz sér vera sifelt mál at gánga þarfinda sinna, en litit eitt verdr ágengt',[20] which means: 'Afbindi: used when there is a continuous straining at stool with little result'. This must be taken as a direct description of the painful 'tenesmi ad anum' and it is natural to think of dysentery. The interesting thing about the word 'abbindi' is that it is unquestionably derived from the Anglo-Saxon 'ebind', and the word therefore must

---

[19] *Grettis Saga Ásmundarsonar, herausgeg. von R. C. Boer.* Halle, 1900, pp. 274 ff.
[20] *Rit þez Komúngliga Islenzka Lardóms–Lista Félags*, Copenhagen, 1788 [1789], ix, 185.

have been taken up in Old Norse as a mere literary word together with the disease it describes. Accordingly, we must assume that the disease dysentery came to this country from England in the Viking Age. This view is supported when we read what the Danish professor Steenstrup says about the 'saga of the Norsemen's forces destroyed by dysentery'.[21] This event was supposed to have taken place in the year A.D. 845. Further, Saxo Grammaticus talks about 'profluvium ventris' during the Viking raid of Ragnar Lodbrok on Bjarmeland (that is, the land by the White Ocean), probably about A.D. 700, an event which is now believed to have been merely legendary. A Latin narrative of the disease of A.D. 845 calls it simply 'dysenteria morbus', and it goes on to say that an untold number of Norsemen brought the disease back with them when they returned home. Also, it is known that Ansgar, called the Apostle of the North, who was, however, never in Norway, died from a bloody flux. It should be noted that he died in Bremen. All these facts point to the belief that dysentery in the Viking Age was a common disease in Norway. It was known in the early centuries of the Christian era and is especially described by Aretaeus of Cappadocia. What is of peculiar interest to us in this connexion is that we presumably imported the disease to Norway from England in the Viking Age, a supposition which in itself is not unreasonable, even though there is no historical proof. The word 'abbindi', derived from the Anglo-Saxon 'ebind', makes this view probable, however, since the name leprosy, 'likþrá', from the Anglo-Saxon 'þrowere', points in the same direction. But, as we shall now see, there is more historical proof in the case of leprosy than in the case of dysentery.

Let us now look a little more closely at the history of leprosy in Norway, since the disease was probably imported from the British Isles in the Viking Age. In support of this view we have first of all the Old Norse name for the disease, 'likþrá', and the adjective 'likþrar', leprous. This word is taken directly from the Anglo-Saxon 'likþrowere'—one who suffers from 'likþrá', or a leper. The fundamental meaning of the adjective 'likþrowere' is 'he who suffers on his body', from the word 'þrowian', to suffer. It is worthy of note that the word 'likþrá' is not found in any of the Edda poems or the ordinary Sagas, while it is found in two places in the famous *Kongespeilet* (*Speculum regale*),[22] which was written in Norway about 1250. In one place the word is used to describe the disease by which Job was struck by God. Of greater interest is a mention of the large marine animals found near Iceland. This reads as follows: 'It is also said that if a man could get hold of its sperm (*rörhvalens*, or in Old Norse, *reydr*) without his knowing that it came from this whale or from other whales, then this sperm would be the surest medicine both for the eyes, and for leprosy and fever, as well as headaches and all diseases by which Man is afflicted.' The remedy mentioned is what in Old Norse is called 'hvals-auki' (that is, spermaceti). But it is more probable that the reference is to ambergris, as in the corresponding Danish word 'hwalsøky', which in the thirteenth-century medical work of the Dane Henrik Harpestreng is simply called 'amra'. This is a preparation made

[21] J. C. H. R. Steenstrup, *Normannerne*. 4 vols. Copenhagen, 1876–82, vol. i, pp. 97 ff., and specially p. 102, note.

[22] *Konungsskuggsjá*. Kristiania, 1848, p. 32.

from the gut of the cachalot whale, and in the Middle Ages it was a medicine of high repute. Otherwise the word 'likþrá' appears repeatedly in the Sagas of the Icelandic Bishops where their lives, covering the years A.D. 1056 to 1330, are described. There are frequent references to the treatment of diseases in these Sagas. Several cases of leprosy are dealt with more extensively, as in the following example: 'Tjörve a man was called. He suffered from a bad disease in his hands. They grew stiff and leprous in such a way that he could not straighten any of his fingers, and this condition had lasted fifteen years.'[23] Here one may accept the diagnosis even though the description is very incomplete.

We believe the word 'likþrá' is quite a frequent one in the Old Norse and Icelandic literatures. The Norwegian professor Alexander Bugge has the following statement on the passage of leprosy from the British Isles to Norway: 'In England and especially in Ireland the Norsemen got to know leprosy as a terrible disease, which they had to try to combat by all means. As early as 921 when King Gudröd of Dublin plundered Armagh in Ulster, the Irish year-book expressly says that he spared "the houses of prayer where the men of God and the lepers stayed". Evidently little time elapsed before leper hospitals were built around the Irish Sea in the Viking settlements. Further south in Cumberland, where the Furness peninsula juts out into the sea, lies Loppergarth, and here according to the Saga a hospital for lepers stood in olden times. This must have been erected by Norsemen, because Loppergarth is a Norse name, meaning "Lepragaard" (lepers' house). The last syllable is the Norwegian "gaard" (house, property); the first is old Irish "lobran", Gaelic "lobhar", meaning sick, especially leprous. From Iceland and Scotland knowledge of the treatment of lepers spread to the Faeroe Isles, where on the bay of Lobbra on Suder Island there was supposed to be a leper hospital.'[24]

This statement of Bugge is in favour of the view that the Vikings at an early stage of their invasions became acquainted with leprosy, and of the probability that the disease was brought to the western part of Norway from the British Isles by this route. The whole question is dealt with by Norwegian, Icelandic and Danish authors, and it is not possible to go further into detail in this article. A most comprehensive treatment of the whole question exists in a manuscript dealing with *The History of Leprosy in Norway* by the late H. P. Lie, the well-known Norwegian leprosy specialist who was formerly Secrétaire générale pour l'Occident de la Societé internationale de Leprologie. (The manuscript is not yet printed, but it is in the possession of the author of this article, and extracts from it were sent to the Congress in Cairo in 1938 under the title of 'From the History of Leprosy in Norway'. It is hoped that the manuscript will be printed *in extenso* at a later date.)

In conclusion it may be worth while to emphasize the fact that Cockayne, even in his time, could instance the direct use of the Old Norse language and Old Norse expressions in the Anglo-Saxon language. For example, in the preface to his *Leechdoms* he says: 'Perhaps in dissecting the curious mosaic work of this Leechbook, we may be as much struck by the Old Dansk,

---

[23] *Biskupasögur.* 2 vols. Kaupmannahöfn, vol. i, 1858, p. 115.
[24] Alexander Bugge, *Vikingerne.* Copenhagen-Christiania, 1904–6, vol. ii, p. 340.

or as people now say, Norse element in the words Torbegete, Rudniolin, Ons worm, and the herb Fornets palm, as by its Irish admixture, or its Greek and Latin basis, or its fragments from King Ælfreds handbook.'[25] Let us look more closely at some of these words. The first syllable 'Tor' of the word 'Torbegete' is found in combinations of words in the Old Norse language[26] and the whole word means 'difficult to get'. More interesting are the two names of plants, 'Rudniolin' and 'Fornets palm'. The first is the plant *Polygonum hydropiper*; 'nioli' means a hollow stalk, and 'rud' means 'red'. The plant is called in Norwegian 'vasspepper' (water pepper), and it has a burning taste of pepper. In English it is called 'Redshank' or as the Norwegian, 'Water pepper'. In the *Leechdoms* (III, 1, viii) it is recommended 'against temptation of the fiend.' It should be worn or placed under the pillow and over the door of the house. Then no evil spirits can cause any harm. In other words, a purely magic 'medical advice'. 'Fornets palm' is probably *Orchis maculata*. The name is derived from an Old Norse giant called Fornjotr.

A parallel state of affairs is seen when we consider Old Danish writings. The Dane Marius Kristensen[27] referred to many Danish medical expressions derived from Anglo-Saxon. The word 'blotætæræ' comes from the Old English 'blodlætere', and refers to the person who performs 'årelating' (blood-letting). 'Bryn' is Anglo-Saxon 'bryne', that is, a disease of the body, and in Danish the word means a more or less serious wound. Compare also the word 'gund' from Old English 'Gund' (pus, mucilage). Also, names of several medical herbs are directly transferred, such as 'Thung', the Anglo-Saxon 'þung', which means hellebore. A peculiar expression for the name of a disease, 'Anaþyrm', that is Ons Worm, is also found in the Anglo-Saxon *Leechbook*. As Cockayne showed, it refers to a narrative in the *Ynglinge Saga* (chapter 25),[28] which deals with a king called Aun or Aane who ruled over the Swedes. He is said to have sacrificed his nine sons, one after another, to Oden. As he was about to sacrifice his tenth son in order to prolong his own life, the Swedes refused to grant his request and Aane died. Concerning this, Cockayne writes: 'It was afterwards called On-sickness when a man died from old age without agony.' This story must have passed over to Anglo-Saxon from Norwegian.

All this evidence strongly indicates that Norway very early received distinct traces of a popular medicine, partly from magical and partly from more practical sources. Unfortunately, there is no definite evidence for this thesis. What is obvious is that the active relations between Norway and the British Isles left deep impressions on the popular medicine of both countries. Another question is whether any traces of Graeco-Roman medicine flowed into Norway through her relations with the British Isles. If we ignore the period of the migrations, this route would be the only one possible for the spread of such an influence. With reference to these migrations, Norwegian

[25] Cockayne, *op. cit.* (13), vol. ii, p. xxxii.

[26] *Old Laws of Norway*, Glossary, p. 647.

[27] M. Kristensen, *Fremmedordene i det ældste danske Skriftsprog (før omtrent 1300).* Copenhagen, 1906, p. 23.

[28] Snorre Sturlason, *Kongesagaer*, trans. G. Storm. Kristiania, 1900, p. 27.

warriors unquestionably played a part in the invasion of South Europe by the Teutonic tribes. It is possible that returning warriors may have brought with them fragments of the old medical art of the citizens of the Roman Empire. But on this point there is no evidence whatever, and any opinion must be the merest guesswork.

GENERAL MEDICAL PRACTICE IN ANGLO-SAXON ENGLAND

by

WILFRID BONSER

THE Anglo-Saxon period stretches from the middle of the fifth century to the middle of the eleventh. Conditions, and our knowledge of them, naturally vary considerably during these six hundred years. For the earlier period Bede is almost our only authority, but fortunately he gives most valuable information on cures effected in his day. But since the manuscripts containing those prescriptions which have survived date mostly from the tenth and eleventh centuries, the picture of Anglo-Saxon medical practice will be truer and more complete for these than for the earlier periods.

The art of curing the sick as well as the duty of caring for them was almost entirely in the hands of the Church in Anglo-Saxon times.

One may assume from the words of Bede that medical manuscripts—if not Hippocrates and Galen, certainly Isidore who derived from them—were among those which Benedict Biscop brought with him from Rome to enrich his two monasteries of Monkwearmouth and Jarrow. Others had no doubt found their way to this country, thanks to the zeal of men like Saint Wilfrid, to be stored in other monasteries. It follows that the Church possessed the book-knowledge of medicine that existed at the time. It was therefore natural that it had power and authority where the practice of medicine was concerned, even though the folk possessed the practical knowledge of herbal and other remedies which had been handed down verbally from one generation to another.

Thus the Church gave official sanction to medical practice, and made it effective in the eyes of the patients, both lay and clerical. Its prayers were requisitioned for the sick, its blessing was attached to prescriptions, its relics were used as media for cures, and wells had to be blessed by it before their water could be used for healing purposes.

It was inculcated by the Church that disease was a punishment incurred as the result of sin. As one of its functions was for the forgiveness of sin after due repentance, it followed logically that it was for the Church also to remove and to cure the disease. A typical description of such an illness and cure occurs in the anonymous *Life of St. Cuthbert*: 'There came some women bearing a certain youth who lay on a litter; they carried him to . . . the holy bishop . . . adjuring him in the name of our Lord Jesus Christ that he would bless him with his holy relics and would utter a prayer for him to the Lord, beseeching God's pardon for the sins by which he was bound and on account of which he endured punishment. So the bishop . . . prayed . . . and blessing the boy, he drove away the disease and restored him to health.'[1]

As disease was regarded as a supernatural visitation, supernatural means were naturally used to avert and cure it. It was a function of a saint, following

---

[1] B. Colgrave, *Two Lives of Saint Cuthbert*. Cambridge, 1940, pp. 117–19 (*Vita auct. anon.*, iv. 5). It will be noted that the disease from which the youth was suffering is not given a name. The motive of the writer was to portray the power and holiness of his saint; the medical aspect was of no importance to him.

in the footsteps of Christ Himself, to cure the sick. The pages of Bede, Eddius Stephanus, and others show that the Anglo-Saxon saints nobly did their share in this work. The most successful cures were probably those of functional disorders, and were accomplished by means of faith and suggestion. A blessing at the hands of a living saint, such as Saint Cuthbert, Saint Guthlac, or Saint John of Beverley might well be sufficient in such cases to effect a cure; or it might be accomplished by a priest of less pronounced personality and reputation through the instrumentality of relics and rites. Each cure would naturally be regarded as a miracle, and as such it directed the attention both of the patient and of the onlookers to the spiritual side. It may be also that men like Cuthbert, after a life of extreme asceticism and contemplation, possessed sympathetic powers which amounted to a kind of hypnotic influence.

But in some cases a saint would use practical common-sense in addition to any call upon the faith of his patient. For instance, Bede gives details of the cure of a case of aphasia by Saint John of Beverley by means of mechanical exercises. 'The bishop . . . caused the poor man to come in to him, and ordered him to put his tongue out of his mouth and show it to him; then laying hold of his chin, he made the sign of the cross on his tongue, directing him to draw it back into his mouth and to speak. "Pronounce some word", said he, "say gae" [yes] . . . He immediately said what was ordered.' The bishop then made him say all the letters of the alphabet, followed by syllables, words and finally sentences, continuing the exercises all the day and the next night.[2]

Relics were the usual instruments employed by the Church for curative purposes; the success of this means depended still more on the amount of faith possessed by each patient. Sometimes the cure seems to have been complete, as, for instance, in the case of a saintly-minded priest who, according to Bede, was restored to health through communion with the spirit of Saint Cuthbert. He prayed for recovery from a long illness at Saint Cuthbert's tomb, and 'felt that he had received throughout his body such a great power from the saint's incorrupt body that he rose from his prayer without exertion and returned to the guest-house without the aid of his attendant or of his staff. A few days later he proceeded on his journey *roborata ad integrum virtute*.'[3]

As the Anglo-Saxon period advanced, healing by means of relics became a stereotyped 'business'. A technique was evolved both for the preservation of the bodies of saints, that is, the relics themselves, and also for extracting 'virtue' from them so that they might be used for healing purposes. Eddius Stephanus, speaking of the death of Saint Wilfrid at Ripon, says: 'They put up a tent outside the monastery, bathed the holy body, and emptied the bath on to the ground in the same place. The people who inhabited the monastery afterwards built a wooden cross on the spot, and the Lord used to perform many marvels there.'[4] The earth, hallowed by the water in which the saint's body had been washed, had become endowed with healing 'virtue' and thus became the medium for future cures. Similarly,

[2] Bede, *Ecclesiastical History*, v. 2.
[3] *idem*, *Life of St. Cuthbert* [in prose], 44.
[4] Eddius Stephanus, *Life of Bishop Wilfrid*, 66.

Bede tells how 'many took up the dust of the very place where [Saint Oswald's] body fell, and putting it into water did much good with it to their friends who were sick. This custom came so much into use that, the earth being carried away by degrees, there remained a hole as deep as the height of a man '.[5]

At the end of the period many places in England must have played the part which is now played by Lourdes. Such were the shrines of Saint Alban at St. Albans and Saint Swithun at Winchester. Ælfric gives many details of cures at Winchester. 'Within ten days two hundred men were healed, and so many within twelve months that no man could count them. The burial ground lay filled with crippled folk, so that people could hardly get into the minster; and they were all so miraculously healed within a few days, that no one could find there five unsound men of that great crowd'. He speaks of the votive offerings in the church: 'The old church was hung all round with crutches (*mid criccum*), and with the stools of cripples who had been healed there, from one end to the other on either wall, and not even so could they put half of them up.'[6]

Apart from functional disorders, which might have been those most amenable to treatment by the means at the Church's disposal, there was one disease whose cure was its special function. There were seven orders of priests, to one of which, exorcists, was assigned the duty of expelling 'devils' from those possessed by them. A series of prayers was prescribed for this purpose. If exorcism was of no avail and the devil was obstinate, more drastic measures were taken. A recipe in the third *Leechbook* (§ xl) prescribes: 'If a man be *mónaþ-seóc*, take the skin of a porpoise, make it into a whip, beat the man with it: he will soon be well.'

In the earlier part of the Anglo-Saxon period relics were resorted to if exorcism was of no avail. Bede mentions a cure effected by the instrumentality of those of Saint Oswald. There came a guest to Bardney Abbey 'who was wont often in the night to be on a sudden grievously tormented with an evil spirit. He was hospitably received, and after supper lay down on a couch. Then he was suddenly siezed by a devil and began to shout and grind his teeth, and to foam at the mouth, and he began to twist his limbs with all sorts of movements. None being able to hold or bind him, a servant ran and . . . acquainted the abbess. She . . . calling a priest, desired he would go with her to the sufferer. . . . The priest chanted and recited exorcisms and did all that he could to allay the fury of the wretched man; but he produced no effect in spite of all his exertions'. The abbess then sent a servant for some of the dust on which had been spilt the water in which Saint Oswald's bones had been washed, and as soon as it arrived in the room, 'he was suddenly silent and laid down his head as if released for sleep, stretching out all his limbs at rest'. After a time he fetched a deep sigh, and said that he was restored to his senses. 'Then the abbess gave him a little of that dust'—presumably in case of a relapse—'and the priest prayed for him, and he spent

⁵ Bede, *op. cit.* (2), iii. 9.   Also, W. Bonser, 'The Magic of St. Oswald'. *Antiquity*, 1935, ix, 418–23.
⁶ Ælfric, *Lives of the Saints*. Ed. W. W. Skeat. Oxford, vol. i, 1881, § xxi, ll. 149–55, 431–34.

a most quiet night. Nor from that time onwards did he suffer any fear or vexation from his ancient enemy.'[7]

There was, however, one branch of the profession which did not appertain to the Church, and that was surgery. *A sanguine abhorret Ecclesia.* Bede's story of the illness of Saint Etheldrida illustrates the separation of the Church from the practice of surgery. He states that the *medicus* Cynifrid was called in by the ecclesiastics, and performed the operation on the saint which the ecclesiastics themselves could not perform. He therefore must have been a layman.[8]

The names of at least four leeches—in addition to Cynifrid—who practised in Anglo-Saxon times are known. The most distinguished was Baldwin of Chartres, who became 'royal physician' to Edward the Confessor. At least one cure at his hands is recorded, that of Leofstan, abbot of Bury, who was suffering from paralysis. The others are Bald, the possessor of the first two *Leechbooks*, whose name occurs in the colophon of the second; Oxa, who prescribed a recipe for the disease called *þeór-ádl* in chapter 47 of the first *Leechbook*; and Dun, who prescribed one for lung disease in chapter 65 of the second *Leechbook*. But whether the last three were clerics or laymen is not mentioned. The occurrence of the word *læce-feoh*—a physician's fee—suggests the beginning of the craft, if not yet the profession, of medicine.

What has been said so far seems but to demonstrate the prevalent ignorance with regard to medicine, and also the futility of most of the measures prescribed. Anglo-Saxon medicine belongs to the Dark Ages, when the spirit of enquiry which had prevailed in classical times had given way to barren formulae. Most leeches were content to copy dead material without questioning its value or its authority. 'It is the wondering and questioning of men like Alfred', says R. H. Hodgkin, 'which was to lead mankind through the accumulated rubbish of unscientific ages to knowledge.'

Two difficulties faced the leeches of that pre-scientific age; firstly, ignorance of causation, and secondly ignorance of the right methods of treatment. The Anglo-Saxons derived their etiology chiefly from classical and post-classical and from native Teutonic sources, apart from what it derived from the body of Church medicine already spoken of. Dr. Singer has written at length of these theories in his paper on *Early English Magic and Medicine*, which I heard him deliver to the British Academy in 1920, and which was my first introduction to this subject. He there says that the 'philosophical basis' of the medicine of the Dark Ages 'is the doctrine of the four elements and the four humours; a view which finds ample illustration in English manuscripts. In the belief of the men of the Dark Ages there was a close relation between the external and the internal world, the macrocosm and the microcosm; and so they discerned a parallel between the four ages of man and the four seasons, between the humours of the body and the solstices and equinoxes, between the four elements and the four cardinal points, and so on'. To amplify the above quotation, the Anglo-Saxons retained among their ideas of the constitution of the human body the Hippocratic doctrine of the four humours, blood, phlegm, black and yellow (or red) bile (*cholera nigra*

---

[7] Bede, *op. cit.* (2), iii. 11.

[8] *idem, ibid.,* iv. 19.

and *cholera rubra*). The predominance of any of these influenced a man's temperament; that of the first-named inclined him to be sanguine in his nature, that of the second to be phlegmatic, that of the third to be melancholic, and that of the fourth to be choleric.

Combined with the four humours, two and two in each case, were Aristotle's four fundamental qualities, the hot, the cold, the wet, and the dry. Physiology and even diet were considered to be governed by such formulae; thus digestion involved the combined operation of the hot and the wet. Section xxvii of the second *Leechbook* deals with 'the various nature of the *wamb* (stomach) and its imperfection, how a man may recognise it.' It deals with the *wamb* when it is hot, cold, or moist. The first condition digests food well, the third has a good appetite for meat but not a good digestion, but a cold *wamb* engenders disease of the brain (*brægenes-ádl*) and madness.

MS. Hunter 100, in Durham Cathedral Library, which dates from a few years after the close of the Anglo-Saxon period, has much to say on the practice of medicine as governed by these philosophical principles. Folio 16v. contains an elaborate diagram of eight intersecting arcs within a circle, designed to show the correspondence of the elements, seasons, humours, and the four ages of man.

'Native Teutonic medicine', to quote again from Dr. Singer's paper, 'may be distinguished from imported elements . . . by the presence of four characteristic elements: the doctrine of *specific venoms*, the doctrine of the *nines*, the doctrine of *the worm* as the cause of disease, and lastly the doctrine of *the elf-shot*.' He quotes the *Lay of the Nine Healing Herbs* from § 45 of the *Lacnunga* as showing how the first three of these occur therein together. These verses tell how Woden smote the serpent, and how the Nine Diseases arose from the nine fragments into which it was severed. The presence of Woden at least indicates a non-classical origin for this lay.

The source to which a great many diseases, rightly or wrongly, were ascribed in Anglo-Saxon times was worms. Apart from intestinal worms, of which a great many different varieties are mentioned in recipes, *wyrm* may be the cause of disease in the hand, in the eye, in the ear, or in the teeth. There is a collection of remedies in the first *Leechbook* (§ vi), 'if a worm eat the teeth.' In one case a candle is to be made of acorn meal and henbane-seed and wax, and lighted; 'let it smoke into the mouth; place a black cloth underneath: then the worms will fall on to it.'

The doctrine of the elf-shot is also one of the chief characteristics of Finnish magic. The Anglo-Saxons attributed the sudden attack of disease to the arrows of elves; infection—in contrast—was considered to be caused by 'flying venom'. Apparently the elves were especially addicted to shooting their arrows at the domestic animals. There are various charms for horses that have been elf-shot. In the *Lacnunga* (§ 60) is the charm: 'If a horse or other beast be shot (*gescoten*), take seed of dock and Irish wax, let a mass-priest sing twelve masses over them, and put holy water on them, and put it on the horse or what cattle soever it may be.' The word *stice* has been translated 'stitch' when used for a disease which was caused by the shots of elves or of witches. Since, however, *stice* also means 'puncture', I suggest that it signifies the hole made in the victim by the elf-shot. § liv of the second

Leechbook gives two recipes, one *wiþ instice* and the other *wiþ stice butan innoðe sie*. Possibly in the former case the elf-shot has penetrated the skin, while in the second it has failed to do so. 'The white stone', says another passage in the second *Leechbook* (§ lxiv), 'is powerful against *stice* and against flying-venom, and against all unknown maladies' —unknown, because caused by supernatural agencies or by witchcraft. The most realistic verses in the *Lacnunga* (§ 76) describing the onset of witches and their discharge of 'little spears' are a charm against *fǽr-stice* ('sudden puncture').

When Christianity came, the elves of heathendom were equated with demons, and therefore diseases caused by them were thought to be the same as demoniacal possession. The charms were therefore modified to suit, and it became necessary 'against elf-disease' to dip the herbs in hallowed water, to lay them under the altar, sing psalms and masses over them, and perform other Christian ritual —often in addition to the older heathen rites —before the drink or salve might be safely administered.[9]

The doctrine of elf-shot as a cause of disease is akin to the classical theory that pestilence was occasioned by the arrows of irate gods, and especially of Apollo. Another Anglo-Saxon theory of the cause of pestilence was also derived from the classics. Galen describes pestilence as 'a disease which attacks all, or the greater number, arising from corruption of the air with the result that great numbers perish'.[10] Bede also speaks of pestilence as being produced from the air when it has become corrupted.[11] He may have derived his idea from Galen, but more probably through the intermediary source of Isidore of Seville,[12] with whose writings he is known to have been familiar.

Perhaps another source of trouble with which the Anglo-Saxon leech had to contend arose from the agency of the disease itself which was regarded as having volition and personality. The story told by Bede of the little boy at Bardney who was suffering from *lencten-ádl* contains an example of this. One of the monks instructed him to 'go into the church, and get close to St. Oswald's tomb'. The boy did as he was bid, 'and the disease durst not affect him as he sat by the saint's tomb, but fled so absolutely, that he felt it no more'.[13] Akin to this idea is devil-possession, already mentioned. The Church formulated various theories as to how a devil might find entrance into a man. One was that he might draw it in in breathing, another that it might enter when he was asleep. Or possibly it might be absorbed with food. The following story from the *Exempla* of Jacques de Vitry illustrates this last possibility: 'Saint Gregory tells of a nun who ate a lettuce without making the sign of the cross, and swallowed a devil. When a holy man tried to exorcise him, the devil said: "What fault is it of mine? I was sitting on the lettuce, and she did not cross herself, and so ate me too" '.[14]

Since the cause of disease was in general unknown, it follows that the Anglo-Saxons were very weak with regard to diagnosis. They had no specific knowledge of the internal organs of the body or of their diseases, and in

[9] W. Bonser, 'Magical practices against elves'. *Folk-Lore*, 1926, xxxvii, 350–63.

[10] Galen, *Definitiones medicae*, cliii. Kühn, xix, p. 391.

[11] Bede, *De natura rerum*, 37 (*De Pestilentia*).

[12] Isidore of Seville, *Etymologiae*, iv. 6. § 17.

[13] Bede, *op. cit.* (2), iii. 12.

[14] Jacques de Vitry, *Exempla*, cxxx. (Folk-Lore Soc.) London, 1890.

consequence but seldom took matters in hand until, judging from the descriptions given of the symptoms, the patient was already dying and human aid was too late.

Such 'diagnosis' as there was in those days was based on written formulae and not on an understanding and consideration of the symptoms of the patient. The Durham manuscript mentioned above gives instructions for the doctor to follow, and the experienced doctor was the one who was *au fait* with the formulae. It was thought that the four humours must be maintained in a state of equilibrium in order that a man might keep in a healthy condition. 'Whenever any one of these humours increases too much', says the manuscript, 'then it causes lengthy sickness—that is, if the doctor is inexperienced or negligent, or if he does not understand the cause or [perceive] through which humour the sickness has originated. But if the doctor is discerning and is cognisant of the cause of the sickness, then he is able to be of use. If, however, he is negligent or has not understood, then he will prolong the period of the sickness until the season-during-which-that-humour-prevails shall have passed and until another of the humours has acquired control : then the influence of the humour through which the sickness was caused is removed'. In other words, the discerning doctor is able to diagnose at once what any sickness may be merely by ascertaining at what hour it began, since it must have been caused by an excess in his patient's system of the humour then dominant. He has but to counteract the excess of humour by applying the opposite as an antidote. 'If blood be the cause, then since blood is sweet, wet and hot, it is necessary that it be counter-balanced by the opposite, that is to say, cold, bitter and dry,' and so on. 'Thus,' the passage happily concludes, 'the doctor becomes experienced, and the sick man is quickly restored to health'.

A patient who found himself in the hands of the leech had but a poor chance of a speedy recovery unless possessed of a strong constitution, since the actual remedies then prescribed were not such as might be expected to be of much avail.

Isidore, speaking of the practice of medicine in general, says that 'there are three kinds of cures in all. The first is the dietetic; the second the pharmaceutical; the third the surgical. Diet is the observance of the law of life. Pharmacy is curing by medicine. Surgery is cutting with the knife; for with the knife is cut away that which does not feel the healing of medicines'.[15] This threefold division obtained in classical Greece,[16] and continued during the Dark and Middle Ages including the Anglo-Saxon period.

A great many Anglo-Saxon prescriptions and recipes have survived. The most important have been printed by Cockayne in his *Leechdoms, Wortcunning, and Starcraft of Early England* (3 vols., 1864–6) and are contained in the *Anglo-Saxon Herbal*, the three *Leechbooks*, the *Lacnunga*, and περὶ διδάξεων. These prescriptions exhibit an extensive acquaintance with medical lore. The long lists of the parts of the body occurring in the *Lorica of Gildas*[17] seem to indicate at least a superficial knowledge of anatomy, and the number of

---

[15] Isidore of Seville, *op. cit.* (12), iv. 9. § 3.
[16] Cf. Pindar, *Pythian Odes*, iii. ll. 52–54.
[17] *Lacnunga*, § 34.

herbs that occur in prescriptions and in glossaries is very great. But the inability to make any practical use of this knowledge is shown by the fact that not one drug in a hundred has the physiological action attributed to it. Ill effects must often have resulted from remedies thus ignorantly, but none the less explicitly, prescribed. One prescription ends with the words, 'with God's help no harm will come'.[18] The phrase might well have been added in most other cases.

The large number of drugs in each prescription is a feature of this material, and is in striking contrast to the practice of the Hippocratic authors. A considerable number of the drugs used in classical times remained in the pharmacopœia of the Anglo-Saxons, but this was owing to the glamour of their origin and not from any experience of their efficacy.

Sigerist notes that the only remedies known in the early Middle Ages— and therefore to the Anglo-Saxons—were small surgical operations (such as blood-letting and cupping) and drugs.[19] The literature of remedies consists of two forms, antidotaries and herbals. In Anglo-Saxon times, the same person, the leech for want of a better name, would use both. Later, the former would be the text-book of the practitioner and the latter that of the pharmacist.

Each prescription specifies purpose, ingredients with weights required, and how it should be administered—if, for example, in the morning, in the evening, before or after meals, after a bath or at what season of the year. The quantities sometimes varied according to the age, sex or strength of the patient. Antidotes are administered in powders, pills (*posel, posling*), decoctions or infusions. Herbs were usually dried and rubbed to powder, or pounded and then mixed with other ingredients such as fat or honey so as to make them adhere. The two following prescriptions will illustrate this. 'If a man's body be hardened, then take plantain, pound (*gecnuca*) it with grease (*smeru*) without salt and work it to a *clam*, lay it on where it is hard'.[20] 'For all swellings, take the flowers of . . . cabbage, pound them with old fat (*rysel*) as you would work a poultice (*clýfa*), put it on a thick linen cloth, lay it to the sore'.[21] *Sealf* is a salve or ointment. The word is found in compounds according to its nature, for example, *smeoru-sealf*, a grease salve and *ele-sealf*, an oil salve; or to the area to which it is to be applied, for example, *eág-sealf*, a salve for the eye and *neb-sealf*, face cream. Two Benedictiones unguenti occur at the end of the *Lacnunga*.

Wine is often prescribed as the liquid in which drugs are to be taken, since its digestive virtue was known in the Dark and Middle Ages. John of Gaddesden, quoting Averroes, says that 'it prevents the food from swimming about the stomach, dispenses the flatulence, provokes the urine and the sweat, and helps nature to expel excess matter'.

Perhaps the chief remedy for all ills until the advent of modern medicine was blood-letting (A.S. *blód-lǽswu*). As Sir Norman Moore has neatly

[18] *ibid.*, § 13.

[19] H. E. Sigerist, *Studien und Texte zur frühmittelalterlichen Rezeptliteratur.* Leipzig, 1923, p. 168.

[20] *Anglo-Saxon Herbal* (Cockayne, vol, i), ii. 11.

[21] *ibid.*, cxxx. 1.

summed up, it was employed 'nearly always, nearly everywhere, and nearly for everything'. In the days before the discovery of the circulation of the blood, it was supposed that the blood was stationary. The particular vein from which blood was to be taken was therefore important, and certain veins were specified so as to cure certain diseases.

The theory that excess of blood was the chief cause of disease originated with Erasistratus of Chios in the third century before Christ. The diminishing of the local supply by blood-letting, though not used by his school, was therefore the logical treatment of a local disease, and was the most popular one both in his time and in the succeeding Dark Ages. It persisted till, and beyond, Anglo-Saxon times. Unfortunately, it was applied without consideration of the patient's condition, and according to prescribed formulae rather than according to reason, so that many who were in a weak condition must have died in consequence.

Blood-letting seems to have been connected with the doctrine of the humours; an evil humour could be eliminated from the system as the blood carried it away. Blood-letting had to be employed at intervals so as to draw off the evil humour as it accumulated, thus keeping the body in a healthy condition.

Bede, in his *De minutione sanguinis, sive de phlebotomia*—if indeed it is his —begins by saying that the best time for blood-letting is from 25 March to 26 May, 'because then the blood is undergoing increase'. The greater part of his tract deals with the parts of the body from which blood should be drawn for pains in various places, and specifies which days of the moon are dangerous in each month. In the last paragraph, however, Bede points out that phlebotomy may be practised at all times, 'si necessitas urget'.

The use of baths for medicinal purposes was derived by the Anglo-Saxons from the Romans. Bede says that Britain 'has both salt and hot springs, and from them flow rivers which furnish hot baths, proper for all ages and sexes, and arranged accordingly'.[22]

The Anglo-Saxons had other means than baths for producing warmth for the benefit of the sick and infirm. The second *Leechbook* prescribes as a recipe for the patient who has a 'stomach which is of a cold or moist nature' that it is 'helpful to him that a fat child should sleep by him, so that he should always put him near his stomach'.[23] The same treatment was prescribed by Oribasius and by Paul of Ægina. The first book of Kings opens with a passage describing the treatment of David in his old age in a similar way.

Emetics and purgatives are constantly prescribed in Anglo-Saxon recipes; the phrase 'drink a strong drink that will run up and down' seems to denote one that will be effective for both purposes at once.

Cauterization was used as a remedy not only in connection with wounds, but also when it could have had no practical utility. An eleventh century manuscript in the Sloane collection in the British Museum contains a kind of primitive anatomical atlas indicating where the cautery was to be applied.[24]

Cupping was practised to draw off secretions as well as blood. An instance

---

[22] Bede, *op. cit.* (2), i. 1.   [23] *Leechbook*, ii. xxvii.
[24] MS. Sloane 2839, fols. iv–3, 'Liber cirrurgium cauterium Apollonii et Galeni'. See L. Thorndike, *History of magic and experimental science*. New York, vol. i, 1923, p. 723.

occurs in the second *Leechbook* in connexion with treatment for a swollen liver: the secretion is to be drawn off at intervals 'with glass or horn' (*teóh mid glese oþþe mid horn*).[25] Presumably the horn of an animal would be used.

The number of animal remedies employed was but few compared with the number of herbal remedies. The *Medicina de quadrupedibus* of Sextus Placitus, of which the vernacular Anglo-Saxon version is printed in the first volume of Cockayne's *Leechdoms*, is arranged under the animals from which the remedies were derived and not under the diseases which were to be cured; it was therefore useless to the practitioner for ready reference. So that the various parts of an animal may be drunk or applied, the instructions are that they should be mixed with oil, wine, vinegar or honey, so as to dissolve them or to make them into a salve. But the methods employed can hardly have disguised the ingredients, which, considering their extreme nastiness in many cases, must have been most obnoxious to the patient. Many would have been more useful as emetics than as medicine.

But by far the largest number of the remedies prescribed were herb remedies. They occur all through the three volumes of Cockayne's work, though the first volume, the *Anglo-Saxon Herbal*, deals especially with them. Plant after plant is described—illustrated in bright colours in the manuscript (Cotton Vitellius C III)—the various uses (useful and otherwise) to which it should be put are elaborated, together with many magical rites to be performed when gathering or administering.

The numerous green herbs that were used may well have been beneficial, however, by reason of their antiscorbutic properties; and since they were employed in the early spring, they may have helped to correct that alteration of the blood from which our forefathers were liable to suffer after a winter's diet in which salt meat and dried peas predominated.

Enough has been said concerning superstitious and magical practices to show that the medicine of those days, whether Church or lay, was steeped in them. Both the magic and the medicine of the Anglo-Saxons were largely derived from Pliny, and from late classical writers such as Marcellus Empiricus who derived from him. Speaking of magic, Pliny says: 'Of the fact that it first originated in medicine, no one entertains a doubt, or that under the plausible disguise of promoting health, it insinuated itself among mankind, as a higher and more holy branch of medical art. Then in the next place, to promises the most seductive and the most flattering, it has added all the resources of religion, a subject upon which, at the present day, man is still entirely in the dark'.[26]

Certain diseases lent themselves more than others to treatment by means of magic. Such were insanity, already mentioned in connexion with Church 'magic', and obstetrics, both a complete mystery in those days. Magic was, however, associated with most branches of medicine, thereby ousting the healing art itself. The magical attributes of objects then used for effecting cures were those which had most value in the eyes of the Anglo-Saxons.

The assessment of what was of value for healing purposes was entirely different from what it had been in classical Greece and from what it is to-day.

[25] *Leechbook*, ii. xviii.   [26] Pliny, *Hist. Nat.*, xxx. 1.

TEXTES MÉDICAUX CHARTRAINS
DES IXe, Xe ET XIe SIÈCLES

par

ERNEST WICKERSHEIMER

IL y a longtemps de cela — c'était avant la première guerre mondiale — j'avais commencé de rechercher les textes médicaux dans les manuscrits latins antérieurs au XIIe siècle, ceci en vue d'une enquête générale sur les oeuvres des médecins du moyen âge qui n'auraient pas encore subi d'influences arabes.

Comme de juste, je me tournai en premier lieu vers les bibliothèques françaises et c'est ainsi que, prenant pour base de départ leurs catalogues imprimés, je parvins à dresser une liste de 94 manuscrits s'échelonnant du VIIe au XIe siècle et dont la moitié exactement appartient à la Bibliothèque Nationale.[1]

Reims y était représenté par huit manuscrits, Angers par cinq, Laon par quatre, Orléans et Vendôme par trois, Dijon, Montpellier, la Mazarine et Rouen par deux, Autun, Cambrai, Douai, Poitiers, Saint-Omer et Valenciennes par un manuscrit.

Après la Bibliothèque Nationale,[2] le plus fort contingent était fourni par la Bibliothèque de Chartres. Je n'y avais pas relevé moins de dix manuscrits datant du IXe, du Xe et du XIe siècle et qui, d'après le catalogue contenaient peu ou prou de textes médicaux. Provenant tous d'anciennes bibliothèques chartraines, huit du chapitre de la cathédrale, deux de l'abbaye bénédictine de Saint-Père-en-Vallée, ils figurent au plus récent catalogue imprimé[3] sous les nos 53, 62, 70, 74, 75, 76,[4] 102, 110, 111 et 193.

Tout cela n'existe plus.

M. Maurice Jusselin, Archiviste honoraire d'Eure-et-Loir, a bien voulu me donner des précisions sur la catastrophe où a péri la Bibliothèque à la gestion de laquelle il consacrait depuis 1909 une partie de son activité.

Au début de la guerre, en 1939, il avait pris l'initiative d'expédier au château de Villebon, à vingt kilomètres au sud de Chartres, manuscrits, incunables et autres livres particulièrement précieux. Le simple bon sens eût exigé qu'ils y restassent jusqu'à la fin des hostilités.

Or, le 7 novembre 1940, une lettre de Bernard Faÿ, que le Gouvernement de Vichy venait de placer à la tête de la Bibliothèque Nationale, annonçait

---

[1] On en découvrira sans doute d'autres au fur et à mesure de la publication du *Catalogue général des manuscrits latins*, dont les deux premiers tomes, parus en 1939 et 1940 sous la direction de Philippe Lauer, contiennent les notices des manuscrits 1–2962 du fonds latin.

[2] Où deux manuscrits médicaux, lat. 9332 et lat. 10233, de IXe et du VIIe siècle, sont venus de Chartres où ils avaient appartenu au chapitre de la cathédrale. Ils ont été étudiés et utilisés par A. Molinier pour son édition des anciennes traductions latines d'Oribase : cf. Oribase, *Oeuvres*, texte... traduit... par... Bussemaker et Ch. Daremberg, 1873, V et 1876, VI. Hermann Stadler s'est servi du ms. lat. 9332 pour son édition de « Dioscorides Lombardus », *Romanische Forschungen*, 1901, XI, pp. 1–121. Molinier a attribué à ces deux manuscrits une origine italienne. Suivant d'autres opinions, ils auraient vu le jour en Orléanais, sans doute à l'abbaye de Fleury; cf. MacKinney, *Early medieval medicine, op. cit.* (6), p. 112 et *passim*.

[3] *Catalogue général des manuscrits des bibliothèques publiques de France; départements, tome XI, Chartres...*, par... Omont, Molinier, Couderc et Coyecque, Paris, Plon, 1890, in-8°, LI, 571 pp.

[4] Ainsi qu'on le verra tout à l'heure, le ms. 76 ne contient rien de ce qui nous occupe ici.

au Conservateur de la Bibliothèque de Chartres la prochaine visite du Dr Wermke, chef du Service des Bibliothèques auprès de l'administration militaire allemande.[5] Wermke y était présenté en ces termes : « Nous avons eu l'occasion de nous louer des services qu'il a rendus à la Bibliothèque [Nationale]. Je n'ai donc pas besoin de vous demander de lui réserver l'accueil le plus courtois. Vous voudrez bien lui faciliter l'accomplissement de sa mission, qui est de protection, en lui faisant les honneurs de votre dépôt. »

On va voir les conséquences de cette mission... de protection. Laissons la parole à M. Jusselin.

« M. Wermke est venu le 3 décembre 1940. Le même jour, 3 décembre 1940, le Feldkommandant, d'après les instructions de Wermke, ordonnait au maire de Chartres de faire rentrer tout ce qui était à Villebon. Nous avons voulu gagner du temps, essayer d'éluder cet ordre, mais, le 11 décembre, le maire recevait un nouvel ordre, plus impératif, au sujet du retour sans retard de notre dépôt de Villebon. Il fallut s'exécuter.

« Nous avons été bombardés quarante-sept fois. Le centre de la ville n'était ni visé, ni atteint ; nous pensions que l'Hôtel-de-Ville et la Bibliothèque, dans le même corps de bâtiment, serait épargné. Or, en 1944, la D.C.A. allemande avait un chef très habile. Un groupe de bombardiers passait sur la ville et menaçait le champ d'aviation. L'avion de tête, celui du chef d'escadrille sans doute, fut touché. Ses mouvements furent sans doute mal interprétés ; ses bombes tombèrent, peut-être involontairement. Tous les autres lâcherent alors leur chargement qui tomba sur le quartier de l'Hôtel-de-Ville. Le feu prit et en un quart d'heure toute la Bibliothèque fut embrasée. La vraie cause du feu est encore discutée, mais le résultat est là. Ensuite dix-neuf pompes françaises et allemandes ne purent que noyer les décombres et achever le désastre. Cela s'est passé le vendredi 26 mai 1944, à 18 heures et quelques minutes ; le personnel de la Bibliothèque, venant de partir, a ainsi échappé à la mort.

« Rien n'est assuré. On a retiré des décombres des parchemins brûlés, déchirés et décomposés et des parties de livres. Les parchemins ont été envoyés à la Bibliothèque Nationale pour essai de reconstitution, mais on ne sauvera que des fragments guère utilisables. Ce ne seront que des souvenirs ».

Ce récit simple et émouvant se passe de commentaires. Mais il n'y a pas qu'à Chartres que les vainqueurs du moment tirèrent de leurs abris des richesses irremplaçables pour les exposer à la fureur des combats ; à Strasbourg nous en savons quelque chose. Pourquoi cette hâte, pourquoi ces exigences ? C'est que les dirigeants du Reich voulaient persuader le monde et se persuader eux-mêmes qu'en 1940 la guerre était finie, que leur victoire était définitive.

Depuis que je les ai eus en mains, les manuscrits médicaux de Chartres ont été étudiés par MM. MacKinney[6] et Tribalet.[7] M. MacKinney en cite même deux qui m'avaient échappé, le ms. 105, du Xe siècle, dont il ne dit

[5] Wermke était, en 1939, Directeur de la Bibliothèque de la Ville de Breslau.

[6] L. C. MacKinney, « Tenth-century medicine as seen in the Historia of Richer of Rheims ». *Bull. Inst. Hist. Med.*, 1934, II, 347–75 ; et *Early medieval medicine with special reference to France and Chartres.* (Publications of the Inst. Hist. Med., Johns Hopkins University, 3rd series, vol. iii.) In-8°. Baltimore, 1937, 247 pp.

[7] Jacques Tribalet, *Histoire médicale de Chartres jusqu'au XII siècle.* Thèse de médecine de Paris, 1936. In-8°. Paris, Vigot, 1936, 154 pp.

pas ce qu'il contenait de médical,[8] et le ms. 80 du IXe siècle où il a découvert, aux fol. 45-7, un texte « De etate hominis »[9] qui ne figure pas au catalogue et qui, comme les deux fragments entre lesquels il se trouvait inséré, pourrait bien avoir été extrait des *Étymologies* (lib. XI, cap. 2) de saint Isidore de Séville.

Notons enfin que M. Thorndike a signalé *Spera Apuleii Platonis*, dans le ms. 113 de Chartres, du Xe siècle provenant du chapitre de la cathédrale où on la trouve à la suite d'opuscules d'Alcuin.[10] Il s'agit d'une de ces combinaisons de chiffres au moyen desquelles le pronostic d'une maladie est déduit du nom du patient et du jour lunaire où celui-ci s'est alité.

J'ai largement tenu compte des travaux de MM. MacKinney et Tribalet. A part quoi, ces notes sont publiées presque sans changement, à peu près telles qu'elles ont été prises il y a environ quarante ans.

I

Ms.53.   XIe siècle.   Provenance : chapitre de la cathédrale.

Recette contre la migraine.

[Fol. 88v°]   Contra migraneam.   Pioniae radix cocta in oleo vetustissimo roseo, que percocta eliciatur tortura lintei, et sic, ubi dolor est, inliniatur sepius, sine dubio juvabit, ita tamen ut infusio sepius capiti imposita precedat vel subsequatur ex suco abrotani cum eadem herba trita in aceto fortissimo cum salis manipulo, et si balneum vis, cum herbis boni odoris in eodem coctis, id usita.   De abrotano factam galeam bene coctam et calidam, capiti impones donec potiris balneo, et de ipsa aqua quaere mane et ultimo effundes caput, et sic ex predicto oleo iterum unge.   Si sedule id egeris, nichilominus proveniet et sic ex predicto.

Les premiers mots, avec quelques variantes insignifiantes, au recto du même feuillet.

II

Ms.62.   Xe siècle.   Provenance : chapitre de la cathédrale (et non abbaye de Saint-Père, ainsi qu'il a été dit.   *Catalogue*, p. 30).

1. *Soranus*, Isagoge in artem medendi.

[Fol. 1]   Horus ysagogus.   Soranus filio karissimo salutem.   Quoniam frequenter plerique nescientes quatenus egrotanti manus tenere debeant... Medicinam quidem invenit Apollo... [Fol. 16]... et valde contrarium naturae paulatim vero ad unamquamque rem venire utilissimum est.   Explicit peri sfigmon ysagogus.

Cf. Tribalet, p. 32-42 ; facsimilé du fol. 1, p. 90.

C'est, attribué à Soranus, une sorte de catéchisme médical par demandes et par réponses, combiné à un *De pulsibus* attribué au même.   Voir l'édition de ces deux ouvrages par Valentin Rose (*Anecdota graeca et graecolatina*, 1870, t. II, p. 241-74 et 275-80), dont chacun des incipit se retrouve au fol. 1 du ms. 62.   A rapprocher de l'adaptation française de notre texte par Tribalet (p. 89-150).

[8] MacKinney, « Tenth-century medicine », *op. cit.* (6), p. 356, note 24.

[9] *idem, Early medieval medicine*, p. 190.

[10] Lynn Thorndike, *A history of magic and experimental science during the first thirteen centuries of our era*.   New York, t. I, 1923, p. 692.

2. *Galien.* De medendi methodo ad Glauconem.

[Fol. 16] Incipit Galieni proaemium ad Glauconem. — [Fol. 16 v°]
Quoniam quidem non solum communem omnium hominum fisin id est
naturam... [Fol. 17] Incipiamus ergo. I. De diversitate febrium. II. De
effemera febre... [Fol. 17 v°]... LVI. De emetritaciis febribus. LVII. De
numero horarum creticorum dierum. LVIII. De prognosticis sanitatis.
LVIIII. Prognostica mortis. LX. Inditia secundi libri. Explicit.
Explicit. — [Fol. 18] Incipit liber primus Galleni didascali de diversitate
febrium. I. Incipiam nunc febrium dicere diversitates... — [Fol. 36 v°]...
LVII. De numerum horarum creticorum dierum. Ut in hoc numerum
horarum quidem accedentium aut minuentium... et urina testentur quamvis
et libro non parva prognostica subjecerit et subinde. Nunc enim de
prognosticis aliquid dicamus. — [Fol. 38] Incipit prognostica. Utile est
etiam hoc nosse ut prognostica vel bona vel mala... Incipiunt signa mortifera
juxta Yppocratis sententiam. Unde scias si quis aegrotae sineque eum
vigiliae longiores turbaverunt... eos morituros, unde finem faciam dicendi
in hoc libro superius de aliis dicturus causis in alium incipiam. Explicit
Galieni didiscalia liber secundus. — [Fol. 40 v°]... Incipit liber quartus.
O Glauco optimum duxi ut et in hoc tertio petendi tibi de ceteris prope
modum omnibus certe de maximis causis quae in corporibus nascuntur
humanis... [Fol. 53]... De aelifatiacos. Elifatiosus autem autem eodem
modo et ipsos curabis ut cancros, quia ut dixi... Inveniuntur etiam haec
tales causae in Germania et Cappadocia et Missia... [Fol. 53 v°]... dum
omnium curationem causarum quanta possum scientiam manifesta ratione
conscribam. Explicit procluna Galieni.

A noter la division en quatre livres, alors que le traité original n'en compte que
deux. Analyse par Tribalet (p. 17–21). Le même texte se trouve plus ou moins
complet dans trois mss. des Xᵉ et XIᵉ siècles : Montpellier 185, fol. 119–40 (copié dans
le ms. 429 de l'Académie de médecine, fol. 58–85, 104–53 v°); Poitiers 184, fol.
1–26 v°; Vendôme 109, fol. 8–35 v° (copié dans le ms. 430 de l'Académie de médecine,
fol. 5–212).

3. *Âges de l'homme.*

[Fol. 37] Infantia VII ann., puericia VII, adolescentia VII, juventus
ter VII, senectus quater VII.

4. *Vertus de la pimprenelle.*

[Fol. 37] Nomen herbe pinponilla. Vires ejus mirabiles precium
transcendunt, nam laqueus draconis ipsa est. Si conmastigata in os ejus
proicitur, statim moritur. Ipsi eciam homines qui inter dracones et serpentes
morantur, si pinponillam biberint, nihil eis nocebit. Confectio contra omnia
venena serpentium et maleficas pociones. Recipe hec : pinponille majoris
radices siccabis ad solem in septembri, genciane, alliorum, ortolanorum,
centauree, cinnamomi. De his omnibus fac pulverem, de pinponilla drachmas
duas, de aliis unciam. Singulas conficis cum melle dispumato et uteris
ad causas predictas. Probatum est ad potiones venenatas et fricdores et
demonium expellit ab homine et spleneticum sine mora sanat. Si vermes nati
fuerint ex aliqua parte mala in homine aut in pecore, pinponilla colligis cum

oratione dominica, dabis bibere per dies octo in aceto et vino cum oleo et ad febres in aqua calida. Probatum est.

A la suite : « Artis definitio secundum Ful. » ; non médical.

5. *Macrocosme et microcosme.*

Figure occupant tout le verso du fol. 37. Elle rapproche les quatre points cardinaux, les quatre éléments, les quatre saisons, les quatre humeurs et les quatre âges de l'homme. Des notes détaillées couvrant ses marges énumèrent les caractères et les effets des vents. Après l'avoir présentée avec d'autres figures médico-astrologiques des IXe, Xe et XIe siècles au XVIIe Congrès international de médecine (Londres, 1913), j'en ai publié un calque dans le *Janus*, 1914, XIX, p. 162. Reproduction dans Tribalet, p. 22.

6. *Du pouls et des urines dans les fièvres et dans diverses maladies.*

[Fol. 38] Incipit liber tertius pros Claucon. Dum esset difficilis ratio nonnullas febrium dimissiones... — [Fol. 41 v°]... quae cum arenas mingit initium cauculum ostendit.

Interpolé dans le texte décrit ci-dessus du *De medendi methodo ad Glauconem* de Galien. On le retrouve dans le ms. 185 de Montpellier [Fol. 130–35 v°], copié aux fol. 86–101 du ms. 429 de l'Académie de médecine.

7. Galien. *De simplicibus medicamentis ad Paternianum.*

[Fol. 54] Incipit virtus eorum quibus causis proficiunt Galieni dogma. Vera haec est virtutis demonstratio omnium medicamentorum qui ad artis medicinae scientiam pertinet, quae si plenissime intellegant hi qui artem medicinae profitentur servare eos medicina per omnem adjutorium in omnem curam adjuvat... [Fol. 54 v°] Incipit alfabetum Galieni ad Paternum. I. Aer ustum. II. Agatia. III. Aerugo. IIII. Amoniaco. V. Aloes... XXXVIII. Alosacine. Expliciunt capitula de A.I. Aer ustum fit maxime de clavis cupreis et vetutis... [Fol. 59 v°]... Explicit de C. Incipit de D. Diptamnum... [Fol. 73 v°]... VI. Yhacantum tursulum herba levem, flos purpureum, folia et radices quasi vulvi tot herba viribus et adfectum stiptica est. Explicit qualitas omnium herbarum.

Ouvrage apocryphe, également attribué à Gariopontus, à tort selon Max Neuburger, *Geschichte der Medizin*, 1911, t. II, p. 285.

8. *Esculapius.* Chronia.

[Fol. 74] I. De cefalea. II. De scotomaticis. III. De epilenticis... [Fol. 74 v°]... XLVI. De podagricis. Expliciunt capitula. Incipit prologus. Quoniam superior liber de capitis vitia usque cervices, secundus de signis earum, tertius vero de cura omnium causarum, nunc quartum exponimus de chronicis, hoc est tardarum passionum, quod per temporalia spacia remorantur, unde nomina acceperunt chronica, hoc sunt temporalia, que passiones gignuntur et fiunt ex flegmate et felle nigro. Oxea id est acutae passiones quae fiunt ex sanguine et felle rufo, quae aut celerius transeunt aut in momento occidunt. In chronicis causis, id est temporalibus, grandis diligentia adhibenda est, quoniam dificillime acutae causae liberantur... [Fol. 109]... contra humidum siccum et alia similia omnium, secundum hunc morem curari, vel apponendum, similiter evacuanda.

Texte anonyme dans lequel MacKinney « Tenth-century medicine », *op. cit.* (6), p. 353) a reconnu *Chronia* d'Esculapius imprimé sous le titre *Demorborum, infirmitatum,*

passionumque corporis humani origine, descriptionibus et cura liber unus à la suite de
Physica de sainte Hildegarde, Argentorati, apud Joannem Schottum, 1533, in-fol.;
quelques chapitres transposés. Par suite de l'intercalation dans l'édition d'un
chapitre absent du manuscrit « quid sit podagricis sequendum », décalage dans la
numérotation des chapitres, 46 au lieu de 47. Prologue non reproduit dans
l'édition, mais dont l'incipit est cité d'après un ms. de Bruxelles par V. Rose (*op. cit.*,
t. II, p. 175). Facsimilés du fol. 74 v° dans Tribalet (p. 32) et dans MacKinney
(*Early medieval medicine, op. cit.* (6), p. 216–17), qui commet une double erreur
en le présentant comme le fol. 14 et en y voyant le début de l'*Aurelius*.

A rapprocher aussi du ms. 175 de Vendôme, du XIe siècle, fol. 47–94, copié dans
Académie de médecine 431, fol. 205–340, où manquent toutefois les chapitres
« XXXVII. De diabitis » et « XLIIII. De psialgicis » du ms. de Chartres, tandis
qu'on y trouve deux chapitres « De peripleumonicis » et « De pleuresis » qu'ignore
celui-ci.

Georg Helmreich (*Mitteilungen zur Geschichte der Medizin*, 1919, XVIII,
p. 24–32) a montré comment le livre d'Esculapius a été incorporé au *Passionarius*
de Gariopontus.

9. *Recettes.*

[Fol. 109] Ad scapularum dolorem rutam in aceto... Ad calculum et ad
petras eiciendas per urinam saxifragam... Item ad calculos et ad eos qui
sanguinem mingunt, certum remedium...

Tribalet (p. 30) traduit la formule d'un emplâtre « micanicum » qu'il a trouvée
« insérée en papillon dans le ms. 62 »; il ne dit pas où. Au sujet de mots que Richer
aurait tiré duprésent manuscrit, cf. MacKinney, « Tenth-century medicine », *op. cit.*
(6), p. 361, 363, 366.

III

Ms.70. IXe siècle. Provenance : chapitre de la cathédrale.

1. *Fragments de pathologie et de thérapeutique.*

[Fol. 126] Ad apostemas quod Greci steotomas apellant, id est genera vel
nomina et loca abent pluris sed unaquaqua per se origine, natura et loca
manifestantur. Alia in cutanuis quod grece aderoma vocant, alia in pectus super
reticulo quod grece empiema apellant, alia in pulmonis vel ejus vicinitatem quod
grece encatalapsis vocant, alie in epate quod grece anaprosis dicunt, alia in splene
vel latere quod grece mesopleoron vocant, alia in stomacho vel testinis quod
grece apostasis apellant, alia apostaema est in testinos majores quod grece
anfinbolam vocant, alia in renis vel in lumbos quod in visica faciunt virificia
quod grece catuetis dicunt. In cutanea apostema sic intelligis : habens in se
grossam et albam et nimis saniosa in similitudinem adipes et cancrena putridinis
carnium... [Fol. 127] Alius dies addis post ipse vulnus intellegis crepuisse
aut per ore aut per annum aut per urine meatus et cum purgare ceperit et
veniunt in site, da eis antedotum Urribaxio qui facit ad apostemas forinsecas
vel intrinsecas. Item ad apostema vino vetus... [Fol. 128] Ad apostema qui
nascitur inferioris partis ventris, id est in stentinis aut longaonem sive visicae
vel eorum vicinitatis, secundum Filomino, dicta illas apostemas periculosa sunt,
quia acuta febris est et nimis anorexia faciunt... Ad longaonem quod grece
tenismon vocant, id est passio intestinorum, causam qui sine colica passione

laborant, id est desiderium ventris cum magno pondere reomatismo et ventris obstrusio cum spissa mucilenta aut sanguinolenta stercora redunt, adsellationem ventris deficultatis ejessionem cum magno labore et aliquando sine morso sunt, sic intelligis, intestinus est crastus, collegens in se flegma frigida pro haec causa, stercus officio suo gerre non possit, sed magis in flegma frigida collegatus est. Evenit haec causa maximae in frigdore nimio ex indejessione vel frigidis potionis. Curatio eorum talis est adhibenda, sicut Galienus ad Claudionem scripsit lavacra calida et unguenta et constrictis cibis, utende sunt catartica et antidota quod huic causa prodesse cognoveris, ut est tiriaca aut adrianum, aut filonium, aut trociscus diaspermato et, si haec minime senserint, catapodias clisteria forcioris adhibenda sunt, ut ad intrinsicas passionis scripsemus... [Fol. 128 v°] Ad anum. Anus enim multa abet nomina. Alii edram dicunt, alii podicem, alii stalem, alii conodoon, alii fincteri vocant; anum dicimus propter inanicionem ventris et corporis et a balano retunditatem nomen accipit et est circulus ductilis et rectum recipit longaonem, et per ipsum stercora sund egerenda et restrictiva, et in ipso orificio ani multas fiunt causas, id est ragadas et hiantis glandolas, cumdolomatas, agrocordenas, verugas, emorruidas et ibi poscias diversorum genera in magnitudinem granorum fave vel pisis aliquando ut avelane fiunt, aliquando tumor eminens ut ipso orificio claudere videantur pro his omnibus superscripta passionis adhibenda sunt adjutoria. Cum causa in turpissimo loco et indecore sunt positi et non curati precadunt, non solum ipse anus tumescit, sed et alia membra que prope sunt et veretri immunda vulnera et sordida, vel maligna inde fiunt, si medice propter turpitudinem vel fetorem ipsas immundicias non extergunt, diligenter curando aut palpando, non succurrunt egrotum. Tunc manifestabitur anticorum dicta: ex talis medicis multi sunt advocati, sed in opere pauci sunt onesti. Curatio super memoratas passiones ani intelligis sic: si ex longaonem, quod grece stalem dicunt, evenit dolor... [Fol. 129] Alia ad scabilia vel ulcera quod grece ragadias apellant, mittit oleo roseo cum ove albumen mixto unguis loca sic collectionis facis et eruperit mox de absimicio inpone, quod si fistolaverit cum sulfor inflammabis aut cumburis, sicut in Cirorgicis scripsemus... Item ad ano qui vermis cabit ex ipso natus pulmone calidum moxsullatum anum inposito, statim vermiculi in pulmone adirgunt, cum extraxeris remitte sepius, colerius mundat. Ad ossa vel nervorum aut musculorum dolorem... [Fol. 130] Ad clisterem quod grece ipoteon vocant, alii puderiton, idem injectaturium per anum multis perforatis caverna abet in longo spacium digitorum IIII, clunibus cervigale subpositum sic subtus memoratas eminas inicienda sunt per clisterem. Enema utilissima maxime neofreticis : marrubio, absentio, malvas, betas... [Fol. 130 v°] Ad fico. Corale, aloe, amoniaco... [Fol. 131] Ad omnis humoris expurgandum : bittonica, salvia, balsemita, anite semen... Ad flegma nimia congregata in stomacho. Galienus auctor quendam hominem invenit cum labore cibum sumendi, nisi tantum ut suavis agrimonies ad edendum quidem utilis aut inutilis accepisset... [Fol. 132 v°] Cura reumatismi qui in ventrem vel intestinis descendere solet, sicut Galienus ad Claudionem scripsit lavacra, calida et constrictiva curatio... Ad variola quas grece flectinas vocant, haec papulas volaticas dicunt pro eo quod de homine in homine transiunt. Curationis eorum diversi sunt. Andragorum flectinas vel postulas inicium passionis si bene intellexerit medicus per fleotomia liberati sunt. Si haec neglexerit, vissicas habundanter infundunt, et si crepuerint, vissicas lavacra sepius visitare jubebis et cum aqua mulsa frequenter omnia loca perunguis... [Fol. 133] Ad scabias quas grece lapidas invocant veteris auctoris dua esse genera dixerunt : una est squamosa, fusci coloris, quidem corticosas squamulas in cuti ostendunt, unde nomen a grece lepra accipit, nascitur ex melancolico humore et deficile curentur; alia vero nascitur simplex ex humore agro et salso que facile curantur... [Fol. 133 v°] Ad proriginem quod grece evismonem dicunt, idem scabia minuta. Nascitur ex antecidentis humoris agridinis, quibus curatio haec est adhibenda; lac aseninum sive ovillum cum mel mixtum... [Fol. 134] Ad manus et pedes ut non albiant ... Ad asso balnium vel pluris asso balnio sic facis : artemisia, ruta, tanacita ... Alio asso balnio sine aqua facias. Carbonis de sarmentis ipsius carbonis unius mittis in calderia feria, ipsa calderia ponis in cuba bene coperta. Cum egrotus sudare cepit, abeat lentiolus mundus, unde extergat de se sudorem cum manu, sudat, alium mittat. Efficacissimum ad omnis passionis... Ad cacexia qui multa habet nomina... [Fol. 135]... ad hidropem veniunt per ventositatem, cacexia ideoque eorum curas et his adhibendi sunt cacectilis utilissimis ad pr.

Il est traité dans ces fragments des apostèmes, du ténesme, des affections de l'anus, des clystères, de la purgation, de la variole, des maladies de la peau, des bains, etc. Oribase, Philumenos et Galien (*Ad Claudionem*, c'est-à-dire *Ad Glauconem*) sont cités.

2. *Régime pour les douze mois de l'année.*

[Fol. 135] Ad cibum vel pocionis quod per singulis mensis visitare oportet — Mense Marcio dulciamen jejunus comedat et primum mere dulce bibat, agramen coctum, radicem confecta, assum balneum visitet, sanguinem noli minemare, solucionem non accipiat, quia [i]psa solucio frigoras generat.— Bonum est mense Aprile sanguinem minimare, pocionem bibere, carnis recentis manducare et radicibus abstinere, sanguinem intercutaneum minemare, calidum usitare, dolorem stomachi purguare, unguentum calasticum usitare et, si factum fuerit, omnia menbra sanare debeant. — In mense Madio nullo penitus caput comedat, calido bibat, calido usitit, capite purgit quia talis in calore precordia ponis pro frigitudinem. Lucit in mense Madio vena epatica incide et potione contra officationem accipiat. — In mense Junio omne die mero de aqua jejunus bibere debet cervisa, nec metus noli bibere, lactucas usitare et calidum bibere debet. — In mense Julio Veneris non utatur, sanguinem non minimetur, potionem ad solvendum non accipiat, salvia et ruta usitet. — In mense Augusto nullo penitus malvas et caulus non manducet et agramen manducet, cervisa et metus nullo poenitus non bibat. —In mense Septembri bucellas in lacte infusas jejunus comedat cotidie et omnia que vis accipere debet, quia omnis escas cum tempore et fructa confecta sunt. — In mense Octubri porrus pluris usita quomodo vis mane, cotidie racimus usita, musto bibe, musto usita, quia corpore sanat et solucionem facit. — In mense November a balneo abstine, capita omnium ne comedas. — In mense December a caulis absteneat; si hoc studiose observaberis, sanitatem non indigebis. — In mense Januario jejunus bibat tres gluppus vini cotidie, nullo penitus sanguinem minimare debet, in pocionem contra officationes et electuarium accipere debet. — In mense Februario betas nec comedat [Fol. 135 v°] de police sanguinem minimare debet, sic tamen ut antea accipiat ad deponendum d[i]agridium confectum est, quomodo ipsa potione bibat... [illisible], balneum intrare debeat et quomodo omnia membra... [illisible] cum vino bibere debet. Cataplasma in capite inpone... [illisible] sanare debeant.

Texte semblable ou apparenté à ceux qu'on rencontre dans les mss : Laon 426 bis, fol. 117v°–118, IXe s.; Bibliothèque, Nationale lat. 2849 A, fol. 23v°, Xe s.; Bibliothèque Nationale, lat. 11.218, fol. 56v°–57, IXe s.; Saint-Gall 225, fol. 136–7, VIIIe s. Dans ce dernier qui m'a été signalé par Monseigneur Andrieu, doyen de la Faculté de théologie catholique de Strasbourg, il est attribué à Hippocrate.

Un texte assez voisin se trouve au fol. 129v° du ms. lat. 2825 de la Bibliothèque Nationale, du Xe siècle, où il a été ajouté à un opuscule traitant du même sujet, mais différent et qui appartient au même groupe que Laon 426 bis, fol. 118–9v°; Montpellier 185, fol. 160–160v°, Xe ou XIe s. (copié dans Académie de médecine 429, fol. 167); Poitiers 184, fol. 67v°–68, Xe ou XIe s.; Reims 438, fol. 30, Xe s. et le texte imprimé dans *Experimentarius medicinae* (Argentorati, apud Joannnem Schottum, 1544, in-fol., p. 247). S'y rattache aussi la brève note qui suit.

3. *Potions pour les douze mois de l'année.*

[Fol. 135 v°] Ratio quisque mensis qualis pocionis usitare debes. Mense Januario gingiber et reopontico. — Mense Februario agrimonia et apii semen. — Mense Marcio ruta et livestico. — Mense Aprilis bettonica et pipenilla. — Mense Madio absintio et fenuculo semen. — Mense Junio salvia floris et savina. — Mense Julio floris de apii et de uva[?]. — Mense Augusto pullegio. — Mense September costo et grano mastice. — Mense October cariofole et piper. — Mense November spico.

4. *Recettes pour la confection des apozèmes.*

[Fol. 135 v°] Apocima ad omnes passiones refrigerandum et sitem tollendum ... Apocimas ad humoris mellancolicas temperandas... Ad nefreticorum causa, Latini renium dolorem dicunt, hac sunt signa...

IV

Ms.74. Xe siècle. Provenance : chapitre de la cathédrale.

1. *Recettes.*

[Fol. 1] Electuarium ad tissim, sive ad pectus, ad omnem infirmitatem stomachi quae de frigore... Antidotum quod facit ad omnem accessionem febris cotidiane, terciane, quartane... Electuarium qui facit ad pectoris dolorem... Electuarium ad raucitudinem... Item electuarium secundum Uribasium...

2. *Poids et mesures médicinaux.*

[Fol. 1] Incipit ratio ponderum vel mensurarum diversorum medicinalium. Siliqua...

Traduit par Tribalet (p. 26). Des textes différents, relatifs aux poids et mesures en médecine, se trouvent dans des mss. contemporains ou plus anciens de la Bibliothèque Nationale : Lat. 6862, fol. 3, Xe s.; lat. 6882A, fol. 15–18, 24–24v°, Xe s.; lat. 9332, fol. 179v°, IXe s.; lat. 11218, fol. 42–42v°, IXe s., copié dans Académie de médecine 421, fol. 58–59; nouv. acq. lat. 203, fol. 3–3v°, viie ou viiie s.; nouv. acq. lat. 1619, fol. 178–178v°, viie ou viiie s. Voir aussi *De ponderibus et mensuris* par Dardanius philosophus dans Montpellier 185, fol. 136–136v°, x^e-xie s., copié dans Académie de médecine 429, fol. 103–4.

Les « Notes sur les qualités du corps » mentionnées dans le *Catalogue* (p. 38) n'ont rien de médical.

V

Ms. 75. x^e ou xie siècle. Provenance : chapitre de la cathédrale.

Hippocrate, Aphorismi cum commentario.

[Feuillet collé à l'intérieur du plat postérieur de la reliure]... longinquitas et reparare qui post egritudinem non poterit continuo sed tardius. — VII. Si quis in egritudine cibum accipiens non convalescat, signum est quia multo utitur cibo. Si autem cibum non accipientibus hoc contingat, signum est quia omnia inagnitionem habent corpora. Ipocrates dum dicit causam curam, significat intellectus vero istius aforismi talis est. Si quis post egritudinem ad salutem revertens... — VIII. Oportet cum voluerit quis purgari molitare debere. In isto loco multi multa senserunt... — VIIII. Quae non pura sunt corpora, quanto magis nutriuntur, plus nocent. Intellectus istius talis est, ut si quis putredinem in se habens... — X. Facile est repleri potuque cibo. In isto loco alii alia senserunt... — XI. Quae relinquuntur in morbis post solutiones iterationes faciunt. Nunc Ypocrates ammonet ut si quis post egritudinem habebit reliquias humoris... signa precedentia, id est capitis dolor dige.

Aphorismes 7–11, avec commentaire, du livre II, correspondant à 8–12 des éditions, telle celle de l'*Articella*; les mots précédant 7, appartenant sans doute au commentaire de 6. Tribalet, en décollant le feuillet a mis au jour un nouveau fragment qui d'après le facsimilé (p. 48) semble ne pas s'adapter exactement au texte précédemment connu. On n'y reconnait que la fin du commentaire de l'aphorisme 12, et les aphorismes 13–17, d'après la numérotation du présent manuscrit.

Même commentaire dans les mss. : Montpellier 185, fol. 1v°–98, x^e ou xi^es.; Bibliothèque Nationale lat. 7021, fol. 18–118v°, xe s.; Bibliothèque Nationale lat. 7027, fol. 67–175, xe s.; Vendôme 172, fol. 11–72v°, xie s. Dans ce dernier, ainsi que dans l'édition de Jean Gonthier d'Andernach (Parisiis, ex off. S. Colinaei, 1533, in–8°), le commentaire est attribué à Oribase. Commentaire sous le nom d'Oribase dans lat. 4888, fol. 105–27 et lat. 7102, fol. 33–96 de la Bibliothèque Nationale, l'un du xiie, l'autre du xiiie siècle. Les variantes du ms. 185 de Montpellier ont été reportées par Daremberg sur une copie du ms. 313 d'Einsiedeln qui se trouve à l'Académie de médecine, ms. 428, fol. 2 et suiv.

VI

Ms. 76. xie siècle. Provenance : chapitre de la cathédrale.

Les rédacteurs du *Catalogue* (p. 40) ont signalé sur une feuille de garde du xie siècle, un fragment d'un traité de médecine. C'est une erreur dont Tribalet (p. 52) a trouvé l'origine : « L'erreur vient de ce que certains mots semblent s'appliquer, qui aux sciences naturelles, qui à la médecine. Ils figurent à titre d'exemple pour expliquer la notion d'opposition (« Socrate est en bonne santé » a un contraire: « Socrate est malade » etc...). Cet ensemble se rapporte plutôt à un traité de métaphysique ou de logique ».

VII

Ms. 102.   Xe siècle.   Provenance : chapitre de la cathédrale.

Recettes.

[Fol. 88v°]   Ad cauculos.   Rafani cortices ex aqua decocti aut in vino aut in aqua sepius potui data ad mensuram trium cocta[?] et cauculum sanat, etiam mulierem, si cauculum habet, sanat. — Ad profluvium mulieris.   De capillo Venere potionem facis et mireris effectum. — Ad dencium dolorem erugine eraminis in aceto infundis et cum linteolo dentem involvis isti. Item acetum cum oleo et solphure coque et mitte in ore dolentis. — Oculorum dolorem vel inpedivit vel sanat.   Radices lava ter super genua et in olla nova coques, deinde ollam ferventem in drappo involverit, exscat et super genua teneas ipsam ollam et super vaporem oculos apertos teneas eos. — [D'une autre main :]   Cornum cervinum et cornu de capra et testis de ovis unde pulli scludiuntur, saponis veteris plenum ovum.

VIII

Ms. 110.   XIe siècle.   Provenance : abbaye de Saint-Père.

1.   *Vertus du béryl.*

[Fol. 95]   De berillo lapide.   Berillus lapis hic magnus etiam et lucidus est, subviridis, clarus, similis oleo Apollinis, sculpis in eum locustam marinam et sub pedes ejus corniclam et sub gemma ponis herbe savine modicum, auro inclusum consecratum gestato et amorem conjugis et majorum omnium facit. Preterea proficit hic lapis ad oculorum vicia et omnem valitudinem si eum in aqua miseris et ipsam aquam potui dederis, ruptos autem spiritu aut suspiriosis et epaticis dolores liberat.

> Précédé d'un commentaire mystique d'*Apocalypse*, XXI, 19–20, où sont décrites les douze pierres sur lesquelles repose la Cité céleste, commentaire différent de celui de Marbode (*Patrologia latina*, CLXXI, c.1771–74).

2.   *Lapidaire avec applications médicales.*

[Fol. 97]   Est autem circa graciam et amiciciam conciliandum obtimus. De jaspide carcedo.   Jaspis, lapis qui et carcedonius, si sanctificatus est, circumligatus aquaticos curat.   Preterea qui portaverit eum a puericia, nunquam mergetur neque vexabitur.   Pulcrum quoque facit gestantem et fidelem, et potentem et omnia perficientem.   Sculpere oportet in eo Martem armatum, aut Virginem stolatam cum veste circumfusa, tenentem laurum. Consecratum est enim per perpetua consecratione. — De topazo.   Topazos lapis tutamentum obtimum est ad divinationes equales, aptissimus est autem. Quod si quis uvam marinam biberit et insaniat, trito eo lapide super cuticulam cum aqua dat furioso, deinde aptatus idem lapis circa collum sanabitur. Sacrificatus etiam tibi, propiciante Deo, utilis est.   Suasionem enim habet secum et impetrationem et gratos facit gerentes se, sanctificatus per perpetuam consecrationem. — De smaragdo.   Smaragdus lapis pulcherrimus est et valedissimus, etiam ad omnem aquariam divinationem persuasionemque habet in omni negotio, portatusque auget substanciam et corpore et sermone castitati aptus, maxime autem subvenit et liberat a tempestatibus, nam quicunque perfecte conservaverit eum, omnimodo impetrabit libertatem. Oportet autem eum perficere sic.   Adeptus lapidem jubes sculpere scarabeum, deinde sub ventre ejus stantem sipticem, postea aper tendatur in longitudinem, tunc in aurea fibula missus discooperta consecratus est, et fac locum quendam bonum preparari, et ornaberis tu et cetera que tua sunt, et videbis gloriam lapidis, quantam ei Deus concessit. [Fol. 97v°] — De corallio.   Corallius lapis maximas habet vires in magica tractacione et in majori negocio moventibus. Est enim tenax et omnia repellit somnia et ludibria suo remedio, maximum autem testamentum adversus iram dominorum est.   Sculptum nomen noctiluce, hoc est agatae, signat autem Gorgone personam.   Portans autem eum numquam capietur a nullo medicamento nec a fulminea umbra immissa. In beluam quoque et pugnam maximum adjutorium est et invictus et efficax et inpetrabilis sine timore, sine tristicia securum facit gestantem et facile impetrantem et introitus faciles.   Preterea consecratus et contritus et seminatus cum frumento aut ordeo aut aliquo fructu, ammovet de terra grandinem et omnem perniciem et tempestatem, insuper in vineis aut olivetis dispersus, repellit omnes odiosos impetus ventorum.   In domum autem positus conservat ab omni maleficio et umbris demoniorum et vana somnia et fulminum ictibus. Malis vero locis si habueris eum, multo efficax erit, resistit autem ventis et tempestatibus et turbidini.   Tanta sortitur potentia iste lapis contra adversas partes.   Consecratur vero a Deo et sanctis locis hoc tutamentum, ut sit maximum die ac nocte, hora diurna vel nocturna, bonumque presidium corallius lapis. — De carcedonio.   Carcedonius lapis pertuso aptatus fertur. Qui eam portat, vincit causas.

Des lapidaires traitant, au moins accessoirement, des vertus médicales des gemmes se trouvent dans les manuscrits de la Bibliothèque Nationale: lat. 2328, fol. 95v°–96, IXe s. et lat. 7028, fol. 140–143v°, XIe s., ce dernier ayant beaucoup de points de contact avec les passages des *Étymologies* de saint Isidore de Séville où il est question de pierres précieuses.

IX

Ms. III.   IXe ou Xe siècle.   Provenance : chapitre de la cathédrale.

1.   *Formule contre l'hémorragie.*

[Feuillet collé à l'intérieur du plat antérieur de la reliure]   Ad sanguinem stringendum pone has litteras super pectus pacientis. S.P.IX.I.B.C.P. OH.A.U...[fin illisible].

Complété par Tribalet (p. 52), par « Q. Amen. »   Une formule magique, mais toute différente, contre l'hémorragie se trouve au fol. 139v° du ms. 689 de Cambrai, du Xe ou du XIe siècle.

2.   *Vers sur la diète.*

[Fol. 92]   De dieta ejusdem.

Prandia lauta modis inturbant plerumque dietae.
Indulges stomacho, mentem male crapula vexat.
Si parcas epulis, sequitur detractio vel laus.
Ut medium teneas labor est et valde cavendum
Ne tibi tristiciam pariat sicut suus est mos.
Si possis igitur prorsus haec prandia vita

At si non liceat hilaris cautusque recumbe et
Ciba cuncta parum tua quae tibi regula dictat
Nec summam nimiam conjectent multa minuta.

À la suite d'un petit traité anonyme *De septem miraculis mundi ab hominibus factis.*

X

Ms.193.   XIᵉ siècle.   Provenance : abbaye de Saint-Père.

Recettes.

[Fol. 187]   Confectio pulveris ad pectus : germandria, acrimonia, silmontanus, gentiana, edera terrestris, radicem de basilisco, sistra, pionia, antena, yva, salvia, ysopus, sarreia, betonica, radicem de livestico, melsega, civerium, artemisia, sal gemma, omnia pigmenta et piper, et bacchas, et ciminum, et peretrum.   Ad balneum : presogom., de edera boscarensi radicem et folia, viscum, savina, apium, salvia, grana de junipero, marrubium album, ysopum, radicem de ebla.

En tête du ms., cette sentence : « Omnis homo primum bonum vinum ponit.» Tribalet qui la reproduit (p. 52), dit qu'elle « témoigne au moins d'un respect modéré pour les principes hygiéniques de Fulbert. »

IBN JAMĪ' ON THE SKELETON

by

C. RABIN

INTRODUCTION

HIBATALLĀH ibn Zain Ibn Jamī', the Jew, was physician to Sultan Saladin of Egypt (A.D. 1138–93). He was very highly esteemed both as a practical physician and as a teacher. His master granted him the high titles 'Sun of Authority' and 'Victorious in Faith' (*Shams al-riyāsa, Muwaffaq al-dīn*). He wrote several minor works, as well as a handbook of medicine, entitled *Kitāb al-irshād li-maṣāliḥ al-anfās wal-ajsād*, 'Guide to the treatment of mind and body', which was put into its final shape by his son Ismaʿīl.[1]

The *Irshād* is an attempt to present the subject-matter of the weighty tomes of Haly Abbas (d. 994) and Avicenna (980–1037) in a much smaller book. This was indeed a pressing need in an age when students learned their text-books by heart. A secondary purpose in writing this book may have been to produce a medical text-book that would pass the criticism of linguistic purists, always a powerful element in the Arab world. The works of most Arab scientific writers were in a style tending towards the colloquial.[2] Ibn Jamī', we are told,[3] never lectured without having before him a copy of Jauharī's *Ṣaḥāḥ*, that most conservative of all Arabic dictionaries. As our text proves, Ibn Jamī' certainly paid more attention to correct grammar than to consistent medical terminology.

Originality was neither demanded nor lauded in writers of that period,[4] and would indeed have been impossible in a subject like anatomy, where research on the object was out of the question. We must consider it meritorious that Ibn Jamī' did not merely copy out his great predecessors, but went back to the source of all medical wisdom, Galen, whose *De ossibus ad tirones* he used for the account of the joints, and probably elsewhere. The translation of that work, made by Ḥunain b. Isḥāq (809–77),[5] seems to have been much studied, judging from the number of manuscripts preserved, both of the full work and the Alexandrine abridgment,[6] but few definite traces of it appear in the great medical writers.

The question of the literary sources of the great writers, Rhazes, Haly Abbas, and Avicenna, has not yet been studied, as far as I am aware. As far as term-inology goes, Haly Abbas has forms closest to the Greek, i.e. drawn directly

---

[1] Cf. G. Sarton, *Introduction to the history of science*. Baltimore, vol. ii, 1931, p. 432; C. Brockelmann, *Grundriss der arabischen Literaturgeschichte*. 2nd edition. Vol. i, 1943, p. 489; M. Meyerhof, *Isis*, 1929, xii, 123.

[2] Cf. A. Müller, *Sitzungsb. d. königl.-bayer. Akad. d. Wissensch., philos.-philol. Kl.*, 1884, pp. 888 ff.

[3] *Ibn Abī Uṣaibiʿa*, ed. A. Müller. Königsberg, 1884, vol. ii, p. 120.

[4] Cf. Brockelmann, *op. cit.* (1), vol. i, p. 284.

[5] Cf. Bergsträsser, 'Ḥunain ibn Isḥāq über die syrischen und arabischen Galen-Uebersetz-ungen'. *Abhandl. f. d. Kunde d. Morgenlandes*, Leipzig, 1925, xvii, 2 (German text, p. 6).

[6] Cf. Diels, 'Die Handschriften der antiken Aerzte I'. *Abhandl. d. preuss. Akad. d. Wissensch.*, 1905, Abhandl. iii, p. 67; to this add one copy of the *Abridgment* in Istanbul, cf. Ritter and Walzer, *Sitzungsb. d. Preuss. Akad. d. Wissensch., phil.-hist. Kl.*, 1934, p. 821.

from translations of Galen's works; Rhazes often deviates sharply, while
Avicenna's terminology appears to be the result of an inner-Arabic (?)
development of the Greek terms, incorporating also many native Arabic terms
ignored by the translators. But we may possibly go one step further. In
several passages our text agrees closely with Avicenna's, and yet differs from it
in points which would be inexplicable if Ibn Jamī' had copied the Avicenna
text which is before us. We must either assume that in the twelfth century
the text of the *Canon* was rather different from that of the manuscripts used by
the editors of the prints (an assumption for which we have no material basis),
or that both Avicenna and Ibn Jamī' used the same source. From the samples
in our text this appears to have been a conflation of various Galenic works of
the type of the Greek *Introductio seu medicus*, or the Arabic-Latin *Anatomia
vivorum Galeni*. The peculiarities of Avicenna's terminology may then in
part be due to this intermediate compendium. On our second assumption it
would also be easy to account for the instances in which Ibn Jamī' has a
better text of a statement in Avicenna than Avicenna himself. We can
hardly doubt that Avicenna, whose martial and political activities, combined
with riotous living, can have allowed him little time for independent research,
relied for his *Canon* heavily on literary borrowing. It seems pretty certain
that the *Abridgment* of *De ossibus* was much used by Avicenna. It is,
however, not identical with our hypothetical source.

The main interest of our text lies in its terminology. Occasion has been
taken in the notes to penetrate behind the scenes of Arabic medical nomenclature. The etymology of the words has been studied wherever possible,
and some remarks made on the history of terms within the course of Arabic
medical writing, a subject which would merit a wider treatment. Special
attention has been paid to the many instances of contradiction between medical
terminology and ordinary literary Arabic usage, as codified in the native
lexica, notably Ibn Sīda and the *Lisān*. These differences are, of course, due
to the fact that Ḥunain and his collaborators were Syriac Christians who had
learned Arabic as a foreign language, and had at Baghdad little opportunity to
discover the finer points of Bedouin anatomical nomenclature. Sometimes,
where the Arabic term was vague or otherwise unsuitable, the translators may
purposely have preferred new terms translated from the Greek.

The translation of the text is based on two Oxford MSS.: Hunt. 19 (=A),
that published here, and Hunt. 242 (=B).

It gives me special gratification to be able to contribute my modest effort to
this volume, since it was Professor Singer who first directed my attention to
the subject of medieval medicine and in many pleasant hours initiated me into it.

TRANSLATION OF THE TEXT
Chapter VII : The Bones

§ 1   The bones (1) are the rigid structures which support the other organs
of the human body. Some are to the body like the basis on which a
thing is built (2), as a ship is erected on its keel (3); others are like
protections and guards, such as the parietal bone (4); others again are
like weapons by which any object likely to knock against the part and
to harm it is repelled, such as the thorns of the spine (5), which are

الفصل السابع في العظام وهو ابتداء القول في تشريح الاعضاء البسيطة
العظام هي الاجسام الصلبة التي عليها مبنى سائر اعضاء بدن الانسان ومنها ماقياسه من البدن
قياس الاساس الذي يبنى عليه الشي كما تبنى السفينة على الخشبة التي في اسفلها ومنها ماقياسه الجنة قياس
والوقاية كعظم اليافوخ ومنها ماقياسه قياس السلاح الذي يدفع به المصادم المؤذي مثل شوك
الصلب الذي يدعى سناسن ومنها ما هو حشو بين فرج المفاصل مثل العظام السمسمانية وجملتها
الا الشاذ منها متجاورة متصلة بعضها ببعض وجملة تركيبها تسمى الجثة وتركيبها بعضها الى بعض
اما على جهة التجاور ويسمى مفصلا واما على جهة الاتحاد ويسمى التحاما والمفصل تجاور طبيعي
بين عظمين والاتحاد التحام طبيعي بين عظمين والعظام التي بينها المفاصل منها ماله لواحق
في اطرافه كالعظم العضد في طرفه الاعلى ولعظم الزند الاسفل ولعظم الفخذ في طرفيه معا ومنها
ماليس له لاحقة كعظمي اللحي الاعلى وبالجملة فان اللواحق توجد لاكثر العظام الكبار منها ولا يوجد
لاكثر الصلبة منها ومن هذه العظام ماله زوايد كالعظم اللحي الاسفل من طرفيه اللذين يليان
الراس والفرق بين اللاحقة والزايدة ان اللاحقة عظم اخر متحد بالعظم الذي هو لاحقة له
والزايدة جزء من العظم نفسه الذي هو زايدة له وما كان من الزوايد ينتهي الى طرف غليظ
مستدير سمي عنقا ويسمى طرفه المدور راسا ونقر العظام التي تدخل فيها روس عظام اخر ما كان
منها عميقا سمي حقا وما كان منها قليل العمق سمي عينا والمفاصل منها سلس ومنها غير سلس ويسمى الموثق
والمفصل السلس هو الذي لاحد عظميه عند الاخر حركة بينة كمفصل المرفق ومفصل الموثق
هو الذي ليس لاحد عظميه عند الاخر حركة بينة كمفاصل عظام الرسغ والمفاصل السلسة فمنها المرفق
ومنها المطرف ومنها المداخل والمغرق هو الذي لاحد عظميه عنق طويل والاخر حق والمطرف
هو الذي لاحد عظميه عنق قصير والاخر عين والمداخل هو الذي لكل واحد من عظميه راس
مهندم في نقرة من الاخر والمفاصل الموثقة فمنها المدروز ومنها المركوز ومنها الملصق فالمدروز
هو الذي لكل واحد من عظميه اسنان وتحاريز تتهندم بعضها في بعض كمفاصل عظام القحف
وتسمى شانا ودروزا والمركوز هو الذي لاحد عظميه زايدة تتهندم في نقرة من الاخر كمفاصل
الاسنان مع العظام التي هي مركوزة فيها والملصق هو الذي يتصل احد عظميه بالاخر على خط
مستقيم كمفصل عظمي الزندين او على سطح كمفاصل الفقرات السفلى من الصلب والذي على جهة
الالتحام منه التحام العظمين بلا واسطة واكثر ما يوجد في العظام المتخلخلة اللينة واما
بواسطة فالواسطة اما غضروف ويسمى الالتحام الغضروفي واما رباط ويسمى الالتحام الرباطي
واما لحم ويسمى الالتحام اللحمي والعظام منها ما هو مصمت لا تجويف فيه كاكثر العظام الصغار ومنها
ما هو مجوف والمجوف اما ان يكون التجويف فيه واحدا عظيما كعظم الفخذ والعضد وما كان منها
كذلك ففيه مخ واما تجاويف كثيرة صغار كالتجاريف كالعظام المتخلخلة اللينة وبالجملة
فما كان من هذه العظام انما يحتاج اليه للوقاية والدعامة فقط ولا يحتاج اليه لتحريك شي
من الاعضاء فانه خلق مصمتا وان كان فيه المسام والخلل والفرج وما كان يحتاج اليه منها

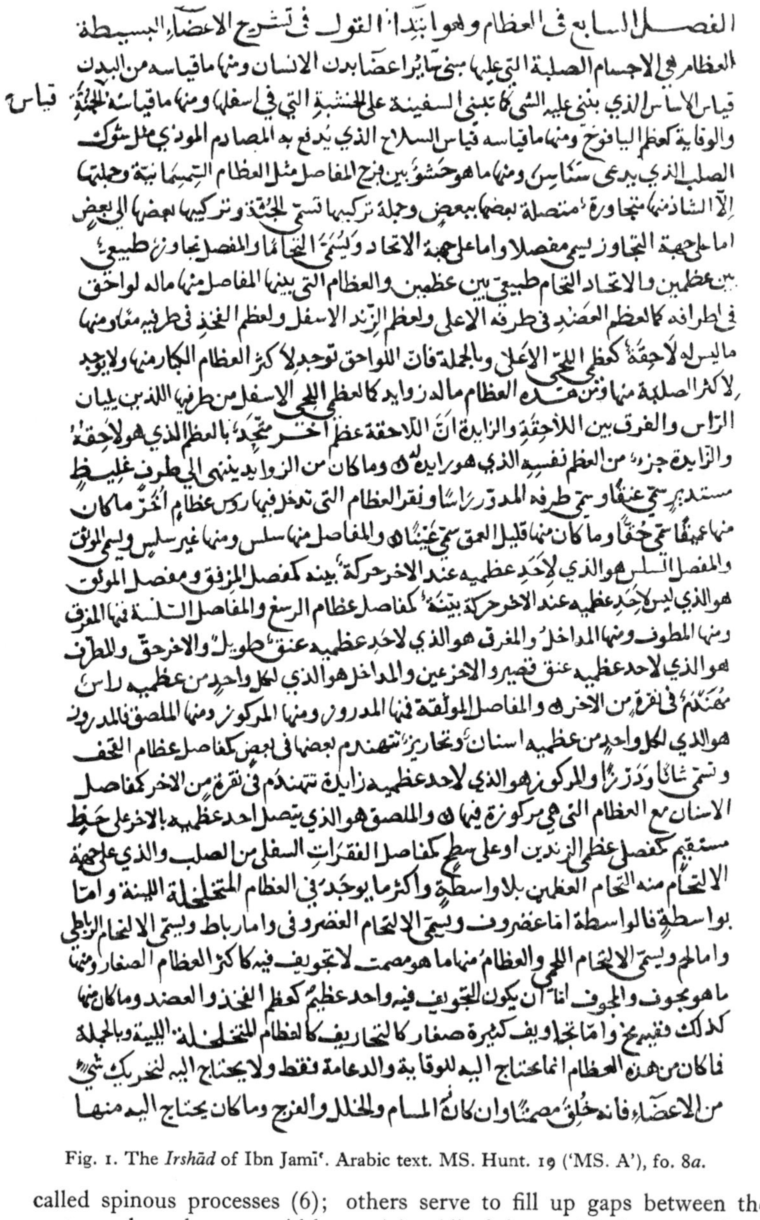

Fig. 1. The *Irshād* of Ibn Jamīʿ. Arabic text. MS. Hunt. 19 ('MS. A'), fo. 8*a*.

called spinous processes (6); others serve to fill up gaps between the
§ 2 parts, such as the sesamoid bones (7). All of them, with few exceptions, adjoin and are connected with each other. All (7*a*) bones together are called skeleton (8). Their junctures with each other are either by juxtaposition (9), when they are called joints (10), or by unification (11),

when they are called symphyses (12). A joint is a natural juxtaposition of two bones, while a symphysis is a natural unification of two bones (13).

§ 3 The bones meeting in a joint either have epiphyses (14) at their extremities, such as the humerus (15) at its upper end, and the ulna (16) and the femur (17) at both ends, or they have no epiphyses, such as the two bones of the superior maxilla (18). In general, epiphyses are found in most of the large bones (19), and are not found in most of the hard bones. Some of these bones possess apophyses (20), such as the two bones of the inferior maxilla (21) at the two ends adjoining the skull. The difference between an epiphysis and an apophysis is that the epiphysis is a separate bone unified with the bone to which it is attached, while the apophysis is a part of that bone itself (22).

§ 4   An apophysis which terminates in a thick round end is called a neck (23); the round end is called head (24). The cavities (25) of bones into which other bones enter, if deep, are called box (pyxis) (26), if shallow,

§ 5 eye (27). Joints are either loose or not loose (28), the latter being called firm (29). Loose joints are those in which the bones move visibly against each other, as in the elbow (30); firm are those joints in which there is no visible relative movement of either bone, as in the joints

§ 6 between the bones of carpus or tarsus (31). Loose joints are divided into immersed (32), contacting (33), and interlocked joints (34). Immersed are those joints in which one bone has a long neck and the other a pyxis; in the contacting joints one has a short neck and the other an eye; in the interlocked joint each bone possesses a head symmetrically

§ 7 inserted (35) into a cavity of the other. Firm joints are either serrated (36), implanted (37), or adherent (38). In the serrated suture each bone has teeth (39) and notches (40), symmetrically inserted into each other, as in the joints of the skull bones (41). Such a suture is called *sha'n* (42) or *darz* (43). Implanted is the joint in which one bone has an apophysis inserted in a cavity of the other, as the joints of the teeth with the bones in which they are implanted. Adherent are those joints in which both bones touch along a straight line, as in the joint of ulna and radius (44), or along an even surface, as in the case of the joints

§ 8 of the vertebrae (45) in the lower part of the spine (46). The welded joints (47) either consist in the welding of two bones without any intervening substance, which mostly occurs in soft porous bones, or with some intervening substance. This may be cartilage (48), called therefore cartilaginous welding [primary synchondrosis], or a ligament (49) called ligamentous welding [secondary synchondrosis with ligaments], or muscular tissue (50), called muscular welding [secondary synchondrosis with fibro-cartilage] (51).

§ 9   Some bones are solid, without any cavities, as most of the smaller bones. Others are hollow (51a). These may either have one large cavity, as the femur or the humerus. Bones that are like this contain

§10 marrow (52). Or they may have many small cavities, like hornets' nests (53), such as the porous (54) soft (55) bones. In general (56), those bones which are required only for protection and support, not for moving one of the limbs, are created solid, though they contain some

لاجل الحركة نقد يزيد في مقدار جويفه وجعل نجو ليفد في وسطه واحدا ليكون جرمه غير
محتاج الى مواقف الغذاء المتفرقة فيصير رخوا بالصلابة جرمه وجعل غذاؤه وهو المخ زيفه
فغاية زيادة التجويف ان يكون اخف وفائدة توحيد التجويف ان يكون جرمه اصلب
وفائدة صلابة جرمه ان لا يكسر عند الحركات العنيفة وفائدة المخ فيه ليغدوه ويربطه
دائما ويكون وهو محروف كالمحبت فالتجويف يقل اذا كانت الحاجة الى الوثاقة اكثر ويكثر
اذا كانت الحاجة الى الخفة اكثر والعظام المشاشية خلقت كذلك لامر الغذاء المذكور
مع زيادة لحاجة بسبب بجبات يكون ينفذ فيها كالرايحة المستنشقة مع المواد في عظم الصفا
ولفضول الدماغ المدفوعة فيها وجميع العظام التي في بدن الانسان سوى عظم ربه حرف
اللام في كتاب اليونانيين موضع عند الحنجرة وعظم يوجد في القلب وعظام صغار وتعرف
بالسمسانية لصغرها تختش خلل مفاصل الاصابع مايتا وثمانية واربعون عظم النطاق الراس
تسعة وخمسون عظاما وفي اليدين ستون عظاما وفي الرقبة والصدر وما يليه تسعة وثلاثون
عظما وفي الرجلين ستون عظما والتي في الراس هي اثنان في اعلاه وهما جمجمتا القحف واربعة
تحتها للحيدران وجوانبها الاربعة وفي عظم الجبهة والعظم الذي يقابله من خلف والعظمان
اللذان في جنبتيه اللذان فيهما الاذنان ويسمان المجزرين واحد كالقاعدة يجمعها ويسمى
العظم الوتدي واربعة في الصدغين في كل صدغ اثنان ويسميان عظمي الروح واربعة عشر
في اللحي الاعلى وفي هذه الاربعة عشر عظم الوجنتان وعظما الانف واثنان اللحى الاسفل
وهما عظما الفكين واثنان وثلثون سنا وهي اربع ثنايا واربع رباعيات واربعة انياب
وعشرون ضرسا والتي في الرقبة والصدر وما يليه في لثلث نقرة سبع للرقبة واثنتا عشرة
للصدر وحمز للكتفن وثلث للمجز وثلث للعصص وسبع عظام القص وفي عظام الزرور وفيه
وعشرون وصلمان منها اربعة عشر سمي اضلاع الصدر وعشرة تدعى اضلاع الخلف وعظا الكتف
واثنان بيسان رايي الكتفين والتربان وعظا العانة وهذا المظا ان لكل منه اجزا ثلثه
جزء الى الجا الى الوحشي من البدن ويسمى المحرفة وعظم الخاصرة وجزء الى الجانب الاسى منه
ويسمى الا سم العام عظم العانة وجزء الى الورك ويبتى جزء الى الورك والذي في اليدين اثنان
في العضدين واربعة في الساعدين وستة عشر في الرصغين وثمانية في المشطين وثلثون
في الاصابع كل اصبع ثلثة والذي في الرجلين اثنان في الفخذين واثنان على مفصل
الوكبتين وتسميا الرصفتين واربعة في الساقين وستة وعشرون في كل قدم مر
عقبت وكعبت وزو رقي واربعة في المشط وخمسة في الرسغ واربعة عشر في الاصابع
كل اصبع ثلثة ظاهرة واثنان خفية فاحد الظا مر يقال له الاكليلي وهو يتقدم
يفصل بين عظم الراس والجبهة مقوس هاكنا ☐ والاخر قطول الراس هكذا يقال له
سهودي واذا اعتبر باضافتها الى الاكليلي حتى يصير هاكنا ☐ قيل له سهم لانه
يشبه قوسا في مُسْطِد سهم والفات يفصل بين الراس من خلف وبين قاعدته

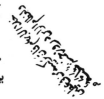

pores (57), hollows (58), and openings (59). Those bones that are required
for movement (60) have a larger degree of hollowness. Their central
cavity is one, so that their body (61) should not require many different
inlets (62) for nourishment and thus become weak (63); their body is
hard and its nourishment—that is the marrow—placed in its centre (64).

§11 The purpose of the greater degree of hollowness is that it is easier to
move such a bone. The purpose of giving it a single hollow is that its
body should become very hard. The purpose of making its body hard
is that it should not break through violent movement. The purpose
of the marrow in it is to nourish it and to keep it always moist (65), so
that, though hollow, it is like a solid bone. The degree of hollowness

§12 decreases where the need is more for strength, and increases where it
is more important that the bone should be light. The spongy (66) bones
have been created like that for the sake of nourishment, as has been
mentioned, as well as owing to the greater need for some stuff (67) that must
penetrate it, as the odour sniffed in with the air penetrates the ethmoid
bone (68) and the superfluities of the brain are expelled through it.

§13 The number of the bones in the human body—apart from a bone
formed like the Greek L (69) which is placed near the glottis, a bone
found in the heart (70), and certain small bones known as sesamoid (71)
because of their small size, which fill the gaps of finger and toe joints—is
248. Of these, 59 are in the head, 60 in the arms, 69 in the neck, chest,
and adjoining parts, and 60 in the legs (72).

§14 The bones of the head are: two at the top, called bowls of the
cranium (73); four underneath them like walls at their four sides (74),
namely the frontal bone (75), the one corresponding to it at the back (76),
and the two bones at the sides in which the ears are, called petrous
bones (77); one bone like a pedestal (78) joining them (or articulating
with all of them), called the sphenoid (79); four on the temples (80),

§15 on each temple two, called bones of the zygoma (81); fourteen in the
upper jaw, among them the cheek bones (82), and the nasal bones (83);
two in the lower jaw, namely the maxillary bones (84); and thirty-two
teeth : four anterior incisors (85), four posterior incisors (86), four canines
(87), and twenty molars (88).

§16 The bones in neck (89), chest (90), and adjoining regions are: thirty
vertebrae (91), of which seven of the neck, twelve of the chest, five of the
lumbi (92), three of the sacrum (93), and three of the coccyx (94);
seven bones of the sternum (95), which are the pectoral bones (96);
twenty-four ribs (97), of which fourteen are called pectoral (98) and ten

§17 pseudo-ribs (99); two scapulae (100); two bones called head of the scapula
(101), and two clavicles (102); the two pubic bones (103), each of which
consists of three parts: one on the outer side as seen from the body,
called ilium (104) or loin bone (104a), a part on the inner side, called
by the same name as the whole, pubic bone, and a part adjoining the
thigh, called box of the thigh (105).

§18 The bones of the arm are: two in the upper arms (105a) and four in the
forearms (106), sixteen in the carpus (107), eight in the metacarpus (108),

§19 and thirty in the fingers, in every finger three. The bones of the legs are:

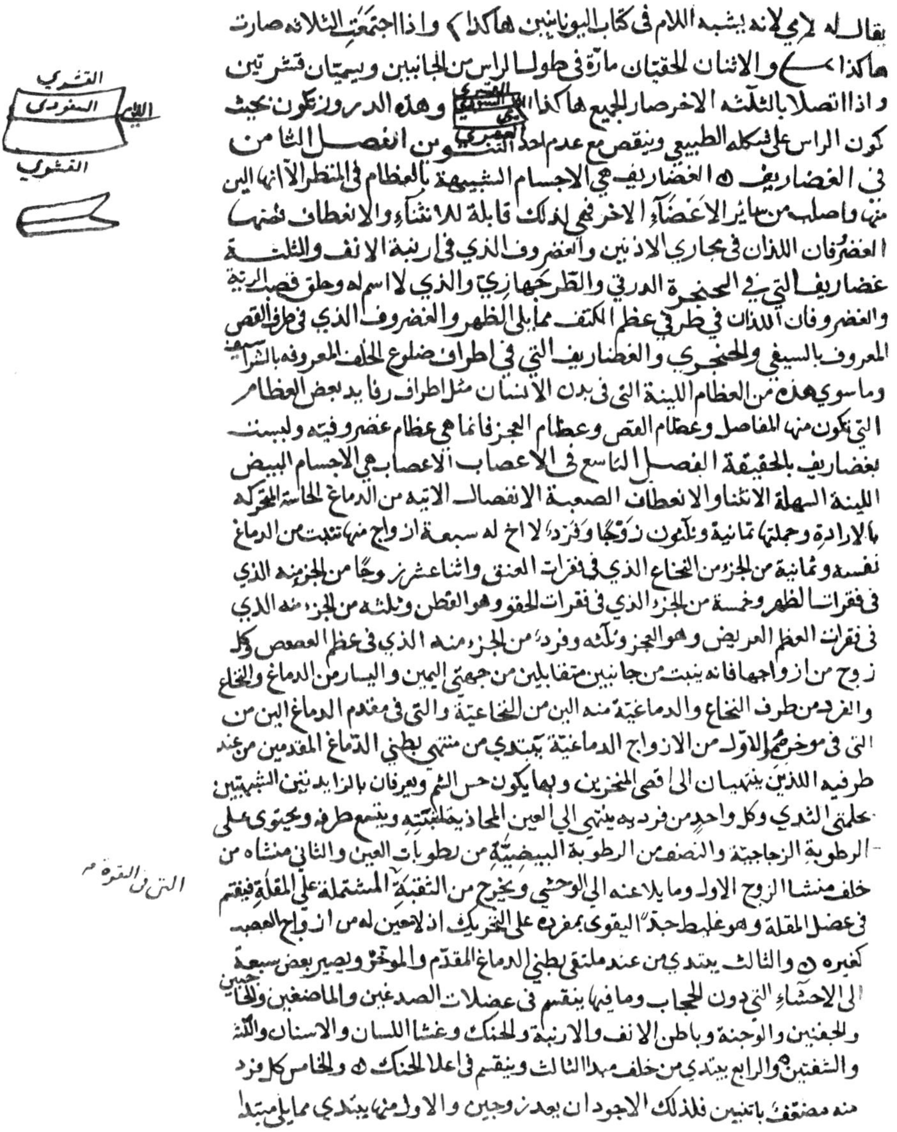

بقاله لاي لانه يشبه اللام في كتاب اليونانيين هاكذا⟩ واذا اجتمعت الثلاثة صارت
هاكذا ⟨⟩ والاثنان للعينان في طولها الراس مائة في طولها الراس من الجانبين ويبقان قشرتين
واذاتصلا بالثلاثة الاخرصار للربيع هاكذا ⟨⟩ وهذه الدرز يكون بحيث
كون الراس على شكله الطبيعي وينقص مع عدم احدى الثلاثة ... من انفصال الثامن من
ذي الغضاريف ... الغضاريف في الاجسام الشبيهة بالعظام في النظر الا انها الين
منه واصلب من سائر الاعضاء الاخرفي لذلك قابلة للانثناء والانعطاف ضفها
العضروفان اللذان في مجاري الاذنين والعضروف الذي في ارنبة الانف والثلثة
غضاريف التي في الحنجرة الدرقي والطرجهاري والذي لا اسم له وطرف الصابية
والعضروفان اللذان في طرفي عظم الكتف ما بلي الظهر والعضروف الذي في اسفل القص
المعروف بالسيفي والخنجري والغضاريف التي في اطراف اضلع الخلف المعروفة بالشراسيف
وما سوى هذه من العظام اللينة التي في بدن الانسان مثل اطراف ارنبا بعض العظام
التي يكون منها المفاصل وعظام العص وعظام الجزء فانما هي عظام عضروفية وليست
بغضاريف بالحقيقة الفصل التاسع في الاعصاب الاعصاب في الاجسام البيض
اللينة السهلة الانثناء والانعطاف الصعبة الانفصال الاتية من الدماغ لحاسة الحركة
ما الارادة وجملة ثمانية وتكون زوجها وفردا لا اخ له سبعة ان واحد منها تنبت من الدماغ
نفسه وثمانية من الجزء للنخاع الذي في فقرات العنق واثنا عشر زوجا من الجزء الذي
في فقرات الظهر وخمسة من الجزء الذي في فقرات المقو وهو العظم وثلثة من الجزء ... الذي
في فقرات العظم العريض وهو الجزء ولكنه وفرد من الجزء الذي منه الذي في عظم العصص وكل
زوج من ازواجهما فانه ينبت من جانبين متقابلين من جهتي اليمين واليسار من الدماغ والنخاع
والفردمن طرف النخاع والدماغية منه اليمن من الخاصية والتي في مقدم الدماغ الين من
التي في موخرها الاول من الازواج الدماغية يتادي من منتهى بطني الدماغ المقدمين مرعند
طرفيه اللذين يشميان الى في العينين وبهما يكون حس الشم ويعرفان بازايدتين الشبيهتين
بحلمتي الثدي وكل واحدمنه وفرد به منتهى الى العين المجاذ بعظمتيه ويتسع طرفه ويحوى على
الرطوبة الزجاجية والنصفين والرطوبة البيضية من رطوبات العين والثاني منشاه من
خلف منشا الزوج الاول وما يلاعنه الوحشي ويخرج من الثقبة المشتملة على المقلة فيقم
في عضل المقلة وموضعها طحجة اليقوى بمعرفة على التحريك اذلا عين لهم ان زوج العصب
كثيره ... والثالث يبتدى من عند ملتقى بطني الدماغ المقدم والموخر ويصير بعض سبعة
الى الاحشاء التي دون الحجاب ومافيها ينقسم في عضلات الصدغين والماضغين وكل
والجفنين والوجنة وباطن الانف والارنبة والحنك وغشا اللسان والاسنان واللثة
والشفتين والرابع يبتدى من خلف هذا الثالث وينقسم في اعلا الحنك ... وللخامس ... وزد
منه مضغف باثنين نلذلك الاجودان بعد زوجين والاول من يبتدى ما لي مبتدا

Fig. 3. The *Irshād* of Ibn Jamīʿ. Arabic text. MS. Hunt. 19 ('MS. A'), fo. 8c.

two femora (109), two over the knee joints (110), called patellae (111),
four in the lower leg (112), and twenty-six in each foot, namely calcaneum
(113), astragalus (114), navicular (115), four in the tarsus (116), five in the
metatarsus (117), and fourteen in the toes, in each toe three, except in
the big toe, which is composed of two bones.

§20   The bones of the head have five sutures (118), three visible (119) and two invisible (120). Of the visible ones, one is called coronal (121) and is at the front of the head separating the head-bone (122) from the front (123). It is curved thus: ⌊ [*sic*] (123*a*). The second runs along the head and is called skewer-like (124). If it is considered in conjunction with the coronal suture, with which it forms this figure:

╠── it is called sagittal (125), because the whole resembles a bow and an arrow across its middle. The third suture separates the head (126) posteriorly from its base (127), and is called lambdoid (128) because it resembles the L in the Greek script, thus ⟨ . When the three come together, they form this figure: ╠─⟨ . The two hidden sutures pass along the length of the head from the corners of the forehead (129) and are called scales (130). All these sutures, taken together, give this picture: ⟨═⟨ . These sutures exist when the head has its natural form, but there are less when one of the two protuberances (131) is lacking.

NOTES TO THE TEXT

Bibliographical Abbreviations

Abridgment   The Abridgment (*jawāmiʿ*) of Galen's *De ossibus*, quoted from British Museum MS., *Or. Add.* 23407.

Abulcasis   *Albucasis de Chirurgia, Arabice et Latine, cura J. Channing*. Oxford, 1778.

Avicenna   *Canon*, Arabic text quoted according to the translation by P. De Koning, *Trois traités d'anatomie arabes*, Leyden, 1903, pp. 432–780, where the Arabic terms are given in footnotes. Where De Koning does not indicate the Arabic, this is tacitly supplied from the printed Arabic *Canon*, Rome, 1590.

Brockelmann   *Grundriss der vergleichenden Grammatik der semitischen Sprachen*. Berlin, 1908–13.

De Koning   *Trois traités*, etc., see under *Avicenna*.

Dhorme   *L'emploi métaphorique des noms de parties du corps en hébreu et en akkadien*. Paris, 1923. (*Extrait de la Révue Biblique, 1920–3*.)

Dozy   *Supplément aux dictionnaires arabes*. Leyden, 1881.

Fagnan   *Additions aux dictionnaires arabes*. Algiers, 1923.

Fonahn   *Arabic and Latin anatomical terminology, chiefly from the Middle Ages*. Kristiania, 1922. (*Videnskapsselskapets Skrifter, II, Hist.-filos. Klasse, 1921, No. 7.*)

Galen   Quoted according to the edition of Kühn. Leipzig, 1821–33.

Haly Abbas   Edited and trans. by De Koning, *Trois traités*, etc., pp. 90–431.

Holma	*Die Namen der Körperteile im Assyrisch-Babylonischen, eine lexikalisch-etymologische Studie.* Leipzig, 1911.
Hyrtl	*Das Arabische und Hebräische in der Anatomie.* Vienna, 1879.
Ibn Hashshā'	*Ibn al-H'achcha (xiiie siècle J.C.), Glossaire sur le Mans'uri de Razès, texte arabe...par G. S. Colin et H. P. J. Renaud.* Rabat, 1941.
Ibn Duraid	*Jamharat al-lugha* (one of the oldest Arabic lexica). Hyderabad, A.H. 1344–51
Ibn Sīda	*Kitāb al-mukhaṣṣaṣ* (a classified word-list in 20 vols.). Būlāq, A.H. 1316–21.
Lisān	Ibn Manẓūr (1232–1311), *Lisān al-'arab.* Būlāq, A.H. 1300. (This is the best Arabic lexicon. It does not record the words used in the Arabic prose of its day, but those considered correct for use in poetry. It is based on the Bedouin language of the first centuries A.H.)
Peñuela	*'Die Goldene' des Ibn al-Munāṣif, ein Beitrag zur medizinisch-arabischen Lexikographie,* etc. Rome, 1941.
Rhazes	*Almansor,* chapters edited and trans. by De Koning, *Trois traités,* etc., pp. 2–89.
Sbath and Meyerhof	*Le livre des questions sur l'œil de Honaïn Ibn Ishāq.* Cairo, 1938. (*Mémoires de l'Institut d'Égypte, I, 36*).
Simon	*Sieben Bücher Anatomie des Galen.* Leipzig, 1906. (The Arabic translation of *De anat. admin.* On the identity of the translator, cf. G. Bergsträsser, *Hunain ibn Isḥāḳ und seine Schule.* Leyden, 1913, p. 41.)
Singer and Rabin	*A prelude to modern science, being a discussion of .... the Tabulae Anatomicae Sex of Vesalius.* Cambridge, 1946. (Publications of the Wellcome Historical Medical Museum, n.s., No. 1.)
Sudhoff	*Ein Beitrag zur Geschichte der Anatomie im Mittelalter.* Leipzig, 1908. (Studien zur Geschichte der Medizin, 4.)

NOTES

(1) The whole of this paragraph is almost identical with Avicenna, p. 452; both are obviously based on the *Abridgment.*

(2) The *Abridgment* and Avicenna add 'such as the spine (*faqār al-ṣalab*)'.

(3) Literally 'the piece of wood which is erected in it first'; The *Abridgment* and Avicenna have 'the piece of wood in its bottom'. Galen (*De ossibus,* introd.; Kühn ii. 733) compares the bones in general to foundation-stones (*themelia*); Aristotle (*De part. anim.* ii. 9; 654.b.30) to the solid framework of a clay figure. In Assyrian the keel was called 'spine of the ship', *eṣenṣēru elippi* (Holma, p. 51; but Dhorme, p. 97, thinks it means the deck).

(4) *'aẓm al-yāfūkh.* In non-medical Arabic *yāfūkh* or *ya'fūkh* denotes sinciput and occiput (cf. *Lisān* iii. 482; Peñuela, p. 59), in medical language only sinciput, Greek *bregma.* Galen in *De ossibus* (Kühn ii. 744 f.) calls the parietals *osta tou bregmatos* in the plural, but in the part of *De anat. admin.*

which is preserved only in Arabic (Simon i. 13) he says: 'the whole bone lying between the two temporal sutures, that is the bone called *yāfūkh*, which is one on both sides'. In medieval Latin *ifek*, *iefec*, etc., denotes the sinciput. For other names of the parietals, see notes 41, 73, 122, 126. The *Abridgment* has here '*qihf* of the head' (cf. note 41).

(5) Avicenna: 'Like the bones called *sanāsin*, which are for the defence of the back, like thorns.' *Shauk al-ṣalab* translates Greek *akantha tōn spondylōn* (Simon i. 24, etc.). It appears to have been coined by the Ḥunain school of translators to replace the native *sanāsin*, which in the *Abridgment* is given as a gloss to it. *Shauk* = thorn, spur, enters also into the term *al-shaukī* 'the spur-bone' = astragalus, in medieval Latin *alsochi* (Singer and Rabin, p. 27). *Ṣalab*, *ṣulab*, or *ṣulb* is said in *Lisān* ii. 14 to mean (*a*) the spine, (*b*) a vertebra (in the plural 'spine'), (*c*) the back. A passage in the Mohammedan traditions, 'He created them when they were in the *aṣlāb* of their fathers', shows that the word was used for loins (cf. 'kings shall come out of thy loins', Gen. xxxv. 11). Perhaps the first meaning of the word was 'sacrum'. The root means 'to be hard', and the sacrum was considered the hardest bone in the body (cf. note 94). The sacrum looks like a cross (cf. German 'Kreuzbein'), and thus we can explain Mishnaic Hebrew *ṣelūbh*, Syriac *ṣelībhā*, Ethiopic *ṣalbō* 'cross'. For the change from 'sacrum' to 'loins' cf. the relation of Assyrian *arkatu* 'back' to Arabic *warik* 'loin' (note 104*a*). *Ṣalab* is used for the spine by all Arabic medical writers except Rhazes, who gives no name for the whole spine.

(6) *sanāsin*, sing. *sinsin*, apparently a reduplication of *sinn* 'tooth', which latter is also said to mean 'spinous process'. The other word for tooth, in the form *ḍarīs* (cf. note 88) is also said to mean 'vertebrae of the back'. The *Lisān* (xvii. 93) does not give the meaning 'spinous processes' for *sanāsin*, but says they denote (*a*) the rims (*ḥarf*) of the dorsal vertebrae, (*b*) the costal cartilages. The meaning (*a*) is probably intended in the verse 'what dost thou think of a raid that leaves of me but *sanāsin* looking like the ring of a shield?' In medical Arabic *sanāsin* only = spinous processes, but not used by the Ḥunain school. *Sinn* is reserved for the odontoid process of the axis. The transverse processes are called *ajniḥa* (sing. *janāḥ*) = wings. In medieval Latin the word appears as *senasen*, *simenia*, *adsenascem*, etc. In Alpago's glossary to the Giunta Avicenna of 1527, we find: 'senasene . . . id est marginis concavitatis spondilium', i.e. the meaning (*a*) above. As this does not appear in medical writers, we must assume that Alpago, who spent many years in the East, used the native lexica in preparing his vocabularies.

(7) *al-ʿiẓām al-simsimāniyya*, a translation of Galen's *sēsamoeidē osta* (Kühn ii. 778); derived from *simsim* 'coriander seed', Assyrian *shamashshamu*, Mishnaic Hebrew *shumshūm*, Syriac *shaushĕmā*. The derivation in -*ānī* suggests that the term is formed in imitation of some Syriac technical term *shaushemānā* (as *jismānī* 'bodily' is an imitation of Syriac *gushmānā*). In Latin writers the word appears as *sesamina*, *simenia*, etc., often confused with derivatives of *sanāsin* (note 6) and of *sulāmiyāt* 'phalanges'.

(7*a*) §§ 2–8 are a reproduction of a passage in *De ossibus* (Kühn ii. 734–8). The *Abridgment* rearranges the material, but its terminology is identical with that found here.

(8) *juththa* is said in the native lexica to mean 'body of a person sitting or lying down' (*Lisān* ii. 432; Peñuela, p. 39). The poetical quotations in the *Lisān* attest, however, not this meaning, but that of 'corpse', which is found also in Mutanabbī (died A.D. 965; ed. Dieterici, p. 550) and in modern Arabic. In the *Arabian Nights*, on the other hand, *juththa* means a body in any position, cf. the phrase *dhū juththa*=possessor of a body, 'corpulent' (Dozy, s.v.). The root-verb means 'to cut off at the roots', so that we may assume the following stages in the development of *juththa*: felled tree—corpse—prostrate living body—body. A similar development seems to have taken place in Assyrian, where *gishshu* (=Proto-Semitic *guththu*) is the region of the hip (Holma, p. 135; Albright in *Revue d'Assyriologie*, xvi, 180). None of the meanings of *juththa* given above justifies its use for 'skeleton', and it was not adopted by later writers. Modern Arabic uses *haikal*=structure, for the skeleton.

(9) *tajāwur* (MS. A. *tajāwuz*) 'action of being neighbours to each other', corresponding to Greek *syntaxis*. Avicenna (p. 454) employs *tajāwur* or *mujāwara* for articulation in general, distinguishing synarthrosis as *mujāwara bilā lāḥiqa* 'syntaxis without epiphysis'.

(10) *mafṣil*; from *faṣala* 'to divide, space', Aramaic *pěṣal*. Semitic words for 'joint' are derived either, as here, from roots meaning to divide, as Mishnaic Hebrew *pereq*, and perhaps Assyrian *buānu* (Holma, p. 4) if connected with *byn* 'to separate'; or from the ideas of connexion, as Hebrew *aṣṣīl* (cf. Arabic *waṣala* 'to connect'), or insertion, as Ethiopic *mabwā'et* (*bō'a* 'to enter'), or from that of movability, cf. *mirfaq*, note 30.

(11) *ittiḥād*, root *wḥd*, translating Greek *henōsis*.

(12) *iltiḥām*. Galen has *sym-physis* 'growing-together'. The Arabic term occurs first in Haly Abbas (p. 106): 'juncture by soldering means that the bones are soldered together precisely ('alā hindāmin=Greek *akribei synthesei*, Galen, Kühn iii. 689). At the point of juncture a white substance is placed like solder (*liḥām*), so that the bones are united (*ittaḥada*). Examples of this are the two bones of the inferior maxilla united at the chin, and the way in which epiphyses are united with the bones at many diarthrodial joints'.

(13) Literal quotation from Galen (Kühn ii. 734).

(14) *lawāḥiq*, sing. *lāḥiqa*, fem. partic. of *laḥiqa* 'to adjoin'. In medieval Latin *luhac, laguahic*, etc., cf. Hyrtl, p. 164.

(15) *ʿaḍud, ʿaḍd*. The word is not found in other Semitic languages, but was borrowed in medieval Hebrew as *ʿeṣedh* (transcribed in the *Fabrica* as *hasad*), and thence probably into Latin as *aseth* (Singer and Rabin, p. 24). Confusion with Latin derivatives of *al-sāʿid* 'forearm' (note 106) was inevitable. From the dual *al-ʿaḍdān* such forms as *alhasran* were derived.

(16) *ʿaẓm al-zand al-asfal* 'the lower firestick'. According to the dictionaries *zand* or *zinād* is the upper one of the sticks by friction of which the desert Arabs produced fire, the lower one being called *zanda* 'female zand'. Such niceties of Bedouin usage were hardly known to the Christian translators of Baghdad; it is interesting that they adopted these slang names rather than the literary names of radius and ulna, *kūʿ* and *kursūʿ*. The latter words were, however, applied in medical texts to the distal extremities of the two bones (Fonahn, p. 81). The Latins rendered *zand* by *focile* 'tinder' (as they used

flints, not sticks, for making fire) and called radius and ulna either *focile superius* and *inferius* or *focile minus* and *majus*. The same names were applied to tibia and fibula.

(17) *'aẓm al-fakhidh*, cf. note 109.

(18) *'aẓmā al-laḥy al-a'lā*. *Laḥy* denotes, in non-medical Arabic, only the inferior maxilla, as do the cognates Hebrew *lĕḥī* (in the Septuagint *siagōn*), and Assyrian *lakhū* (Holma, p. 31). See further note 84. Galen (Kühn ii. 749) treats the superior maxilla as two bones because of the suture along its middle, which exists in apes, but not in man (Singer and Rabin, p. 40). Ibn Jamī' is as inconsistent as Galen in the division of the upper jaw, cf. note 82.

(19) Galen (Kühn ii. 735): 'Most large bones have epiphyses towards other bones.' The source of the statement about hard bones is the *Abridgment*.

(20) *zawā'id*, sing. *zā'ida*, fem. partic. of *zāda* 'to be more, to overhang'.

(21) *'aẓmā al-laḥy al-asfal*. On *laḥy* see note 18. The apes dissected by Galen, especially when young, have a mandible more easily separable at the point of synosteosis than man's (Galen, Kühn ii. 754; cf. Singer and Rabin, p. 33).

(22) Galen (Kühn ii. 733): 'an apophysis differs from an epiphysis in that the latter is a unification of two distinct bones (*heterou pros heteron*) while the former is part of the bone'. Of Arab medical writers, only Ibn Jamī' observes this distinction. Haly Abbas knows only *zawā'id* of various kinds, Avicenna only *lawāḥiq*. Ibn Jamī' probably found this distinction in *De ossibus* (not in the *Abridgment*), but the Ḥunain school was by no means consistent. In the Arabic *De anat. admin.*, *lāḥiqa* does not occur, and *zā'ida* is often used where apophyses are described.

(23) *'unuq*, *'unq*, Greek *auchēn* (Galen, Kühn ii. 736). See also note 89.

(24) *ra's*, Greek *kephalē*.

(25) *nuqra*, translating Greek *koilotēs*, means a small round hole in a rock, as the Hebrew *niqrath ha-ṣūr* (Exod. xxxiii. 22; Septuagint *opē*). It is used in the *Abridgment* as here (*a*), but in the writers edited by De Koning it does not seem to occur with the meaning of socket of a joint, though it is recorded thus by Ibn Hashshā' in his vocabulary to Rhazes (p. 85). Haly Abbas speaks of *ḥufra* 'fossa'. *Nuqra* had wide anatomical currency in other senses: (*b*) hollow of the neck, in Latin *nocra* (confused with *nuca* from *nukhā'* 'spinal cord', cf. Peñuela, p. 70); (*c*) orbit of the eye; (*d*) acetabulum (all from *Lisān* vii. 87); (*e*) jugular fossa; (*f*) glenoid cavity (both Fonahn, p. 103); (*g*) articular convexities of vertebrae; (*h*) orifices of veins in the uterus (both De Koning, p. 829).

(26) *ḥuqq* 'small bowl of wood or ivory', from a root meaning 'to hollow out', translating Greek *kotylē*. According to *Lisān* xi. 340 it denotes acetabulum and glenoid cavity. Cf. also note 105.

(27) *'ain*, translating Greek *glēnē*. In actual Arabic anatomical usage, *'ain* is not applied to a cavity but to a projection: (*a*) *'ain al-katif*=*oculus scapulae* for the spine of the scapula, as early as the Arabic *De anat. admin.* (Simon i. 309; cf. Singer and Rabin, p. 22); (*b*) *'ain al-fakhidh* 'eye of the femur', for some part of the back of that bone (Ibn Sīda ii. 49); (*c*) *'ain al-rukba*= *oculus genu* for the patella (*Abridgment*; Rhazes, p. 22; Avicenna, p. 510), but for this cf. note 111 at end; (*d*) *oculus adjutorii* for the trochlea and capitulum

(Hyrtl, p. 9), no doubt also of Arabic origin. Arabic 'ain has numerous meanings, one of which is 'bud'. It may be this meaning which has given rise to the strange terms.

(28) *mafṣil salis*, opposite *ghair salis*, cf. *salas al-baul*, 'inability to retain urine' (Ibn Ḥashshā', p. 121) and Mishnaic Hebrew *shallesh, shalshel* 'to let a thing hang loosely'. It is not a translation of *diarthrōsis*, to which it corresponds. The terminology of §§ 5–7 is of a much more independent character than the general run of Arabic terms created to render Greek ones. The reason may lie in the impossibility of reproducing the elements of words like *diarthrōsis* and *arthrōdia* in Arabic.

(29) *muwaththaq*, corresponding to *synarthrōsis*, passive partic. of *waththaqa* 'to make firm', cf. also *muwaththaq al-khalq* 'firm of build, sturdy'.

(30) *mirfaq, marfiq*, cf. Mishnaic Hebrew *marpēq*. The root means 'to be easy (to move)'. Ethiopic has a verb *rafaqa* 'to lie down', which is probably derived from 'elbow', though *mirfaq* is not used in Ethiopic (cf. Latin *cubitus* and *cubare*).

(31) *rusgh*, see note 107.

(32) *mughraq* or *mugharraq*, pass. partic. of a root meaning 'to sink'; corresponds to Greek *enarthrōsis*. Of Arabic writers known to me, only Ibn Jamī' knows these names of the classes of diarthrodial joints. Haly Abbas enumerates them without naming them.

(33) *muṭṭarraf* (for *mutaṭarraf*, cf. Wright, Arabic Grammar i. § 111), literally 'touching the extremities (*ṭaraf*) of each other'; Greek *arthrōdia*.

(34) *muddākhal* (for *mutadākhal*), cf. *tadākhala* 'to mix socially'; Greek *ginglymos* 'joint'. Haly Abbas does not recognize this class.

(35) *muhandam*. The verb *handama* 'to dispose, arrange' (cf. Dozy) is post-classical, being derived from *hindām*, a loan from Persian *andām* 'body, stature, proportion, symmetry'. The school of Ḥunain used it to render Greek *akribei synthesei* (cf. note 12).

(36) *madrūz*, pass. partic. of *daraza* 'to sew', cf. note 43, is like the next two terms apparently taken from Avicenna. The *Abridgment* has *alladhī tarkībuhu bi-darz* 'what is joined by suture'. Haly Abbas has *al-mafāṣil allatī 'alā jihati l-durūz* 'joints after the manner of seams', both closer to the Greek *rhaphē* 'seam'. In Latin writers *medaruzan* (Fonahn, p. 51, s.v. *derezi*) a confusion between *madrūz* and the dual, Latin *direzan* (cf. note 43).

(37) *markūz*, pass. partic. of *rakaza* 'stick a lance, etc., in the ground', corresponds to Greek *gomphōsis*, from *gomphoō* 'fix with a peg'.

(38) *mulṣaq*, from *alṣaqa* 'to glue'; in Greek *harmonia* 'joining by a clamp'. Avicenna has the synonym *mulzaq*, Haly Abbas (p. 106) *'alā jihati l-iltiṣāq*. The *Abridgment* MS. is corrupt here, but seems to have read *mulzaq*.

(39) *sinān*, pl. of *sinn*, corresponds to Greek *exochē* 'protuberance' (Galen, Kühn iii. 689). This and the next word also in Avicenna (p. 454); they are not found in the *Abridgment*.

(40) *tahāzīz*, pl. of *tahzīz*, verbal noun of *hazzaza* 'to notch'.

(41) *'iẓām al-qiḥf* here denotes the outer bones of the cranium, as also in the *Abridgment*. In Avicenna (p. 460, cf. de Koning's note 2) it applies to the parietals alone. The word *qiḥf* means also a drinking-bowl (like *jumjuma*).

This is probably the primary sense, as *qaḥafa* means 'to wash away'. That the meaning 'skull' was felt to be a derivative is shown not only by the statement in the dictionaries that a cranium can only be called *qiḥf* when separated from the other bones, but also by the usage of the Ḥunain school, who rarely use it without a defining attribute, such as '*qiḥf* of the head' (Simon i. 353; *Abridgment*); '*qiḥf* of the brain' (Sbath and Meyerhof, p. 90), cf. also German 'Hirnschale'. (There is no basis for the assertion of Hyrtl (p. 189, quoted Peñuela, p. 72) that Avicenna uses *qiḥf* for the occipital. In the passage he adduces there is no *qiḥf*, only *qamaḥduwa* 'protuberantia occipitalis'.)

(42) *sha'n*, pl. *shu'ūn*, used already in the *Abridgment*. The Arab lexicographers describe these as tear-ducts, referring to the belief that tears emerge from the brain through the sutures; Abū 'Amr (died A.D. 775) even applies the name to the lachrymal ducts, of which he gives a reasonably correct description. One might be tempted to seek here the origin of this word, as I did in Singer and Rabin, p. lxxxiii. The derivation proposed there is, however, not possible. I would suggest connecting it rather with the common Semitic word for 'laced boot', Hebrew *śĕ'ōn* (Isa. ix. 4), Ethiopic *sha'n*, etc., so that we would have a comparison of the suture with the lacing of such a boot (which it does in fact resemble more than a seam). The word seems to have been transferred from the sutures to the bones at a very early date, as *shu'ūn* means 'top of the head' in a Mohammedan tradition (*Lisān* xvii. 96). Arab medical writers constantly confuse bones and sutures, and their tradition is continued in the use of the Latin *soonia*, *alsunam*, *asoan*, etc. (cf. Singer and Rabin, p. 29).

(43) *darz*, pl. *durūz* 'seam', a Persian borrowing (cf. *darzī* 'tailor'). The word seems to be an innovation of the Ḥunain school, being a closer rendering of Greek *rhaphē* than *sha'n*. Only *darz* appears in the Arabic *De anat. admin.* The Arab writers use the two side by side. The word has been borrowed by the Latins (a) in the singular as *alderazi*, *derezi*, (b) in the plural as *adorez*, *adoren*, etc., (c) in the dual as *direzan* (Fonahn, p. 53), the last perhaps first in a term for the temporal sutures, *al-darzāni al qishriyyāni* (cf. note 130).

(44) '*azmā al-zandain*, lit. the two bones of the 'two firesticks' (cf. note 16). The forearm is called *al-zandāni* sometimes even in non-medical Arabic.

(45) *faqarāt*, see note 91.

(46) *ṣalab*, see note 5.

(47) § 8 reproduces precisely Galen's account (Kühn ii. 738 ff.).

(48) *ghḍdrūf*, metathesis for *ghurdūf*, which is derived with geminate-dissimilation (cf. Brockelmann i. 243) from a root meaning 'to be soft', cf. *ghaḍaf* 'softness in the upper part of the ear', *ghaḍif* 'lop-eared'. The word means, according to the *Lisān* (xi. 173, 175): (a) upper rim of auricle, (b) 'the bone at the edge of a vertebra', i.e. the intervertebral disc?, (c) the nasal cartilage, (d) the cartilage, also called *nughd*, at the top of the scapula in the horse. *Iltihām ghuḍrūfī* translates Greek *synchondrōsis*.

(49) *ribāṭ*, also *rābiṭa*, from a root meaning 'to tie'. *Iltihām ribāṭī* is Greek *synneurōsis*.

(50) *laḥm* 'meat, flesh'. Haly Abbas (p. 200) distinguishes three kinds of *laḥm*: muscles, non-muscular flesh (=muscles of spine and buttocks), and 'soft flesh' or glands.

(51) Here ends the extract from *De ossibus*. It is interesting to contrast Galen's classification of joints, as reproduced by Ibn Jamīʿ, with those of Haly Abbas (pp. 104-8) and Avicenna (p. 454).

Ibn Jamīʿ	Haly Abbas	Avicenna	
		name	*example*
A. joint	A. joint	A. loose:	wrist
1. loose	1. loose		
a. immersed	*a*. short process	B. tight, not	
b. contacting	*b*. long process	firm:	metacarpus
c. interlocked	*c*. unrounded process		
	d. with epiphysis		
2. firm	2. firm	C. firm:	sternum
a. suture	*a*. suture		
b. implanted	*b*. implanted	D. implanted:	teeth
c. adherent	*c*. adhering	E. suture:	cranium
B. soldering	B. soldering	F. adherent:	radius and ulna,
1. cartilaginous			lower vertebrae.
2. ligamentous			
3. muscular			

It is obvious that Haly Abbas' and Avicenna's classifications are not independent of Galen's, nor can they be considered developments of the latter. They make the impression of being abridged systems brought about by imperfect tradition. Was it Ibn Jamīʿ's distinction to have gone back to pure Galenism; and if so, what were the secondary sources the earlier writers used?

(51a) *mujawwaf*, a passive participle from the root of *jauf* 'belly, cavity'. From the same root we have *al-warīd al-ajwaf*=vena cava, which Vesalius (*Fabrica*, p. 376 *bis*) still knew to mean '*vena ventrem habens*' (though he falsely ascribes this meaning to the Hebrew *ha-nābhūbh*).

(52) *mukhkh*, from a root meaning 'to be fat, full of sap'; Hebrew *moăh* (Job xxi. 24: Septuagint *myelos*). In Syriac the word means 'brain'; in Assyrian it has gone a stage further to mean 'cranium', 'top' of anything (Holma, p. 12).

(53) *takhārīb* (MS. B), so also the *Abridgment*; MS. A has *tahārīf*, which might make sense if it could mean 'probe-holes', cf. *miḥrāf* 'surgeon's probe'.

(54) *mutakhalkhala*, cf. Mishnaic Hebrew *kĕlī mĕḥulḥāl* 'a container with perforated walls', *ḥalḥēl* 'to ooze through'. The root is closely related to that of *khalal*, note 58.

(55) *layyina*, lit. 'pliable, flexible'.

(56) §§10-12 are almost identical with Avicenna, pp. 452-4.

(57) *masāmm*, cf. also *sumūm*, *simām* 'apertures of the face', *summa* 'opening of the vagina'.

(58) *khalal*, sing. *khalla*, lit. 'defect', cf. note 54.

(59) *furaj*, sing. *furja* 'interstice, gap'. Avicenna: 'though they contain such pores and openings as are inevitable'.

(60) Avicenna: 'also for movement'.

(61) *jirm*, a rather obsolete word for 'body', frequent in anatomical usage, cf. Fonahn, p. 73. The word means 'bone' in Hebrew and Aramaic, but in the latter language is used for 'self' (as Hebrew *'eṣem*). South-Arabian *grb*, Tigre *garob* is 'person'. The word is used for the 'body' of a bone in the *Abridgment*, corresponding to *sōma* in Kühn ii. 759, line 15.

(62) *mawāqif*, sing. *mauqif*, lit. 'standing-place', also 'occasion, meeting, start for races', etc. The sense needed here is not recorded elsewhere.

(63) *rakhw*, lit. 'relaxed'.

(64) Avicenna: 'its food . . . is concentrated in its stuffing (*hashw*)'.

(65) Avicenna adds: 'and does not become brittle by the desiccating action of movement'. The desiccating effect of movement is mentioned by Galen, *Ars medica* xxv (Kühn i. 373).

(66) *mushāshiyya*, i.e. like *mushāsh* 'soft, spongy earth'. The choice of this to render *spongoeidēs* may have been due to the circumstances that the sponge and its later name, *isfanj*, were not known at Baghdad in the time of the translators. They sinned, however, against Arabic usage, as (according to *Lisān* viii. 239) *mushāsh* means (*a*) marrow (thence *mashsha* 'to suck marrow from a bone') and (*b*) articular cartilage. The Prophet is described as *jalīl al-mushāsh* 'with prominent joints'. Ibn Ḥashshā' says (p. 72) that the bones of the sternum are *mushāshiyya*, i.e. cartilaginous. Avicenna (or the source common to him and Ibn Jamī') seems to have drawn here on *De usu partium* viii. 7 (Kühn iii. 652), where Hippocrates is quoted as describing the ethmoid as *spongoeidēs*.

(67) *ma'a ziyādati ḥājatin bi-sababin yajibu an yakūna yunfidhu fīhā*. For *sabab* 'thing, substance', see Dozy, s.v. Our text is here better than that of the Avicenna editions, which read . . . *li-sababi shai'in yajibu* . . . translated by De Koning: 'ils ont encore besoin de cette disposition pour une autre raison ayant rapport à quelque chose qui les doit pénétrer'. MS. B reads *bi-sababi an yakūna*, which makes no sense, but like the Avicenna corruption is due to the copyist's taking *sabab* in the usual meaning of 'cause'.

(68) *'aẓm al-miṣfāt* 'strainer bone', in Haly Abbas (p. 310) 'the bone resembling a strainer', as *ēthmo-eidēs*.

(69) *Lambdoeidēs* for the hyoid occurs only in *De musc. diss.* (Kühn xviiiB. 957) and in the Arabic part of *De anat. admin.* (Simon i. 70). It is the only Greek form known to the Arabs (Rhazes, p. 23, Avicenna, p. 452), who, however, had a native name for it, *al-fā'iq*, in Latin *alsaich*, etc. The human hyoid is U-shaped: the Λ-shape is animal, as well as the Y-shape described by Galen's term *hyoeidēs*.

(70) It is typical of the purely literary character of Ibn Jamī''s anatomy that he omits to mention the fact, expressly stated by Galen (*De anat. admin.* vii. 10; Kühn ii. 619) and Avicenna (p. 690), that this cartilaginous bone is not found in man.

(71) *simsimāniyya*, cf. note 7. The same list in Rhazes (p. 23) and the *Abridgment*.

(72) This is the number given by the *Mishnah* (*c.* A.D. 200) and all Arab writers (cf. Singer and Rabin, p. 28). Rhazes (p. 23) says that it is arrived at by counting after the manner of Galen. The latter only says (*De foet. form.* vi; Kühn iv. 694) that there are more than 200 bones. The number 248 is,

however given in the pseudo-Galenic *Abridgment*. Modern text-books count 200 bones in all. The difference is mainly due to our counting only 22 bones in the head and 52 in the trunk.

(73) *jumjumatā al-qiḥf*. *Jumjuma* has in the lexica the same meanings as *qiḥf* (note 41): parietals, cranium, skull, drinking-bowl. Since it seems to be cognate to Hebrew *gulgoleth* (cf. Golgotha), Assyrian *gulgullu* 'skull', the meaning 'drinking-bowl' would be secondary (it also occurs in Assyrian: Holma, p. 12), while in *qiḥf* the meaning 'bowl' is primary, and that of 'skull' added after the model of *jumjuma*, as so often in slang. In medical language *jumjuma* is rarely and vaguely used. Abulcasis (i. 16) identifies it with the occipital. The dual occurs only in a difficult passage of Avicenna (p. 630), where a branch of the internal jugular is said to enter the skull at the junction of 'the two *jumjumas* of the skull'. The site probably meant is that of the two parietal foramina, which lie between the parietal eminences. In fact one MS. reads *ḥajmatā al-qiḥf*, *ḥajma* being (*Lisān* xv. 6) a protuberance of a bone which can be felt through the skin. If this was the original reading then we must accuse Ibn Jamī' not only of having employed a corrupt Avicenna text, but of having misunderstood it. Strangely enough the same corrupted term, in Hebrew translation, reached Vesalius by oral tradition as *qadhroth ha-moāḥ* 'the bowls of the brain' (cf. Singer and Rabin, p. 29: the interpretation and emendation there given is thus void). In Latin *jumjuma* is represented by *gingia, gangama*, cf. Hyrtl, p. 146,

(74) The idea of the cranial bones as walls and base does not occur in Galen, and is apparently due to Avicenna (p. 460). In Assyrian the occiput is called *kutallu* 'wall' (Holma, p. 14).

(75) *'aẓm al-jabha* (also in Avicenna, *loc. cit.*, and Haly Abbas, p. 112), translating Galen's *to kata metōpon ostoun* (*De oss.* i; Kühn ii. 745).

(76) Like Avicenna, *loc. cit.*, Ibn Jamī' does not name here the occipital, though he has a name for it (note 127). The Greek *inion* is vaguely rendered by the Arabs as *mu'akhkhar al-ra's* 'back of the head'.

(77) *al-ḥajariyyāni*, from *ḥajar* 'stones'. Ibn Jamī', like Rhazes (p. 52) and Avicenna (*loc. cit.*), follows the pseudo-Galenic *Introductio seu medicus* (Kühn xiv. 721); only Haly Abbas follows Galen (*De ossibus* i; Kühn ii. 745; and the *Abridgment*) in restricting the application of the term to the petrous portion.

(78) *qā'ida*; in Avicenna *qā'idat al-dimāgh* 'pedestal of the brain'. The sphenoid is described as support of the head by Galen (*De usu part.* xi. 19; Kühn iii. 934). The medieval Latin *os basilare* may either be a translation of this, or a corruption of *os paxillare* 'wedge bone' (cf. Singer and Rabin, p. 32). On *qā'ida*=occipital, see note 127.

(79) *al-'aẓm al-watadī* 'the tent-peg bone', from *watad, watid, watd* 'tent-peg'. Rhazes (p. 16) says simply *al-watad*. The Latin forms *alguededi, alguateda, getedi* come from the Arabic (*gu=w*), but *geteth* may be due to the influence of the Hebrew *yĕthēdhī* (Old Spanish *g* was pronounced like *y*).

(80) *ṣudghāni*, sing. *ṣudgh*; Syriac *ṣedh'ā*, Mishnaic Hebrew *ṣedha'*. The word is used in the Arabic *De anat. admin.* and in Avicenna (p. 462) for the region of the temples, by Haly Abbas (p. 112) for the squamous portion of the temporal bone. The Latin *os temporale* goes back to the pseudo-Galenic *Introductio seu medicus* (Kühn xiv. 720; but cf. xviiiA. 430).

I   N

(81) *'azma al-zauj.* Normally Arabic *zauj* (like its Syriac and Mishnaic Hebrew cognates), though borrowed from Greek *zygon,* denotes not a yoke but a pair. This explains why in Latin our term was rendered as *ossa paris.* The name was used confusedly. Ibn Jamī', like Avicenna (p. 460), follows *De ossibus* (Kühn ii. 746) in taking the zygomatic arch (malar plus zygomatic process of temporal) as one bone. Galen himself in *De usu part.* (Kühn iii. 936) restricts the name *zygōma* to the zygomatic process. This Hippocrates (Kühn iii. 170) describes as a separate bone. He is followed in this by Haly Abbas (p. 114).

(82) *'azmā al-wajnataini. Wajna,* in Latin *ugene, gena,* translates in Simon i. 63 Greek *mēlon*=region of the upper cheek, i.e. the portion covering the malar bone. But our term certainly does not denote the malar. Ibn Jamī' gives here a rather arbitrary selection from a well-known list, which is found in full in some copies of Avicenna's *Canon* (cf. De Koning, p. 464 and Peñuela, p. 120). It seems also to have been known to Rhazes (p. 17). It is based on two enumerations of Galen: *De ossibus* iii (Kühn ii. 751, analysed by De Koning, p. 783) and *De usu part.* xi. 20 (Kühn iii. 936). There we find a bone 'containing the cheeks (*mēla*; Kühn writes *myla*) and almost all teeth', which De Koning identifies as the superior maxilla proper, after deduction of the upper portions and of the intermaxillary (of animals and foeti), while Daremberg and Ruelle translate 'portion externe ou zygomato-faciale du maxillaire supérieur'. Possibly this list is another bit of our hypothetic common source, perhaps based upon, but different in arrangement and expression from, the list of 14 bones found in the *Abridgment.* Ibn Jamī' seems to have had a better version of it than Avicenna, as he names the nasal bone, while Avicenna speaks of the 'two bones limited by the longitudinal and transverse sutures'. Haly Abbas (p. 116) adopts the alternative division into eight bones as in *De ossibus* (Kühn ii. 748), calling the 'cheek bones' *'azmā al-khaddain. Khadd,* Latin *alchad,* denotes the soft part of the cheek covering the maxilla proper (Peñuela, p. 121), and is thus a more suitable term than *wajna.*

(83) *'azmā al-anf,* also in the *Abridgment* and in Haly Abbas (p. 116), not in Avicenna. *Anf* 'nose' is common Semitic.

(84) *'azmā al-fakkaini.* Syriac *pakkā* is 'cheek'. The *Lisān* (xii. 364) explains *fakk* as 'place at the temples where the maxillae meet' and as 'upper or lower maxilla'. Avicenna (p. 462) calls the upper maxilla *al-fakk,* the lower *al-fakk al-asfal.* Haly Abbas (p. 118), however, calls the lower maxilla *al-fakk.* Here the name is applied to each half of the inferior maxilla as separated by the anterior symphysis (note 18).

(85) *thanāyā,* sing. *thaniyya,* derived from the root for 'two', Latin *dentes duales.*

(86) *rubā'iyyāt,* sing. *rubā'iyya,* lit. 'possessing four of something' (*Rubaiyat* =four-line poems), Latin *dentes quadrupli.* I cannot account for these names. The name for the incisors, *qattā'a*=Greek *tomeis* is used by the *Abridgment* and Haly Abbas, but appears neither here nor in Avicenna.

(87) *anyāb,* sing. *nāb;* cf. Syriac *nībhā,* Assyrian *naiābu.* Perhaps connected with the Hebrew *nūbh* 'to grow', *nībh* 'produce'.

(88) *adrās,* sing. *dirs.* While medical writers from Ḥunain onwards (Simon i. 65) use *dirs* for molar, non-medical Arabic (*a*) uses it as synonym of

sinn 'tooth' (*Lisān* vii. 422; Ibn Ḥashshāʾ, p. 93), and (*b*) has no separate word for molar, but divides the molars into two groups varying in proportion, the posterior one being mostly called *ṭawāḥīn* 'grinders'=Greek *myletai* (cf. Peñuela, p. 149). In Ethiopic and Syriac (*'ershā*) the cognates of *ḍirs* mean definitely molar (in Exod. xxi. 27 the Ethiopic Bible translates Hebrew *shēn* as 'molar or tooth'), and we may assume that the translators of Ḥunain's school, who were mostly Syriac speakers, were influenced by their mother tongue in choosing *ḍirs* to render 'molar'.

(89) *raqaba*. In the Arabic *De anat. admin.*, *raqaba* is reserved for the neck of the body, while the synonym *'unuq* (note 23) is applied to 'necks' of organs or bones. In other medical texts this distinction is not made any more than in Greek.

(90) *ṣadr*.

(91) sing. *faqra, fiqra, faqāra*; plur. *fiqarāt, fiqirāt, fiqrāt, fiqar, fiqār, faqārāt*. Rhazes uses instead *kharazāt* 'strung-up beads', and it is likely that *faqra*, etc. meant originally the same, as according to *Lisān* xiv. 143 *mufaqqar=mukharraz* 'strung-up'. Mishnaic Hebrew *ḥulyōth* means 'links in a chain', while the Greek word for vertebra, *spondylos* 'whorl', visualizes only the individual vertebra.

(92) *qaṭan*. According to *Lisān* xvii. 222 this meant, besides 'loins', the rump of a bird, which perhaps accounts for its apparent derivation from the common Semitic root meaning 'to be thin'. The name 'vertebrae of the chest' for the dorsals is Rhazes' (p. 16) and Avicenna's (p. 482), while Haly Abbas (p. 124) keeps Galen's 'vertebrae of the back'. The *Abridgment* gives both names together. The name 'vertebrae of the back' is in Rhazes applied to dorsals and lumbars together. Native Semitic divisions of the spine differed considerably from Galen's. The early philologist Abū l-Haitham (*Lisān* vi. 369) enumerates: six in the neck, six in the interscapulary region, six of the back (associated with the false ribs), one called *al-qaṭāt* 'the sand-grouse', six in the sacrum, the last of which is called *al-quḥquḥ*. The Jews (*Mishnah Oholoth* i. 8) counted nine in the head, eight in the neck (dorsal), six in the 'key of the heart' (cf. Assyrian *pī libbi*, Egyptian *r-ib* 'mouth of the heart'= abdomen), five at the excretory organs (=sacrum). The numbers given for the sacrum are thus more correct than Galen's, cf. Singer and Rabin, p. 43.

(93) *'ajuz, 'ajiz, 'ajz, 'ujz, 'ijz*; cf. Mishnaic Hebrew *'ākhūz* 'posteriors'. Perhaps the word is connected with Ethiopic *'agasha* 'to be permanent', so that it means 'the indestructible bone', cf. next note. In Latin *hagiz, alharis, alhovius, alhagiagi* (cf. Singer and Rabin, p. 43). The sacrum of three vertebrae is simian.

(94) *'uṣ'uṣ, 'aṣ'aṣ, 'uṣuṣ, 'aṣuṣ*; cf. Hebrew *'āṣeh* (Lev. iii. 9). Names for sacrum and coccyx in Greek and Arabic offer many problems. In Arabic the coccyx is denoted by many names, some of which were certainly slang terms for the anus: *quḥquḥ, fanīk* (=junction of the jaws), *'idrīṭ* (=gullet, or perhaps 'wind-breaker'), *baus* (=gaudy), *nāq* (=she-camel?), *tha'laba* (=vixen), etc. (cf. *Lisān* iii. 388). Perhaps Greek *kokkyx* 'cuckoo' was also a slang term for the anus. Quite different is the case with *'ajb al-dhanab* "*'ajb* of the tail' for coccyx. The name *'ajb* is said by the lexica to denote a vertebra at the top or bottom of the sacrum, and appears to be an old name for the whole sacrum,

perhaps including the coccyx. The Hebrew cognate *'aghābhōth* is the place where the feet of the foetus lie (i.e. the sacrum?), cf. Babylonian Talmud *Niddah* 30b. From *Lisān* viii. 321 we learn that the *'uṣ'uṣ* or *'ajb* is the first bone formed in the foetus and the last to disintegrate in the corpse; others say it never disintegrates. The Jewish Rabbis believed that the 'almond of the spine' (=sacrum?) never disintegrated, and would be used on the day of resurrection as starting-point of the new body (cf. Hyrtl, p. 165 ff.). Saint Isidore in the seventh century A.D. still knew that the sacrum was held in magical reverence by pagans (*Etymologiae* ii. 1). Cognates of *'ajb* are Arabic *'ajiba* 'be struck with wonder', Hebrew *'āghabh* 'have sexual desire', Syriac *'aggebh* 'to paralyze', all words of obvious magical content. It thus means 'the magic bone', exactly like Greek *hieron ostoun*. The *Abridgment* also gives the name *al-'aẓm al-a'ẓam* 'the greatest (awful, powerful) bone'. To *'us'us* corresponds in Latin *alhosos, alhaos, alazpaz, abhaum, abhaus*, etc.

(95) *qaṣṣ*, sometimes spelled *qass*, in dictionaries also *qaṣaṣ* and *qaṣqaṣ*. In non-technical Arabic it denotes the middle breast, for which there were many different names (cf. Ibn Sīda ii. 20). It may be a cognate of Ethiopic *gaṣṣ* 'face' (=front of body), or of Assyrian *siqqat* (*sikkat, siggat* ?) *ṣēli* (Holma, p. 50), which probably=sternum, and may literally mean 'pin of the ribs' (cf. Aramaic *sikktĕhā*, Mishnaic Hebrew *sikkāh*, 'pin, thorn'). In Latin it appears as *cassos, alcaz*, etc. (Hyrtl, p. 88; Singer and Rabin, p. 22). The seven segments are a simian feature.

(96) *'iẓām al-zaur*, occurring only here, though parallel to Rhazes' term (p. 18) *'iẓām al-ṣadr*. *Lisān* iv. 422, *zaur* is said to mean the upper breast. The 'daughters of the *zaur*' are the ribs; the 'daughters of the *ṣadr*' the interstices of the ribs (Ibn Sīda ii. 20). The root means 'to be crooked, hollow', cf. Ethiopic *zaur* 'circle', Syriac *zĕwārā* 'hollow hand'. Our word may be the same as Talmudic Aramaic *zairā* 'perforated vat', just as Greek *thōrax* is derived from a root meaning 'to contain'.

(97) *aḍlā'*, sing. *ḍila', ḍil'*, common Semitic. The root seems to have meant 'to be crooked', cf. also the synonym *maḥniyyat al-janb* 'crooked thing of the flank' (*Lisān* x. 94). On other usages, cf. Fonahn, p. 52.

(98) *aḍlā' al-ṣadr*. So in Haly Abbas and Avicenna. The *Abridgment* calls them *al-aḍlā' al-khāṣṣa* 'the special, proper ribs', to which the next term may be the antonym.

(99) *aḍlā' al-khalf* (*khilf*?), with *khalf* as noun in the genitive, in all writers from Ḥunain (Simon i. 28) onwards. The *Lisān* (x. 95) calls the asternal ribs 'ribs of the sides' and adds that the lowest only is called *al-dil' al-khalf* (in x. 440 *al-khilf*), which may mean 'the rib which is left over' or 'the rib given in exchange'. This looks as if it were a reminiscence of the Biblical story of the creation of Eve. Note that the *Lisān* speaks of one rib, not two. Thus Ḥunain both misunderstood the form, turning an adjective into a noun, and wrongly extended its use. Avicenna (p. 490) has a name rendering the idea of Greek *pleurai nothai* 'false ribs': *al-aḍlā' al-kādhiba* 'the lying ribs'. The equivalent *aḍlā' al-zūr* 'ribs of falseness', used by the *Abridgment* and Avicenna, may have orginated in a misunderstanding of the name *aḍlā' al-zaur* 'ribs of the chest' (cf. note 96) for the true ribs (Ibn Sīda ii. 20). Avicenna also invented the 'true ribs', *al-aḍlā' al-ṣādiqa*, in Latin

costae verae. I have not found the source of *al-aḍlāʿ al-khullaṣ* 'the sincere ribs' (Fonahn, p. 52), which, rather badly translated, appears in Latin as *costae perfectae* (Singer and Rabin, p. 33).

(100) *ʿaẓmā al-katfaini*. *Katif, katf, kitf* can, according to *Lisān* xi. 202, also denote the humerus. Haly Abbas (p. 130) calls the scapulae ʿthe two bones of the *katif*', as if *katif* denoted both scapulae together, cf. the relation of Assyrian *arkatu* 'lumbar region' to Arabic *warikāni*, Hebrew *yĕrēkhayim* 'the two loins' (Dhorme, p. 98). In Biblical Hebrew two words, *kāthēph* and *shĕkhem*, are confusedly used for both scapula and clavicle. Mishnaic Hebrew and Aramaic agree with Arabic in using *kāthēph, kathpā* for scapula.

(101) *raʾsā al-katfaini*, i.e. the acromion. Galen (Kühn ii. 766 and iv. 128) reckons it as a separate bone. Only the *Abridgment* renders *akr-ōmion* precisely as *ẓāhir al-katif* 'prominent part of the scapula' and restricts *raʾs al-katif* to the acromio-clavicular cartilage. Other Arab writers use *raʾs al-katif* vaguely for that cartilage (Avicenna, p. 492), the ridge of the scapula (Haly Abbas, p. 132) and the acromion itself. It was further confused with *al-akhram* 'the flat-nosed' and *minqār al-ghurāb* 'crow's beak' (Latin *rostrum corvi*, Sudhoff, p. 35), both of which probably properly referred to the coracoid (cf. Singer and Rabin, p. 21).

(102) *al-tarquwatāni*, sing. *tarquwa*. The word is in general use, but its etymology is enigmatic, since there is no root *trq* or *rqw*. Perhaps it is connected with Assyrian *tikku* 'neck', the *r* being due to geminate-dissimilation (Brockelmann i. 243). The ending -*uwa* occurs also in *qamaḥduwa* 'external occipital protuberance'. Latin *alrathutan*, etc.

(103) *ʿaẓm al-ʿāna*, used from Ḥunain (Simon i. 87) onwards. The dictionaries say *al-ʿāna* is pubic hair. It appears to be a slang term, derived either from *ʿāna* 'she-ass' (cf. French *chatte* 'pubis' and the words for anus in note 94), or from an archaic dialect word *ʿāna* 'water tank'.

(104) *al-ḥarqafa*. This is the native Arabic word for the part, but of medical writers only the *Abridgment* and Avicenna (p. 507) give it. According to *Lisān* x. 391 it means either the iliac crest ('which becomes prominent with emaciation'), or the pelvis plus acetabulum. The word may be connected with *ḥqf* 'to be crooked, bend the body', with an *r* due to geminate-dissimilation (cf. Brockelmann i. 243). In Latin *alhatafar, alharta, alharcafa*, etc., perhaps also *althavorat* (Singer and Rabin, p. 34).

(104a) *ʿaẓm al-khāṣira*. This term, translating *lagōnōn osta*, was probably created by the medical translators to replace *al-ḥarqafa*. *Khāṣira* is the region between iliac crest (*ḥarqafa*) and the lowest rib (*al-quṣairā*; *Lisān* v. 322). The root means 'to contract', cf. *khaṣr* 'waist', and Ethiopic *khaṣīr* 'small', Syriac *ḥeṣrā* 'little finger', Assyrian *eṣīru* 'small'. It is more difficult to connect it with the other Semitic words for 'loins': Aramaic *ḥarṣā*, Hebrew *ḥālāṣayim*, Assyrian *khinṣu*.

(105) *ḥuqq al-warik*. For *ḥuqq* see note 26. *Warik* or *wark* is 'the bone that is to the femur as the scapula to the humerus' (Ibn Sīda ii. 41), i.e. Galen's *ischion* (so in Simon i. 28). In the *Abridgment* and in Haly Abbas (p. 140) the ischium is *ʿaẓm al warik*; the acetabulum Haly Abbas calls *ḥuqq al-warik*, the *Abridgment ḥuqq al-fakhidh*. Avicenna (p. 506) transfers *ʿaẓm al-warik* to the lower ilium, calling the acetabulum *ḥuqq al-warik*, and (p. 508) the ischium *ḥuqq al-fakhidh* 'box of the femur'. Ibn Jamīʿ seems to have

confused Avicenna's terms still further by trying to apply them to Galen's division of the innominates. Through ignorance of the lines of ossification all ancient divisions were necessarily arbitrary (cf. Singer and Rabin, p. 34). Rhazes (p. 18) does not subdivide the innominates (which he calls *'aẓmā al-khāṣirataini*, cf. note 104a), but on p. 20 betrays knowledge of the Galenic division. The word *warik* is common Semitic, denoting at first (in Assyrian) the lumbar region of the back (Dhorme, p. 99), then (in Hebrew and Arabic) the flanks and hips, and finally even the femur, as in 'root of the *warik*'= acetabulum (*Lisān* xi. 341). On the other hand, in Ibn Sīda ii. 41 the *ghurābāni* 'two crows'=tops of the iliac crests are described as 'heads of the two *warik*'.

(105a) *'aḍudāni*, cf. note 15.

(106) *sā'idāni*, sing. *sā'id*. This is said by Jauharī (d. 1003) to mean the upper arm, by Fīrūzābādī (1329–1414) the forearm. The latter is the meaning with which it is used in anatomy, where it completely ousted its synonym *dhirā'* (Haly Abbas, p. 134). In Ibn Sīda i. 166 *sā'id* is said to be= radius, and *dhirā'*=ulna (the latter also in the *Abridgment*). All this bears a surprising resemblance to the fate of the Greek equivalents. In Plato *brachiōn*=upper arm, *pēchys*=forearm. In Aristotle both mean forearm. Pollux fixes for *brachiōn* the meaning forearm. Later *pēchys* became 'ulna' (cf. Singer and Rabin, p. 24). *Sā'id* means 'supporter', which was translated into Latin as *adjutorium*, but applied to the humerus. In the meaning 'forearm' it was taken over as *asaid, alseid, absceid, alcadid*, etc.

(107) *rusghāni*, sing. *rusgh, rusugh* 'wrist or ankle'. In Latin *rasga, rascha, raseta, recepta*, etc.

(108) *mishṭāni*, sing. *mishṭ, musht, mashṭ* 'comb' (cf. Ethiopic *mashaṭa* 'to tear out'), translating Greek *kteis*, translated into Latin as *pecten*. Following Galen (Kühn iii. 203) the Arabs excluded the metacarpal of the thumb from the metacarpus, thus giving the thumb three phalanges. Latin *mastalcaf* is *mashṭ al-kaff* 'metacarpus of the hand'.

(109) *fakhidh, fakhdh, fikhdh*; cf. Syriac *puhdā* 'sinew of the thigh', perhaps also Hebrew *paḥadh* in Job xl. 17 (which would then, because of the sound-change dh-d, be an Aramaic loan). The 'head of the femur' means in Arabic medical literature the same as with us, but in ordinary language the patellar end (*Lisān* xi. 21).

(110) *mafṣil al-rukba*; cf. Biblical Aramaic and Mishnaic Hebrew *arkhubbāh*: the other Semitic languages have forms of the type *birku*. Its original meaning seems to have been similar to the German *Schoss*, since Mishnaic Hebrew *arkhubbāh* includes the femur (cf. *Mishnah Ḥullin* iv. 6), Arabic *rakab* denotes the pubis, Assyrian *birku* the penis, *burku* the lap.

(111) *raḍafa, raḍfa*, connected perhaps with a Yemenite Arabic verb meaning 'to lay out cushions' (Ibn Duraid, *Jamhara* ii. 364, cf. Dathina colloquial Arabic *raḍaf* 'place on top of each other'). In *Lisān* xi. 21 *al-raḍf* is described as 'a cluster of bones in the knee, holding each other like fingers', i.e. the whole joint, and said to be beneath *al-dāghiṣa* 'the choker', described as 'a small bone on top of the knee, covered in flesh and fat', i.e. the patella. The medical translators seem thus to have misunderstood Arabic usage. The form *raṣfa*, given by De Koning and Fonahn, does not exist, though *raṣafa* is one of the tendons attached to the patella (*Lisān* xi. 20). In Latin *radfa* is represented

by *alresafe, aresfatu,* etc., often confused with derivatives of *rusgh* (Hyrtl, p. 201). The frequent medieval term *oculus genu* translates Avicenna's *ʿain al-rukba* (p. 510), which originally denoted not the patella, but the cavities behind it (Ibn Sīda ii. 51).

(112) *sāq*; common Semitic (in Assyrian it covers the femur including knee and genitals, cf. Holma, p. 134 and notes 8, 110). Tibia and fibula are in Arabic called by the same names as radius and ulna (note 16). Haly Abbas (p. 142) follows *De ossibus* (Kühn ii. 774) and the *Abridgment* in calling the tibia *sāq*.

(113) *ʿaqib*; common Semitic. In Latin *achib, abrip, aldip,* etc. (Hyrtl, p. 5).

(114) *kaʿb* (perhaps cognate with Eth. *kĕʿūb* 'double'), though denoting in medical works the astragalus, is in common Arabic the malleolus, usually in the dual (cf. Ibn Sīda ii. 56 and *Koran* v. 8). Confusion between the two goes back to the Greeks (Galen, Kühn xviiiB. 756; cf. Singer and Rabin, p. 26). Originally the word seems to mean 'knot of a reed'; in the *Abridgment* it is also used of phalanges of thumb and toes. In Latin *cahab, caib, alcahab,* also *cahabin* 'malleoli'; the last named may be from the curious irregular plural *kaʿābīn,* found in the *Abridgment* for 'phalanges'.

(115) *al-zauraqī,* translating Greek *skapho-eidēs,* from *zauraq,* the Persian name of the round Tigris boats, a familiar sight at Baghdad where the early translators worked.

(116) *misht,* cf. note 108. Rhazes (p. 22) counts only three tarsal bones and 25 in the whole foot. For the name of the cuboid see Singer and Rabin, p. 28).

(117) *rusgh,* cf. note 109.

(118) *durūz,* cf. note 48.

(119) *al-durūz al-zāhira.*

(120) *al-durūz al-khafīyya;* only here. Avicenna (p. 458) calls them *kādhiba* 'false', the *Abridgment* and Haly Abbas *al-qishriyyāni,* translating *lepido-eidēs* (cf. note 130).

(121) *al-iklīlī,* translating Greek *stephaniaia,* from *iklīl* 'diadem', a loan from Aramaic. Already in the Arabic *De anat. admin.* and the *Abridgment.*

(112) *ʿazm al-raʾs.* This rather vague term for the parietals (viewing them as one bone!) comes apparently from the *Abridgment.* It is not found in the great medical writers, but reached Vesalius in the Latin form *os capitis* (Singer and Rabin, p. 29). For other names see notes 4, 41, 73, 126.

(123) *al-jabha* (without *ʿazm*), cf. note 75.

(123a) The curious shape with corners is also found in the MS. of the *Abridgment* which I use.

(124) *saffūdī,* from *saffūd,* 'broach, spit' (cf. Syriac *shappūdhā*), translates *obeliaia* of the pseudo-Galenic *Introductio seu medicus* (Kühn xiv. 720 prints *oboliaia*). It is still unknown to the *Abridgment.* In Avicenna (p. 458) *saffudi* and *sahmi* have erroneously changed places.

(125) *sahmī,* from *sahm* 'arrow', already in the *Abridgment al-shabīh bil-sahm* 'resembling an arrow'. Galen calls it 'the straight lengthwise one'=Arabic *al-mustaqīm.* This *sahmī* is the source of Latin *sagittalis.*

(126) *al-raʾs,* a further contraction of *ʿazm (muʾakhkhar) al-raʾs* (note 122), also used in the *Abridgment.*

(127) *qā'ida.* This word, used by Avicenna for the sphenoid (note 78), does not occur with the meaning 'occipital' in the great Arabic writers, but the Latin *os basilare* has also the meaning 'occipital' (Fonahn, p. 107, cf. Hyrtl, p. 143). Haly Abbas, p. 112, uses *qā'ida* for the meeting-place of sphenoid and occipital, our 'base of the skull', and this seems to have been done already by Galen, since in the Arabic *De anat. admin.* (Simon i. 7) the arteriae fossae or profundae are said to arise at the *qā'idat qiḥf al-ra's* 'base of the skull'.

(128) *al-lāmī,* translating *lambdo-eidēs,* though the Arabic letter *lām* has no similarity with Greek lambda.

(129) *al-jabīn,* denotes the region of the temporal surface of the frontal bone, between eyebrow and forelock (*Lisān* xvi. 236). The root means 'to be crooked', so that the Syriac *gẹbhīnā* 'eyebrow' may represent the earlier meaning. Occasionally in Arabic *jabīn*=forehead. Haly Abbas uses *'aẓm al-jabīn* for the temporal bone, as if *jabīn* meant 'temple' (*ṣudgh,* note 80).

(130) *al-qishratāni;* perhaps we should read *al-qishriyyāni* (cf. note 120), from *qishra* 'scale'. In Latin *corticalis,* due to misunderstanding of the Arabic where *qishra* also means bark (cf. Singer and Rabin, p. 39).

(131) *al-nutū'āni,* sing. *nutū'* or *nutuww,* (wrong points in MS.), i.e. sinciput and occiput. This sentence hints at Galen's speculation, *De usu part.* ix. 17 (Kühn iii. 752) which is reproduced in full in the *Abridgment;* cf. also Avicenna, p. 458.

INDEX OF TERMS

(The numbers refer to the notes)

(a) Arabic Terms

THE MASTERS OF SALERNO AND THE ORIGINS OF PROFESSIONAL MEDICAL PRACTICE

by

H. P. BAYON

THE writings of the *Magistri Salernitani* are worthy of reconsideration at the present time, because there is still much misunderstanding regarding the 'School' of Salerno itself, the women who were supposed to have taught medicine there, and the manner in which the doctrines of a *Magister* differed from the practice of a *medicus*, who might be a cleric or a simple lay medical adviser. The inception of academic study during the eleventh century led to a remarkable alteration—still unrecognized—in the development of the medical profession. In the improvement of medical education the Salernitans played an important role, since they introduced the scholastic method of study. It must be admitted that in the course of time strict adherence to Scholasticism was a hindrance to progress, but, nevertheless, it was an unavoidable stage in the advance of knowledge.

It should be said that in studying the Salernitan texts it is often difficult to distinguish between a genuine original document or a faithful copy of such a document on the one hand, and copies showing later emendations on the other. This is particularly the case with respect to the so-called *Regimen Salerni*, which was copied and recopied, altered and expanded, imitated, translated, and later repeatedly printed, so that in its present form it is a work only remotely connected with the Salerno of the eleventh century.

There is considerable doubt regarding the origin of the School of Salerno. Its supposed foundation by the Roman emperors is mentioned in a contract alleged to have been concluded in 1147 between the City of Salerno and Count Roger, but Kristeller,[1] for reasons fully discussed in his interesting study, considers this assertion to be a spurious interpolation in a privilege granted by Alfonso I in 1442. In this essay it has, therefore, seemed advisable to base any conclusions on a comparative study of the earliest available manuscripts, even though these are few in number and not easily accessible.

The Present Position of Salernitan Studies

A century ago August Henschel examined a sheaf of old manuscripts in the library of the Magdalene Gymnasium at Breslau. This collection bore the title *Codex herbarius*, and he found it to consist of thirty-five medical treatises by different authors. The results of Henschel's studies appeared first in 1846 in *Janus*,[2] and four years later he published a paper on another manuscript.[3] They were soon followed by the two monumental works[4, 5] of

---

[1] P. O. Kristeller, 'The School of Salerno: its development and its contribution to the history of learning'. *Bull. Hist. Med.*, 1945, xvii, 138–94. [p. 164.]

[2] A. E. G. Theodor Henschel, *Janus*, 1846, i, 40–84.

[3] *idem, De praxi medica Salernitana commentatio*. Vratislaviae, 1850.

[4] Salvatore De Renzi, *Collectio Salernitana ossia documenti inediti*. 5 vols. Naples, 1852–9.

[5] *idem, Storia documentata della Scuola Medica di Salerno*. Naples, 1857.

Salvatore De Renzi, which provided most valuable documentary evidence. Though De Renzi's enthusiasm often carried him far beyond the bounds of sober interpretation his work has been a source of admiration to all subsequent students. Among others his conclusions were accepted by Daremberg,[6] Littré,[7] Haeser,[8] and Puschmann.[9] Puccinotti[10] devoted twenty-two chapters of his well-known work to Salernitan medicine. His thesis was somewhat marred by the fact that he stretched the evidence in his attempt to prove that the 'School' had been a monastic or religious institution. Special attention must be directed to Steinschneider's careful and scholarly studies of Constantine the African.[11] Between 1911 and 1923 Karl Sudhoff, frequently through the medium of dissertations by his pupils, published an extensive series of Salernitan studies which will be considered later. Capparoni,[12] by publishing in 1923 the ancient Church Registers in Salerno, brought to light several names which had been overlooked by De Renzi. Apart from these authors all histories of medicine refer to Salerno as a medical centre in the Middle Ages. But historians in general also refer to the ancient city because it is considered to have had the first university in Europe.[13] The views of Sarton on this point may be mentioned. He says: 'Salerno was never a fountain-head, but it was the earliest distributing center of medical ideas in Europe and all later scholars are somewhat indebted to it'.[14] Later he says: 'Salerno was a scientific or professional school, the first of its kind in Christian Europe'.[15]

The latest study is by Kristeller,[1] who has settled certain questions convincingly. He is mainly concerned in proving that the School and the College—two distinct bodies—continued to exist from the thirteenth and fourteenth centuries until the beginning of the nineteenth, when a decree restricted the granting of degrees to the University of Naples and so stopped the examinations by the Faculty of Salerno.

As a result of consideration of these various works and the examination of accessible manuscripts, this study has explained the significant part played by the Salernitan Masters in initiating the medical profession as it now exists in all parts of the civilized world. It is suggested that the following study defines the essential differences between the *medicus* and the *Magister medicinae*. Further, there has emerged a clearer conception of the 'School' in the eleventh and twelfth centuries, and of the later College of Masters in Physic.

There has also emerged a more definite understanding of the position of both these institutions in relation to the oldest universities, such as Bologna (before 1158), Montpellier (1137–60), Paris (1100), Oxford (1140),

[6] Charles Daremberg, *Histoire des sciences médicales.* 2 vols. Paris, 1870.

[7] Émile Littré, *Médecine et médecins.* Paris, 1872.

[8] Heinrich Haeser, *Lehrbuch der Geschichte der Medicin.* Third edition. 3 vols. Jena, 1875–82.

[9] Theodor Puschmann, *Handbuch der Geschichte der Medizin.* 3 vols. Jena, 1902–05.

[10] Francesco Puccinotti, *Storia della medicina.* 3 vols. Leghorn, 1850–66. (The section to which reference is made in the text is in vol. ii, pt. i, 1855.)

[11] M. Steinschneider, *Virchows Archiv,* 1866, xxxvii, 351–410.

[12] P. Capparoni, '*Magistri Salernitani nondum cogniti*'. London, 1923. (Publications of the Wellcome Historical Medical Museum, o.s., No. 2.)

[13] H. Rashdall, *The Universities of Europe in the Middle Ages.* Ed. Powicke and Emden. 3 vols. Oxford, 1936, vol. i, pp. 75–85.

[14] G. Sarton, *Introduction to the history of science.* Washington, vol. i, 1927, p. 699.

[15] *ibid.,* p. 725.

Cambridge (1204), Padua (1222), Naples (1224), Siena (1240). It should be mentioned that the university, in the modern sense of the word, with its several faculties and regular teachers, first originated in the fourteenth century, but this complex question cannot be discussed fully here.

Medical Writings and Practice to A.D. 1200

A rapid glance may be cast on the state of medical knowledge and practice from early times to the twelfth century in those countries that had some direct or indirect contact with Salerno.

In ancient Greece, in the fifth century B.C., it is doubtful to what extent orthodox medicine held the field. It is also not clear to what extent the greatness of even a man like Hippocrates was generally recognized; moreover, in his most authentic writings there are traces of non-Hellenistic influences. For example, Bayon[16] showed that in the *Aphorisms* the pregnancy tests described are of Egyptian origin, and there is no evidence that they are not interpolations by later scribes. The Hippocratic School, with its insistence on accurate prognosis and the simplest types of therapy, could not have made much headway against the miraculous cures by magical charms and votive offerings. In Sicily, in Alexandria, in Rome and in Byzantium, many other schools of medical practice and doctrine prevailed during the period between the fifth century B.C. and the first century A.D., and the practitioners appeared to have belonged to the most diverse classes, ranging from the philosopher or the high priest to the wise old woman or even a slave.

The same may be said of medical practice in the age of classical Rome, from the third century B.C. to the third century A.D. For example, Cato the Censor tells how he treated the members of his household and resented the appearance of the 'Graeculus esuriens' as a medical practitioner. Both Juvenal and Martial indicate that medicine was taught at the bedside by a form of apprenticeship, and from other sources it can be learned that ophthalmologists were an inferior class of practitioners. It is worth-while remembering also that Celsus himself was not a *medicus*. Galen, the most influential of orthodox physicians, frequently ranted against his bungling competitors, who often represented unorthodox schools.

In Alexandria from the third century B.C. to the seventh century A.D. there was a centre of medical learning which trained eminent physicians, who travelled widely but practised mostly in the great cities. Nevertheless, general medical practice among the people must have been mostly of a votive or semi-magical character. The same remarks apply to Byzantium during the sixth and three succeeding centuries. Archiaters were appointed, and in the Metropolis and outlying districts medical practice may well have been on a high level. But it existed side by side with cures wrought by wonder-working shrines and images.

In countries subject to Moslem rule it can be shown that from the seventh century onwards eminent philosophers practised and taught medicine. As physicians they were highly respected, and though they were often officially attached to the courts of princes, they seemed to have treated all classes of the population in hospitals. Their knowledge was based on classical Greek

---

[16] H. P. Bayon, 'Ancient pregnancy tests in the light of contemporary knowledge'. *Proc. Roy. Soc. Med.*, 1939, xxxii (Sect. Hist. Med.), 61–72.

and Latin learning, and the extensive information provided by some of these men enabled them to be recognized later as encyclopaedic philosophers. The fame of Avicenna, Rhazes and Averroës soon spread; but there were other authors who wrote in Arabic who were not Moslems—for example, the Jews and the Nestorian Christians. Some authorities have accepted the theory that Arabic culture was spread by the Saracen pirates who harassed the shores of the Mediterranean. It would appear more likely that the contrary is the case, since these corsairs destroyed the soil on which learning and knowledge would have flourished. It should be remembered that the writings of the Arabic philosopher-physicians extended to countries which the scimitar never reached.

In western Europe during the ninth and tenth centuries every prince or other dignitary had his personal physician, usually a high-ranking clerk in Holy Orders who could read and write and was acquainted with medical treatises, and who in addition might also be versed in astrology. But the popular lay *medicus*, or practitioner of medicine, was illiterate and relied mostly on animal and vegetable substances, which are still employed in the medicine of folk-lore, and he could also provide charms consisting of objects or formulae to which quasi-magical effects could be attributed.

These remarks on the position of the physician may be supplemented by comments on the status of the surgeon and of the obstetrician. It should be remembered that, since the times of both Celsus and Galen, the practice of surgery had nearly everywhere become dissociated from that of physic. The complex reasons for this cleavage cannot be dealt with here; but surgery was itself in a very backward state. The pain in most surgical procedures made many patients resort to wonder-working ointments and salves, and the danger inherent in cutting operations deterred others. Further, monks were not allowed to shed blood, and a similar prejudice prevailed among Moslems who much preferred the cautery. The skill and knowledge of anatomy required for major surgery was not often found, and surgeons would frequently not undertake operations which were fraught with great risk. As an example, the case may be cited of Duke Leopold I of Austria,[17] who fell from his horse and sustained an open compound fracture of the thigh. No surgeon would undertake the amputation of the gangrenous limb and the Duke ordered his servant to chop it off with an axe. This resulted in the death of the Duke.[18] It is true that in India both plastic surgery and the treatment of compound fractures had been practised by men of the potter-caste for centuries before our era; but in European countries the spread of Christianity did not hasten the progress of operative surgery.

In view of the fact that one of the most popular of the Salernitan treatises dealt with obstetrics, gynaecology and cosmetics, a few words may be said on the relation between orthodox medicine and the treatment of women's ailments during the first twelve centuries of our era. During child-birth all women—even queens and princesses—were attended only by women, though a philosopher-physician might be called in to cast a horoscope. The training of these handywomen was obtained by actual experience during an

---

[17] It was Leopold I (not V as Puschmann says) who captured Richard Coeur-de-Lion.

[18] T. Puschmann, *A history of medical education.* Trans. E. H. Hare. London, 1891, p. 270.

PLATE IV

Gon & Caius MS 117/186.

239

Trotula

Fig. 1. Trotula manuscript. Early fourteenth century
(Gon. & Caius College, Camb, MS. 117/186, fo. 239ʳ)
(See note on p. 219)

apprenticeship. Soranus[19] (A.D. 78–117) had written a small treatise, intended for the guidance of midwives, in which he described podalic version and primary suture of the torn perineum, and Aëtius of Amida in the sixth century summarized all previous knowledge of obstetrics but added nothing new. The means at the disposal of handywomen at difficult births consisted of amulets, charms, potions made from herbs, invocations of the saints— especially Saint Margaret—and the employment of the obstetric chair to which remarkable properties were attributed. A piece of coral or a magnet held in the hand of the patient were especially popular.

Sudhoff quoted the following charm:

Ad feminam laborantem de puero pone hec scripta fere ipsam: Maria peperit yesum † elysabebt johannem † anna mariam † eclinia remigium † sator † arepo tenet † opera ratas † Item tere diptamnum et da mulieri con vino et pariet.[20]

This may be compared with the Anglo-Saxon charm which is given by Payne.[21]

The Clerical or Lay 'Medicus' and the Salernitan 'Magister'

From what has been written, it will be appreciated that in Christian countries the medical practitioner or *medicus* was for many centuries a simple craftsman or artisan. In Moslem countries the philosopher-physician was held in high esteem, though the popular 'Hakim' probably practised there also, since they were relatively numerous in Constantinople even in recent times.

Reference to the life and works of Shabbethai ben Abraham ben Joel of Otranto is made by Charles and Dorothea Singer.[22] This physician, usually known as 'Donnolo', was the personification of the legend of the foundation of the Salernitan School by four masters, since he exhibited the influence of Hebrew, Arabic, Greek and Latin learning in his writings. Against this it may be objected that there is no record that Donnolo ever resided, learned or taught at Salerno; moreover, he wrote in Hebrew and his fragmentary writings are considered to represent the remains of the first Jewish medical treatises.

A minor but relative point is that the name Donnolo, by which he is commonly known, means 'a little master'; he was not a *Magister* such as the learned physicians who wrote in Salerno approximately two hundred years later. The Singers refer to some instances in the life of Donnolo which show that, while his treatment differed from that used by the monks, he did not have to come into competition with the Christian layman. We may hence infer that these Christian practitioners were few or not of great standing. De Renzi[23] recalled the names of several medical practitioners which he had traced in documents in southern Italy. Some of these men were clerks in Holy Orders, but there is no evidence that they were connected with the School or Faculty of Medicine or that they were designated as *Magistri*, a title at that time

---

[19] *Die Gynaekologie des Soranus von Ephesus*. Ger. trans., Munich, 1894.

[20] K. Sudhoff, 'Die Salernitaner Handschrift in Breslau'. *Archiv für Geschichte der Medizin*, 1920, xii, 101–48. [p. 145.]

[21] J. F. Payne, *English Medicine in the Anglo-Saxon Times*. Oxford, 1904, pp. 130–2.

[22] C. and D. Singer, 'The origin of the medical school of Salerno'. In *Essays on the history of medicine presented to Karl Sudhoff*. Ed. C. Singer and H. E. Sigerist. Zürich, 1924, pp. 121–38. Also, C. and D. Singer, 'The School of Salerno and its legends'. *History*, 1925, x, 242–6; reprinted in Charles Singer, *From magic to science*. London, 1928, pp. 240–8.

[23] De Renzi, *Storia documentata*, op. cit. (5). See especially the chapter entitled 'Medici Salernitani anteriori al Mille', pp. 156 ff.

reserved for judges and lawyers. Even in Salerno the *medicus* could be an illiterate person. De Renzi also mentions a Jewish *medicus* called Judas, whose name appeared in a document dating from the year 1005.[24] This was apparently the first Jewish *medicus* who practised in Salerno.

The name of Petrocellus appeared in 1035. He was a cleric and a *medicus*, and he left property to his children, for at that time celibacy was not obligatory for priests in the Roman Catholic Church. De Renzi states that he was the author of *Practica Petrocelli Salernitani*, a writing similar in context to the *Passionarius* of Gariopontus. De Renzi also believed that this Petrocellus was the 'Magister Petrus de Salerno' of the manuscript in St. John's College, Cambridge.[25]

Alphanus, a Benedictine from Cassino, was Archbishop of Salerno from 1058 to 1085. He was known also for several medical manuscripts, such as *De quatuor humoribus corporis humani* which has been edited by Capparoni,[26] and *De pulsibus* edited by Creutz.[27] A translation from the Greek of the work *On the Nature of Man* by Nemesius of Emesa had a fairly wide influence in the Middle Ages, though it left little trace in subsequent Salernitan writings. This translation is also attributed to Alphanus.

The fact that Alphanus and certain other clerics each bore the designation *medicus* has been used to support the view that the 'School' of Salerno was a religious foundation. But it seems evident that on the contrary the priests who practised medicine were not attached to any particular school and left no record of their systems of healing. It is possible also that they treated patients by laying on of hands or similar methods. Bearing in mind the meaning of the term *medicus* at that time, it will be understood that the mere presence of medical practitioners in any particular place did not imply an organized medical faculty in that area. The healing art, if not a part of religious practice, was at that time a craft and not a learned profession. It should not be forgotten that the healing of the sick was one of the apostolic duties enjoined in the Gospels. Compare, for example, the rule of the Order of Saint Benedict (A.D. 529) which says: 'Infirmorum cura ante omnia et super omnia adhibenda est.'

That the majority of these men were both clerks in Holy Orders and practitioners (*clericus et medicus*) is understandable, not only because of the close connexion between faith-healing and medical practice, but also because priests and monks supervised the infirmaries. They were, however, often self-taught, and were posted to the infirmary because they were interested in medical matters. Many monasteries adopted this principle. Persons outside the monastery were prohibited by various councils, from that of Rheims in 1131 to that of Paris in 1212, from giving medical treatment and legal advice to its inmates.[28]

Thus though it may seem that the *medicus*, who was a cleric, and the *Magister*, who was a layman, were analogous, this analogy is more apparent than real, and it will be seen that their medicine was quite different.

---

[24] *ibid.*, p. 162.

[25] *ibid.*, pp. 163–6.

[26] P. Capparoni, *Il 'De quattuor humoribus corporis humani' di Alfano I Arcivescovo di Salerno.* Rome, 1928.

[27] R. Creutz, 'Der Frühsalernitaner Alfanus und sein bislang unbekannter *Liber de pulsibus*'. *Archiv für Geschichte der Medizin*, 1937, xxix, 57–83.

[28] P. Capparoni, *op. cit.* (12), p. 19.

The Origins of the 'School' of Salerno

The legendary assertion that the 'School' of Salerno was founded in remote times by a Greek, a Latin, an Arab and a Jew is given by Mazza.[29] This assertion is as credible as many other legends printed about the same time.[30]

The question whether Salerno constituted the first university depends first of all on the meaning attached to the word *universitas*. In the eleventh and twelfth centuries this word did not have the modern meaning. For example, Powicke and Emden mention a *universitas iudaeorum* at Catania before 1283.[31] The word often meant a congregation or merely a group. Hence if the presence of pupils from foreign parts constituted a *studium generale*, then Salerno in the eleventh century was already a university. If, on the other hand, the teaching of the *Trivium* or the *Quadrivium* is the determining factor, then Bologna or Paris were first in the field.

Whether Salerno antedated Bologna as a university or *studium generale* is a matter of definition, since it can be shown that it was only in the beginning of the thirteenth century that logic was taught at Salerno. Medicine was taught at Bologna by Taddeo Alderotti (1215–95), and in 1222 the *Magister in phisica* of Salerno became a *Medicus in phisica* as a result of academic instruction; and about fifty years later the title was changed to *Doctor medicinae*. About the same time there was a *Doctor chyrurgiae*. Originally the title 'doctor'—meaning wise in some branch of learning, usually theology—was not conferred academically. Thus Magister Thomasius Saracenus, *Doctor in phisica*, who died in 1284, was a cleric.[32] In Capparoni's excellent book *medicus* is translated 'doctor', which proves confusing, since the title *Doctor in phisica* did not appear in Salernitan documents until the thirteenth century.

The 'School' of Salerno became known when Petrocellus, Gariopontus and others compiled their treatises and copies reached places outside southern Italy and even the British Isles. It can be assumed that students, such as Adelard of Bath (d. *c.* 1130), came to Salerno to improve their knowledge and to sit at the feet of their renowned teachers. But these teachers were singly independent *Magistri* who were not connected with any organized body, and were probably competing sharply for pupils. Perhaps a century later, when the fame of Salerno had spread widely, these *Magistri medicinae* possibly became united in a corporate guild of teachers of medicine. This association was lost during the siege of 1194; but at a later date a similar association was formed at Salerno, so that mention is made of it, under the name of *curia*, in the edicts of 1231 and 1240. All the documentary evidence supports this view, as is shown by the careful study by Kristeller.[33]

From the work of De Renzi it can be seen that it was after the advent of Constantine the African that the Salernitan authorities began to write and that

---

[29] See A. Mazza, *Urbis Salernitanae hist. et antiq.*, in J. G. Graevius and P. Burmann, *Thesaurus antiquitatum et historiarum Italiae*, etc. Lugd. Bat. vol. ix, 1681, p. 4.

[30] Cf. for example Le Maire's attempt to trace the University of Orleans from a Druid school (*Histoire et antiquitez de la ville et duché d'Orléans*. 2 vols. in 1. Orléans, 1645, vol. i, p. 332).

[31] Powicke and Emden, *op. cit.* (13), vol. i, p. 158.

[32] Capparoni, *op. cit.* (12), p. 45.

[33] Kristeller, *op. cit.* (1).

the title *Magister* was first assumed. It was after this period, too, that the custom arose of quoting extracts from classical manuscripts—a procedure which might justify the designation of Salerno as a 'School'. The Florentine teacher of Bologna, Taddeo Alderotti—Dante's 'Mastro Taddeo'—complained that Constantine 'insanus monacus in transferendo peccavit quantitate et qualitate', but at that time no better Salernitan texts were available. Though Constantine became a monk at Monte Cassino, he neither resided long in Salerno, nor adopted the title of *Magister*. Yet he provided most of the original classical background which laid the intellectual foundation of Salernitan medicine as we know it to-day.

Charles Singer[34] added materially to our knowledge of the life of Constantine in his fundamental study of the fourteenth century manuscript in the British Museum. He discusses our main source of information regarding Constantine, namely, Peter the Deacon (1107–40), who wrote about forty or fifty years after Constantine's death. Singer notes several improbabilities and anachronisms which the story contains, such as the confusing of names of different persons.[35] It can be assumed that Constantine was a Moslem and born at Tunis. He travelled in eastern countries, studied Arabic translations of Greek works and eventually reached Salerno, possibly as a Saracen slave. He became secretary to the Norman Duke, Robert Guiscard, and if this is the case it must have been after 1075. He adopted Christianity and entered the monastery of Monte Cassino, where he lived until his death. He left in manuscript Latin translations of various galenical writings, which he translated from the Arabic text of the Egyptian Jew, Isaac Judeus. Constantine's texts were printed and published at Basel, 1536–9.

The first of the Salernitan Masters about whom there is some definite but scanty information is Guarimpoto, who is also known by the name Gariopontus[36] and variants such as Warimpotus. De Renzi[36] put forward evidence to show that Gariopontus was not a Greek; and it is now accepted that the name indicates that he must have been a northern Italian, and possibly a Lombard. Capparoni[37] traced a 'Guarimpotus subdiaconus' who lived at Salerno about the year 1040.

In the tenth century Salerno was a health resort for pilgrims from northern lands. This is the case despite the fact that a few literary references may be interpreted to imply that, at that date, the Salerno *medici* were known for their practical skill; for example, Adalberus, Bishop of Verdun A.D. 985–8, went to Salerno 'curationis gratia'. In 1095 the First Crusade was proclaimed, but even before then pilgrims had gone to the Holy Land from Mediterranean and Adriatic ports such as Montpellier, Genoa, Marseilles, Venice, Bari and Salerno. Of these only Montpellier and Salerno became important medical centres. We do not know why this happened, but what can be accepted is the fact that from the time of the appearance of the *Passionarius* of Gariopontus[38] several medical

[34] C. Singer, 'A legend of Salerno. How Constantine the African brought the art of medicine to the Christians'. *Bull. Johns Hopkins Hosp.*, 1917, xxviii, 64–9.

[35] Such mistakes occur also in modern biographies of Paracelsus, Servetus and others. The purpose of critical history is to unravel such tangled skeins and evolve if possible a clear pattern.

[36] *op. cit.* (5), pp. 168–72.

[37] *op. cit.* (12), p. 14.

[38] [Gariopontus], *Passionarius Galeni ... aegritudines a capite ad pedes usque complectens.* Lugduni, 1526.

manuscripts can be traced which seem to be the work of some Salernitan *Magister*. Thus arose the fame of the 'School' of Salerno, and though the name may conjure up ideas of class-rooms, it seems more probable that instruction was in the house of the *Magister* and consisted in the pupil being given a text to copy for his own use.

The earliest existing Salernitan manuscripts are those at Breslau. Sudhoff[39] obtained expert palaeographic opinion on these and decided that they were written some time between 1160 and 1170. The variety of medical subjects discussed suggests that they may have been copies of the texts of different authors.

We cannot help sympathizing with De Renzi in his courageous attempt to prove the antiquity of the 'School' of Salerno by making the documentary evidence agree with speculative assumptions. The subject is discussed in many chapters of his work, but one example will be sufficient to indicate his method:

> Ed oltre il titolo *Scuola Salernitana* troviamo nelle più antiche testimonianze citati sempre molti Medici contemporanei. Tale quella di Adalberone che viene a farsi curare dai *Medici Salernitani*; tale Orderico Vitale che la chiama antica Scuola: tale le varie associazioni, delle quali fanno parola le opere di Guarimpoto, di Cofone, de' Plateari, ed un poco più tardi da'Maestri di Egidio Corbeil.[40]

So many useful documents are quoted in De Renzi's books, that he might safely have left them to speak for themselves. These show that Adalberus, Archbishop of Bremen, was attended by Adamatus, a *medicus* from Salerno. Desiderius, the Abbot of Monte Cassino, went there for medical treatment, but there is no mention of a school of medicine. The evidence of Orderic Vitalis, who was born at Shrewsbury about 1075 and who died after 1141, could not be relevant before 1100. Many examples could be quoted to show that at the time when these documents were compiled ('illo tempore'), fifty years might be considered as 'long ago'. Even the testimony of Gilles de Corbeil (*c.* 1198) did not refer to 'a little later' ('un poco più tardi'), but to a century later. In fact, it seems safe to assume that the literary activity of the Salernitan authors was great from the year 1100 onwards, and that their fame was then assured. Their popularity can be explained by the fact that they practised a type of therapy which was practical and straightforward; that they quoted just as much of the classical authorities as would impress the reader and no more; and that their writings were easily understood and their teaching easily applied in practice.

In the year 1194 a great disaster befell Salerno. It was besieged, conquered and sacked by Henry VI of Hohenstaufen, and many of the inhabitants were enslaved. It may have been at this time that the manuscripts went to Breslau. After this event the manuscripts that had been copied kept alive the tradition of the 'School'. Medical practitioners must have again met in Salerno within a couple of decades, because Frederick II (*Stupor mundi*), son of Henry VI, after founding the University of Naples with its medical faculty (1224), made decrees in 1231 and 1240 in which he regulated the granting of degrees by the Masters of Salerno.[41]

[39] K. Sudhoff, *op. cit.* (20), p. 102.
[40] De Renzi, *op. cit.* (5), p. 143.
[41] *ibid.*, p. lxxvi.

After this event the existence of a *Collegium* in Salerno is relatively well documented, though there is no evidence of literary activity. It is known, however, that in the meantime several centres of study had arisen in Naples, Reggio Calabria, Siena, and even further afield at Bologna, Paris, Montpellier and Oxford. It can be assumed that some of these schools obtained a greater variety of good classical texts than Salerno, and so the scholastic era had begun in earnest, and Hippocrates, Galen and the Moslem medical writers soon surpassed anything which Salerno could provide. Thus we find references such as that in the passage in the British Museum manuscript, which originated in northern Brabant in the first three decades of the fourteenth century. Singer translates this passage as follows:—

> Wherefore at Salerno he [Constantine] is regarded as the very first of physicians and there, unto this day, they speak of his works, though now, decayed with age, they are considered by the moderns as in the twilight of science. But that science has been reborn, and a young shoot has gone out from the old vine in the famous city of Montpellier (verbatim: *ad montem pessulanum celeberrime*).[42]

Thomas Aquinas (1225–74), *Doctor angelicus*, wrote that four cities were pre-eminent, Paris for science, Salerno for medicine, Bologna for jurisprudence and Orleans *in actoribus* or for literature. A similar remark was made by Galfridus, who lived about 1250; Orleans became a *studium* about 1255.

Barely eight decades later, Petrarch visited Salerno in 1330 and wrote in one of his letters: 'Fuisse hic medicinae fontem fama est, sed nihil est, quod non senio exarescat'. Incidentally, by quoting only a part of Petrarch's statement some writers have made him say that Salerno was a fountain-head of medicine; but, actually, Petrarch qualifies this statement.

Kristeller[43] quotes fully documentary evidence regarding the organization in 1442 of a 'Collegium seu publicus conventus magistrorum medicinae et doctorum phisicalium', and he deals also with the Faculty of Medicine in Salerno. His evidence shows that both the Faculty and the College continued to exist—however precariously—till the granting of degrees was restricted to Naples by a decree dated 29 November 1811. But De Renzi,[44] writing in 1857, mentioned the existence of a 'Liceo' with teachers of anatomy, physiology, pathology, legal medicine, clinical and practical surgery, obstetrics and operations, so that even in his day some semblance of medical tuition was still preserved.

The 'Regimen Sanitatis Salerni' and its Probable Inception

By far the most popular and wide-spread of Salernitan writings is the medical poem which usually begins with the line 'Anglorum regi scripsit tota scola Salerni'. Sudhoff made a careful study of the manuscript copies of this and similar poems which he had discovered in German libraries, and by comparing them with the versions quoted by J. B. M. Baudry de Balzac,[45] he came to the following conclusion:

> Völlig einwandfrei und unwiderleglich hat meine Nachforschung aber das Ergebnis zutage gefördert: Mit der eigentlichen Ruhmesperiode von Salerno, mit

[42] Singer, *op. cit.* (34), p. 68.   [43] Kristeller, *op. cit.* (1).
[44] De Renzi, *op. cit.* (5), p. 608.   [45] Died 1848.

PLATE V

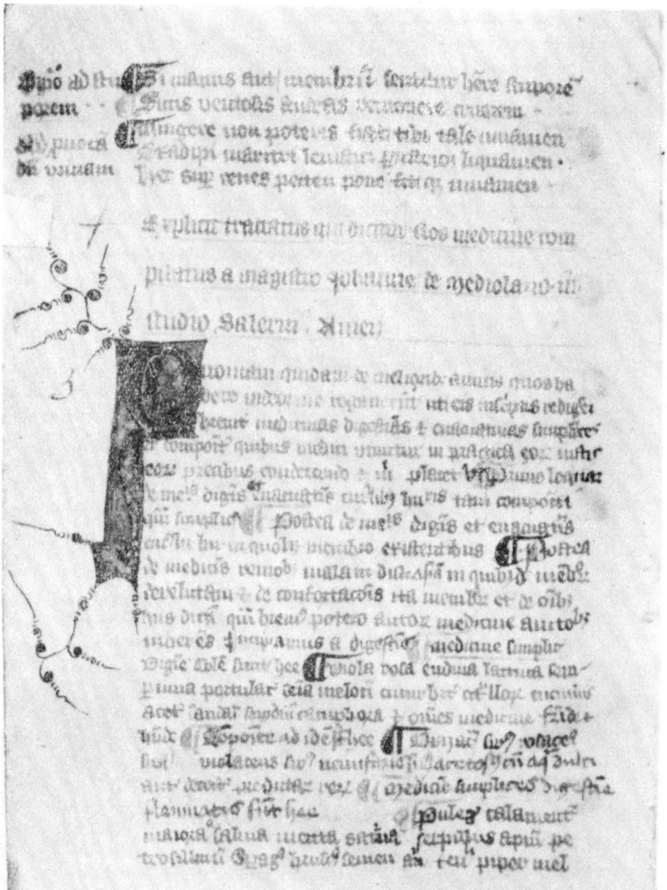

FIG. 2.   Manuscript of the *Flos medicinae*
(Brit. Mus., Sloane MS. 3468, fo. 22**v**)
(See note on p. 219)

PLATE VI

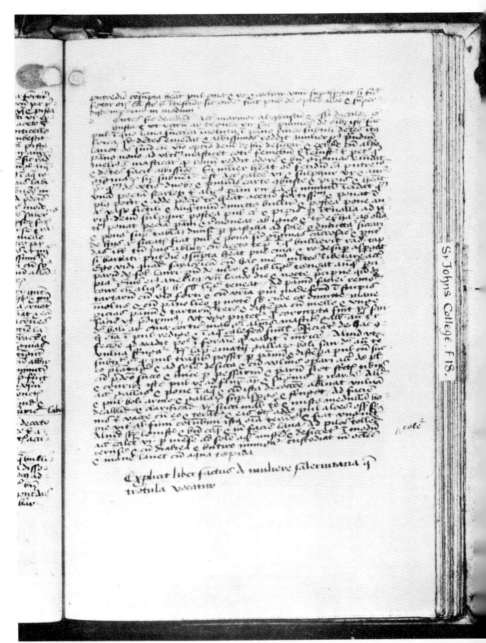

FIG. 3.   Trotula manuscript
(St. John's College, Camb, MS. 155, tract 14, *explicit*)
(See note on p. 219)

dem Salern des 12. Jahrhunderts, mit Hochsalerno also hat das landläufige 'Regimen sanitatis versificatum' (Arnaldi) als Ganzes auch nicht das Mindeste zu tun.[46]

Sudhoff puts forward the following arguments in favour of this sweeping assertion: (a) No manuscript of the *Regimen* is older than the early fourteenth century. It is true that the earliest copy in the British Museum dates from the fourteenth century, and so also do the opening lines which have been scribbled in the manuscript book in St. John's College, Cambridge. (b) The *Regimen* was not mentioned in the *Epistola Theodori philosophi ad imperatorem Fridericum* which was written in 1240. Sudhoff concluded that if it had been known at that time it would have been quoted, but it is difficult to see the reason for this opinion.[47] (c) Little verse came from Salerno at the zenith of its fame, which Sudhoff believes to have been in the middle of the twelfth century.[48] This is a debatable objection, since verse was commonly written in southern Italy before and after the twelfth century. (d) In some instances John of Milan is quoted as the author, and in one copy the poem is dedicated to Charlemagne.[49] (e) Several other objections are mentioned in Sudhoff's series of papers on the subject; but a particularly conclusive objection is that he quoted an excerpt from a report by an Aragonese ambassador, who wrote that in August 1301, in the villa 'La Scorzola' of Pope Boniface VIII, Arnald of Villanova prepared a small book on the rules of health for the use of the Pope, who greatly admired it.[50] Sudhoff concluded that this fact confirmed that Arnald was the author of the version of the *Regimen seu flos medicinae*, which was eventually printed under his name. The *Flos medicinae* is a long poem which contains observations on medical matters unknown in twelfth-century Salerno. But many shorter versions exist, and these reveal the rudimentary knowledge of hygiene which could be expected from Salerno of that period. It does not seem reasonable to consider the simpler poems as excerpts from the longer version. It should be mentioned that Arnald was connected with Montpellier, and at one time was court physician to Pedro III of Aragon (1239–85), surnamed ' el Grande'.

If it is conceded that the expanded version was written by Arnald in 1301 and the fame of Salerno was no longer what it had been, the dedication to the *Anglorum rex* presumably was made because such was the custom in the short versified address. It has been suggested that the *Anglorum rex* was Robert, Duke of Normandy (1054–1134), who passed through Bari in 1096 on his way to the Holy Land, and returned through that port, at which he married Sibilla, daughter of Geoffrey de Conversana, Count of Salerno. Robert of Normandy was a claimant to the throne of England and was treated as a sovereign in southern Italy. He was suffering from a poisoned wound in the arm which possibly developed into chronic sepsis. The devoted wife sucked it and died as a result.[51]

---

[46] K. Sudhoff, 'Zum Regimen Sanitatis Salernitanum'. *Archiv für Geschichte der Medizin*, 1920, xii, 149–80. [p. 180.]
[47] *ibid.*, p. 164.
[48] *ibid.*, p. 161.
[49] *ibid.*, p. 160.
[50] *ibid.*, p. 167.
[51] Capparoni, *op. cit.* (12), p. 13.

De Renzi's 'Medichessa Trotula' and the 'Mulieres et Nobiles Salernitanae'

The most readily available Salernitan treatise in manuscript form is that ascribed to the person called 'Trotula', and usually entitled De passionibus mulierum. It was printed and reprinted several times, first at Strassburg in 1544.[52] The main texts correspond to the manuscripts, such as that in Caius College, Cambridge, but the editor added alchemical matter, which evidently dates from a period later than the twelfth century. A good translation of a printed text was published by Mason Hohl in 1940.[53]

The De passionibus mulierum was the first gynaecological treatise composed for the instruction and guidance of male practitioners of medicine in the east or west. It thus differed from the work of Soranus which was clearly addressed to midwives or handywomen. The chapters dealing with cosmetics often form a separate manuscript bearing the title Trotula de ornatu mulierum; these consist of a formulary of aids to beauty, of which many examples are known, from the time of ancient Egypt to the present day.

In this country there are at least twenty-seven manuscript copies of Trotula. There are three in Cambridge colleges, one each at Caius, St. John's and at Trinity. The copy in the University Library at Cambridge is an excerpt from the Thesaurus pauperum. In Oxford there are fourteen copies in the Bodleian and various colleges. The British Museum has eight or nine, while two are in the catalogue of the Hunterian Library at Glasgow. Spitzner[54] in 1921 mentioned twenty-one copies of 'Trotula' in German, Belgian and French libraries. It is, therefore, evident that this small treatise must have been well appreciated in the thirteenth and fourteenth centuries. It appeared in print in 1544, 1547, 1555, 1556, 1586, 1597. There may have been other editions, but those I was able to trace after the sixteenth century dealt with the text from the historical standpoint.

The authorship of the 'Trotula' De passionibus has been hotly contested. De Renzi[55] asserted strongly that it was part of a much larger treatise, embracing the whole of medicine, written by the 'Medichessa Trotula'. There is little evidence to support this assumption and what does exist is weak. Hiersemann[56] made the alternative suggestion that De passionibus was the work of a man called Trottus who also wrote part of the Breslau Codex, on the margin of which he left marks such as 'Trot', or 'tt'. Against this it may be said that, though documentary evidence supports the existence of several Salernitan women called Trocta or Trotula,[57] there is no mention anywhere of a man called Trottus. Again, the remedies recommended for gynaecological ailments in Trotula and the 'Trot' manuscript in Breslau are different. It may further be said that the manuscript copies of De passionibus which I have examined state

[52] The editio princeps is in the following collection: Experimentarius medicinae. Continens Trotulae ... Aegritudinum muliebrium .... Ed. Geo. Kraut. 3 pts. in 1 vol. Argentorati (Jo. Schottus), 1544.

[53] The Diseases of Women, by Trotula of Salerno. A translation of 'Passionibus mulierum curandorum', by Elizabeth Mason Hohl. Hollywood, Calif., 1940.

[54] Hermann Rudolf Spitzner, Die Salernitanische Gynäkologie und Geburtshilfe unter dem Namen der Trotula. Leipzig, 1921.

[55] De Renzi, op. cit. (5), pp. 194–208.

[56] Conrad Hiersemann, Die Abschnitte aus der Practica des Trottus in der Salernitanischen Sammelschrift 'De aegritudinum curatione'. Leipzig, 1921.

[57] Capparoni, op. cit. (12), p. 39.

quite clearly that the work was undertaken at the instigation of a matron, who noted with sorrow how often her sex suffered from many serious maladies. The text also mentions how Trotula dealt successfully with a case of ventosity of the womb. The text says that 'Trotula vocata fuit'. If Trotula had been the author, the sentence would presumably have read: 'Et ego autem, Trotula, vocata fui'. Thus in the chapter on cosmetics it was written: 'Et ego autem vidi quadam Saracenam cū hac medicinā multa liberare'. Here the first person is employed though not the name. However, it may be doubted whether a Salernitan *Magister* would condescend to recommend the prescription for a mouth-wash used by a Saracen woman. It should, however, be remembered in connection with the authorship of such doubtful manuscripts that in the Middle Ages it was uncommon for authors to write their works. They were usually dictated and copies were then made.

In the library at St. John's College, Cambridge, there is a manuscript *Trotula de morbis mulierum* (No. 155–14) which begins 'Cum auctor' and ends 'lauet cum aqua tepida'. This manuscript has an important colophon: 'Explicit liber factus a muliere salernitana q̄ trotula vocatur'. This shows that in the fourteenth and fifteenth centuries *De passionibus* was thought by some to be the work of a Salernitan woman. My own view is that Trotula probably inspired *De passionibus* and contributed to the chapters 'De ornatu mulierum'.

As to the text itself, though it can be praised for reviving suture of the perineum and its support during child-birth, it can be criticized for not recommending the suckling of babies by their mothers, and for advising instead the choice of a wet-nurse.

More or less veiled references to abortifacients are a feature of similar classical writings. It can be said that Trotula deals professionally with the drugs recommended 'ad provocanda menstrua', whilst other writings such as *Thesaurus* reveal to the medical eye abortifacients which were well known in ancient times. The same attitude is seen in a brief section dealing with sterility due to a relaxed womb and the methods suggested to remedy the condition. In printed editions these have the sub-heading 'Ut corrupta apparet virgo', an intention which is emphatically disclaimed in the manuscript text which I have seen. It can thus be said that the text reveals an improvement in professional outlook when compared with other classical writings of the same nature.

In *De ornatu* a lip-salve is recommended for those whose lips have been cracked by too passionate kissing by their lovers. This may be considered a peculiarly feminine remark. There are many other prescriptions, but no magical love philtres, though some aphrodisiacs are mentioned.

Admittedly, in difficult or slow births Trotula recommended the holding of a piece of coral or a magnet in the hand. This savoured of magic, though in other matters it is difficult to say where magic ends and organotherapy begins.

Thus Thorndike says: 'Trotula is no longer believed to have been a woman, and we have to judge the women of Salerno mainly by what others have to say of them'.[58] He then quotes from a commentary of Master Bernard of Provence, whom he suspects to be Bernard Gordon of Montpellier, to the effect that the 'mulieres Salernitanae' recommended the eating of acorns from the gizzards

[58] Lynn Thorndike, *A history of magic and experimental science*. New York and London, vol. i, 1923, p. 740.

of doves to increase the retentive faculties and so cure sterility. Thorndike also notes that they gave their husbands excrements of asses 'in crispellis' for the same purpose, and he considered that these prescriptions savoured of magic. De Renzi[59] quoted from the Salernitan *Circa instans* of Johannes Platearius and the *Practica brevis* fourteen examples of remedies recommended by 'mulieres Salernitanae', but added the remark: 'E vero che molte di queste pratiche si riferivano ad usi volgari di medicina domestica comuni a tutti i popoli'. Therefore, even De Renzi, who wished to prove the existence of Salernitan 'donne scienziate', had to admit that their remedies were those of vulgar, not classical medicine.

An answer to the question whether the woman Trotula was the actual author of *De passionibus* would decide whether she can be considered the first woman professor; because it is evident that the Masters of Salerno did not teach *ex cathedra* but through their writings.

The Doctrines of Salernitan Medical Texts

The writings of the early Salernitan Masters such as Petrocellus, Gariopontus and the authors of the Breslau collection, were those of physicians pure and simple. No major surgical interventions were recommended, apparently because plasters and ointments would give the same result as the scalpel and cautery. For example, a marvellous 'Unguentum ossicroceum' would further the healing of broken bones; drugs could dissolve bladder stones without recourse to lithotomy; and wounds and fistulae could be healed by wonderful ointments, without the painful intervention of cautery or knife.

The first Salernitan surgical treatise was by Roggero Frugardi, written about 1170. It became known as *Summa Rogerii*, and was later edited by Roland of Parma and incorporated into the *Glossulae quatuor magistrorum*.

The frequent use of the actual cautery in surgery must have discouraged patients from consulting the surgeon, though the 'spongia somnifera' was described in the printed *Antidotarius Nicolai* of 1471. Von Brunn[60] decided that the 'spongia somnifera' was first prescribed by Ugo di Lucca and not by Nicolas the Salernitan. De Renzi[61] states that this work existed in manuscript under the name of Magister Maurus. Whatever its authorship it was a work often consulted, and the Cambridge Statutes of 1396 required medical undergraduates to read this *Antidotarius* of Nicholas in addition to the usual works.

Another small but significant Salernitan writing should be mentioned. This is the *De adventu medici ad aegrotum* which is in the Breslau Collection. Though not printed till it appeared in De Renzi,[62] it reveals the beginnings of professional etiquette by laying down rules of behaviour towards patients. It should be recalled that Withington[63] mentions King Gram sitting in a tattered garment disguised as a *medicus* among the menials.

Among the latter Salernitan authors is Magister Matteo Silvatico. He

[59] De Renzi, *op. cit.* (5), pp. 206–7.

[60] Walter von Brunn, 'Die Stellung des Guy de Chauliac in der Chirurgie des Mittelalters'. *Archiv für Geschichte der Medizin*, 1920, xii, 94.

[61] De Renzi, *op. cit.* (5) pp. 284–90.

[62] De Renzi, *Collectio Salernitana, op. cit.* (4). Naples, vol. ii, 1853, pp. 74–80.

[63] E. T. Withington, *Medical history from the earliest times.* London, 1894, p. 225.

presumably lived sometime between 1297 and 1342, since De Renzi[64] quoted documents of those years in which the name of Matteo Silvatico occurred. He was the author of a pharmacological treatise. In the printed version of 1541 entitled *Pandectae Medicinae* he quotes Avicenna on the distillation of opium with oil of roses for the purpose of preparing a soporific.[65] This Matteo Silvatico, who is also known as 'Mantovano', is thought to have been Mastro Mazzeo della Montagna of Boccaccio's *Decameron*, who calls Mastro Mazzeo 'grandissimo medico in chirurgia'. The story describes how the surgeon prepared a clear distillate of opium ('addoppiata') to deaden the pain of operation for the removal of a gangrenous bone from the leg of a patient. The wife's lover drank the potion by mistake and fell in a dead sleep lasting twenty-four hours.[66]

Boccaccio was probably wrong in saying that the opiate was clear and tasteless as water, for both mandrakes and opium were mixed with wine to mask the taste and enhance the effect.[67] Apart from this comprehensible inaccuracy, Boccaccio can be believed, for he had lived in Naples and would be well acquainted with local gossip. Therefore, it can be accepted that a Salernitan *Magister*, whose existing writing is a pharmacological compilation, was in practice predominantly a surgeon, since the *Decameron* said that Mastro Mazzeo was called as far afield as Amalfi to attend wounded in a street brawl. De Renzi[68] did not admit that Matheus Silvaticus was a Mantuan by birth or cognomen, since the family name Silvatico was common in Salerno and in documents which he examined a 'Matthaeus Salernitanus' was named. It may be right that Boccaccio should call him 'della Montagna', which later authors made into 'Mantovano'. In Italian, Matteo and Mazzeo are the same name.

Achievements of the Salernitan Masters in the Middle Ages

The outstanding merit of the Salernitans was that they provided practitioners of medicine with small, easily understood, simple compilations from classical authors. Moreover, by their example and their writings they advanced the idea that medicine in all its branches, instead of being practised on votive or religious principles, could, for those able to read and write, be the subject of academical study, and could be taught by teachers who had a knowledge of the classical authors. Indeed, it seems probable that instruction consisted in the teacher handing out compilations to be copied by the pupils.

From De Renzi onwards many authors—for example, Guthrie[69]—held the view that Salernitan medicine bears little or no trace of Arab influence. Such dogmatic statements are possibly misleading, especially in view of the fact that Copho and others employed Arab anatomical terms, that eastern drugs were freely prescribed in the medical writings, and that Constantine was

[64] De Renzi, *op. cit.* (5), pp. 527–8.

[65] Matheus Silvaticus, *Pandectae medicinae*. Lugduni, H. à Porta, 1541, cap. cxv, fo. xlix.

[66] *Decameron*, fourth day, tenth story (*Everyman*, i, 285).

[67] Cf. Lynn Thorndike, *The herbal of Rufinus*, New York, 1946: 'Mandragora—D(ioscorides) herba est cuius cortex vino mixta ad bibendum datur eis quorum corpus propter curam secandum est ut soporeti dolorem non sentiant' (p. 178). Also (of opium, p. 215): 'Macer illius in vino currat decoctio sumpta'. Also: ' . . . gustu amarissimus . . . das bibere cum aqua calida' (p. 214).

[68] De Renzi, *op. cit.* (5), p. 528.

[69] Douglas Guthrie, *A history of medicine*. London, 1945: 'It is now generally accepted that Salernitan medicine bears little or no trace of Arab influence' (p. 103).

a Saracen who translated from the Arabic manuscripts. Bearing in mind also the fact that Saracen women ('Saracenae') are mentioned in Trotula, one may reasonably ask: What is meant by Arabic influence?

Certain guiding principles emerge from a perusal of various Salernitan manuscripts, and for convenience these will be briefly summarized.

In the first place, disease was not considered to be due to Divine chastisement, but was the result of natural causes such as the deficiences of certain humours. This fact constituted a definite break with monastic or votive medicine.

Secondly, references to Sacred Writings are restricted to the Old Testament. Thus Trotula begins with a quotation from Genesis; in *De adventu medici* the practitioner was advised to approach the patient like the Angel that guided Tobias. It is true that this manuscript ends with the valedictory salutation 'vade in pace, Christo duce', but this is an example of common usage. Similarly, in serious illness the visit of a priest was recommended, and this is still usual among Roman Catholics. Complete absence of any invocation to the saints is also remarkable, for such invocations were recommended even as late as the Byzantine authors. For example, Aëtius of Amida (sixth century) advised the following incantation to extract a bone hastily swallowed: 'As Lazarus from the grave and Jonah out of the whale, Blasius, the martyr, servant of God saith: Bone come up or go down!' The invocations to Saint Margaret designed to hasten labour did not appear in Trotula, but are mentioned much later by Rabelais. It can be assumed, therefore, that the Salernitans obtained some of their knowledge from Hebrew sources.

Thirdly, though Galen was not free from astrological fancies and several Moslem authors were great promoters of the art, astrological conceptions do not appear in Salernitan medicine. To-day this absence is praiseworthy, but at the time it may have been due to lack of the knowledge necessary for casting a horoscope. It may, of course, have been due to the teaching of Jewish translators, since it is known that learned Hebrews abhorred astrology, magic and witchcraft—for example, Maimonides (1135–1204).

Fourthly, incantations or magical formulae for staunching blood or hastening delivery in child-birth are not mentioned in Salernitan texts, though they are often noticeable in additions to manuscripts in a later script. It is true that Salernitans recommended substances, like the heart of a stork for epilepsy, whose therapeutic action seems to us to be nil; but in the state of knowledge at the time they may well have been held to be effective, without being magical.

Thus the *Magistri Salernitani* by their example and writings introduced from the East a system of professional medical practice and education that has evolved and been continued to the present day, spreading progressively to all parts of the civilized world.

Though the claim that Salerno represented the first university in western Europe is not easily established, yet it can be said that the writings of the Salernitan Masters did make an approach to the study of medicine on the basis of a knowledge of the ancient classical authors. It thus heralded the advent of Scholasticism, which though it was superseded by the New Philosophy propounded by Vesalius, Galileo, William Gilbert and Harvey, yet in its time represented a necessary stage in the progress of Science.

NOTES ON THE ILLUSTRATIONS

FIG. 1.   *Trotula manuscript (Camb., Gon. & Caius MS. 117/186, fo. 239ʳ).* Early fourteenth century.   This is probably the earliest Trotula manuscript in existence.

'Cum auctor universitatis Deus in prima origine mundi rerum naturas singulas juxta humanum genus distingueret conservavit sibi dignitatem super aliorum animalium conditionem, scilicet rationis et intellectus libertatem quia eius perpetuam volens sustinere generationem . . . [l. 21] Quoniam ergo mulieres viris debiliores sunt natura et quia in partu sepissime molestantur hinc est quare in eis sepius habundant egritudines et maxime circa membra operi nature debita et ipse conditionem sue fragilitatis propter verecundiam et ruborem faciei egritudinum suarum que in secretiori loco accidunt, medico angustias revelare non audent.   Earum igitur miseranda calamitas et maxime cujusdam mulieres gracia animum meum sollicitans impulit ut circa aegritudines earum evidencius explanare sanitates ex libris.'

[When God, the creator of the Universe, in the first beginning of the world distinguished the individual natures of things according to the human race, he granted it a dignity superior to the condition of other animals, that is, freedom of reasoning and intellect.   Desiring to continue their generation perpetually . . .   Since therefore women are by their nature weaker in their powers, and because they are frequently injured in child-birth, it follows that they suffer more often from sicknesses and especially in their limbs owing to the effect of nature; because of the same frailness they do not dare to reveal to a physician, for shame and blushing, their maladies in secret parts.   Therefore, their miserable condition, and especially for the sake of these women, has induced me to explain more clearly from books the [rules of] good health.]

FIG. 2.   *Brit. Mus., Sloane MS. 3468, fo. 22ᵛ.*   Ending of the *Flos medicinae.*

'Explicit tractatus qui dicitur flos medicine compilatus a magistro Johanne de mediolano in studio Salerni: Amen.'

[Here ends the treatise called the *Flos medicinae* compiled by *Magister* John of Milan in the *studium* of Salerno.   Amen.]

This is the only known reference to John of Milan, who seems to have been a Salernitan, unless the above statement is a fabrication.   This manuscript dates from the fifteenth century, but in the original form the verses are probably much earlier. The remainder of the page is the beginning of another, irrelevant, treatise.

FIG. 3.   *Trotula manuscript (Camb., St. John's Coll. F 18).*

At the end the scribe wrote:

'Explicit liber factus a muliere salernitana q̄ trotula vocatur.'

[Here ends the book made by a Salernitan woman who (? which) is called Trotula.]

It is unfortunate that the 'q' is not completed, since it is not clear whether it refers to the authoress or the book.

A LA RECHERCHE DE MARGUERITE D'YORK

par

J. J. TRICOT-ROYER

« LE nom de Marguerite, *La Grande Madame*, doit surtout nous rappeler à nous Belges, celle qui, fixant sa résidence à Malines, ne s'y fit connaître que par ses bienfaits. . . . C'est ici que la veuve du Téméraire a coulé les longues et pénibles années de son veuvage; c'est également ici qu'elle se choisit sa dernière demeure dans l'église des Récollets, dévastée et transformée en magasin de fourrages. Et nul ne songe aujourd'hui à visiter ou à retrouver sa sépulture sous le foin et la paille, le jour où dans la Métropole déserte on célèbre encore son anniversaire.» Ce sont quelques fragments d'une requête adressée au Conseil communal de Malines en 1892. Cette requête, et plusieurs autres dans la suite, dont la nôtre, demeurèrent sans résultat.

Or, le 7 septembre 1936, nous fûmes assez surpris d'apprendre qu'un archéologue malinois avait reçu l'autorisation de fouiller, et les moyens de le faire, dans l'église des Récollets, à la recherche de Marguerite d'York, troisième femme du duc Charles de Bourgogne, dit le Téméraire. Le 10 octobre suivant nous fûmes agréablement surpris de recevoir, des autorités communales, la mission d'étudier les ossements trouvés, *aux fins d'établir avec plus ou moins de certitude leur identité.* J'acceptai et demandai alors que me fût adjoint mon collaborateur ordinaire, le Dr. Sondervorst, auquel fut adjoint le Dr. Van Doorslaer de Malines.

Les travaux entrepris dans l'axe du sanctuaire avaient abouti à la mise au jour d'un caveau double contenant dans l'un de ses compartiments des ossements appartenant à trois personnages. Après nombre de séances, les os sont rigoureusement discriminés et les charpentes des squelettes sont rajustées aussi parfaitement que possible. En conclusion nous enregistrons le résultat suivant, qui constituera le fond de notre rapport :

Le squelette A serait celui d'un homme adulte de la taille de 1m. 64.

Le squelette B de sexe indéterminé, âgé d'au moins 50 ans, de la taille de 1m. 57.

Le squelette C pouvait être celui d'une femme de 50 à 60 ans, de la taille de 1m. 54.

La grêle élégance de l'ossature, les faibles reliefs des attaches musculaires, la largeur de l'échancrure ischiatique, et l'absence de dents de sagesse permettent cette hypothèse. Par contre, l'épaisseur des os crâniens, à moins d'être pathologique, plaiderait pour le sexe masculin. Cependant, constatation singulière, chez les trois personnages les os longs accusent une longueur plus grande à gauche qu'à droite, ce qui fait penser à un caractère de famille.

Enfin, notre entourage attachait grande importance à certaines particularités anatomiques propres à la famille des Plantagenets d'où est issue Marguerite. Or, les seuls termes de comparaison dont on dispose de ce point de vue se bornent aux enfants d'Edouard IV, roi d'Angleterre, frère de la duchesse, et dont, naguère l'identification fut établie par les savants Lawrence Tanner et William Wright, lors du transfert des malheureux princes de la Tour de Londres à Westminster. M. le Professeur Charles Singer voulut bien nous mettre en rapport avec les savants anglais, dont l'examen se borna à déterminer l'âge

PLATE VII

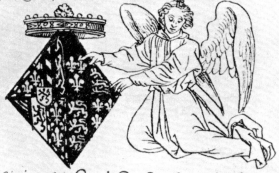

des enfants. Ils ont cependant attiré notre attention sur la présence, chez eux, d'os wormiens dans l'articulation occipito-pariétale. Ce signe, auxquels ils attachaient de l'importance, ne put être décelé dans le cas présent. Quant au roi Edouard IV, exhumé au siècle dernier de dessous le dallage d'une église anglicane, il ne fit l'objet d'aucune description morphologique.

La duchesse avait elle-même désigné l'endroit exact de sa sépulture comme il appert de son épitaphe. Nous en donnons la plus ancienne copie à nous connue. L'auteur est un savant épris d'art et d'archéologie qui a consigné ses observations en un manuscrit richement enluminé, propriété de la Bibliothèque Nationale à Paris. Les monuments mentionnés, encore existants de nos jours, nous sont garants de la rigueur de ses descriptions. La date du manuscrit doit se situer entre 1550 et 1560, donc presque immédiatement avant les troubles destructeurs. Nous avons fait prendre une photographie de la page qui nous intéresse (Fig. 1). Entrant donc aux Cordeliers voici ce que note le curieux visiteur:—

> Sur l'huis du cœur en une arcure est haulte et puissante dame Madame marguerit de Yorck sœur d'Edouard . . . . . . du nom Roy dangleterre femme iiie de Charles duc de bourgôgne, laquelle est à genoux présentée par saincte marguerite. Et de l'aultre costé du dit huys Icelle dame couche morte sur une natte enveloppée dung suaire, une couronne sur son chief avec trois cordelliers l'administrans. Le tout faict d'allebastre, et y a ung ange, tenans ses armes en Lozenge. Lepitaphe en lame de cuyvre est tel.

> Sub limine ostii hujus chori Illustrissima et Serenissima d̄n̄ā margareta de Anglia ducissa burgundie pia humilitate corpus suum condi mandavit serenissimorum principum Edouardi et Ricardi regum anglie soror, Uxor quondam Inclyte memorie Carolj ducis burgundie et Brabantiae et Comitis flandrie Arthesie etc domini mechlinie etc Juris, Religionis, Reformationis, pietatis, mire fautrix mechlinie oppido suo dotalico novembris die vicesima tertia anno domini millesimo quingentesimo tertio. Orate pro ea.

Nous croyons bien que c'est la seule relation directe d'un témoin oculaire qui nous soit parvenue.

Nous comprenons donc qu'il existe deux groupes d'albâtre: l'un sur le portique du chœur, face à la grande nef, le second de l'autre côté du portique, face au Maître-Autel. La duchesse a recommandé de placer son corps *sub limine ostii hujus chori*. Il est naturel qu'elle occupe la profondeur du vestibule entre les deux sculptures, placées l'une à la tête (nef), l'autre à ses pieds (chœur). Quant à la lame de cuivre portant l'épitaphe, nul ne peut dire si elle recouvrait directement la tombe, encastrée dans le pavement, ou si elle fut simplement appliquée à l'une des parois du porche. On peut même supposer dans ce cas qu'elle avait en vis-à-vis les armoiries en losange soutenues par l'ange qui figure au centre de la page du manuscrit. Ce texte porte bien *sub limine* (sous le seuil), tandis que la plupart des auteurs postérieurs disent *sub lamina* (sous la lame), qui nous séduit beaucoup moins. Mais tous sont d'accord pour situer sous le jubé l'endroit précis de la sépulture dont il ne reste plus rien à leur époque.

Quelle fut donc la destinée des monuments et tombeaux de la Duchesse? Le tout périt soit au mois d'août 1566 lors des exploits des iconoclastes malinois, soit le 2 octobre 1572 quand les Espagnols livrèrent la ville au pillage; soit enfin le 9 avril 1580 et jours suivants quand la ville fut victime du saccage dit 'Engelsche furie', dont les auteurs transportèrent en Angleterre des bateaux chargés de monuments ou de simples pierres funéraires. Plusieurs chroniqueurs relatant les faits en furent les témoins, ou tout au moins les contemporains. Une phrase d'un document copié, je ne sais où, par M. le Chanoine van Caster dit notamment: *Sed reliquias affoderunt et disperserunt Geusii.* Sanderus, dont la première édition est de 1659, alors que survivent encore nombre de témoins oculaires, écrit:

Defunctorum autem corporum reliquias per diserta loca spargentes, a suis sepulchris, in quibus per longa tempora tumulata jacuerant, fundibus eruerunt; ita ut illustr. D. Margaritae Caroli Audacis Ducis Burgundiae uxoris nec aliorum insignium Personarum, quas hic sepultas fuisse, ante retulimus, reliquiarum aut monumentorum ullum vestigium appareat.

Il se comprend que notre rapport désola le Conseil communal de la ville, mais devant l'intérêt incontestable du grand nombre de tombes mises à jour, il fut décidé de continuer les fouilles. Il me fut alors dit: «C'est à vous et à votre rapport que nous devons notre succès.» Notre mission nous parut donc élargie et nous résolûmes dès lors d'étudier le problème *ab ovo*. Nous ne tardâmes pas à constater que les fouilles étaient basées sur un mauvais départ. Les deux cercles archéologiques rivaux de Malines croyaient que l'église du treizième siècle, complètement détruite (rasée?) au seizième siècle, avait été rebâtie sur les fondations anciennes. Or la largeur primitive fut portée de 10 mètres à 25 mètres, d'où il résulte que l'axe de l'ancien sanctuaire doit être reporté vers le sud à une ligne correspondant à peu près à l'alignement des colonnes du côté épître. Il en résulte que toutes les tombes mises à vue jusqu'à ce jour sont postérieures à 1610. Nous mîmes au courant les édiles malinois, et j'écrivis à M. le Professeur Armstrong qui s'intéressait aux fouilles, lui faisant part de mes doutes décevants sur la possibilité de découvrir quoi que ce fût du tombeau de Marguerite.

Sans perdre courage cependant l'on se remit à creuser dans le nouvel axe. Or le 16 octobre 1937, à 19 heures, la radio de Bruxelles annonçait *urbi et orbi* le grand succès des fouilles de Malines: on venait de découvrir, l'après-midi même, le squelette de Marguerite d'York, et plus avant, vers l'autel, comme il convenait, celui de Florent Berthout de Malines, un géant de plus de deux mètres! Le lendemain 17 la commission se réunissait au complet sur les lieux mêmes, et, effectivement, entre les fondations des deux premières colonnes, en une tombe assez vaste et bien construite, gisait un squelette de femme en position anatomique parfaite, et dont l'élégance du geste des bras croisés sur le torse était preuve que jamais il n'avait subi de heurt intentionnel direct.

Malgré le précision des textes relatifs à la profanation des sépultures dont nous en avons cité quelques-uns, il y avait là de quoi troubler le plus sceptique. Je recommandai à mon collaborateur M. Sondervorst de prélever un os long pour l'évaluation de la taille, les os du bassin pour la détermination assurée du sexe; les os du crâne, aux fins d'y repérer d'éventuels os wormiens. Je lui avais recommandé en plus de fouiller avec soin la voûte sous-jacente où pouvaient se trouver des menottes, des charnières et des clous du cercueil.

En place de tout cela M. Sondervorst ne fut pas peu surpris de rencontrer un second squelette, masculin celui-ci. C'était sans doute le tombeau d'époux réunis dans la mort, par l'effondrement de deux cercueils superposés.

Dans le voisinage immédiat on mit à découvert quelques tombes identiques et toutes semblables à celles du chœur, d'où nous concluons qu'elles sont toutes de la même époque.

Pour être complet, il convient d'observer que les termes « sur l'huis de cœur », qui sont contemporains, et « Sub oxali ut vocant », qui n'apparaissent que 76 ans après la destruction de l'église, ont donné lieu à une interprétation différente. Certains ont prétendu, alliant les deux textes, que le jubé des Récollets s'ouvrait dans le mur sud, faisant suite aux bâtiments claustraux, et que c'est sous la porte permettant le passage du cloître dans le chœur qu'il fallait rechercher les restes illustres.

Répondons immédiatement que l'auteur du manuscrit de Paris, dont nous reproduisons la page intéressante, décrit les objets tels qu'il les voit en entrant dans l'église, comme les retrouvera le lecteur, et que ce n'est donc pas par la « clôture » qu'il y a pénétré.

Néanmoins on creusa à l'endroit désigné, et on réclama même les lumières d'un sourcier. Un squelette fut trouvé à la profondeur normale, sous l'ancien pavement. Il est, hélas, incontestablement du sexe masculin. Le sourcier avait déclaré qu'on trouverait là des ossements humains (comme partout ailleurs) et inspectant le mur il désigna l'endroit où s'étalait il y a 350 ans une plaque de cuivre !

L'on s'est demandé pourquoi, en 1892, après le vote unanime du Conseil communal en faveur de l'exhumation de Marguerite, il ne fut plus question de ce projet. Un archéologue avisé n'en aurait-il pas démontré l'inanité ?

BAHA'-UL-DOULEH AND THE QUINTESSENCE OF EXPERIENCE

by

CYRIL ELGOOD

IT is generally held that Arabian Medicine in the lands of the Eastern Caliphate (by which is meant Greek Medicine through Arab spectacles, as Sarton so well puts it) is no longer worthy of study after Arabic ceased to be the scientific language of all Islam, and after the last Caliph had been trampled to death by the Mongols. It is true that all 'Iraq drops out of the story. But even in the Golden Age the Persians had played a prominent part in the scientific life of Baghdad. With its fall they, and they alone, were in a position to carry on the traditions of the great clinicians of the Baghdad School of Medicine. To say, therefore, that Arabian Medicine is not worthy of study after the middle of the thirteenth century is to condemn as profitless the study of all the scientific work of medieval Persia. This is an overbold statement. A Nation and an Age which produced Hafiz and Sa'di among the poets, which produced the miniatures of Behzad and the carpets from the royal looms of Shah 'Abbas the Great, such a Nation and Age was not likely to be deficient in great men in the sister Art of Medicine. The tradition of Firdausi was preserved in the writings of Hafiz: the tradition of Rhazes in the work of Baha'-ul-Douleh.

That Baha'-ul-Douleh is quite unknown to Europe may be ascribed to two factors. In the first place, the few orientalists who were also doctors and capable of appreciating medical literature have all been Arabic scholars and not Persian. One thinks of Professor E. G. Browne as the great exception. He was a professor of Persian and Arabic and also a Fellow of the Royal College of Physicians. But I doubt if he ever read a Persian medical manuscript written after the fall of Baghdad. One thinks of Dr. Max Meyerhof. But his interests were entirely Syrian and Egyptian. Even Germans, like Wüstenfeld, have dealt exclusively with Arabic-writing Persians. It is sufficient to read through the excellent bibliography which Fonahn has added to his *Quellenkunde*[1] to realize the truth of this statement.

In the second place, manuscripts of Baha'-ul-Douleh's work are rare. I know of three only: one in the India Office (No. 2955), one in the Bibliothèque Nationale, Paris (No. Suppl. 1161), and one in my private possession. This last was transcribed in the year 1052 A.H. (i.e., A.D. 1642) and finished on a Tuesday, being the twelfth day of the month of Zi-ul-Q'adat, by a writer whose name has been erased. This erasion is a common feature of Persian manuscripts and signifies, I think, that the manuscript was at some time stolen and the writer's name erased to prevent identification. This copy of mine consists of 355 folios, each containing twenty-two lines of a rather small but well written text. The part of the page occupied by text measures 4¾ in. by 7½ in. There are no illustrations. The beginning of each new paragraph is marked by a red line over the first word; the beginning of a new subject by the initial word being in red ink.

---

[1] Adolf Fonahn, *Zur Quellenkunde der Persischen Medizin*. Leipzig, 1910.

A short couplet completes the book:

> *Har keh khwanad dua tam' daram*
> *Zankeh man banda gunahkaram*
> *Een navishtam ta bamanad yadigar*
> *Man namanam khat bamanad rozagar,*

which I translate

> O Reader, a prayer I desire
> Lest I pay for my sins in Hell-fire
> I make my memorial this my endeavour,
> I live not, but my words will live on for ever.

There must be other copies of Baha'-ul-Douleh's work in smaller and private libraries to which I have not had access, as his work was popular both in Persia and in India. That great compendium of medical opinion, the Iksir-i-'Azam (lithographed at Lucknow in 1289 A.H., i.e., A.D. 1872) quotes him several times. 'Ali Afzal Qati' of Qazvin, a physician of the late Safavid period, writing to his brother who has just started medicine, recommends to him for his study only two Persian medical writers—al-Jurjani (*floruit* eleventh century) and Baha'-ul-Douleh. Finally, the *Quintessence* was lithographed in Teheran in A.D. 1866.

I can hardly believe that Baha'-ul-Douleh wrote nothing except the *Quintessence*. Most writers of those days were prolific. Yet I have found no reference to any other work of his. It must be remembered that the book which forms the subject of this essay is known under two titles. Some call it *Khulasat-ul-Tajarib* or *Quintessence of Experience*: others refer to it as the *Khulasat-ul-Hikmat* or *Quintessence of Wisdom*. These are one and the same work.

Of the author extremely little is known. His full name is Muhammad Husayni Nurbakhshi Baha'-ul-Douleh. His father was named Mir Qawam-ul-Din and was a citizen of Ray, a town close to the modern Teheran and the birthplace of the great Rhazes and the theologian Fakhr-ul-Din. I am inclined to think that he was a doctor, both because it was extremely common in those days for a son to follow his father's footsteps, and also because there is found in the text of the *Quintessence* an unnamed person, whose doings and sayings Baha'-ul-Douleh frequently quotes with an intimate knowledge and reverence which suggests more than the relationship between teacher and pupil. In any event his brother was also a doctor, for he mentions him by name, calling him Shah Shams-ul-Din, and recounting his successful cure of an impotent man, who was enabled through his treatment to take two wives and have a son by each. Baha'-ul-Douleh himself was also a married man and had several children. He says that he experimented on them with the various methods of curing otorrhoea.

Baha'-ul-Douleh was born about the middle of the fifteenth century. I know of no evidence to give a more accurate date. Persia was then under the rule of Shah Rukh who had made Herat his capital. He made his medical studies in Ray and later in Herat under Persian and Indian teachers. At first he worked in the household of Sultan Husayn Mirza, the Prince-Governor of Herat; and, doubtless, it was on the death of that prince that

I   P

he returned to Ray and soon became the leading physician of that city. Here he very nearly died of an attack of dysentery, and here in the year A.D. 1501 he composed the only book that he is known to have written. Hajji Kjalifa says that he died in Ray in 1507. He must have been the last great man which that city produced. For even in his lifetime the city was decaying, and very soon after his death it was completely abandoned and left in ruins.

The *Quintessence of Experience* is exactly what the title implies. It is the quintessence of a life of clinical experience, a summary of the observations of a man trained in that wide School of Medicine which only Islam could produce. His quotations show the breadth of his reading. The name of Hippocrates appears twelve times, of Galen thirty-seven times, of Avicenna twenty-seven times, and of Rhazes ten times. Besides these, he quotes Sabit ibn Qurra, Sayyid Isma'il al-Jurjani, Ibn ul-Baytar, and many Indians and others of lesser repute.

Baha'-ul-Douleh himself must have been a keen observer. Scattered through his work are observations which a physician of to-day can neither accept nor deny. They have not been noted. Thus, Baha'-ul-Douleh asserts that stammerers never become bald, that a black and lustreless pupil in a state of health signifies a short life, that as long as a splenomegalic complains of pain in the left side there is hope of a cure, that a fruit-eater is very prone to catarrh, and that the appearance of pigmentary patches on the face or body of an epileptic heralds the cessation of the fits.

In addition to minor aphorisms which are scattered throughout his book, there are several original contributions to the clinical study of disease. He was the first to record (as far as I know) the spontaneous cure of cutaneous leishmaniasis after twelve months of ulceration.[2]

Earlier in this same chapter he describes three varieties of rash which I have found in no other treatise on medicine. I have given a full translation for what it is worth.

'Know then that chicken-pox (*humayqa*) is a condition mid-way between measles (*husba*) and smallpox (*jidri*). For the signs and symptoms of this disease are like the signs and symptoms of those diseases, but in all respects it is less dangerous.[3]

'Now there are three other kinds of eruptions which I have seen in this country whose signs and symptoms also resemble measles and smallpox in more than their appearance. The first is known as *Tayghak* (or the Little Sword) from its resemblance to a thorn. This is a small eruption with a sharp point, like a soft thorn. It is raised above the skin so as to be appreciable when stroked. The colour of the eruption is a little redder than normal skin. It is slightly irritating. There is no fluid, no increase in size, and no tendency to form crusts. It will of itself disappear.

'The second kind of eruption is called *Khashkhāshak* (or the Little Poppy), again on account of the resemblance. This is a small white eruption like a poppy-seed, raised a little above the level of the skin. There is no fluid, no irritation, and no crust formation. It tends of itself to disappear.

---

[2] Baha'-ul-Douleh, *Quintessence*, Elgood MS. (abbrev. 'Q' in following notes), ch. 7, f. 146 *a*.
[3] This is Avicenna's wording. See *Canon*, iv. 3. 1.

'The third kind is called *Mardārayk* (or the Little Pearl), again from the resemblance. The rash consists of discrete pimples similar to pearls. They are very small and raised above the skin . . . [I make no sense of the next ten words] . . . There is no itch, no vesicle formation, though they are brighter than the vesicles of well developed smallpox, no crust formation, and no increase in size.

'All these three rashes are relatively benign and come to an end sometimes soon, sometimes late.'[4]

In his terminal paragraph to the chapter on diseases of the eye, he is undoubtedly describing what is now popularly called hay fever, which was not recognized in Europe until 1819.

'I have seen many persons whose brains have become heated in the spring by the smell of red roses. They get a catarrh and a running of the nose. They also had an irritation of the eye-lids, which when this season passed subsided together with the catarrh and the nasal discharge. These people benefitted very little by treatment.'[5]

In this connexion it is only just to point out, even at the cost of diminishing Baha'-ul-Douleh's fame, that this description is probably not original. The fact is not mentioned in the *Quintessence*, but we know from Ibn abi Usaybi'a that Rhazes wrote a monograph (now lost) which he called *A Dissertation on the Cause of Coryza which occurs in the Spring when the Roses give forth their Scent*. The verbal resemblance is so close that it is almost impossible that Baha'-ul-Douleh should have made an altogether independent observation of this particular form of allergy.[6]

His description of an epidemic cough, however, which occurred at Herat while he was there, can be nothing else but the earliest account of whooping cough. This disease was not recognized in Europe until the end of the sixteenth century, and was not described until Willis wrote his monograph in 1658.

'Coughs and such diseases as arise from excess of damp air, sometimes also arise from infected air on account of the aversion of the spirit and the lungs to inhale infected air. I have several times proved this. Twice while I was at Herat, there was a mild infection of the air, which caused a universal cough without catarrh. The cough became so severe that it did not cease until vomiting occurred. Patients grew weak: children lost consciousness. Many people, old and young, fainted from the violence of the cough, and in some cases during the first epidemic even died. At last an Indian physician ordered people to eat every day a few ounces of raw ginger dissolved in warm water. The second epidemic occurred in the spring and there were fewer fatal cases. The treatment was venesection, laxatives, feeding with powdered ginger, and so forth. I and all my household caught the cough, but by these methods of treatment it subsided in a couple of months. But it did not completely disappear until we had made a change of air.'[7]

His description of syphilis is the earliest known account of the disease to be written outside Europe. That others had already written on the subject

---

[4] *Q.*, ch. 7, f. 126 *a*.   [5] *Q.*, ch. 9, f. 394 *b*.
[6] Ibn abi Usaybi'a, *'Uyūn al-Anbā*, 'Classes of Physicians'. Ed. A. Müller, 2 vols. Königsberg, 1884, vol. i, p. 319.
[7] *Q.*, ch. 13, f. 215 *a*.

we know from the preliminary remarks to the monograph on syphilis which
'Imad-ul-Din wrote some fifty years later.[8] In the *Quintessence* Baha'-ul-Douleh
devotes four pages to this disease,[9] about one-third of this being concerned
with the source of infection, the signs, and the symptoms, and the remaining
two-thirds being concerned with treatment.

A little earlier in the same chapter he describes its introduction into
Persia. 'The Armenian sore arose in Europe. From there it spread to
Constantinople and Arabia. In the year 1498 it appeared in Azerbaijan.
Then it spread to 'Iraq, Persia, and so on. Many people both here and there
caught it and are still catching it.'[10]

The symptoms, he says, are similar to those of smallpox. Hence it is also
known as Abileh-i-Farang or European pox. As it is associated with a burning
sensation, others know it as *Atishak* or the Little Fire, through a confusion
with anthrax or *Ignis Persicus*. Besides the rash the patient may complain
of sore throat. 'I saw a woman once who complained of a sore throat for
some time and suddenly came out in the rash of the European pox.'[11] Or
nervous symptoms may predominate. 'Sometimes the pain is so great
that the patient wishes that he were dead: sometimes he falls to the ground.
I once saw a woman who had lost the use of her feet for a period, just as though
she were paralysed.'[12]

Treatment consists in cleansing the body by suitable purges, by venesection
and appropriate food. The usual polypharmacy is to be employed. Various
ointments are advocated. At the very end of the section he makes this
cryptic remark: 'In short by these methods equilibrium and health are
restored until the time of perfect coction. Then the salve known as The
European Pox Medicine can be used as prescribed until perfect health is
restored. This is the most potent method of treatment.'[13] He does not say
what this salve contained. A few lines later he speaks of giving an electuary
of mercury. The constituents of this electuary (which he says is his own
invention) he gives in the terminal chapter of the *Quintessence*.[14] Later in
the same chapter he gives two more prescriptions which contain mercury
'being the compositions of European doctors.'[15] I think, therefore, that his
use of mercury was not chance, but frankly borrowed from the experience
of Europeans.

Baha'-ul-Douleh was no surgeon. On the contrary, he recommends all
physicians to hand over their surgical cases to a Master Surgeon. His
digressions into surgery show that surgical technique was very highly
developed and that the range of operative interference was very wide. Over
and over again he stresses that the patient must be given an anaesthetic
before the operation. 'Do not fail to understand', he writes, 'that every
treatment which involves severe pain or discomfort requires first the
administration of a strong drug to the Faculties. After this has taken effect,
begin the operation. Otherwise fear may set up another disease.'[16]

The word here used is *Mukhadir*. This means 'intoxicant' or 'drug',

[8] See my translation entitled 'A Persian Monograph on Syphilis'. *Ann. Med. Hist.*, 1931,
n.s. iii, 465–86.
[9] *Q.*, ch. 7, ff. 131 *b*–133 *a*.   [10] *Q.*, ch. 7, f. 126 *b*.   [11] *Q.*, f. 132 *a*.
[12] *Q.*, f. 131 *b*.   [13] *Q.*, f. 132 *b*.   [14] *Q.*, ch. 28, f. 349 *a*.
[15] *Q.*, f. 352 *a*.   [16] *Q.*, ch. 7, f. 144 *a*.

and is the word that Avicenna uses.[17] Examples of such drugs are mandragora, hemlock and best of all opium.

Baha'-ul-Douleh also uses the word *behush kardan*,[18] which simply means 'to render unconscious'. In another instance he speaks of a Habb-ul-Shifa' or Healing Pill which can be used as an anaesthetic. This pill contains ginger, rhubarb, and datura.[19] This pill was not always taken by the mouth, but occasionally powdered and snuffed up the nose. It was therefore a vague groping towards inhalation anaesthesia.

Historians of surgery will be surprised to learn that he describes a case of laparotomy with drainage for a peritoneal abscess,[20] and suprapubic cystotomy for removal of vesical calculi and retention of urine. He was not unaware of the difficulty of getting the wound to close in this last case, but, as he shrewdly remarks, 'it is better to live with it open than die with it closed.'[21] Even more remarkable is his statement that the usual treatment of cancer was an extensive amputation, but that in his opinion no treatment was of any use, excepting the application of a theriacum of aqua fortis in which lead had been dissolved.[22]

His story of a successful skin-graft is worth translating. 'A certain patient suffered from a severe impetigo (*s'afa*) which involved the whole head. No treatment was of any use. So a Master Surgeon named 'Ala-ul-Din, an Indian who lived at Ray, gave him an anaesthetic and excised the whole of the skin of the scalp and replaced it by the fresh skin of a dog. He stitched the wound up tight, rubbed in salves and creams at the edges, and then applied a poultice. He gave the food proper to a surgical case. After a while the flesh united. This case was published in the court of Sultan Husayn ibn Bayqara,[23] and truly it is a marvel.'[24]

Throughout each chapter stories of patients, his own or his father's, are scattered to illustrate his points. Their clarity and accuracy resemble the clinical accounts in the *Continens* of Rhazes: their vividness makes the book far more readable than the *Canon* of Avicenna. An occasional humorous story makes the book interesting even to the non-medical reader. For example, he recounts the unexpected cure of a hernia (or more probably of a hydrocœle, the Persian word is indefinite) in an elderly merchant. A certain unfortunate man, he says, had a rupture as big as a melon. To contain it he had made a special bag which he rested upon his saddle-bow when riding to and from the city. One day he met on the road a rascally Turcoman, who demanded to know what the bag contained. He naturally refused to believe what he was told and thought that the merchant was trying to deceive him. He raised his staff to attack and rob him. The poor man, dodging the blow aimed at his head, received the full force of the staff on the rupture. He fell from his horse unconscious and the Turcoman made off. A surgeon was hurriedly called and stitched up the scrotal wound. The wound healed perfectly, and the man found to his joy that he was completely cured of his tumour.

---

[17] Avicenna, *Canon*, i. 4. 30.   [18] e.g., *Q.*, ch. 7, f. 129 *a*.   [19] *Q.*, ch. 27, f. 347 *a*.
[20] *Q.*, ch. 17, f. 249 *a*.   [21] *Q.*, ch. 22, f. 288 *b*.   [22] *Q.*, ch. 7, f. 139 *b*.
[23] For a discussion on the court of ibn Bayqara, see E. G. Browne, *A literary history of Persia.* London, 1902–20, vol. iv, p. 63, etc.
[24] *Q.*, 7, f. 129 *a*.

The era of Baha'-ul-Douleh was the last of Persian isolation. It also coincided with the last of the great medieval shahs. With Tahmasp on the throne, who succeeding as a boy of ten reigned for fifty-two years and died in 1576, the period of European penetration into Persia may be said to have begun. Papal envoys indeed had found their way into the interior many years before. But now came missions with less exalted ideals. The Doge of Venice sent military proposals for an alliance against the Turks. Queen Elizabeth of England sent her merchants to seek new trade routes and fresh markets. The arrival of the East India Company, with its own physicians and novel medical ideas, meant the final overthrow of the school of thought in which Baha'-ul-Douleh learned and taught.

To what extent the writing of Baha'-ul-Douleh contributed to the keeping alive of Avicennan Medicine after its contact with the new Harveian School it is extremely difficult to say. The writers with whom I am acquainted who wrote after the publication of the *Quintessence* very rarely (as is usual) quote any authority for their statements. Conservatism and respect for authority was no less strong in the sixteenth and seventeenth centuries than it had been in the thirteenth and fourteenth. Thus, as is to be expected, Baha'-ul-Douleh's contributions made very little impression on his successors. The standard, too, of his writing is so uneven. His sparkling contributions of true medicine are so buried among frank magic, that he cannot justly be said to have done very much to hinder that decline into astrology and gross superstition into which doctors of the succeeding period fell. His importance in the story lies not so much in his influence on succeeding generations as in his almost unique position as a clinician, in a century which produced great pharmacists, encyclopaedists, and collectors of the sayings of others. I set him forth not as a link in a chain, but as the singer of the swan-song of Persian Medicine.[25]

[25] Since this essay was written I have presented my MS. of the *Quintessence* to the library of the Royal College of Physicians.

JOHANNES HARTLIEB'S GYNAECOLOGICAL COLLECTION AND THE JOHNS HOPKINS MANUSCRIPT 3 (38066)

by

HENRY E. SIGERIST

THE Library of the Johns Hopkins University possesses very few medieval manuscripts,[1] but among them is a fifteenth century German medical manuscript which is interesting and important in many respects. It contains several gynaecological treatises, translated and adapted from the Latin into German by Dr. Johannes Hartlieb between 1460 and 1465. Six other manuscripts of the same texts are known,[2] but the collection has not been published so far nor has it been examined adequately.

There can be no doubt that a critical edition would be very desirable from the linguistic point of view as well as for the content of the texts. Since the Johns Hopkins manuscript is a very good one, it will have to be consulted when an edition is prepared and, as the manuscript seems to be practically unknown, I wish to give a brief analysis of it, discussing at the same time some of the problems involved.

I. Dr. Johannes Hartlieb, an Early German Humanist

Johannes Hartlieb[3] was more a courtier than a physician. His entire life was spent in the service of several ruling houses, and of his many books—translations and adaptations from the Latin—only two dealt with medical subjects. He was born in the beginning of the fifteenth century of parents who were probably servants of Lewis VII, Duke of Bavaria-Ingolstadt. At the instigation of Lewis, he wrote at Neuburg in 1430 his first book, *Kunst der gedächtnüsz*, a treatise on mnemonics.

Soon thereafter he went to the University of Vienna, where Lewis supported him by providing for him the revenues of an Ingolstadt parish. In 1433 he graduated as bachelor, then became a magister and later a doctor of medicine. In 1434 he wrote an astrological treatise, *Über die Erhaltung des Sieges*. Having gained access to the court of Albert VI, of Habsburg, he translated for his new patron the *Tractatus amoris* of Andreas Capellanus.

From 1440 to 1468, the year of his death, Hartlieb was in the service of the Dukes of Bavaria-Munich. He served them as a courtier, as physician-in-ordinary and occasionally on diplomatic missions. He was particularly close to Albert III, whose daughter, Sibylla, he married. Sibylla was the child of Albert and of the famous Agnes Bernauerin, the beautiful daughter of a barber who, married secretly to Albert in 1432, was tried for witchcraft by Albert's father, Ernest, and was drowned in the Danube in 1435. After

---

[1] Seymour de Ricci, *Census of Medieval and Renaissance Manuscripts in the United States and Canada*. New York, 1935, vol. i, pp. 753–5.

[2] Cgm. 261; Cod. pal. germ. 480, 488; Wolfenb. 69, 8°; Berlin MS. germ. 928; Dresden 314.

[3] The most exhaustive study on Hartlieb is Karl Drescher, 'Johann Hartlieb. Über sein Leben und seine schriftstellerische Tätigkeit'. *Euphorion*, 1924, xxv, 225–41, 354–70, 569–90; 1925, xxvi, 341–67, 481–564. R. Newald's article in Wolfgang Stammler, *Die deutsche Literatur des Mittelalters, Verfasserlexikon*, col. 195–8 is mostly based on Drescher.

the death of Albert III in 1460, Hartlieb was in the service of his son and
successor, Sigismund.

As a writer, Hartlieb was not in any way original. He translated or adapted
from the Latin the kind of books that his noble patrons or their wives or
relatives wished to have, but his translations were written in good taste. In
the beginning he followed the Latin originals rather closely, while he appears
much freer in his later books, omitting dull passages and adding picturesque
details. In his early works he revealed a strong predilection for occult
subjects, but after 1451, when he had come under the influence of Nicolas
Cusanus, he condemned them and became very devoted to the church. This
did not prevent him from translating books that would satisfy the erotic
curiosity of his patrons.

Besides the works already mentioned, Hartlieb wrote versions of the stories
of Alexander and of St. Brandan, adapted the *Dialogus miraculorum* of
Caesarius of Heisterbach, and compiled a *Buch von der hand*, a treatise on
chiromancy that was printed in 1473.[4] He also compiled a *Buch aller
verbotenen kunst* and made a collection of notes on geomancy.

Apart from the gynaecological collection, Hartlieb touched medical subjects
only once, when he translated Felix Hemmerlin's treatise on hot baths.
The translation was never printed but is preserved in the Munich manuscript
(MS. germ. 732) of 1474.

II. *The Gynaecological Collection*

Hartlieb's gynaecological collection is usually referred to as being a
translation of the *Secreta mulierum* of Albertus Magnus with a commentary
by Tortula (!).[5] The text, however, consists of several different books thus
forming a collection of gynaecological treatises, translated and adapted from
the Latin into German.

The books are dedicated to Sigismund, Duke of Bavaria-Munich,
Count-palatine of the Rhine:

> Seytt nun dw aller hochgelobtister furst herrtzog Sigmundt pfaltzgraffe bey
> Rreyenn ecc. in deiner pluenntnn jugenntt inn allem wollust des irdischenn paradeys
> im obernn paierlanndt. . . . [6]

Sigismund succeeded his father in 1460 and Hartlieb died in 1468. This
permits us to conclude that the book was written between 1460 and 1468.
Born in 1439, Sigismund was twenty-one years of age in 1460 and twenty-nine
in 1468. Hartlieb's reference to the 'flourishing youth' of his patron sets
the date of the translation closer to 1460 than to 1468. It is very unlikely
that the book could have been written before 1460. Drescher has already
pointed out[7] that Hartlieb would never have dared to dedicate such a book
to Sigismund as long as the old Duke was still alive.

In 1465 Sigismund had an interview with the Emperor, Frederic III, and
a special copy of Hartlieb's book was made for the Emperor. It is still
preserved (Berlin MS. germ. 928) and is remarkable for the fact that Hartlieb

---

[4] A facsimile edition was published by Ernst Weil in 1923, *Verlag der Münchner Drucke*.
[5] Both Drescher and Newald, *op. cit.* (3), spell 'Tortula'.
[6] The quotations unless otherwise indicated refer to the Hopkins MS.
[7] Drescher, *op. cit.* (3), xxv, 239.

re-wrote his preface dedicating the book to Frederic.[8]   It is very probable that this copy was made as a result of the conversations that Sigismund had with the Emperor, and this would mean that the translation was made before 1465.   We can, therefore, safely date the book as having been written between 1460 and 1465.

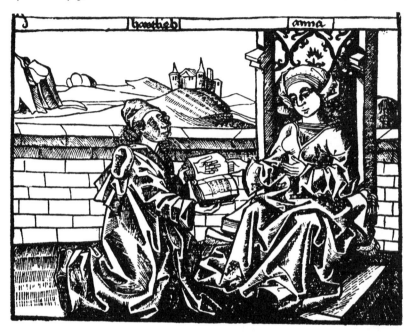

Fig. 1. Hartlieb presenting his book on chiromancy to Anna, wife of Albrecht III of Bavaria. From *Buch von der hand*, Augsburg, 15th century.

Like many members of the Wittelsbach family, Sigismund was weak, sensuous and extravagant.   Throughout his life he dressed in the same colour combination of black, red and white.   A handsome youth, beloved by women, he never married but had illegitimate children, probably many more than were ever recorded.   A contemporary chronicler said of him: 'He felt at home with beautiful women, with white doves, peacocks, guinea pigs, birds and all kinds of strange animals, and also loved string music'.[9]   Hartlieb was close to him in spite of the great difference in age, for Hartlieb's wife was, after all, his step-sister.   Hence it is no wonder that the doctor was his adviser, not only in general medical but also in sexual matters, in all questions concerning *secreta mulierum*.   The repeated exhortations that the information given in the book was only for married people, and should not be misused for licentious purposes, were strangely out of place in a book addressed to a bachelor of Sigismund's character.   They rather emphasized the importance

[8] Drescher published the preface, *Euphorion*, 1925, xxvi, 341 ff.
[9] See *Allgemeine Deutsche Biographie*. Leipzig, 1892, xxxiv, p. 283.

of certain prescriptions, while covering them up with a veil of respectability. The intimacy between the two went so far that they used a secret code for the recording of particularly delicate matters.[10] The reference to Ovid's tragic fate shows that Hartlieb was fully aware of the fact that his book was not so much a medical treatise as rather an *ars amatoria*.

The bulk of the first part consists of a German version of an extremely popular book, *The Secrets of Women*, attributed to Albertus Magnus. The popularity of the book is evidenced by the large number of manuscripts preserved. Thorndike[11] lists twenty-four and Wickersheimer[12] fifty-five manuscripts containing the Latin text. The book was printed in forty-seven editions in the fifteenth century[13] and many times thereafter.[14]

Much has been written about the book and, since it discusses a rather delicate subject, it was thought that it could not have been written by so worthy a Dominican as Albertus Magnus, a very unhistorical consideration. The Middle Ages had a very detached attitude toward matters of sex, and Thorndike has very justly pointed out[15] that a number of similar books were written at that time by lay and ecclesiastical writers. Most of the content of the book can be found in other writings of Albertus Magnus, and if he did not compose it himself, it was probably compiled from his writings by one of his students.

The *Secrets of Women* was translated into vernacular languages, and from 1531 a book appeared in Germany in numerous editions, issued under some such title as *Die Heimlichkeyten Alberti Magni, allen Hebammen und Kindtbaren Frawen dienlich* or *Von den Geheimnissen der Weiber*.[16] The titles, however, are misleading, and Christian Ferckel demonstrated long ago[17] that these German prints are not translations of *De secretis mulierum* and have nothing in common with the Albertinian treatise. They are compilations from various sources, chiefly from the *Rosengarten* of Eucharius Rösslin[18] and from the *Fasciculus medicinae* of John of Ketham.[19] We can, therefore, discard them here entirely.

The Latin treatise *De secretis mulierum* was, however, translated into German, and such a translation is preserved in the fifteenth century Einsiedeln manuscript 297 (pp. 387–440).[20] There is no doubt that there must be

[10] See Drescher, *op. cit.* (3), xxv, 238.

[11] Lynn Thorndike, *A history of magic and experimental science*. New York, vol. ii, 1923, pp. 749–50.

[12] E. Wickersheimer, 'Henri de Saxe et le *De Secretis Mulierum'. Proc. Third Internat. Congr. Hist. Med.* Antwerp, 1923, pp. 253–8.

[13] Klebs 26; *Gesamtkatalog*, 719–66.

[14] L. Choulant, 'Albertus Magnus in seiner Bedeutung für die Naturwissenschaften'. *Janus*, 1846, i, 127–60.

[15] Thorndike, *op. cit.* (11), pp. 742 ff.

[16] The editions are listed in Hugo Hayn, *Bibliotheca Germanorum, gynaecologica et cosmetica*. Leipzig, 1886.

[17] C. Ferckel, *Die Gynaekologie des Thomas von Brabant*. Munich, 1912.

[18] Eucharius Rösslin, *Der swangern Frauwen und Hebammen Rosegarten*. [Strasbourg, 1513.] First edition. A facsimile edition was published by Gustav Klein in Munich, 1810.

[19] See C. Ferckel, 'Zur Gynäkologie und Generationslehre im Fasciculus medicinae des Johannes de Ketham'. *Arch. f. d. Gesch. d. Med.*, 1913, vi, 205–22; also H. E. Sigerist, 'Eine deutsche Übersetzung der Kethamschen Gynäkologie'. *ibid.*, 1923, xiv, 169–78.

[20] H. E. Sigerist, 'Deutsche medizinische Handschriften aus Schweizer Bibliotheken'. *Arch. f. d. Gesch. d. Med.*, 1925, xvii, 237 ff.

PLATE VIII

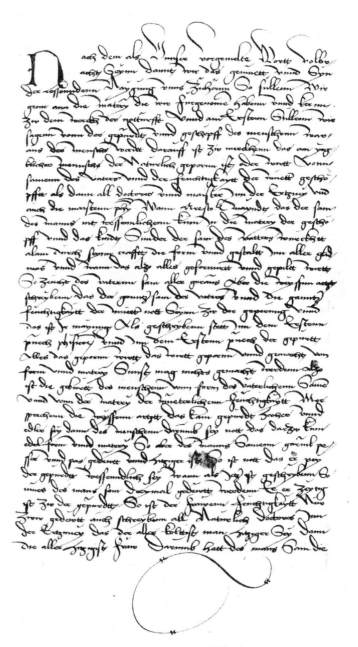

PLATE IX

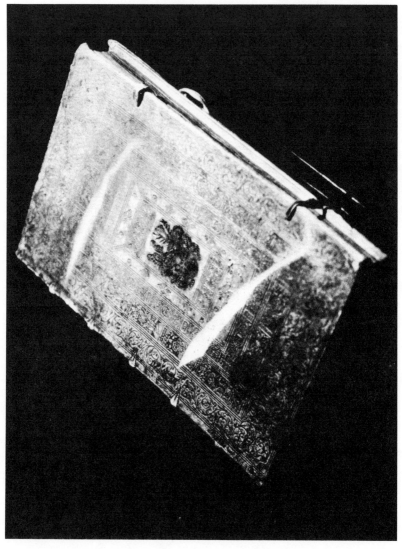

Fig. 3.   The Johns Hopkins Manuscript 3 (38066)

·other manuscripts of it, but I cannot ascertain at the moment whether this translation was ever printed.

Hartlieb's version contains much more than a mere translation.   The fact that the Latin treatise has 13 chapters, the Einsiedeln translation 24 and Hartlieb 70 does not mean much because the division into chapters was very arbitrary.   But Hartlieb himself tells us that his book is a compilation:[21]

fol. 1ʳ: Here begin the chapters of the book Secreta mulierum, Macrobius, Trotula and Mustio, Gilbertus, and many other abstracts from many secret writings of the natural masters, on the nature of women and what is peculiar to them in all matters.   Also how a man shall live and deal with women so that true love and friendship may not be destroyed between married people.

And in the preface Hartlieb tells us more about his sources:[22]

fol. 5ʳ: Item Albertus Magnus has made the book Secreta mulierum and has put into it many matters of nature but not as coherently and clearly as the masters of medicine have said.   (fol. 5ᵛ): For Avicenna has said explicitly of what complexion women are, and how the semen becomes one with their moisture, also about the nourishing, the structure and the whole life of the embryo; also how long it shall lie in the mother's body and how the womb opens up through the will and at the command of the Almighty God.   Then he says how one shall medicate and nourish the child.

Item Mustio, a great master from Greece, also wrote, for the benefit of an emperor called Gamaliel, a book on child-birth and the going out of the embryo. This book teaches and says that child-birth and the going out of the infant occur in eighteen ways, but only two ways are safe and good without aid, the other ways are all deadly or at least cause great worry.   He has also reported and written how such mistakes[23] of nature might be corrected by the instructed midwives, with medicines and skilfull procedures.   Yes, praiseworthy Lord, believe me that there was a great need for this book in German lands.

Also, a very great master in matters of nature called Macrobius, in his book on the interpretation of the dreams of Scipio, has written explicitly on the conception of children and also how woman and man must be skilled so that they make perfect and healthy children; and also what complexions belong together that children result; and more about mistakes when two persons come together who are not of the same nature in respect to children, how one must prepare them that they have children together.   He also says in this connexion that a woman and a man may come together who have not the right love for one another.   He also gives all kinds of advice how this may be changed and overcome by instructed and faithful people.   And he says that such a condition may be recognized from the complexion.   Thereupon he says that there is a book that gives advice and instruction how to create great love and friendship between man and woman through manifold devices (fol. 6ʳ) that are natural and not at all sinful, but that this book has not to be revealed lest it be used for illicit love and licentiousness.   This book was hidden until the time of a king called Egwant[24] who had a very loyal and clever man and doctor called Gilbertinus.   He opened up the book for the benefit of his lord, the king, and the book begins thus:

There is nothing more harmful than anger and enmity between married people

[21] The German text is given later in this essay.

[22] See later for German text.

[23] The German text has *irrung in der natur*.   Drescher, *op. cit.* (3), xxvi, 343, suggests the reading *perung* instead of *irrung*, but I do not see any necessity for changing the text.

[24] The Berlin MS. has *ain Küng in Engcnland der hyesz eguart.*

because great harm results from it.   Hence I will reveal for the sake of married people only the secret book of Macrobius which tells how true love, loyalty and faithfulness may be created between married people.   But if someone wishes to practise and use this art for illicit licentiousness and extra-marital love, I pray that God Almighty in dire wrath may stifle his art and make it ineffective.   Oh, praiseworthy Lord, believe me; should the use of the book be permitted for extra-marital licentiousness, it would have grave results.[25]   And truly all that is said in it has nothing to do with magic but deals with herbs and ointments, roots, griffons, as has been written very clearly in this book.

There is also a book that has been written by a queen by name of Trotula.   This book tells about many secret matters of women, namely, how they may become pregnant and how they shall behave during pregnancy; also how they shall purify themselves in childbed.   The book also tells of all infirmities of women which cause displeasure to men, be they infirmities of the vagina, of the hands, mouth, teeth, or skin.   It gives such great remedies that it seems a real miracle that a woman can acquire so much beauty.   It is certainly true that Galen, Rhazes, and Avicenna have written in their books about cosmetics of women and they called this art Gummeras,[26] but this is all little compared to what Trotula has written and taught.

My most gracious Lord, it is certainly true that Albertus Magnus has written much in his book Secreta mulierum, but he has not touched any of these things nor has he given information about them.   His book is an instruction about legitimate secret matters only.   This is why he concealed such things and did not mention them, and no one should say that he did not know them for he was undoubtedly a very skilful master.   And I think that he left these things out, because he was afraid that these deep secrets and art be misused and be applied and used for illicit love and licentiousness, for he prepared and wrote many books on spiritual subjects, and he prepared and wrote this book when he was old and in his years of decline.

My most gracious and praiseworthy prince and lord, if you should arrange to have only the text of the book Secreta mulierum translated into German, it would be fragmentary and very unintelligible and would bring no benefit to the readers. If, however, the above mentioned books are also included and thoroughly worked in, then I do not think that any book has ever been written in the world that could be more useful and more amusing for all married people . . . .

In the preface to the Berlin manuscript Hartlieb describes his method of compilation in more detail:[27]

wann aber die obgenanntten puecher auch dartzu getragen und geschriben, und ausz iglichem das dan jn igliches capittel gehort, getzogen nach dem besten als ich dan gethon hab, wann iglichs gar öfft gemelt wirt, das doch nit not ist, so offt ze schreyben wann der recht kern und grunt aller jn trottula geschryben ist. . . . .

In other words, Hartlieb added to the various chapters of the *Secrets of Women* corresponding passages from the other sources; not all of these, because this would have caused endless repetitions, but only the most appropriate passages.

There has been a good deal of discussion as to whether Hartlieb compiled his books from various Latin sources, or whether he simply translated Latin compilations from single manuscripts.   The latter was undoubtedly true in

---

[25] The Berlin MS. adds *wan kein weyb so hoch oder so nyder ist, sy mocht durch die kunst verlaydt werden.*

[26] Other MSS. have *summa rasis, gumerasses, gumeras.*

[27] Drescher, *op. cit.* (3), xxvi, 344.

the case of his Alexander Book, as Hans Poppen has demonstrated convincingly,[28] but it is equally true that his *Buch aller verbotenen kunst* was an original compilation,[29] and I think there can be not the slightest doubt that our book was an original compilation also.   We do not know of any similar Latin compilation and, moreover, we have Hartlieb's explicit testimony. There is no reason why we should not take it at its face value.

While the major portion of the book, namely fol. 1[r] to fol. 69[r], is based on the *Secrets of Women*, the second part (fol. 70[r]-110[v]) contains primarily an adaptation of the Salernitan treatise of Trotula.[30]

The third and shortest part, fol. 112[r]-123[r] (fol. 111 is blank) contains excerpts, recipes, quaestiones and responsiones from various sources which will have to be ascertained from case to case.

III. *The Johns Hopkins Manuscript*

In the following I shall give a brief description of the book with excerpts long enough to permit an opinion on its content and quality.

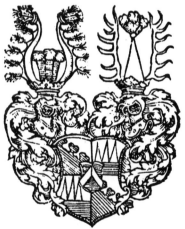

Chriſtophorus Baro à VVolckbenſtain, *& Rodnegg, etc.* M. D. XCIIII.

Fig. 4. Book-plate in the Johns Hopkins MS.

MANUSCRIPT 3 (38066).   Late 15th century.   Paper.   125 leaves, 300 × 195 mm.   One column, 200-215 × 140 mm.   23-27 lines.
Gatherings.   [VI-1] +9 VI +[IV-2].
Signatures.   None.
Script.   See Fig. 2.   Careful late 15th century script.   Chapter headings in red.

[28] H. Poppen, *Das Alexanderbuch Johann Hartliebs und seine Quelle.* Inaug. Diss., Heidelberg, 1914.

[29] J. Hartlieb, *Buch der verbotenen Kunst.* Herausgegeben von Dora Ulm. Halle, 1914.

[30] About Trotula see H. R. Spitzner, *Die salernitanische Gynäkologie und Geburtshilfe unter dem Namen der 'Trotula'.* Diss. Leipzig, 1921; also K. C. Hurd-Mead, 'Trotula'. *Isis,* 1930, xiv, 349-67.

Binding. Ornate Renaissance binding (see Fig. 3), with the coat of arms. of Baron von Wolckenstain und Rodnegg impressed in gold.

History. The manuscript has a book-plate according to which the book was in the 16th century in the collection of Christophorus a Wolckenstain et Rodnegg etc. (see Fig. 4).

Catalogue. Seymour de Ricci, *Census of Medieval and Renaissance Manuscripts.* New York, 1935, vol. i, p. 753.

CONTENT

1. fol. 1ʳ–69ʳ: SECRETA MULIERUM CUM ADDITAMENTIS

[Table of Content]

fol. 1ʳ: Hie hebenn sich ann die Capittel v̈ber das puech Secreta mulierum macrobium Trottula vnnd Mustio Gilbertum vnnd gar vil ander auszug die gezogenn sein aus maniger gehaim der Natürlichenn maister vonn aller Natur der frawenn vnnd was denn frawenn zugehörtt inn allenn dingenn. Auch wie ain man mit frawenn lebenn vnnd thunn sol das Rechte lieb vnnd fründschafft zwischenn Eleutenn nit zerstörtt werdenn mag.

Item zw dem Erstenn gar ain schönne Vorred wie vnnd wem das puech getewtztt sey vnnd wie man die gros gehaim sol verpernngenn vnnd nit offenn unwirdigen personn [5ʳ]

Item das erst Capittel der Textt alberti mangny hatt das puech durch seines gesellenn pett willenn getewtztt [7ʳ]

Item das ander Capittel sagtt wie arestolis vnnd annder physici schreybenn wie vnnd was all gepurtt sein [7ᵛ]

Item das dritt Capittel sagtt wie all thir inn dr specy vnnd gestaltt Ewig sein vnnd nit in irem Leiben vnd personn [7ᵛ]

Item das viert Capittel Sagt wie der menschenn gebertt Edler vnnd höcher sey dann aller thier vnnd geschöpff [8ʳ]

Item das fünfft Capittel sagt Seytt mal Lautter gesagt ist das des menschenn geburtt die aller edlist ist So ist pillich das mann sagtt wie der mensch geschopfftt empfangen vnnd gepornn werde [8ᵛ]

Item das secht Capittel sagtt wie all red vorred sein vnnd vonn vil fragem wie die menschenn werdenn [8ᵛ]

Item das sybennt Capittel sagtt wie vor Troy menschenn vnnd rissenn aus faulen tämpffenn der erd vnnd infliessenn der sterrnn vnnd planetten an vatter vnnd ann muetter vermischung gewachssnn Sein [9ʳ]

Item das acht Capittel sagt wie vonn Sölher vnnd annder Irrung der Natürlichenn maister nit vil zw schreybe sy das (1ᵛ) ainfaldig Lewtt nit dadurch inn Irrung vallenn [9ʳ]

Item das Newtt Capittel hebtt erst recht ann zw sagenn vonn der gepurtt des menschenn [9ᵛ]

Item das zehennt Capittel sagtt wie die geburtt vnnd geschöpff Empfanngen werdt in mueter leyb [10ᵛ]

Item das aidlifft Capittel sagtt wie offtt ain fraw die empfanngenn hatt durch grossenn Lust der mynn die erstenn geschöpff verderbt vnnd wie das zugett [11ʳ]

Item das zwelft Capittel sagtt was die Natur vnnd feuchtigkaytt sey ⟨das⟩ in der myn vonn der frawenn gett vnnd vonn wann die selb feuchtigkaytt kem vnnd wie sy vonn denn frawenn get [11ᵛ]

Item das drayzehenntt Capittel sagtt von vil fragem der frawenn menstrua vnnd wie sy sol kumen vnnd was farb sy sain soll [12ᵛ]

Item das vierzehennt Capittel sagtt vonn wannen denn frawen ir menstrua fliessnn vnd auch vonn welher stat [13ʳ]

Item das fünffzehenntt Capittel sagtt warumb all monad die frawenn denn flus der menstrua habenn vnd wo sy sich sameltt vnnd auch vonn ettlichenn manenn die auch denn pluett flus habenn [13ᵥ]

Item das sechzehenntt Capittel sagt vonn wanne denn frawenn ir Natur kum in der mynn so sy schwanger sein vnnd so die mueter ist beschlossnn [14ᵛ]

Item das sibenzehennt Capittel sagtt warumb die schwanngernn frawenn Nach dem Erstenn monadt der myn vast begernn vnnd mer dann vor vnnd man das an inn merckenn vnnd erkennen soll [15ʳ]

Item das achtzehenntt Capittel sagt wie die gepurtt vnnd geschöpff inn muetter Leyb geformett werdtt [16ʳ]

(2ʳ) Item das Newnzehennt Capittel sagtt Wie all philosophy schreybenn das der menschs vnnd alle ding aus denn vier Elementtnn gemacht werden [17ʳ]

Item das zwantzigist Capittel Sagtt wie der mensch auch die Natur der planettnn vnd sternn Aigenschafft gewingenn vnnd wie inn tag vnnd nacht xxiiii stundt sein vnnd wie all stundt ain planett Regiret [17ᵛ]

Item das ainunndzwanzigist Capittel sagtt was Natur vnnd aigennschafft des gestirnns planettnn vnnd die zaichenn ydem menschenn inn sunderhaytt vnnd in gemaynn gebenn [19ʳ]

Item das xxii Capittel sagtt die glidmas die ygklicher planett denn Kindenn geb Namlich Saturnus [19ᵛ]

Item das xxiii Capittel sagtt was glidmas Jupitter vnnd mars den kindenn gebenn sol [20]

Item das xxiiii Capittel sagtt was glidmas Vennus vnnd mercurius [vonn] ⟨vnnd⟩ der mon denn kindenn gebenn sol [21ᵛ]

Item das xxv Capittel sagtt wie ygklichs glid ann dem menschenn der zwelff zaichenn ainem zugeaygenrt werdt Als das Hauubt dem aries der hals Thawro die arm geminis [22ʳ]

Item das xxvi Capittal sagtt was glid denn drewenn zaichenn Leo cancerus vnnd virgo zugehörnn [23ᵛ]

Item das xxvii Capittel sagtt was glid denn dreyenn(!) zaichenn Libra vnnd scorpio zugehörnn [24ᵛ]

Item das xxviii Capittel sagtt was glid denn dreynn zaiche Capricornnus Aquarius vnnd pisce zugehornn [25ᵛ]

Item das xxix Capittel sagtt wie maister albertus Demonstrat das die zaichenn gewaltt habenn v̈ber die gelid [26ʳ]

(2ᵛ) Item das xxx Capittel sagtt Wie all siechtagenn sich merernn nach denn vier quatternn des mans [27ʳ]

Item das xxxi Capittel sagtt warumb der monscheynn so schedlichenn sey vnnd doch der Sunenn scheynn vil stercker ist [28ʳ]

Item das xxxii Capittel sagtt was Natur vnnd mayung ygklicher planett geb dem ganntzen menschenn vnnd am Erstenn vonn saturnno [28ᵛ]

Item das xxxiii Capitell sagtt Was Natur Jupiter geb seinenn kindenn vnnd was ir aigennschafft Sey [30ᵛ]

Item das xxxiiii Capittel sagt vonn dem mars vnnd vonn denn kindenn die daruntter gebornn wordenn was Natur sy seynn [31ᵛ]

Item das xxxv Capittel sagtt Vonn der Sunenn was Natur vnnd aigennschafft sy denn kindenn geb [32ʳ]

Item das xxxvi Capittel sagt was natur vennus kinder Seynn vnnd was inn zugehörtt [33ʳ]

Item das xxxvii Capittel sagtt was Natur Mercurius seinenn kindenn geb [34^r]

Item das xxxviii Capittel sagtt was der monn seinenn kindenn geb vnnd was Natur sy Seynn [36^r]

Item das xxxix Capittel sagtt warumb der monn inn der mydt ain schwartz mayl hab vnd wie das zugee [36^r]

Item das xl Capittel sagtt inn welher mas die sternn vnnd planettnn dem menschenn ir Natur vnnd aigenschafftt gebenn [37^r]

Item das xli Capittel sagtt wie die unvolkumen thierenn geporenn werdenn [38^v]

(3^r)   Item das xlii Capittel sagtt Vonn der sundflus Wie die werd [40^r]

Item das xliii Capittel sagtt wie inn der mueter der frawenn mer dann ain feucht werdenn mag [40^v]

Item das xliiii Capittel sagtt warumb ettlich thier vil feucht geberenn vnnd ettlich night [41^v]

Item das xlv Capittel sagt warumb vnnd vonn der gepurt in mueter leib vnnd vonn des kindes ausganng [43^r]

Item das xlvi Capittel sagtt wie die feucht aus mueter leyb gee vnnd zw welher zeytt [44^r]

Item das xlvii Capitell sagtt wie offtt die frawe misperet vonn dem thonner [44^v]

Item das xlviii Capittel sagtt vonn ettlichen fragenn vnnd auch vonn dem thonner [46^v]

Item das xlviiii Capittel sagtt warumb vnnd in welhem monadt die kindt am pestenn zw der geburtt sein [47^r]

Item das l Capittel sagtt wie sich die schos vonn göttlicher hilff vnnd besundernn genadenn auff thun [48^r]

Item das li Capittel [Capittel] sagtt vonn ettliche fragenn von wannen denn kindenn in muetter Leyb die Narrunng kum davonn es lebtt [48^v]

Item das lii Capittel sagtt vonn denn wundernn vnnd tadelhafftigenn kindenn wie das zugett vnnd geschech [49^v]

Item das liii Capittel sagtt wie die monster vnnd wunder gepornn werdenn vonn anndernn sachenn der frawenn vnd des mans [51^r]

Item das liiii Capittel sagtt wie auch vonn übrigenn samenn die monster werdenn [52^r]

Item das lv Capittel sagtt aber vonn Ettliche wundern vnnd monnsternn [53^v]

(3^v)   Item das lvi Capittel sagtt wie im denn gaistlichenn dingenn die mit dem leyb alain sunder auch die sel berürnn auch wunder vnnd monster werdenn [54^r]

Item das lvii sagtt vonn pildernn vnnd herttenn stamenn fundenn saindt [55^r]

Item das lviii Capittel sagtt von denn zaichenn wann ain fraw schwannger sey oder nydt [56^r]

Item das lviiii Capittel sagtt ob ain fraw ains Suns schwannger sey oder ainer tochter [57^r]

Item das lx Capittel sagtt vonn der Keuschhaytt der Iunckfrawenn [57^r]

Item das lxi Capittel sagtt wie man sich huette sol vor den frawenn wann sy ir wochenn habenn [58^r]

Item das lxii Capittel sagtt vonn ettliche zaichenn wie man ein Iunckfraw erkenn sol [59^r]

Item das lxiii Capittel sagtt vonn ettliche siechtagenn die denn frawenn vonn ir muetter vnnd menstrua kumenn [60^v]

Item das lxiiii Capittel sagtt vonn der ursach vnnd ordung der fruchtparkaytt vnnd was ir das offtt ain fraw oder ain mann unfruchtper vnnd unperhafft ist [62^r]

Item das lxv Capittel sagt vnnd lernntt wie man denn unperhaffttnn lewttnn zw hilff kum das sy perhafft werdenn [63^r]

Item das lxvi Capittel sagtt vonn dem samenn vnnd natur des mans vnnd der frawenn [65^r]

Item das lxvii Capittel sagtt wie der mennschs die edlistenn vnnd pestenn dewung hab [66^r]

Item das lxviii Capittel sagtt was die sperma des mans vnnd der frawen Sey [67^r]

(4^r)   Item das lxviiii Capittel sagtt vnnd gibtt dem puech Enndt vnnd Erzeltt was gesagt sey vnnd er pitt das übel gesagtt sey zustraffenn [68^r]

Item das lxx Capittel sagt wie man Gott lob Ere vnnd dannck sagenn sol inn allenn dingen etc.

[Introduction]

(5^r)   Albumaser schreybet inn seinenn hochenn Engaung in die astronomey des gleichenn schreybt auch pthomeus in seinem quatriperdes mit dem paidenn sagtt vnnd hiltt auch Auerorus inn dem Erstenn Comenntt über das puech vonn der hochenn Natur das mann nenntt methaphisica die redenn all geleich hellennd alzo wann sich der mennsch naigt vnd kertt zw der verstantnus der verunfft vnnd weyshaytt so nachenntt er gott vnd geleicht sich seinenn Enngelnn vnnd vertt sich vonn der statt der vnvernufftigenn thiern vnnd vichenn.   So aber der mensch sich naigtt vnnd kertt zw leybs lust vnnd fleucht die weyshaytt So nachennt er denn vnvernufftigenn thieren vnnd verfertt sich vonn gott vnnd seinenn Engelnn.   Darumb ist weyshaytt vnd vernufft zubegernn vor allenn dingen.   Seytt nun dw aller hochgelobtister furst herrtzog Sigmundt pfaltzgraffe bey Rreyenn ecc. in seiner pluennttnn jugenntt inn allem wollust des irdischenn paradeys im obernn paierlanndt zw volkumennhaytt aller leyplichenn lufft über genntt vnnd vollenndt ist an mich doctor harttlieb des hochverporgenn puech die gehaym der frawenn das albertus mangnus mit grosser müe vnnd arbaytt gesamlett vnnd gemacht hatt vonn Latey-nischer Zungenn inn teutsche sprach zw pringenn So ist ye das ain wortt zaichenn das dw kunst vnnd weyshaytt lieb hast vnnd doch dem pleunntt jugennt nit latein vnnd kernn last zw vnnsittenn vnnd fleyslichenn wollustenn das sich pillich alle weytte lanndt vnnd lewtt freyenn sullenn.   Ey was ist pesser vnnd hocher wann ains furstenn weyshaytt.   Als Solomonn spricht ains furstten weyshaytt ist seynnenn vnnterthann pesser vnnd fruchtpar dann ain fruchtber abennd Regenn.   Darumb hochgelobter Furst so dem gepott sich zeuchtt zw Nutz zu frumer deinenn Erenn vnnd vnderthann so pin ich willig vnnd gehorsam das puech zw teutschenn inn mass als hernach geschrybenn stett.   Item das puech Secreta mulierum hatt gemacht Albertus mangus vnnd hatt dareynn gesetztt garvil natwrlich ding doch nit so gemain vnnd lauter als dann die maister in der Ertzney gesagtt haben. (5^v) Wann Avicenna hat gar aigenntlich gesagt von was Connplexionn die frawenn Sein vnnd wie sich der sam vereinst inn ir feuchtigkeytt auch vonn der Narrung, zw samenn fuegung vonn allem lebenn der frucht Auch wie lanng sy ligenn sol in der mueter leib vnnd wie sich die schlos auff thun vonn des hochstenn gottes willen vnnd gepiett.   Darnach wie man ain yglich frucht Erzneynn vnnd nerenn sol.   Item mustio ain hocher maister aus kriechenn der hatt zu lieb ainem Kaysser genantt gamaliel auch geschribenn ain puech vonn der geburtt ausganngk der Frucht das selb puech lernett vnnd sagtt das die gepurdt vnnd ausganng der kindt ist achtzehennerlay vnd sindt alain Nur zwenn weg die ann mittel glucklich vnnd guett seynn die andernn weg sindt all todlich oder aber vast sorgklich.   Darpey hatt er auch gemeltt vnnd geschribenn wie man der selbigenn irrung in der natur mit Ertzney vnnd Kunstenn zw hilff kumen sol durch die gelertenn heffamenn. Ja hochgelobter furst glaw das dis puech geteutscht ain grosse Notturfft wäre inn teutschenn lanndenn.   Item gar ain vast grosser Naturlicher maister genandt Macrobius der hatt geschrybenn inn seinem puech vonn der auslegung der träwm Schippionis gar aigenntlich vonn Empfachung der kinder auch dabey wie fraw vnnd man sollenn geschicktt sein das sy volkumen vnnd gesuntte frucht machenn.

Mer welhe Conplexionn zw samenn gehörnn das sy kindt machen vnnd mer vonn Irrung wo zwo personn zusamenn kumen die da nit ainer Natur sindt zw kindenn. Wie man die berayttnn sol das sy Kinder miteinander habenn. Er sagtt auch dabey das woll ain fraw vnnd ain man zusamenn kumenn die kain rechte lieb zusamenn mugenn habenn. Er geytt auch gar mangerlay rad wie man durch gelertt vnnd drew lewtt das wenndenn vnnd vnnterkumen sol. Unnd sagt das sölichs inn der Conplexionn woll zurecht kumenn sey. Darnach sagtt Er wie ain puech sey das Ratt vnnd Lere geb wie man zwischenn man vnnd weyb Grosse lieb vnnd freuntschafftt mach gar mit mangerlay dy(6^r)ngen die Naturlich ann alle Sündt zugenn. Aber das selb buech sy nit zuoffennwarnn durch der vnzimlichenn lieb vnnd pulschafftt willenn. Das selb puech ist verporgenn gewesenn Bis auff ain Küng genanntt Egwannt der hat gehabtt gar ein vast trewen kunstreichenn man vnnd doctor gehaissenn Gilbertinus der hatt das puech zw lieb seynem herren dem Küng geöffnnett vnd das puech hebt sich also ann: Es ist nichts schedlichers dann vnwillenn vnnd feynntschafftt zwischen Eleyttenn wann es kumbt dauonn grosser schadt. Darumb will ich alain durch die elewtt offennwarnn das gehaim puech Macrobii Wie recht lieb trew statt werdt zwischenn Elewttenn werr aber die kunst treybenn vnnd Nutzenn will zw vnnzimlicherr puelschafftt vnnd lieb aus de Eee So pitt ich das der almechtig gott mit sainem grymenn zornn sein kunst wennde vnnd nit gefallenn las. O Hochgelobtter Furst glaub mir soltt das puech aus der Eee zupulerey sein Erlaubt das gros ding damit volbracht werdt vnnd inn warhaytt alles das darynn stett das ist kain zauberey vnd gett als zw mit krewternn vnnd salbenn wurtzenn greyffenn als dann inn dem selbenn puech gar lautter geschribenn stett. Item Es ist ain puech das hatt gemacht ain künigin genantt Trottula das selb puech sagtt von mangerley gehaym der frawenn Nämlich wie sy sullen schwannger werdenn vnd wie sy sich inn der tracht halttenn sullenn. Auch wie sy sich in der Kindelttpett Rainigen sullenn auch dapey sagtt das puech vonn allenn dätllnn der frawenn die dann dem manenn vnlust machenn. Es sey ann der guldenn porttenn an henndenn an munndtt an zenntt vnnd allenn farbenn. Es gett auch dapey so hoche Ertzney das gros wunder ist wie ain weyb sölich gross hübpschhaytt müg Ergründenn. Item es ist woll war das Galienus Rasis vnnd Avicenna in irenn puechernn vonn der frawenn zier geschribenn habenn vnnd sy hayssenn die kunst Gummeras aber Es ist alles klain (6^v) gegen dem das Trottula geschribenn vnnd gelertt hatt. Mein aller genädigister herr Es ist woll war das albertus mangnus in seinem puech Secreta mulierum garvil geschribenn hatt aber der sach kaine berürtt vnnd gemellt doch sein puech ist Nuur ain anweyssung zw der gerechttenn verporgenn gehaym. Darumb er solichs verschwigenn vnnd nit gemellt hatt. Da mag Nyemannt sprechen das ers ⟨nit⟩ gewist hab Wann an zweyffel er ist gar ain grosser kunst Reicher mag⟨ister⟩ gewessen. Vnnd ich main Er hab darumb das gelassenn das Er besorgtt hab die hoch gehaym vnnd kunst wurdt misprauchtt vnnd zu vnzymlicher mynn vnnd pulchaff gebraucht vnnd genütztt wann er garvil puecher gaistlicher gemacht vnnd geschribenn hatt vnnd hatt das puech Erst ym altter vnnd Seynem abnemenn gemacht vnnd geschreybenn. Mein aller genadigister hochgelobtter furst vnnd herr ir sullet Nun das puech Secreta mulierum allain nach dem Textt schaffen zw teutschenn So wirtt es beschrottenn vnnd vast vnverstentlich auch es prachtt denn lesernn kainen frümen. Wan aber die obgenanten puechernn auch darynn getragenn vnnd grüntlich geschribenn werdenn So glaub ich das kain ainig puech in der Natur nye gemacht wurdt das puech wirtt nutzer vnnd lustiger allenn Elewttenn. Aber ain vast gros sorg ist darauff das disse gehaym haymlichenn gehalttenn werdt. Wann solttenn die grossenn gehaym werdenn ganntz offennware das wär ymer schad. Gott wurdt es auch vngerochenn nicht lassenn. Wann Arestolis schreybt werr die gehaym der offennwartt vnnd vnwirdigt der ist ain zersterer der haymlichenn haymligkaytt, So schreybett auch Orienus der hochmaister in der Natur alzo wer offennwartt vnnd Ent deckt die haimligkaytt dem werdenn die götter gehaissig vnnd legenn an inn ain straff. Wer wist tugennthaffter hochgelobter furst das Ovidius der hoch poett vonn denn frawenn Etlich haimligkaytt offennlich geschribenn hatt Darumb warett er gesannt inn (7ʳ) das Ellennd vnd Ewigklichenn verprantt vnnd vertrybenn von dem glüchsäligenn Kaysser augusto. Darumb hochgelobet furst weltt ir das puech inn haymligkaytt habenn vnnd nit offenwarnn so will ich das Ewer fürsttlich genadenn gernn Rechtt vnnd woll zw teutschs machenn wann ich sy in meiner gewaltt hab. Woltt aber E. f. g. das puech offennwarnn vnnd gemaynn machenn So ist kain guett genad forcht noch Nott so gros das ich das alles zw teutschs machenn woll. Wann was hulff mich aller weltt reichtung so ich gottes vngenandt vnnd zornnliche straf täglichenn leydenn muest.

[First and last chapter of text]

(7ʳ)   Item das Erst Capittel sagtt denn Warnn Text wie albertuus mangnus das puech durch seins gesellenn gepett gesamelt hatt.

Merung der rechtenn Weyshaytt geb euch gott inn dissem lebenn so Eure günstig vnnd allen danckperkaytt gesellschafftt mich Weysigklichenn gebettenn hatt das ich Euch ettlich grosse gehaym vnnd verporgennhaytt so bey denn frawenn vnnd ir tangen sindt kindett vnnd offennwarett das ich angesechenn hab Eure gepette vnnd flechenn der hatt mich nit gehindertt noch gesaumbtt tragkaytt noch vnwillenn solich klain puechlein zuvolenndenn. Sunder mich hatt gesawbt das kindlich gemuede zw solichenn hochenn vnnd tieffenn kunsten yedoch so will ich Ewr begernn zw willenn werdenn vnnd genug thun vnnd mach Ewch das puech dareynn ir gar vil vnnser begernn vnnd willenn vindt vnnd schreyb darynn nicht anders dann das inn der Natürlichenn kunst vnnd Ertzney Erfundenn wirtt als ver ich dann jetz kann vnnd mir yetz zuschreybenn ist vnnd ich pitt Euch honig suesse gewissenn vnnd Rainigkaytt das ir inn disenn dingenn statt vnnd verschwigenn seydt vnnd vertaugett das alzo inn grosser gehaym das kainem kindt der iar oder weysshaytt zwtayl oder geoffenward werdtt vnnd so ir das trewlichenn haltt vnnd thuett so sprech ich Euch das ich Euch noch will grosser gehaym vnnd verporgenn kunst offenn vnnd lerrnn will als vill dann inn der Ertzney nott ist vnnd mir gett der herr verleucht zw schreybenn vnnd zuoffennwarnn.

. . . .

(68ᵛ)   Das lxx Capittel sagtt wie man gott lob Ere vnd danngk sagenn soll in allenn dingenn

Item als der maister gott genadt vnnd danck sagtt das soltt man thun inn allenn dingen das reden nit alaynn die cristlichenn maister sunder die haydnischenn (69ʳ) maister redenn das auch Als geschrybenn stett durch Arestotilem inn dem puech Etticorum denn gottenn denn maisternn vnnd denn gepottenn mag Nyemantt gering thun das hatt ain gesechenn der maister vnnd hatt im anfanngk vnnd am endt gott lob vnnd danck gesagtt inn Ewigkaytt. Es sprichtt Seneca wer vonn seinenn werckenn gott nit genad lob vnnd dangk sagtt der ist poss willenns vnnd wirtt Nymer in er gehalttenn. Es spricht auch Boecius inn dem Ratt schlag vnnd trostung der philosophy inn dem erstenn puech inn der vierttenn prosa Als offt ainer Seynn arbaytt der weltt zw Rum sagtt vnnd gott nit verains lob vnnd dangk sagtt als offtt hatt er der weltt upigkaytt zw lon. Darumb sag ich genadt vnnd dangk seynnem gottlichenn wessenn vnnd dreyenn person des vaters durch denn guettenn anfangk zw dem andernn mal der person gottes Sun durch das pessa mittel zw dem drittenn der person gottes heyligenn geystes durch das guett Ennd. Die drey personn inn

ainem wessenn sollenn wir im hertzen glaubenn mit dem mundt worttenn vnd
wercknn zw hayl vnnd trost vnnser Sel Amen

2. fol. 70ʳ–110ᵛ: TROTULAE LIBER

[Table of Content]

Item das xxii Capittel sagtt vnnd lerrnntt wie man vnnd frawen lindt an irem leyb werdenn [104ʳ]

Item xxiii Capittel lerrnntt wie die frawenn ir angesicht ziernn vnd schonn machenn sollenn [104ᵛ]

(71ᵛ) Item das xxiiii Capittel lerrnitt wie die frawenn ir angesichtt ziernn vnnd schonn machenn wan sy pissern vnnd schmeckhnn vnd wie man das wendenn sol [108ʳ]

Item das xxv Capittel sagtt vonn dem schmeckhettenn attem mundt vnnd nassenn [108ᵛ]

Item das xxvi Capittel sagtt vonn allem geprechen der zennt wie man das wendenn sol [109ᵛ]

[Introduction, first chapter and end]

(72ʳ) Nun Die Vorred Trottula Was sy bewegtt hatt das puech zw Samelnn vnnd machenn

Durchleuchtigster Hochgebornner Fürst als Ewr fürstlich genadt geschaffenn vnnd gebettenn hatt das puech albertus mangus das man Nennt Secreta mulierum das ist die gehaym der frawenn das ist Nun woll teutschtzt nach dem Textt vnnd geornnd glos vnnd sag doch gar wenig hilff vnnd trost damit man denn frawenn an irenn gehaymen prechenn vnnd siechtagenn wenndenn nit gerattenn.   Darumb hatt Trottula alles gesetztt das denn frawen ann irren gehaimenn stettenn mag v̈bels geschechenn vnnd dapey wie man denn selbenn prechenn wendenn sol.   Wann vil keuscher frawenn vnnd junckfrawen seynt Ee sy ainem man wissenn liessnn irenn geprechenn Ee littenn Sy gros nott als ich dann vil vnnd offt Erfaren han Ee das ain fraw ir gehaym woltt Entdeckhnn vnnd den manenn Enplössnn Ee habenn sy todlichen schmertzenn gelittenn.   Darumb ist woll pillich das Trottula das puech geteutschtt hatt wann vil frawen dadurch getröst werdenn in allenn geprechenn gestalltt vnnd farb vnnd was dadel frawen haben mū(72ᵛ)genn die selbenn werdenn all gewarnnt mit der Lerr Trottula als dann hernach gar lautter gemeltt vnnd geschrybenn stett.

Hie hebet sich ann der Textt vnnd die gehaym glos des puchs Trottula vnnd darynn gezogenn die gehaym macrobii gilbertini vnnd mustio der maister

Das erst Capittel

Da gott der merer vnd schöpffer aller ding in dem anfangkh der weltt alle natur vnd ygkliche inn seynem gesch⟨l⟩echt Beschueff vnnd sy tayltt da wirdigett er menschliche Natur mit hocher wirtt v̈ber all annder Seynn geschöpff vnd gab inn verstanndnus vnnd verunfft vnnd freyenn aigenn willenn vnnd woltt dapey das menschlich geschlechtt durch ir geperung kinder vnnd merrung gebenn das sy Ewigklichenn pliben vnzergenncklich darumb beschueff gott zway geschlechtt frawen vnnd auch man aus inn paiden geperenn württ ir gleich in loblicher würckhung.   So macht er die natur vnd Conplexion des mans warm vnnd (73ʳ) truckhenn vnnd das des mans hitz vnnd truckhenn nit zuvil württ woltt   Er die frawenn habenn kaltt vnnd feucht das sy der mon hitz vnd truckhenhaytt prauchenn in ain gleich temperirtt auch als kaltt vnnd feucht mynder crafftt hatt dann hitz.   Darumb woltt er denn manenn gebenn grosser crafft vnnd würckhung seyd dann die frawen kranckher Natur sindt dan die man So gewingenn sy öffter vnnd mer kranckhaytt wann in der tracht auch gepürtt werdenn die lieben frawenn gar offtt kranck vnnd gelaidigtt vnnd von irer scham wegenn thuenn sy ir kranckhaytt inn ir gehaym denn artzttenn nit sagenn sölich gros laid vnnd leidenn Auch ettlich Erber frawen flechenn vnnd pittenn hatt mich Trottula bewegtt in zw rattenn vnnd helfenn von allenn geprechenn dadeln vnnd ungestaltt der frawenn kostlicher

Ertzney zw hilff kumen vnnd die werdenn dann ausgezogenn aus denn pestenn puechern Ypocras galienus vnnd ander kunst riech ärtztt darumb will ich sagenn vnnd lerrnenn Am erstenn die ursach sölich gehaymer kranckhaytt darnach die zaichenn wie man das Erkennenn sol darnach die Hilff vnd Ratt wie man inn zw trost vnnd stett kumenn sell mit Ertzneynn.

. . . . . .

(110ᵛ)   Hochgelobttr Fürst Nun hatt Ewr genadt das ganntz puech Trottula das da sagtt vonn der gepurtt der kindt vnnd irenn Emppachung dennocht sindtt noch verhannttenn drew puecher macrobius vnnd seynn Comenntt Gilbertinus das die hochenn gehaym sagtt die vast zuverpergen synnd das sy nit annders dann inn der Eee gepraucht werdenn wann Es ymermer schad vnnd schanndt were seltt die gehaym Entdeckhtt werdenn vnnd offenn war seynn sovil grosser sach sindt darynn die zw der myn gehörnn wann was darzw gehörtt das frawenn vnd manenn gar grossnn lust darynn habenn vnnd wie man das wennden sol inn dem Namen der heyligenn drivältigkaytt amen

Deo gracias

3. fol. 112ʳ—123ʳ: EXCERPTA GYNAECOLOGICA VARIA

fol. 112ʳ: *Ut mamille non crescanntt.*

⟨D⟩as die prüst nit wachssnn Nym alaun das krairtt haist wiltt papelnn vnnd zerreyb sy woll vnnd leg sy v̇ber die prüst.   Ain annders Nym mogenn öl kolbenn vnnd senndt inn woll inn Regen wasser vnnd dunckh darynn ain leynnes tuech vnnd leg es drey tag auff die prüst als hays dw es magst Erleydenn.

. . . . . .

fol. 123ʳ: Item Wie wirtt die Verstäntig sel dem kindt inn muetter leyb Eingossenn ob doch der vatter im gepernn schickhtt vnnd . . . die matery zw Empfachenn die verstänntigkeyt als das selb sprichtt Arestotile inn primo de celo et munndo der würckhuntt geb die gestaltt vnnd die zwsamfuegung der Conplexionn Aber ain sölichs ist nit verstänndigkaytt als er das selb Bewartt in Tercio de anima Comento quarto Distinctione prima quid indelectus Die verstannt wirtt dem menschenn zugefuegtt durch die zufuegung vnd inmaiginacio als der heffamen mit dem streff vnnd der selb artickell ist inn dem glawbenn verdampt vnnd darumb so ist die antwortt vnnd ist cristlich vnnd glaubich das der almechtigh gott genugsamigklich die matery die frucht des kinds Eingeist vnnd auch die vernufftt vnnd das spricht Augustinus die selb wirtt inn der schepffung Eingossnn vnnd in dem Eingiessnn So wirtt die geschopff Amenn

Tetragramathonn

THE IDEA OF THE QUINTESSENCE

by

F. SHERWOOD TAYLOR

THE word *quintessence* is one of the many that have passed from medieval science into modern speech. To-day it is a metaphorical term expressing the purest or most perfect form or manifestation of some quality; but in the seventeenth century and earlier it denoted a volatile principle that could be separated from a material substance and possessed its characteristic activity in a high degree. Thus alcohol was termed the 'quintessence of wine'. The term *quintessence* (*quinta essentia; quintum esse*) expresses the belief that it was something over and above the four elements present in the matter from which it was extracted, and this implies that it was not strictly a material substance. On the other hand, it was clearly not a spiritual substance in the sense that we should use the word to-day, nor was it identical with the element that composed the celestial regions. It was regarded as a being intermediate between the material and the spiritual or celestial, and capable of acting as a link by means of which the former could be influenced by the latter. It was, in fact, thought to consist of a *subtle matter*, and this is the first conception we must seek to trace.

The Idea of Subtle Matter in Greek Natural Philosophy

It is only since the time of Descartes that we have divided the world sharply into material and spiritual realms, without any connecting medium. This, the modern view, stands in the sharpest contrast with that of the first natural philosophers. They recognized matter and also mind; but they did not regard them as mutually exclusive. There was gross matter that could be touched and handled; then a series of grades of ever more subtle matter, ranging from mists, cloud and smoke through exhalations, air, ether, and the animal spirits, to the soul and spiritual beings.

Aristotle in the beginning of his *De anima* shows that many of the early philosophers identified 'soul' with 'fire' or 'air'. Heraclitus says that the first principle, the 'warm exhalation' of which everything else is composed, is soul. Anaximenes says that 'just as our soul, being air, holds us together, so do breath and air encompass the whole world'; while Cicero says that Anaximenes regarded air as a god. The Pythagoreans held that a 'boundless breath' outside the heavens was inhaled by the world. Diogenes of Apollonia is more explicit: 'My view is that that which has intelligence is air; the soul is air; everything is a transformation of air.' We must, of course, reject the idea that these men identified the soul with the kind of matter that we to-day call air and describe in our text-books. It is perhaps truer to say that they included air and the soul in the same class of 'spiritual substances'. These spiritual substances were not regarded as immaterial in any sense that we should now give to the word. Real fog that could wet, wind that could blow, were of the same nature as the exhalations of the earth and heavens, and the soul itself; none of these were considered as wholly immaterial in the modern sense of the word, and consequently could be thought of as subjects for physical manipulation.

The idea of a world-soul appears clearly enough in Plato's *Timaeus*, and in the Platonic *Epinomis* its interaction in nature is clearly expressed. 'After the fire we will put the ether and we will admit that of this ether the soul of the world forms living beings which take from this ether a great part of their substance.' Aristotle, most influential of all authors of antiquity, made extensive use of the notion of subtle matter in his system of nature, of which it forms an essential part. The idea that this subtle matter may yet be capable of forming a part of solid stones and metals is found in a famous passage from the *Meteorologica*, which was probably one of the chief roots of the doctrines of alchemy:

> Some account has now been given of the effects of the secretion (ἔκκρισιν)[1] above the surface of the earth; we must go on to describe when it is shut up in the parts of the earth. Just as its twofold nature gives rise to various effects in the upper region, so here it causes two varieties of bodies. For we maintain there are two exhalations (evaporations, ἀναθυμιάσεις), one vaporous (ἀτμιδώδης), the other smoky (καπνώδης), and there correspond two kinds of bodies that originate in the earth, the 'fossils' (ὀρυκτὰ) and metals (μεταλλευτά). For the dry exhalation is that which by burning makes all the 'fossil' bodies, such as the kind of stones that cannot be melted, realgar and ochre and ruddle and sulphur,[2] and other such things. Most of the fossil bodies are coloured ashes or a stone concreted from them, such as cinnabar. The vaporous exhalation is the cause of all metals, fusible or ductile things, such as iron, copper, gold. For the vaporous exhalation being shut in makes all these things, and especially in stones. By their dryness being compressed and congealed into one thing, just like dew or hoar-frost, when it has been separated it generates these things (the metals). Hence these things are water in a sense, and in a sense not. For the matter was that of water potentially, but it is no longer; nor are they from water which has been changed through some affection, such as are juices. For copper and gold are not formed like that, but each of them was formed by the exhalation congealing before water was formed. Wherefore all are affected by fire and have some earth; for they contain the dry exhalation. But gold alone is not affected by fire. This is the general theory of all these bodies, but we must consider each of them in particular.[3]

These exhalations are subtle and volatile entities that can work their way through the solid rock, as the Pythagorean fire at the centre of the Earth was thought to work its fructifying way to the surface. The concept of subtle matter was enormously developed by the Stoics, especially Zeno and Chrysippus, who systematized the theory of *pneuma* or 'spirit'. They conceived of God as being at once mind ('world-reason'), and also original matter, fire, the breath of life or *pneuma*. In their philosophy *pneuma* is at once the original matter from which all things have originated and is the all-pervading, all-ruling creative world-reason. It is matter and the power that creates it and the mind that is manifest in man. It is not identified with, though it is the remote origin of, the crude elements which we regard as

[1] Aristotle, *Meteor.* i. 3 and i. 4. When the sun warms the earth there is an 'evaporation' or 'secretion'. Some thought it to be of one kind, but Aristotle thought it to be of two; one dry, like smoke; and one of a moist or breath-like kind.

[2] These four substances and cinnabar are in continual use by the Greek alchemists of the earliest period, which is probably a testimony to the influential character of this passage.

[3] Aristotle, *Meteor.* iii. 6; 378ᵃ.

matter, but it is that which informs and transforms them. This concept, dynamic and teleological, of *pneuma* working out its own possibilities made a strong appeal to Greek physiologists and physicians. The body was constituted of the four elements which were blended to give the right tempering of the qualities, warm, moist, cold and dry; but the control of bodily functions was vested in the vital principle, the *pneuma*, the breath of life from the world-soul which was the great residue thereof. The function of respiration was to draw in this *pneuma*, which was then distributed by way of the lungs and blood-vessels. Each organ had its own particular *pneuma* by means of which it operated and was controlled, in a manner recalling the functions of the *archaeus* of the Paracelsian school.

This *pneuma* cannot be called immaterial or material. It is the principle of mind on the one hand; yet on the other it can move like a fluid, be drawn in and expelled by the force of the lungs.

Galen, who summed up Greek medicine in his great collection, made extensive use of the idea of *pneuma*, and was followed by almost all the physicians who taught before the later part of the eighteenth century. His *pneuma* was translated by the Latin word *spiritus*, and the English 'spirits'; and when we talk to-day of a man being full of animal spirits we are translating Galen's phrase *pneuma psychikon*. In Galen's system the *pneuma* is drawn into the lungs with the air and passes therewith to the heart, where, by a sort of combustion it combines with the 'natural spirit' extracted by the liver from the chyle, forming the 'vital spirit' which is distributed by the arteries. Part of this is transformed in the brain to the *pneuma psychikon* or 'animal spirit'. This subtle entity traverses the nerves as sunshine passes through air and water, and so operates the muscles. We may note then that Galen's *pneuma* resembles matter in that it has the power of local motion and could be admixed with matter and put it in motion. On the other hand, it is unlike matter in its subtlety, that is, its power of passing through continuous matter without disrupting it. It has, we notice, degrees of subtlety, being transformed from the gross natural spirits to the subtle animal spirits by processes akin to combustion and distillation—an idea of which later authors, to whom distillation was known, were to take advantage.

So the contemporary reader of Greek natural philosophy would have no difficulty in believing that a 'subtle matter' could form the spirit of man, or a solid metal, or indeed any other natural object; for these breaths or exhalations were potentially the matter of all things. He would also regard this *pneuma* as a substance that could move, could be concentrated in a particular organ, and could be prepared from matter and subtilized to the point of becoming the agent of mind.

But *pneuma* was to the ancients not only a potential matter and a physiological medium, but also a directive agency. In the earliest period of natural philosophy the source of motion and change was readily thought of as a kind of life. Thales said that all things are full of gods; the magnet has a soul in it because it moves the iron. Empedocles said, 'Know that effluences flow from all things that come into being', and this directive influence was, of course, prominent in the Stoic philosophy. When astrology gained its great importance, towards the beginning of the Christian era, the supposed influence of the planets upon everything on earth required explanation. This influence could be conceived as something having an intelligent power or as a blind force, but generally it was considered to be a manifestation of this 'spirit'. To quote Diodorus Siculus:

> They[4] say these gods[5] in their natures do contribute much to the generation of all things, the one being of a hot and active nature, the other moist and cold, but both having something of the air; and that by these all things are both brought forth and nourished. And therefore that every particular being in the universe is perfected and completed by the sun and moon, whose qualities, as before declared, are five: a spirit or quickening efficacy, heat or fire, dryness or earth, moisture or water, and air, of which the world does consist, as a man made up of head, hands, feet and other parts. . . . And therefore they called the *spirit* Zeus, which is such by interpretation, because a quickening influence is derived from this into all living creatures, as from the original principle; and upon that account he is esteemed the common parent of all things.[6]

This passage is of great interest, for here appears the clear concept of *pneuma* as a *fifth element and active principle* in all things. The same notion, that there is in things a spirit, akin to and receptive of the influences of the celestial world, is characteristic also of the Hermetic philosophy, which is to be found in such works as the *Poimandres*, and which had a powerful influence in moulding the ideas of the earliest alchemists.

With the spread of Christian ideas it became clear that if the planets exerted any such influence, they did so as intermediaries of the will of God. The Neoplatonists and Christians alike pictured a hierarchical descent of influence from the divine to matter, and certain Neoplatonic Christians, such as the Bishop Synesius of Ptolemais, could think of this divine emanation as a *substance* widely diffused rather than a *directed ray*. Thus in one of his hymns, written before his conversion, he writes:

> For then it was the Good
> Source of the spirit of man
> Was divided without division;
> And immortal mind, efflux
> Of divine parents,
> Descended into matter
> Scanty indeed, but whole and one everywhere,
> The whole diffused into the whole
> Revolved the vast hollow of the heavens
> Preserving all this whole.
> It is distributed into different forms
> Part of it in the courses of the stars,
> Part of it the choirs of angels,
> Part likewise in the heavy bondage
> Found an earthy form,
> And disjoined from its parents
> Drank dark oblivion, blind in its cares
> Wondering at the joyless earth.[7]

---

[4] The Egyptians.
[6] Diod. Sic., *Bibliotheca historica*, i. 2.
[5] Osiris and Isis.
[7] Migne, *Patrologia graeca*, vol. lxvi, col. 1590.

Synesius envisages a noble subtle formative entity coming down from on high; but he also has the concept of the contrary active material principle rising from below:

> Sink beneath the earth
> Trail of the Serpents,
> Sink beneath the earth, too,
> Titan serpent
> Demon of matter
> Cloud of the soul
> Delighting in phantoms
> Cheering on his whelps
> With imprecations.[8]

I have not hitherto alluded to any alchemical author, but I would now point out that we have established in antiquity a very general notion of a substance that could be regarded as a universal agent and patient, something that could act upon everything and become potentially everything; that this was thought to be manifest both as something which came down from the celestial regions—an influence or celestial virtue—and also as that which rises up from the earth to meet it—smoke and vapour; and that it could be conceived of as an active principle and fifth element.   Spiritus, $\pi\nu\epsilon\hat{\upsilon}\mu\alpha$, breath, was that which is common to heaven and earth.[9]

The Idea of Subtle Matter in Alchemy

The originators of the attempt to isolate the quintessences of things were alchemists, and we therefore require to pursue the idea of subtle matter in the alchemical texts.

The first important body of alchemical texts are those written in Greek at dates between *c.* A.D. 100 and A.D. 600.[10]   The greater part of them have been edited by Berthelot,[11] and translated into French.   The translation should be used with caution, since the text is sometimes corrupt and almost always obscure, so giving free rein to the expression of the translator's opinions.

Characteristic of almost all alchemical writings is the manipulation of a substance whose nature is not revealed, but which takes an essential part in that perfection of matter which is the ostensible purpose of the alchemical processes.   The Greek alchemists commonly spoke of this as $\theta\epsilon\hat{\iota}ov$ $\mathring{v}\delta\omega\rho$, *the divine water*, while the alchemists of the Latin west knew it as the *mercury of the philosophers*.   These are always characterized as a subtle, volatile substance, capable of penetrating all things and to be found everywhere.

The practical part of alchemy is clearly designed for the manipulation of what the modern chemist would term volatile liquids.   Thus the greater part of alchemical laboratory practice consists of distillation, and the author has shown elsewhere[12] how the Greek alchemists invented and perfected all the main types of distillation apparatus that were in use up to the nineteenth

---

[8] *ibid.*, col. 1595.

[9] Cf. I John v. 7–8.

[10] F. Sherwood Taylor, 'A survey of Greek alchemy'. *Journ. Hellenic Studies*, 1930, I, 109.

[11] M. Berthelot, *Collection des anciens alchemistes grecs.* 3 vols. Paris, 1887–8. (In the following notes, the references are to the Greek text.)

[12] F. Sherwood Taylor, 'The evolution of the still'. *Annals of Science*, 1945, v, 185.

century. In general, though we hear so much of stills and see pictures of alchemists' laboratories furnished with little else, we are told almost nothing about what was distilled in them. The Greek alchemists speak of distilling sulphur, θεῖον, but every chemist must regard the processes described by them and the design of their apparatus as being quite inconsistent with the distillation of a substance of such a high boiling-point. Furthermore, these distillations were, in Greek alchemy at least, said to produce a liquid, the *divine water*,[13] and not a solid such as would result from distilling sulphur. There is scarcely sufficient evidence to enable us to conclude what was distilled. However, Zosimus[14] describes the distillation of eggs in terms that do actually correspond to what I have observed in distilling eggs, and many of the synonyms for the divine water refer to plants. I would tentatively suggest that the Greek alchemists were engaged in the distilling of living, or potentially living, matter in which the generative spirit of the heavens would be thought principally to reside; they may further have distilled dew, which was thought to be the influence of the heavens in tangible form.

An examination of the texts of the Greek alchemists shows that most of them were greatly concerned with those entities which may be grouped under the name of *pneuma*, of which the Latin equivalent is *spiritus*, and which we will translate as 'spirit'. The word *pneuma* occurs very frequently, and denotes what we would call a 'vapour', and again a sort of 'tingeing spirit' which gave colour to metals;[15] it is something that penetrates metals, as the 'spirits' of Greek physiology pervade the body.[16] Out of a large number of passages, we may note the following typical statement. Spirit is obtained by the expulsion of a 'mercury' from a metallic body.[17] The All has life and spirit and is destructive: he who understands this has gold and silver.[18] The word 'spirit', we are told, signifies a volatile substance and the sublimed vapours (αἰθάλη) resemble the spirit; there is the white vapour, the cloud of cinnabar, and 'a spirit, darker, moist and pure';[19] every vapour is a spirit[20] and so also are the powers of tingeing,[21] 'for this has a sulphurous and caustic nature'. The spirit is in the fume raised in the distillation apparatus or the *kerotakis*.[22] As man is made from liquids and solids and spirit, so also is copper.[23] A liquid can be made by distilling certain yellow substances, yolk of eggs, the 'saffron of eggs', and celidony, in double measure; and after opening the apparatus you will find the herbs burnt, having lost their proper colour, that is to say their proper spirit.[24] The bodies (of metals) receive a spirit and this is the 'fleeing spirit of the pursuing body'.[25] 'Chrysolithos' is

[13] Berthelot, *op. cit.* (11), texte grec, p. 141.

[14] *ibid.*

[15] *ibid.*, texte grec, p. 119, l. 12; p. 126, l. 9; p. 149, l. 12; p. 165, l. 1, etc.

[16] *ibid.*, texte grec, p. 124 § 8.

[17] *ibid.*, texte grec, p. 125, l. 4.

[18] *ibid.*, texte grec, p. 144, l. 6.

[19] *ibid.*, texte grec, p. 150, l. 11.

[20] *ibid.*, texte grec, p. 152, l. 4.

[21] *ibid.*, texte grec, p. 150, l. 12.

[22] *ibid.*, texte grec, p. 165, l. 1.

[23] *ibid.*, texte grec, p. 171, ll. 9, 11.

[24] *ibid.*, texte grec, p. 227, ll. 10–16.

[25] *ibid.*, texte grec, p. 252, ll. 1–7.

a spiritual and airy being.   In the Komarius and Cleopatra text,[26] and also in the Visions of Zosimus, the body-soul analogy is freely used of metals and their tingeing spirits.   The greater part of the former text, as it occurs in the manuscripts, consists of a *Dialogue of Cleopatra and the Philosophers*, which has been thought to be one of the earliest alchemical writings.   Here again we find very clearly expressed the idea of an *anima media*, or spirit, as the agent of the alchemical process:

> Tell us how the highest descends towards the lowest, and how the lowest rises towards the highest, and how the middle element approaches the highest to come and be made one with it, and what is the element that acts on them: how the blessed waters descend from on high to visit the corpses, stretched out fettered and cast down in the darkness and the recesses of the Hades, and how the medicine of life comes to them and awakens them.[27]

Again, of the same substance we are told, 'That is divine, which being made one with divinity, renders the substances divine'.[28]

The sense of *pneuma* in these texts seems to differ from that of *aithale* and *nephele*.   The former is a very common term in Greek alchemy and means 'a vapour or volatile substance obtained by sublimation'.   It is evidently a grosser volatile than *pneuma*, for Mary, cited by Olympiodorus, tells us that 'unless all the bodies are subdivided by fire, and the vapour ($\dot{\alpha}\iota\theta\dot{\alpha}\lambda\eta$), *becoming a spirit* ($\pi\nu\epsilon\hat{\upsilon}\mu\alpha$), rises, nothing will be completed'.[29] The word *nephele* is applied to more gross and visible vapours;   and perhaps *nephele, aithale, pneuma* may be taken as successive grades of subtlety of matter obtainable by distillation, the *pneuma*, as we have seen, being regarded as a link with the 'highest', the 'divine'.

It is quite clear then that both the practical and theoretical parts of Greek alchemy are concerned with raising a 'spirit' from a body by physical processes of distillation and sublimation, and this process was clearly carried out with success.   The insoluble difficulty of the alchemical process was to find a means of incorporating this supposedly tingeing spirit into the 'dead bodies' (metallic compounds) and so converting them into gold and silver. The alchemical process is not, however, our immediate concern, which is rather with the idea of spirit as Quintessence, a term which is not found in Greek alchemy.

The Idea of the Quintessence among the Arabs

It seems improbable that the idea of a fifth element as a *pneuma*, constituting the activity of a body and linking it to the celestial world, should have passed directly from antiquity to the Latin alchemical writers of the early fourteenth century.   We cannot at present trace a direct derivation from an Arabic writer, but we must note the existence of similar ideas in the Arabic world.   Jābir ibn Ḥayyān has left a *Book of the Fifth Nature*[30] (*k.al-ṭabī'a al-ḫāmisa*), the meaning of which term has been discussed by Paul Kraus;[31]

---

[26] *ibid.*, texte grec, p. 293, l. 9.

[27] *ibid.*, texte grec, p. 292, § 8.

[28] *ibid.*, texte grec, p. 296, ll. 6–11.

[29] *ibid.*, texte grec, p. 93, l. 16.

[30] P. Kraus, *Jābir ibn Ḥayyān.* (*Mémoires présentés à l'Institut d'Égypte*, t. XLIV.) Cairo, 1943, vol. i, p. 95.

[31] *ibid.*, vol. ii, p. 153.

its primary meaning appears to be the substance that underlies the forms of the four elements, yet the term *rūḥ*, i.e. *pneuma*, is in one instance applied to it. We may therefore be prepared to entertain the idea that the notion of the quintessence, as held by the fourteenth-century alchemists, was present to the Arabs, who may have been the source of the former's theories.

The Discovery of the Distillation of Alcohol

Hermann Diels in his remarkable paper 'Die Entdeckung des Alkohols'[32] advances evidence that alcohol was occasionally prepared at periods much earlier than the thirteenth century, to which its discovery is commonly assigned, and perhaps as early as the time of the first Greek alchemists, the usual process being the distillation of strong wine with some form of salt. Although doubt has been cast on this view, it appears not improbable though not proven. The Arabs appear to have distilled wine, but not to have thought the product very interesting. Thus the *Liber Servitoris* of Albucasis[33] describes the distillation of 'vinegar for whitening' in a still similar to that in which rose-water is distilled, and then merely tells us that wine can be distilled in the same way. It does not appear that any of the well-known Arab pharmacists employed distilled alcohol as a drug, nor that it was known to the Arabs before the thirteenth century.[34]

In the twelfth century the technical treatises, the *Mappae Clavicula* and the *Liber ad comburendos hostes*[35] of Marcus Graecus, mention the distillation of alcohol from wine, but they describe the product as *aqua ardens*, a water that burns, and not as a medicine. It is thought that the first mention of alcohol as a drug is in the work of Salernus,[36] about 1150, but it is only in the succeeding century that its use becomes general.

Vitalis de Furno and Thaddaeus of Florence (thirteenth century) are spoken of by Kopp[37] as the first to extol *aqua vitae* as a medicament. The relevant passage of Thaddaeus has been published by von Lippmann.[38]

An early reference to *aqua vitae* is found in the Acts of the Dominican provincial chapter at Rimini in 1288.

> Since we have learnt that certain brethren have instruments by which they make the water which is called *aqua vite*, we strictly enjoin all priors within eight days after they have arrived at their convents, to have vessels of this kind destroyed and sold and not to permit water of this kind to be made in our houses.[39]

This suggests that the process of distilling *aqua vitae* was not new in 1288. The prohibition does not imply that the making of this 'water' was sinful, for there are numerous acts prohibiting other secular occupations to the friars.

[32] H. Diels, 'Die Entdeckung des Alkohols'. *Abhandl. d. Königl. Preuss. Akad. d. Wissensch.*, 1913, *Philos.-Hist. Kl.*, Heft iii, 35 pp.

[33] Albucasis, *Liber Servitoris Liber XXVIII Bulchasi Benaberazerin trāslatus a Simóe ianuēse iterprete Abraā iudeo tortuosiēse*. 1471. (Editions of 1479, 1484 and 1491 exist.)

[34] M. Berthelot, *La chimie au Moyen Âge*. Paris, 1893, p. 61.

[35] *ibid.*, p. 117.

[36] E. O. von Lippmann, 'Zur Geschichte des Alkohols'. *Chem. Zeitschr.*, 1920, xliv, 625.

[37] H. Kopp, *Geschichte der Chemie*. 4 vols. Braunschweig, 1843-7, vol. iv, p. 274. (The work he cites exists in MS. at Munich.)

[38] E. O. von Lippmann, 'Thaddäus Florentinus (Taddeo Alderotti) über den Weingeist'. *Arch. f. d. Gesch. d. Med.*, 1914, vii, 379.

[39] *Archivum fratrum praedicatorum*, 1941, xi, 163.

Arnaldus da Villanova,[40] writing about 1309–12, states that it can be obtained from wine or lees of wine by distillation. He extols its curative virtues in all manner of ailments and especially for those associated with old age. He does not, however, treat it as a substance of a spiritual character, or as differing materially from the general class of drugs. The idea that alcohol was of a quasi-spiritual nature, in the sense of being a link between the terrestrial and celestial worlds, first appears in the works attributed to Ramon Lull (1235–1315), but probably written by his followers in the mid-fourteenth century. Conrad Gesner[41] tells us downrightly that Ramon Lull 'was the first man to write of the quintessence, though it was unknown to all the physicians of his time, nor written of in any book nor tried in practice'; and, indeed, there appears to be no mention of the quintessence in works prior to the treatises attributed to him.

Fourteenth-century Treatises on Aqua Vitae

There exists a group of alchemical treatises,[42] dealing with *aqua vitae* and the quintessence, which are attributed to Arnaldus da Villanova, already discussed, Raimundus Gaufredus (Galfridus), Raimundus Lullius and Joannes de Rupescissa. If the *De virtutibus aquae vitae* is correctly attributed to Raimundus Gaufredus,[43] it must belong to the late thirteenth century and be the oldest of these works; but there may well be doubt as to the correctness of the attribution. Joannes de Rupescissa's work must be supposed to date from the first half of the fourteenth century, and if we accept Thorndike's careful survey of the evidence,[44] the earliest of the treatises attributed to Lull belong to the second half of the fourteenth century, some sixty years after the death of Ramon Lull; but some, including the author of this essay, would be inclined to regard them as contemporary with Rupescissa. Rupescissa's works are in some manuscripts attributed to Lull; and the above group of texts will here be considered together, without respect to their conjectural chronology or attributions, and will be referred to as the Lullian texts. The printed editions of the Lullian texts concerning the quintessence do not give an adequate idea of their content; for by far the greater part of the complicated diagrams—trees, circles, intersecting triangles, and so forth—by which their author expresses chemical or alchemical relationships are to be found only in manuscript copies, and are not reproduced in the printed texts.

The most significant of the Lullian treatises for the consideration of the idea of the quintessence is the work entitled *De secretis naturae seu de quinta essentia*. This is divided into three or sometimes four books, but in some manuscripts and printed copies only two are found. It was first printed in 1514, and again in 1518, 1542, 1546 and 1567. The edition of 1546 appears to be the best and fullest. Numerous manuscripts are known, which by reason of the tables and schemes and the drawings of apparatus (Figs. 2 and 3) much exceed the printed copies as sources. It would be a long task to

[40] Diels, *op. cit.* (32), p. 19, note (2).

[41] *Thesaurus Euonymi Philiatri De remediis secretis.* Tiguri, 1553 (see note (76)).

[42] The connexion between alchemy and the making of the quintessence is found in all the Lullian works. Their alchemical process seems to have consisted in the repeated circulation of a liquid in the pelican until it was converted into the stone.

[43] Lynn Thorndike, *A history of magic and experimental science.* New York, vol. iv, 1934, p. 16.

[44] *ibid.*, vol. iv, chap. i; *passim*.

catalogue these, but among those I have consulted I would mention a manuscript written *c.* 1420, formerly the property of George Ripley, Robert Green of Welby, and John Dee, and now in the library of Mr. D. I. Duveen; and also MS. Ashmole 1484, in the Bodleian Library.

The author first tells us what is meant by a Quintessence:

But in this chapter we propose to explain in one brief summary, and tell you that first of all there are three principles, by the knowledge of which the worker of this art performs what he wishes, both in medicine and in metallic and lapidific alchemy, in order that he may compound whatever he wishes, as long as he does not depart from nature.

The first principle which the artist of this work should know is matter; through which principle the medicine or stone receives its existence as a substance, because if the matter is such as nature requires, it will be acceptable to the form, which will not be able to be removed through any defect of impression when the virtue is operating therein, because it is the principal medium between the said matter and other essences, as we shall tell you as this book proceeds.

The second principle is most simple with respect to the first, since it is the medium of the first, by which indeed the first immediately has its perfecting.

The third principle is the quintessences, from which the seven virtues[45] depend, both operatively and informatively in the quintessences in inferior material things, which quintessences are mediated.

The first principle, or matter of the first principle, is quicksilver, with all its metals alterable in that whitening which we will reveal in the third distinction.

The second principle, or the matters of it, are subtle liquors (*limphae*) in which the muddiness of the first principle is resolved in a middle substance and subtle matter, in which the true mineral virtues are at rest.

The matter of the third principle is most essential to the existing therein of the virtues of the stars, fixed and not fixed, and their aspects: and these by daily influences are infused into the matter made proper thereto with the help of the second principle, which immediately rests in the mineral virtue, which is in herbs, in animals and in metals. And so it is the cause of the second principle and is a suitable recipient of the third and of all its virtues descending from the heaven, which virtues are the perfection and form of every generated thing, as is clearly seen by inherent principles. For, indeed, it generates materially from the first principle, whence goes forth the mineral virtue, which is the quintessence of the elements, which is simple matter, and this is truly perfected in receiving a form through the celestial quintessence, which flows into it and impresses it. And so this middle virtue, artificially made pregnant by a sharp virtue, through the material perfecting influence with its virtues of the first principle, puts the matter in its perfect being through the middle mineral virtue, which is the thing common to stones and medicines and metals [p. 22]. . . And so the quintessence is made from the four elements, and in it are, in fact, all the elements with all their acts. But all these are aggregated in it in so subtle a matter and in so subtle a form and in so near a simplicity in their respective fashion. . . .

This nature, my son, the philosophers have called heaven (*cœlum*), wherefore as the heaven pours into us sometimes heat, sometimes moisture and so forth, so does the quintessence in the human body at the pleasure of the artist. . . .

To this *cœlum* we apply its own stars, which are plants, stones and metals, to be life and health to all of us in common.[46]

[45] i.e. of the seven planets.

[46] *Raimundi Lullii Maioricani de secretis naturae, seu de quinta essentia.* Norimbergae, per Ioh. Petreium, 1546.

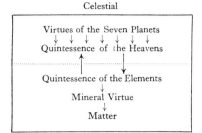

Celestial

Virtues of the Seven Planets
↓ ↓ ↓ ↓ ↓ ↓ ↓
Quintessence of the Heavens
↑ ↓
Quintessence of the Elements
↓
Mineral Virtue
↓
Matter

Terrestrial

Fig. 1. Scheme of the relations of the quintessences, as described in the Lullian *De secretis naturae.*

Thus we may form a scheme as in Fig. 1. It is clear that the quintessence of the elements, if isolated, would be full of the virtues celestial, and by its affinity to the mineral virtue found in all matter could instantly affect it, as our author says, in the same fashion as the eye of the basilisk slays without any sort of mechanical contact.

How was this quintessence, this *cœlum,* to be made? By distillation, and in practice by the distillation of wine. No doubt the reason for the choice of wine was that by distillation it was already known to yield a rare and effective medicine, an *aqua ardens* and *aqua vitae,* but the choice could be justified in other ways for, as a later author tells us, wine is

a liquor clearly divine and celestial, the principal habitation of the dew and celestial moisture drawn from the heaven and the earth through the vine—that wood twisted, uneven and nothing pleasant to the eye; yet unfolded for the benison of the Sun into hanging grapes, whence finally, by pressing and due fermentation, it yields and is digested to a juice, limpid and most friendly to human nature, without which God would not have men be nor can men please God, whether in actions purely spiritual or corporal.[47]

The Lullian work does not justify this choice of material but at once describes the process of making the quintessence. This was not thought to be a mere ardent spirit, but, characteristically, an ardent spirit raised to a higher potency. Here is his description of the process:

And so in the name of our Lord Jesus Christ, take red wine or white, and let it be the best that can be found, or at least take wine which is not at all sour, not too little or too much, and distil *aqua ardens,* as is customary through copper side-tubes (*per cannas brachiales aeris*) and afterwards rectify it four times for a greater rectifying.[48] [Fig. 2.] But I tell you that three times is enough for it to be rectified, and let it be very well shut up so that the burning spirit does not exhale. . . It is an infallible sign for you, my son, when you see that sugar moistened with it and put to the flame is set alight in the same fashion by the water.[49] When you have prepared the water you have therein the matter from which the quintessence is extracted. Take it therefore, and put it in the vessel which is called a vessel of circulation, or in a pelican [Fig. 3], which is called the vessel of Hermes, whose form appears below, and close the orifice very strongly with olibanum or soft mastic, or quicklime mixed with egg-white and put it in dung very hot of its own nature, or in marc,[50] to which no heat is imparted *per accidens*; which, my son, you can do, if you put a large quantity of any of these things in a corner of your house, which quantity may be thirty labourers' loads. This is needed so that the heat of the vessel may not fail, for if the heat were to fail, the circulation of

[47] *D. Johannis Tackii . . . triplex phasis sophicus.* Francofurti, 1673, pp. 19–40.
[48] There is no mention here of the addition of salt or tartar.
[49] *Comburatur similiter aqua.* This is the ancestor of the gunpowder test for proof spirit and probably more exacting. The spirit made was therefore well over proof.
[50] Grapeskins from the wine-press (*vinacea*).

the water would be destroyed, and what we want would not happen, if continuous heat were not administered to it by continual circulations.[51] Our quintessence will be separated, in the colour of the sky, which you can see by a diametrical line dividing the upper part or quintessence from the lower or dregs which are of a turbid colour.[52]

When the circulation had been continued for many days, and the vessel was then opened, a wonderful fragrance would come from it that would attract everybody into the house (apparently overcoming the odour of the thirty loads of dung), or would attract birds to the top of a tower. These were the signs that the quintessence was perfected. The quintessence so prepared was that of wine; but in order to extract their proper quintessences from any animal or vegetable materials, all that was required was to grind them up, let them putrefy (i.e. ferment), distil off a water, rectify it and circulate it as for making the quintessence of wine.

We must suppose that the result of these practical operations would simply be a strong spirit, and that the sky-blue colour mentioned was either a fiction deriving from the affinity of the quintessence to the blue heaven, or else the result of some accidental impurity. The *quinta essentia* of the Lullian texts was, therefore, as far as we can see, a very strong brandy, but was regarded by its makers as a concentration of the heavenly influence fixed in a noble and subtle body.

A substance so remarkable both in practice and in theory could not fail to attract attention, and, indeed, a long series of books deal with its preparation and virtues. Joannes de Rupescissa,[53] Jean de Roquetaillade, according to Trithemius, was a Franciscan friar who lived in Aquitaine in the first half of the fourteenth century. Certain texts are attributed to him in some manuscripts and to Lullius in others, but the *De quinta essentia*, which is printed in a rare volume of treatises[54] on related subjects, is certainly his.

The purpose of Rupescissa is to seek a thing which shall preserve and restore the body until the last day of death at the term fixed beforehand by God. To confer such incorruptibility a thing incorruptible is needed, so none of the four elements can avail. We must seek the thing which bears the same relation to the four qualities of the body as does the heaven to the four elements. This is the quintessence. This quintessence is called *aqua ardens, anima vini seu spiritus*, and *aqua vitae*. It contains 'our sun' and 'our stars', and it influences the body just as the true celestial bodies influence it.

Rupescissa's method of preparing the quintessence is in all important respects the same as that described in the texts attributed to Lullius and described in the last section. Having told us how to prepare an ardent spirit

----

[51] The punctuation of the 1546 edition here seems incorrect, and I have followed the Venice edition of 1542.

[52] The passage quoted is translated from *op. cit.* (41), lib. i, pt. ii, the 2nd canon.

[53] Ferguson, *Bibliotheca chemica*. Glasgow, 1906, vol. ii, p. 305.

[54] *Joannis de Rupescissa qui ante CCCXX annos vixit de consideratione quintae essentie rerum omnium, opus sane egregium. Arnaldi di Villanova epistola de sanguine humano distillato. Raymundi Lullii ars operativa: et alia quaedam . . . Accessit Michaelis Savonarolae libellus optimus de aqua vitae, nunc valde correctus quam ante annos 27 editus. Hieronymi Cardani libellus de aethere se quinta essentia vini.* Basileae, [n.d., but probably 1561]. Another edition appeared at Basle in 1597. The Cardan text is not contained in this work and is cancelled on the title-page. It exists elsewhere.

PLATE X

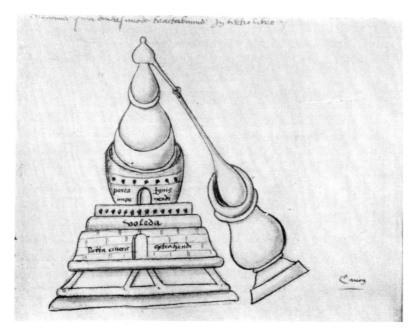

FIG. 2. Distillation of wine, from the Lullian *De secretis naturae*
(Bodleian Library, Oxford, Ashmole MS. 1484, fo. 8ᵛ)

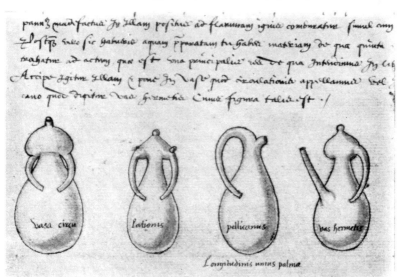

FIG. 3. Vessels for circulation, from the Lullian *De secretis naturae*
(Bodleian Library, Oxford, Ashmole MS. 1484, fo. 10ᵛ)

PLATE XI

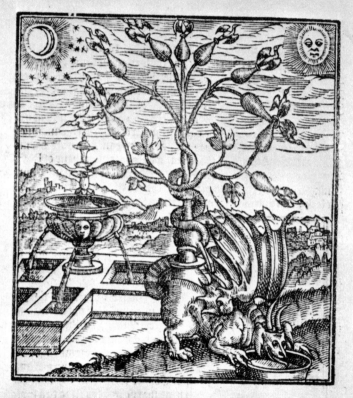

FIG. 4. The vine represented as a kind of still subtilising the mineral moisture to a volatile quintessence in sympathy with the heavenly bodies

(G. Baker, *The New Jewell of Health*, 1576, copied from Turneisser, 1570)

and circulate it, he goes on to describe how we are to fix the 'sun' in the 'heaven', i.e. make potable gold. This he does by repeatedly quenching hot leaves of gold in the *aqua ardens*. The 'heaven' could also extract the heavenly influences which resided in plants, etc., which had been influenced by the stars appropriate to their specific nature. Thus the quintessence could be rendered hot, cold, moist or dry, or could be given medicinal properties, by extracting with it the appropriate plant or animal material having that quality, the result being something—in fact, a solution of various essential oils, etc.—very like a liqueur. It is not unlikely that the complex liqueurs made by religious orders, for example, Benedictine,[55] with their immense variety of plant ingredients, are actual examples of a 'philosopher's heaven' in which have been fixed the stars of so many plants.

Michael Savonarola

The Paduan physician, Michael Savonarola, grandfather of the famous Girolamo, wrote on the quintessence about 1420–30. His work,[56] dedicated to Lionel, Marquis d'Este, was not published till 1532. It was reprinted in 1561[57] and 1598. He gives an excellent first-hand account of the distillation of alcohol from wine. In his time the retort was apparently preferred to the alembic, and the vapours were cooled by passing the condenser-tube through a wooden vessel of water, running water being preferable if large quantities were to be prepared. *Aqua vitae* was evidently beginning to pass from the condition of a heavenly medicine to that of a beverage, for Savonarola tells us:

> I am mindful of the words which that most eminent man, Antonius de la Scarparia, the most famous physician of the world in his time, was often wont to pronounce with a merry heart; for in his eightieth year he used to say '*O aqua vitae,* by thee my life has already been prolonged by twenty-two years!'

He discusses what is a reasonable dose, and mentions 'Giminianus tuus' who joyfully swallows eight ounces a day, and affirms with an oath to all that the taking of it is the reason why he has lived in good health to the age of eighty. Savonarola, however, deplores the levity with which this arcanum is treated, for he says:

> Let not him who desires to be healed by it hastily proceed to take it; but with much veneration, faith, and with the observations of worship, take it as another sacrament. . . How we must laugh at, nay rather pity, the ignorance of people who take it irreverently, and almost only when they have a hang-over (*fere soli crapulantes*).

Doubtless there exist in manuscript numerous fifteenth-century works concerned with distillation which I have not had the opportunity to see. Mention should be made of Joh. Wenod de Veteri Castro who (about 1420) described and figured the cooling of the condenser-tube by a water jacket.[58] I have also been unable to see the first edition of the very rare book of Michael

[55] Benedictine was invented in 1510 by Dom Bernardo Vincelli, who 'dabbled in Chemistry and was devoted to the preparation of medicinal beverages' (*Encyclop. Britannica*, 14th edition, sub 'Benedictine').

[56] Michael Savonarola, *De arte conficiendi aquam vitae simplicem et compositam deque ejus admirabili virtute ad conservandam sanitatem ad diversas humani corporis aegritudines curandas, libellus*. Hagenoae, apud Valent. Kobian, 1532. (Cited by Manget, *Bibliotheca scriptorum medicorum*, vol. ii, pt. ii, p. 161).

[57] *v.* note (54).

[58] Ferchl and Sussenguth, *A pictorial history of chemistry*. London, 1939, p. 50.

Schrick[59] printed at Augsburg in 1474. I have however seen the edition of 1521, and another very rare work by this author,[60] both of which I would regard as practical pharmacological treatises not dissimilar in character to, though much smaller than, Braunschweig's *Kleines Distillier-buch* of 1500.

Distillation Books of the Early Sixteenth Century

The principal place among these is taken by the works of Hieronymus Braunschweig (Brunschwyg, Brunschwick). It appears that his first distillation book, the *Liber de arte distillandi, de simplicibus,*[61] was first published in 1500. This, the *Kleines Distillier-buch*, was translated into English by Laurence Andrewe[62] in 1527. In 1504 Braunschweig produced a much larger book, usually termed *Liber de arte distillandi de compositis*. I have not had access to this edition but have used that[63] of 1519. In 1503 he published his *Medicinarius*,[64] the content of which is similar to that of the 1512 and 1519 editions of the *Liber de arte distillandi de compositis*, though it contains fewer illustrations of apparatus. No attempt is here made to give a complete bibliography of this complex subject, but rather to indicate the progress of ideas concerning the quintessence.

The earlier work begins by telling us what distillation is. In the words of Laurence Andrewe's translation:

> dystyllynge is none other thynge but only a puryfyenge of the grosse from the subtyll/ and the subtyll from the grosse/ eche seperatly from other/ and to thentent that the corruptyble shalbe mad incorroptyble/ and to make the materyall immateryall/ and the quycke spyryte to be made more quycker/ because it shold the soner perce and passe thrugh by the vertu of his great goodnesse and strengthe that therein is sonke and hyd for the conceyvgng of his helthfull operacyō in the body of man/ for distyllacyon is an elementall thyng/ for thrugh the movgng of the naturall Hevynes/ every one must be naturally governed by the bodies above/ lykewyse the body of man thrugh an experte master in medecynes/ and thrughe the waters that there ben devyded from the grossenes of the herbes eche in his substance/ and that to be conveyed to the place most nedfull for helthe and cōforte/ lyke as heafter more dylygently shalbe declared.

It may be noted that the distillate is still thought of as incorruptible, immaterial and living (quick). Lull's analogy of the heavens governing man's body can be traced, but Braunschweig at this period either failed to

[59] Michael Schrick, *Hienach volget eyn nützliche Materi von manigerley ausgeprannten Wassern wie man die nützen und prauchen Soll zu gesuntheyt des menschen.* Augspurg, J. Bämbler, 1474. (Cited from J. G. T. Grässe, *Trésor des livres rares et précieux.* Dresden, 1859–69.)

[60] [Michael Schrick] *Ein nutzlich puchlein von allen gebranntē Wassern Gerectfertiget auss dem newen distillir buch.* [c. 1500–02.]

[Michael Schrick] *Ausgebreñte und distillierte wasser / Wie sie zu jedem gebrestenn des menschēn leibs / und wo zu sunst deren gebrauch fürtregliche dienet / Nach Ordnung mitt grossen fleiss ietz new zusamen bracht und geordnet.* Zu Strassburg bei Christian Egenolphen. In Augst / Des M.D. und XXX Jars.

[61] [Hier. Braunschweig] *Liber de arte distillandi de simplicibus. Das buch der rechten Kunst zu distillieren die eintzige ding.* Ger. durch *Johannes grüeninger: Strassburg, in dem achte tag des mayer 1500.*

[62] *The vertuose boke of the distyllacyon of all manner of waters of the herbes in this present volume expressed with the figures of the stillatoryes, tr. out of duche by L. Andrewe.* London, 1527.

[63] *Das buch zu distillieren die zusamen gethonen ding Composita genant, durch die eintzigen ding, unt das büch Thesaurus pauperum, für die arman, durch experiment von mir Jheromyms Brunschwick aft geklubt und geoffenbart.* Strassburg, J. Grüniger, 1519.

[64] *Medicinarius. Das Buch der Gesundheit. Liber de arte distillandi simplicia et composita. Das nün Buch der rechte Kunst. . .* Strassburg, 1503.

understand it or has slurred its full implications. The author having declared what distillation is, proceeds to develop a very practical treatise on the subject. He mentions the preparation of *aqua vitae* by distillation in the 'pellycane', and at the end makes 'A fayre addycyon of an other master of the vertue of aqua vitae which is made of wyne/ or the feces' (i.e. dregs of wine). Here he gives the test for aqua vitae, found in Savonarola, that if a cloth be wetted with it and the aqua vitae lighted it should set fire to the cloth. The author gives a list of its virtues. It eases the diseases that come of cold, gives 'yonge corage' and a good memory, purifies the five wits of melancholy and of all uncleanness when it is drunk by reason and measure (five or six drops in a spoonful of wine in the morning), and so on. It relieves toothache when held in the mouth.

In Braunschweig's larger distillation book[63] there is a long section on the distillation of the quintessence. His fourth chapter (fo. xx recto *et seq.*) deals with the question of what *quinta essentia* is. It is not a thing composed of any of the four elements, since it is the soul and power and nobleness drawn out of the overplus of the elementary thing. It is not cold nor moist nor dry nor hot as are the other four elements. This question was debated, we learn, at the University of Padua in 1463, and physical reasons are given why the quintessence cannot be an element of air, fire, water or earth. It is a tempered complex which is very close to and above all elementary things, and so can bring man's body to a tempered state; the analogy of the lunar influence is again cited. It is the philosopher's heaven, etc.: in all this he follows the earlier authors. In the fifth chapter he proceeds to the practical details, which are clearly enough explained, but he gives few or no principles that do not appear in earlier manuscripts. The illustrations of circulatory vessels come from the Lullian manuscripts. Braunschweig's work is very practical throughout. He evidently believes fully in what Lull and Rupescissa say of the quintessence, but is not inclined to stress its mystical aspects.

The next distillation book was the *Cœlum philosophorum*[65] of Ulstadius, published at Friburg in 1525. Unlike Braunschweig's work it is principally concerned with the more superstitious aspects of distillation. The theme of the book is set out at the beginning under the heading *Canon generalis*. It reads: 'Stellarum vini, quae coelo philosophico applicantur, Cuiuscunque sint complexionis: naturae, seu proprietatis, ipsum cœlum perfectissime ad se trahit, Lullio, Arnoldo et Rupescissa Authoribus.' The work is far from being original. The figures are all taken from Braunschweig; some large sections of the text are also taken directly from the same source, while others come from earlier authors such as Rupescissa.

The Quintessence in the Works of Paracelsus

It may perhaps be said that the central idea of the writings of Paracelsus is the preparation of what we may term 'spiritual medicines', and the influence of the works we have been discussing, for example, the Lullian treatises and those of Rupescissa, is easily recognizable. His spiritual medicines are

[65] *Cœlum philosophorum seu de secretis naturae. Liber. Denuo revisus et castigatus. Philippo Ulstadio Patricio Nierenbegensi. c. Authore.* Friburg, 1525. (This appears to be the first recorded edition, though the 'Denuo revisus' etc. suggests an earlier issue. There are numerous later editions.)

classed as *arcana* and *quintessences*, but the distinction between his usage of these terms is not obvious. Thus in the *Paragranum*:

> It is not the physician that controls and directs, but heaven by the stars; and therefore the medicine must be brought to an airy form in such a manner that it may be directed by the stars. For what stone is lifted up by the stars? None but the volatile. Hence many have looked for the *quintum esse* in alchemy, which is nothing else but that in this way the four elements are removed from the arcanum, and what then remains is the arcanum. . . It should be known what astrum is in this particular arcanum and what is the astrum of this particular disease and what astrum is in the medicine against the disease.[66]

The stomach is the alchemist that prepares the medicine and makes the astra accept each other: the alchemist is an 'outer stomach' which prepares the medicine for the stars. Thus the medicine is 'directed', and brings about a concordance of the stars and the body.

Again in the *Labyrinthus medicorum errantium*:

> So also it is with medicine, which is made by God, but it is not made ready prepared in its final form, but instead is mixed with dross . . . the dross must be taken away and the medicine is there. That is alchemy.[67]

The third book of the *Archidoxis* is devoted to the Quintessences, and Paracelsus gives a full definition of what he intends by the word:

> The quinta essentia is a *materia* which is extracted bodily from all things, and from all things in which there is life, separated from all impurity and all that is mortal, made subtle and purified from all, separated from all elements. Now it is to be understood that the *quinta essentia* alone is the natural power, goodness and medicine, which is shut up in things without a harbourage and extraneous incorporation; further it may be the colours, the life and the property of the thing, and is a spirit like the spirit of life, with this difference that the *spiritus vitae* of the thing is permanent and the *spiritus vitae* of man is mortal.[68]

In physical fact, of course, nothing resembling such a quintessence can be prepared from the majority of bodies, least of all from the metals. Paracelsus believed he had prepared quintessences from the metals and gives recipes difficult of interpretation, in which the metals are dissolved, presumably in nitric acid or aqua regia, and distilled. The distillate (containing no metal in the majority of cases) was treated with alcohol. The same is true of the recipes for preparing the quintessences of 'marcasites', minerals, precious stones and similar bodies. The quintessences of plants, spices, and suchlike on the other hand are prepared by the traditional method of extraction with alcohol and distillation.

Among the 'magisteries' treated in the sixth book of the *Archidoxis* are the potable metals. These are made by taking *circulatum* (i.e. alcohol circulated by the Lullian process) and circulating this for four weeks with metal leaves—very much the same process as is described by Rupescissa. Paracelsus does not, however, acknowledge his debt to the earlier authors who wrote on the quintessence, for in his work *On the correction of impostures*[69] he condemns

[66] *Theophrast von Hohenheim gen. Paracelsus. Sämtliche Werke herausgeben von Karl Sudhoff.* 14 vols. Berlin, 1923–33, vol. viii, p. 185.

[67] *op. cit.* (66), vol xi, p. 187.

[68] *op. cit.* (66), vol. iii, p. 118.

[69] *Chirurgischer Bücher und Schriften . . . Philippi Theophrasti Bombast von Hohenheim . . . Durch Johannem Huserum Brisgoium.* Strassburg, 1605, vol. i, appendix, p. 55.

the treatises of Arnald da Villanova, of Rupescissa and of Ulstadius as utterly untrue; and it would appear that he did not identify the spirit distilled by their process with his ideal quintessence. It is noteworthy that he does not seem to use the word 'quintessence' to represent alcohol, and it is he who first gave to the latter substance the name of *alcool vini*.

The recipe for the 'magistery of wine'[70] gives perhaps the first account of the concentration of alcohol by freezing. A flask is filled with old wine, sealed, and digested in a dung bed for four months. It is then exposed to the severest winter weather until a part freezes; this is rejected and the rest is then digested on a sand-bath.

In the *Secundum manuale*, which is probably not a genuine work of Paracelsus but contains much of his practice, this recipe appears in a clearer form:

> *On secrets in wine.* Take wine and put it in a stoppered glass vessel in winter in the snow and let it stand overnight to make ice, and make a hole through the ice to the centre of the glass vessel and you will find there red wine not congealed, and it will not congeal. And that is the true quintessence of wine.

This is, of course, a perfectly feasible way of concentrating the alcohol in wine. The same work tells how a German alchemist of fifty years of age made spirit of wine and converted it into potable gold, and was transformed to the form of a youth of twenty. Evidence of popular belief in such feats appears in the letters of Erasmus, who speaks of the Quintessence in terms that seem to have a touch of irony:

> Est hic Medicus nostras, qui praesidio quintae essentiae prodigiosa designat facinora, e senibus iuvenes, e mortuis vivos facit: unde nonnulla spes est ut rejuvenescam si modo liceat Quintam Essentiam degustare!

The Quintessence in the later Sixteenth Century

After the time of Paracelsus we note a double movement of opinion about the Quintessence. The alchemical authors no longer tend to regard it as the physical substance, *aqua vitae*, then becoming familiar to all as a medicine or beverage, but rather to treat it as something far more subtle and hard to discover. The writers on distillation, on the other hand, tend to write plainly and simply about spirit of wine as a physical substance, and to drop the idea that it was a substance of a different order from other liquids.

An example of the former type of work is Leonhard Thurneysser's *Quinta essentia*,[71] which treats of the quintessence with a degree of obscurity that puts it as far out of reach as the philosopher's stone. The idea of the quintessence as a remote arcanum persists for more than a century, as is witnessed by the work of Tackius previously cited.[47] [Fig. 4.]

Leaving aside these arcane writers, we find that Braunschweig and Ulstadius were followed by a host of practical writers upon distillation. The earliest of these was Walther Hermann Ryff, whose work is mainly taken from Braunschweig. Amongst others may be mentioned Bartholome Vogter's

[70] *Archidoxis. Liber sextus. Extractio magisterii in vino.* Huser edition, Basle, 1590, pt. vi, pp. 67–8; also *Opera omnia.* 4 vols. Geneva, 1658, vol. ii, p. 24.

[71] *Quinta essentia Das ist die Höchste Subtilitet | Krafft | und Wirkung | Beider de Furtrefelichisten (und menschlichem gschlecht den nutzlichen) Könsten der Medicina und Alchemia . . . Durch Leonhart Turneisser.* [? Berlin], 1570.

little book, with perhaps the first printed illustration of a still-room as distinguished from pictures of the still itself.[72] Neither this nor the little work of Remaclus Fuchs[73] adds anything to the practice or theory of distillation. They are practical little books unconcerned with the theoretical or arcane aspects of the quintessence.

In 1551 Adam Lonicer published a work which contains a section *De arte distillatoria*.[74] This work is not concerned with the quintessence, but is notable for the fine series of figures of distillation apparatus, most of which appear to be original. It has what I believe to be the first sectional illustration showing the use of a worm-tube in a water-jacket, previous authors showing the condenser as a straight tube traversing the water-vessel. The use of a worm-tube is however probably very early, for a 'serpentinum' is mentioned in the Lullian texts.

We may mention also at this stage the excellent account of distillation apparatus given by Pietro Mattioli in the later editions of his commentaries on Dioscorides.[75] He does not concern himself with the quintessence or *aqua vitae* or potable gold.

Lonicer's work was followed in 1553 by a very popular book by Conrad Gesner, published anonymously as *Thesaurus Euonymi Philiatri*.[76] This was translated into many languages. Peter Morwyng, fellow of Magdalen College, Oxford, translated it into English[77] in 1559, and this translation was re-issued under a slightly different title in 1565.

George Baker's work, published in 1576 and referred to below, is largely derived from Gesner. Gesner follows Lullius and Ulstadius in what he says about the quintessence: he regards the various kinds of *aqua vitae* as drugs of very great potency, but he no longer has anything to say about their

[72] *Wie man alle gebresten und kranckhaiten des menschlichen leibs / ausswendig und ynwendig / võ dem haupt an biss auff die füss / artzneyen und vertreiben soll / mit auss gepranten wassern / Durch den weyt berümbtē Mayster Bartholomeũ Vogter / Augen Artzet zũ Dillingen / bey dem Hochwirdigen etc. Herrn / Herrn Christoffen Bischoff zũ Augspurg / Dem gemainen menschen zũ gũt / Newlich zusamen gesetzt und gezogen.* [Augsburg, H. Steyner, MDXXXI.] This rare first edition and the edition of 1533 are in the Wellcome Historical Medical Library. I have to thank Dr. D. I. Duveen for the loan of the rare 1541 edition.

[73] *Historia omnium aquarum quae in communi hodie practicantium sunt usu, vires, et recta eas distillandi ratio, libellus plane aureus, nunc in communem utilitatem evolgatus, per Remaclum F. Lymburgen. Accessit preterea conditorum (ut vocant) und specierum aromaticorum, quorum usus frequentior apud pharmacopolas, tractatus, omnibus quibus est medicina cordi non minus utilis quam necessarius.* Venetiis. Exc. Venturinus Rossinellus. MDXXXXII.

[74] *Naturalis historiae opus novum quo tractatur de natura et viribus arborum, fruticum, herbarum, animantiumque terrestrium, volatilium et aquatilium: Item, gemmarum, metallorum, succorumque concretorum, adeoque de vera cognitione, delectu et usu esse debet . . . Per Adamum Lonicerum . . . Accesserunt quaedam de stillatitiorum liquorum ratione, eiusque artis et instrumentorum usu atque de peculiaribus medicamentorum simplicium facultatibus.* Francofurti. [Preface dated 1551.] ('De arte distillatoria', pp. 337-49.)

[75] *Petri Andreae Matthioli Senensis medici commentarii sex libros Pedacii Dioscoridis Anazarbei de materia medica. . . .* Venetiis, MDLXV. (Earlier editions do not contain the work on distillation.)

[76] *Thesaurus Euonymi Philiatri, de remediis secretis, liber physicus, medicus, et partim etiam chymicus, et oeconomicus in vinorum diversi superis apparatur, medicis et pharmacopolis omnibus praecipue necessarius, nunc primum in lucem editus.* Tiguri, MDLIII.

[77] *The Treasure of Euonymus conteyninge the wonderful hid secretes of nature, touchinge the most apte formes to prepare and destyl medicines, for the conservation of helth: as Quintessence, Aurum potabile, Hippocras, Aromatical wynes, Balmes, Oyles, Perfumes, garnishyng waters, and other manifold excellent conjections. Wherunto are joyned the formes of sundry apt Fornaces, and vessels, required in this art. Translated (with great diligence and labour) out of Latin by Peter Morwyng fellow of* Magdaline Colleadge *in Oxford.* London, 1559.

immaterial or spiritual character. These liquors were evidently becoming familiar. It would be an impossible task to follow all the mentions of *aqua vitae* made during the sixteenth century, but its degradation from the status of a spiritual arcanum was complete when it became a customary beverage. This seems to have occurred at the end of the sixteenth century. Thus George Baker in his *Newe Jewell of Health*,[78] largely taken from Gesner, tells us that its 'use has grown so common with the neather Germanie, and Flaunders, that freelier then is profitable to health, they take and drinke of it'; and this tendency is again mirrored by the fact that in 1592 the Senate of Nürnberg legislated against certain secret taverns which sold *aqua vitae*, which was the concern of pharmacists alone.[79] Usquebaugh (lit., water of life) is mentioned as an Irish drink at least as early as 1420, but it must be doubted if this was a distilled liquor. The Irish Usquebaugh which is mentioned in 1581 was, however, almost certainly a distilled spirit: and the Scots variety is mentioned very shortly after this date.[80]

Once the public was consuming *aqua vitae* freely they knew just what its virtues were, and the idea of a quintessence as a separate and higher form of matter soon became obsolete. But the word has survived as a metaphor, and the terms *eau de vie* and 'spirits' may serve to remind us of the days when ethyl alcohol seemed to be the link between earth and heaven.

[78] *The New Jewell of Health, wherein is contayned the most excellent Secretes of Phisicke and Philosophie, devided into fower Bookes. In the which are the best approved remedies for the diseases as well inwarde as outwarde, of all the partes of mans bodie: treating very amplye of all Dystillations of Waters, of Oyles, Balmes, Quintessences, with the extraction of artificiall Saltes, the use and preparation of Antimonie, and potable Gold. Gathered out of the best and most approved Authors, by that excellent Doctor Gesnerus. Also the Pictures and maps to make the Vessels, Furnaces and other Instrumentes thereunto belonging. Faithfully corrected and published in Englishe by George Baker, Chirurgian.* London, 1576.

[79] *Leges ac Statuta Ampliss. Senatus Norimbergensis, ad Medicos, Pharmacopoeos et alios pertinentia.* Noribergae. MDXCVIII. (Stat. xxx.)

[80] Since this paper was written there has appeared a *Short history of the art of distillation* by R. J. Forbes, Leyden, 1948. This work gives an admirable account of the later history of the development of the manufacture and use of spirits.

BOOK III

THE RENAISSANCE

THE SCHOOL OF FERRARA AND THE
CONTROVERSY ON PLINY*

by

ARTURO CASTIGLIONI

I

AMONG the writers of classical Latin whose works played an important role in the development of scientific thought in the Middle Ages and the Renaissance, Gaius Plinius Secundus, the Elder (A.D. 23–79), undoubtedly deserves an outstanding place. The history of his life, very well known through the famous letters of his nephew Plinius Caecilius to Tacitus, gives us an interesting and dramatic description of the remarkable activity of this great scholar, passionately devoted to study. He played a role in the history of the great conquests, accompanying or leading the victorious march of the Roman legions in Germany, Spain, and Gaul. Vespasian trusted him with the government of Gallia Narbonensis and later of a province of Spain. He was in Africa and became eventually the Prefect of the Roman Fleet at Misenum, one of the most important naval stations of the Empire. He does not seem to have had any part in the political intrigues of his time; a friend of Vespasian, he enjoyed the confidence of Titus and Augustus, and devoted all his activities to his military duties and to his studies. He surely was, as we can judge from his writings, a man of vast interest in all fields of science, eager to learn and to collect with remarkable diligence matters of interest from all the books he was reading. He was always accompanied by a shorthand writer, to whom he dictated extracts and notes from the works which he was reading. He left his nephew a hundred and sixty volumes in manuscript.

When Vesuvius erupted in A.D. 79—the eruption which subsequently destroyed Herculaneum and Pompeii—Pliny immediately went to the danger area in order to observe the facts. At Stabiae he followed attentively and took notes of the increasing fury of the volcano. On the third day he dined cheerfully, refusing to take shelter or to abandon the place. In the afternoon he lay down to rest. The torrents of lava flowed over the city and the house, and his body was found three days later, uninjured.

The *Historia Naturalis*, the only book by Pliny which has survived, has enjoyed an immense popularity for many centuries. It has been so often studied, discussed and quoted that this is not the place to describe the contents of this work. Books xx to xxxii deal with medical observations, prescriptions, stories, superstitions, and magical beliefs connected with medicine. It has been often said, and it is true, that Pliny is amusing, and pleasant to read; sometimes his ingenuity is fascinating and his remarks astonishing. I think one could say that Pliny was a great journalist: he tried

* The inspiration for this essay came from the scholarly chapter on ' Science under the Roman Empire' by Charles Singer, in his *From Magic to Science* (London, Benn, 1928). Singer has studied with an original conception and with diligent research the period of transition from magic to scientific critical learning, and has written some interesting pages about Pliny, whose book he calls 'the prototype of medical writings for fifteen centuries'. In that chapter he gives a brilliant critical appreciation of Pliny's work.

to collect as much information as possible from different sources, some of which were not very reliable, to put it in order, and then to present the result of his inquiry and of his observations to the attention of his readers, uncritically and without drawing any reasoned conclusions. As a reporter he never assumes the role of a judge, even when he evidently does not accept what he has been told. Often he adds: 'I have been told so', or 'people believe that', or 'this is the general opinion'; but very cautiously he never asserts his own belief, nor does he ever either affirm or deny the statements made by others. The *Natural History* of Pliny is undoubtedly a most complete collection of primitive beliefs, and a magnificent contemporary picture of the state of knowledge in all fields. Pliny had read, extracted and quoted an enormous number of books. He had stored an immense knowledge, and his work, illustrating directly or indirectly the evolution of science from the oldest sources, is invaluable for the historian. During the Middle Ages, Pliny was probably less popular among the physicians than Dioscorides. His book, however, was much sought after, and it was the first to be printed after the Bible, in 1469.

The partly inexact, rarely precise, but very numerous descriptions of plants and seeds, and the great number of therapeutic directions made the book a rich source for students; it was often consulted by the authors of the herbals. Pliny's book was not intended to appeal to physicians or scholars, but directly to the common people. Pliny was an enemy of physicians and did not miss any opportunity of bitterly criticizing their work. He attacked many of them personally and accused them of cheating their patients, taking care only of their own interests. His book was written as a popular encyclopaedia, to which everybody might appeal directly and find some important information, some stories and some advice. The result of this attempt is that the book abounds with descriptions of the customs, the beliefs, the superstitions, and the current ideas of Pliny's day. At that time a definite boundary between superstition and objective experience was practically non-existent, and primitive traditional magical medicine was still flourishing. Observer and naturalist as he was, Pliny declares himself to be an enemy of magicians and wonder-healers, but nevertheless, he accepts and recommends remedies the efficacy of which is evidently founded only on belief in magic. He does not attach any great importance to the doctrines of Hippocrates, and does not even try to analyse or explain his prescriptions. He is neither correct nor original in his botanical descriptions nor in his names for herbs, and he leans heavily on Theophrastus and the minor writers. But it is his fundamental belief that in nature all remedies may be found.

In the field of folk medicine, Pliny's work marked a milestone in medical history. He collected information from all kinds of people and different parts of the world. The continuous ardent thirst for knowledge is the foremost characteristic of his personality.

II

In the fifteenth century, when classical writers achieved the highest honours and all Latin authors appeared worthy of praise and diligent study, Pliny was one of the first to attract the attention of physicians, of naturalists, and

PLATE XII

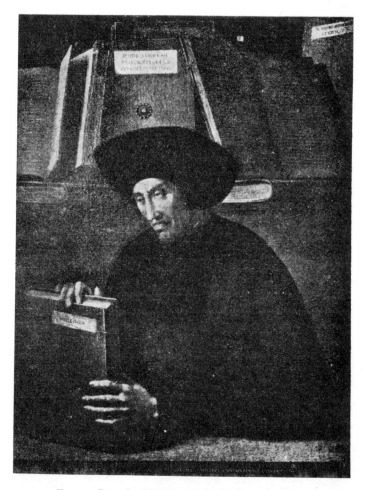

Fig. 1.   Portrait of Leonicenus by L. Costa, in Ferrara

(Published for the first time by P. Capparoni in *Rivista ital. d. storia d. sci. med.,*
1942, xxxiii, p. 5)

PLATE XIII

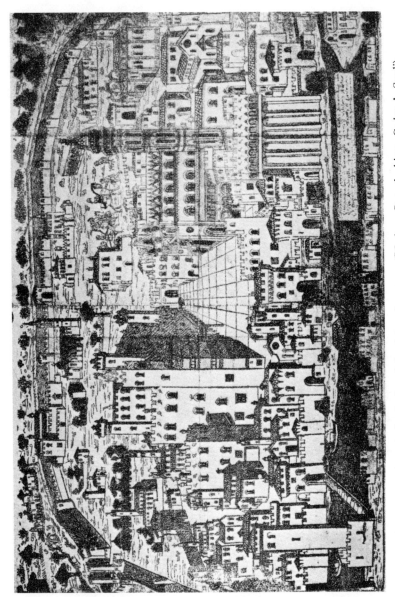

FIG. 2. Ferrara at the beginning of the sixteenth century. (Modena, State Archives, Codex A. Sardi)

especially of *literati*. The revival of Pliny and the enthusiastic welcome given to his work were characteristic of the Italian scholarship of the last decades of the fifteenth century. The *Historia Naturalis* was one of the most popular books, familiar to students and to teachers. It was in fact the easiest to understand and the most amusing to read. The interest in Pliny was only a sign, but one of the most obvious signs, of the new flow of studies in natural history which derived from it. It was, on the other hand, connected also with the increasing reaction against Arabism, which had been in great favour in the Italian universities at the end of the thirteenth century. In the field of natural history it was manifestly necessary to have an indisputable authority, and no classical author other than Pliny could have assumed this role. Pliny was acclaimed as one of the most authoritative teachers of natural science.

It was at the end of the fifteenth century that there began the famous controversy about Pliny which constitutes a significant episode, marking as it does the beginning of the criticism which some have regarded as a decisive revolt against scholasticism. In reality it was at first only a cautious literary attack. The central figure in this episode was Nicolò Leoniceno, professor of medicine at the School of Ferrara. Ferrara had been the centre of humanistic studies since Hugo Benzi, a famous physician and humanist, had been called from the service of Nicolò III of Este to teach at the University. The Council of Ferrara (1437) played an important role in the history of the church and of humanism. Benzi, who was very well versed in Greek philosophy and was considered the prince of classical scholars, took no active part in the meetings of the Council, but in a famous discussion which took place in the house of the d'Este, and which was attended by a great number of high ecclesiastics from all countries, he delivered some memorable speeches which showed his vast erudition and perfect knowledge of the classical texts. The humanistic School of Ferrara had been founded by Alessandro Guarino, a scholar of great renown, to whose lectures students flocked from every part of Europe.

Nicolò Leoniceno (Leonicenus) (1428–1524), born in Lonigo near Vicenza, was surely the most famous of the teachers at the School of Ferrara. He had been a pupil of Ognibene de'Bonisoli, professor of rhetoric and Greek and annotator of Latin and Greek classics. At the age of eighteen he was perfectly familiar with Latin literature. He studied medicine at Pavia, and it is said that he succeeded in answering all the questions at his examination in the classics. It seems that he was then for some time in England, to which country he had been invited by some of the English students whom he had met, but we have no certain information on this point. In 1464 he was called from the service of Borso d'Este, first Duke of Ferrara, to teach at the University. The connexion between medicine and philosophy in the universities of the fifteenth century was so close that Leonicenus began by teaching Greek philosophy; and though he was later appointed to the chair of theoretical medicine, he became an authority in the field of classical medical literature rather than in that of practical medicine. He was a friend of another famous scholar, Valla, who was for some time a professor in Ferrara, and of Erasmus of Rotterdam, who spoke of Leonicenus with admiration. In this group of scholars of Ferrara there was a courageous tendency to criticize the classical texts. In 1490 Leonicenus was a guest of Lorenzo de Medici in Florence. He was welcomed very cordially and he became a friend of Angelo Poliziano, an exquisite poet and Latinist, whose criticisms of the classical texts seem to have inspired Leonicenus' activity. He began to follow the examples of other scholars, such as Coluccio Salutati, who had been the first to emend the texts of Sallust and Varro, and who was followed by Pomponius Mela. Leonicenus was evidently more interested in Pliny and the medical writers. When Politian published his *Miscellaneae* and sent him a copy, Leonicenus dedicated to him the manuscript of his *De Plinii aliorumque in medicina erroribus*. The book was printed in Ferrara *apud Magistrum Laurentium de Valentia et Andream de Castronovo socios* in December 1492. It is a small book of eighteen leaves. It is remarkable that this work, which provoked a literary storm, was not written by a young rebel. Leonicenus was sixty-four years old, a mature scholar, at the time when the work appeared to which he owes a lasting fame, and many bitter sorrows. The text is preceded by a letter from Politian to the author, dated 3 January 1491, in reply to the dedication of the manuscript to Politian. Hence it is obvious, as Thorndyke has admitted, that the work with the dedication to Politian which has not survived, had circulated in manuscript; this may explain the difference in the dates. In his letter Politian, while acknowledging the merits of Leonicenus, does not conceal his regret at the attacks on Pliny, and he quotes one of Leonicenus' criticisms in order to show that the attacks were hardly justifiable.

The book was considered, on account of the importance of the persons involved in the contest and of the controversy which it originated, as a powerful and decisive attempt to attack scholastic dogmatism in the person of one of its most famous representatives. Albrecht von Haller called Leonicenus 'the first who dared, after many centuries, to be acutely critical', and Sprengel, in his *History*, praised Leonicenus as the most courageous innovator of his time: 'His work marks the beginning of a new and very flourishing epoch in the study of medicine, and there is no other work in the history of medicine which deserves comparison with it.' The praise of Sprengel and the earlier eulogy of Haller seem, however, to be exaggerated. In fact, reading attentively the first work of Leonicenus, one immediately sees that there is nowhere even the slightest criticism of Pliny's judgement nor of his medical prescriptions; nor is there any discrimination in the matter of superstitions and legends. The attack on Pliny is chiefly a literary criticism of the text, and an attempt to identify the plants, since Pliny had sometimes confused the Latin and the Greek names. The first attack is therefore of little importance from the scientific point of view; it never starts from clinical observation, and it does not criticize the treatment suggested by Pliny. An important item in the discussion is whether and how far Pliny had consulted and copied Dioscorides and Theophrastus. Pliny is criticized as a learned scholar and not as an expert physician—which he never claimed to be. The criticism turns on the correctness of the definitions. The whole discussion is therefore—especially in the first edition of the book—chiefly philological, in the style of Valla, Politian and other humanists. The opinions of Pliny and his authority are never really considered. Thorndyke correctly notes that Leonicenus himself still accepted many superstitions; for instance,

PLATE XIV

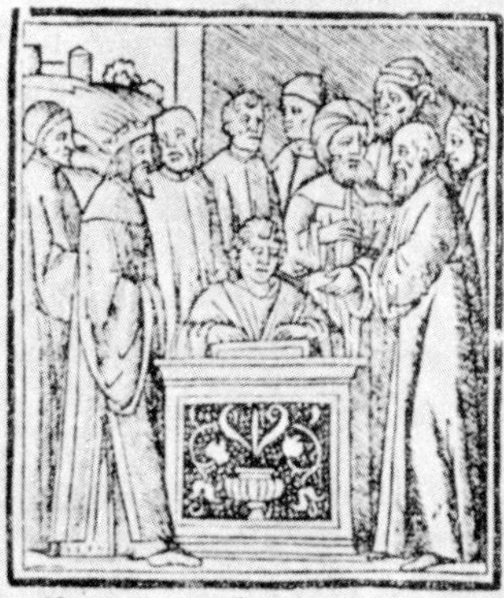

CAII PLINII SECVNDI VERONENSIS NATVRALIS HISTORIÆ LIBER PRIMVS.

C.Plinius Secundus Veronensis.T.Vespasiano suo Salutem.

PRÆFATIO.

LIBROS NATVRALIS historiæ, nouitiū camœnis quiritiū tuorū opus natum apud me proxima fœtura, licentiore epistola narrare constitui tibi iucundissime Imperator (sit enim hæc tui præfatio uerissima, dum maximo consenescit in patre.) Nāq; tu solebas putare esse aliqd meas nugas, Vt obiicere moliar Catullum conterraneum meum (agnoscis & hoc castrense uerbū.Ille.n.ut scis) ꝑmutatis prioribus syllabis duriusculum se fecit,q̄ uolebat existimari a uernaculis tuis & famulis. Simul ut hæc mea petulantia fiat,quod ꝓxime non fieri questus es in alia procaci epistola nostra,ut in quædā acta exeam. Sciantq; oēs q̄ ex æquo tecū uiuat iperiū. Triūphalis & cēsorius tu sextūq; cōsul,ac tribunitiæ potestatis particeps,Et quod his nobilius fecisti,dum illud patri,pariter & equestri ordini præstas,præfectus prætorio eius,omniaq; hæc reipu.Et nobis quidē qualis in castrensi cōtubernio? Nec quicq̄ mutauit in te fortunæ amplitudo in iis,nisi ut prodesse tātundē posses,ut uelles. Itaq; cū cæteris in uenerationē tui pateāt omnia illa,nobis ad colēdū te familiarius audacia sola superest. Hanc igitur tibi imputabis,& in nostra culpa tibi ignosces. Perfricui faciē,nec tamē ꝓfeci,quando alia uia occurris ingens,& longius etiam submoues ingenii facibus. Fulgurat i nullo unq̄ uerius dicta uis eloquentiæ,tribunitiæ potestatis facundia. Quanto tu ore pr̄is laudes tonas? quāto fr̄is amas? Quantus in poetica es? O magna fœcunditas animi. Quēadmodū fratrē quoq; imitareris excogitasti. Sed hæc quis posset intrepidus æstimare subiturus ingenii tui iudiciū,præsertim lacessitū? Neq; enim similis est cōditio publicātiū, & nominatim tibi dicantium. Tum possem dicere,quid ista legis imperator? Humili uulgo scripta sunt,agricolarum,opificum turbæ,deniq; studiorum ociosis. Quid te iudicem facis. Cum hanc operam cōdicerem,nō eras in hoc albo. Maiorem te sciebā,q̄ ut descensurum huc putarē. Præterea est quædā publica etiā eruditorū reiectio. Vtitur illa & M. Tullius extra omnē ingenii aleam positus. Et quod miremur per aduocatū defēditur. Hæc doctissimū + oīum Persiū legere nolo. × Lesiu Decimū uolo. Qđ si hoc Lucilius,qui primus cōdidit stili nasum,dicendū sibi putauit. Si cicero mutuādū,præsertim cum de republi.scriberet,quāto nos causatius ab aliquo iudice defendimur? Sed hæc ego mihi nūc patrocinia ademi nuncupatione. Quamplurimū refert,sortiatur aliquis iudicē,an eligat. Multūq; apparatus itererest apud inuitatum hospitem & oblatū,cū apud Catonē illū ambitus hostem,& repulsis tanq̄ honoribus ✢ ineptis gaudentem,flagrantibus comitiis pecunias deponerēt candidati,hoc se facere pro innocētia,quod in rebus humanis summū esse profitebantur,inde illa nobilis. M.Ciceronis suspiratio. O te fœlicē. M.Porci, a quo rem improbā petere nemo audet. Cum tribunos appellaret. L. Scipio Asiaticus,inter quos erat Gracchus, hoc attestabatur,uel inimico iudici se approbare posse. Adeo summū quisq; causæ suæ iudicem facit, quēcunq; eligit,unde prouocatio appellatur. Te quidem in excelsissimo humani generis fastigio positum,summa eloquētia,summa eruditione præditū,religiose adiri etiam a salutātibus scio. Et ideo immensa præter cæteras subit cura,ut quæ tibi dicantur,cōdigna sint. Verū & diis lacte rustici multæq; gentes supplicant,& mola tantum salsa litant,qui non habent thura. Nec ulli fuit uitio deos colere quoquomodo posset. Meæ quidem temeritati accessit hoc quoq;,q; leuioris operæ hos tibi dedicaui libellos. Nam nec ingenii sunt capaces,quod alioquī nobis perq̄mediocre erat. Nec admittunt excessus,aut orationes,sermonesue, aut casus mirabiles,uel euentus uarios,nō alia iucunda dictu,ac legentibus blanda. Sterili materia rerū natura, hoc est uita narratur. Et hæc sordidissima sui parte,ut plurimarū rerum aut rusticis uocabulis,aut externis, immo barbaris cum honoris præfatiōe ponendis. Præterea iter est non trita authoribus uia,nec qua peregrinari animus expectet. Nemo apud nos quidem qui attentauerit. Nemo apud græcos qui unus omnia ea tractauerit inuenitur. Magna pars studiorum amœnitates quærimus. Quæ uero tractata ab aliis dicuntur, immensæ subtilitatis,obscuris rerum tenebris ꝑmuntur,iam omnia attingenda quæ græci τὰς ἐγκυκλοπαιδείας uocant,& tamen ignota,aut incerta ingeniis facta. Alia uero ita multis prodita,ut in fastidium sint adducta. Res ardua,uetustis nouitatem dare,nouis authoritatem,obsoletis nitorem,obscuris lucem, fastiditis gratiam,dubiis fidem,omnibus uero naturam,& naturæ suæ omnia,itaq; etiam nō assecutis,uoluisse abunde pulchrum atq; magnificum est. Equidem ita sentio peculiarem in studiis causam eorum esse, qui difficultatibus uicti utilitatem iuuandi prætulerūt gratiæ placendi,idq; & in aliis operibus ipse feci,& profiteor me mirari Liuium authorem celeberrimum in historiarum suarum, quas repetit ab origine urbis

aa iiii

FIG. 3. First page of Pliny, *Historia Naturalis*, Venice, 1525
The author is shown writing his book

PLATE XV

Fig. 5. First page of Colleuccio, *Pliniana Defensio*, Ferrara, 1493

Fig. 4. First page of Leonicenus, *De erroribus Plinii*, first edition, Ferrara, 1492

he asserted that a root of cyclamen is so inimical to pregnant women that when a woman with child steps over it, abortion results; that the female viper in conceiving bites off the head of its mate, and that the young gnaw their way out of the body of the mother. One of the questions most discussed concerned the nature of cinnabar. Pliny had upheld the old belief that it was formed from the blood of the dragon and of the elephant mingled in their mortal combat. Leonicenus asserted that cinnabar is a mineral substance, but other authors had already corrected this mistake of Pliny.

We are not able to judge what reaction this book by Leonicenus produced in medical circles; the professors and doctors were silent. But immediately after the work had been published another humanist entered the contest. Pandolfo Collenuccio, a friend of the Dukes Gonzaga and Podestà of Mantua, had no connexion with medical studies. He was a lawyer—*leguleius quidem* as Leonicenus contemptuously calls him without mentioning his name—who published some apologues and comedies. His *Pliniana defensio* was printed in Ferrara by Andreas Bellfortus Gallicus. It is undated, but it must have been published very early in 1493, a few weeks after the publication of Leonicenus' work, because it is quoted by Hermolaus Barbarus in his *Castigationes* published in the same year. Collenuccio is from many points of view better informed and certainly more exact than Leonicenus. It must be admitted that the lawyer's criticism is more rational than that of the professor of medicine. In fact, he made the definite observation that, if anyone wants to judge correctly the importance and efficacy of a remedy, philological discussion is futile. Collenuccio had evidently had the chance to study botany and herbals, and he did not lack some practical botanical experience. He tells of having talked with herbalists in Venice, and he seems to have collected plants and objects of interest in the study of natural history. His answer was prepared rapidly, and, as it appeared three weeks after the publication of Leonicenus' book, it seems probable that he had had access to his manuscript. The work appears to have been the result of a careful study of the subject and shows more than a superficial knowledge of botany. It is in seven books, in the form and style of a legal defence, and his attacks on Leonicenus are sometimes severe.

The second defender of Pliny was less aggressive but more weighty. He was Hermolaus Barbarus, a man of great authority. His work was published in November 1492 in Rome by Eucharius Argentus Germanus, and a second edition by the same printer with some additions and notes by Pomponius Mela appeared in February 1493. Hermolaus Barbarus (1444–93), the author of the *Castigationes Plinianae*, was considered one of the greatest humanists of his time. He had been a student in Padua, where he had obtained his degree in 1477. He published a scholarly commentary on Aristotle, and in 1486 was sent as Venetian Ambassador to Frederick III, and in 1488 to Pope Innocent VIII, who created him Patriarch of Aquileja. He had a vast knowledge of Greek and Latin literature, and it was an important moment when he became a participant in the controversy.

The *Castigationes Plinianae* are superficially a series of corrections of Pliny's mistakes, on the lines of Leonicenus. In fact, Barbarus claimed to have corrected more than five thousand errors, supposedly due to copyists and

I   s

printers; but at the same time he declared that it was impossible to admit that Pliny himself had made mistakes, and that therefore his fame was unassailable. This long book, written in a scholastic vein with many repetitions and sometimes with long discussions about the spelling of a word, is therefore not intended to be essentially an attack on Leonicenus, who is never even referred to by name. However, in different parts of the book the assertions of Leonicenus are contradicted. We now see that this work of Barbarus is a humanistic exercise in a purely literary form. Barbarus had no knowledge of medicine or botany. He tries only to clarify the botanical definitions and to identify some plants; and, at the same time, he strongly defends Pliny's name and reputation against all attacks.

The work of such a man, who enjoyed a great reputation as an outstanding scholar and who was a friend of the Emperor and the Pope, required an immediate answer from Leonicenus. In the same year 1493 the latter wrote his reply to Barbarus, who however died before he could read it. This letter was not published until 1509, and then Leonicenus expressed his reverence for the great scholar and lamented his death; but he justified himself for having dared to attack Pliny. He said that he had done so only to correct verbal slips and errors of description, which he admitted could have been ascribed to copyists. He tried to excuse himself by quoting among others Giovanni Francesco della Mirandola, who had also observed many errors in Pliny. Leonicenus stood by all his former corrections. His behaviour towards Barbarus was very respectful, but towards Collenuccio obviously contemptuous, perhaps because he resented this work, which was an outspoken attack against his medical authority.

But the sorrows of Leonicenus had not yet come to an end. In 1509 Lodovico Bonaccioli of Ferrara, a physician, entered the contest. He published the treatise of Leonicenus with additional comments and discussions. The book was published in Ferrara, *per Ioannem Macciochium.*

A disciple of Leonicenus, Ludovico Pontico Virunnio, arose to defend him against the attack of Collenuccio (Ferrara, 1509, *per Ioannem Macciochium*).

Among other adversaries were the famous anatomists Alessandro Benedetti, Antonio de Ferraris (under the Latin name of Galateus), and Filippo Beroaldo, in a commentary on the work of Barbarus published in 1496. There were many others, among whom are two who were only briefly mentioned by Leonicenus, namely 'a teacher of boys' and 'a grammarian'. In the edition of 1509 the text of *De erroribus* is divided into four chapters and has 98 leaves. It contains many criticisms of Avicenna and other Arabian authors, many corrections of mistakes in anatomical descriptions of Mundinus, and especially a long discussion on the confusion between the pharynx and the larynx. It also contains a very exhaustive discussion on the composition of the theriacum according to different authors, and especially on the role of viper flesh in its composition. Pliny and others had asserted that European vipers were not to be used in this composition, but Leonicenus gives examples to show that their use is advisable. This question, and the discussion on serpents, was again dealt with by Leonicenus later on in his works on serpents (*De tiro seu vipera*, Venice, 1497: *De vipera libellus*, Venice, 1506: *De dipseade et pluribus aliis serpentibus*, Bologna, 1518; Basel, 1532)

PLATE XVI

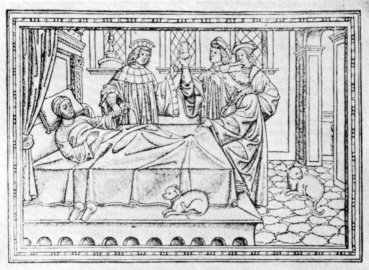

ꝛureum opus ꝛ fublime ad medellã non parum ꝑtile
ℙlinÿ pbilofopbi ꝛ medici itegerrimi.nõnullaꝗ
opufcula ꝑidelicet Joãnis ꝛlmenar:ℕicolai
ℒeoniceni iterpꝛetis fideliſſimi ambobus:
ꝺe moꝛbo gallico ꝑt ꝑulgo dicitur:ꝛn
geli ꟓolognini ꝺ cura ꝑlcerũ ꝑterio
rum:ꝛleꝛãdri ꟓenedicti ꝺe peſte:
ꝛ ꟓominici ꝛꝛcignanei ꝺe põ
deribus ꝛ mẽfuris nuper
inuẽti ad pꝛaꝛim quã/
maꝛie neceſſarÿ
feliciter in/
ℒum gratia   cipiunt.   ꝛ ℙꝛiuilegio.
✠

FIG. 6.   First page of *Aureum Opus Plinii Ad Medellam*, Bologna, 1516, which
contained the work by Leonicenus on Syphilis

PLATE XVII

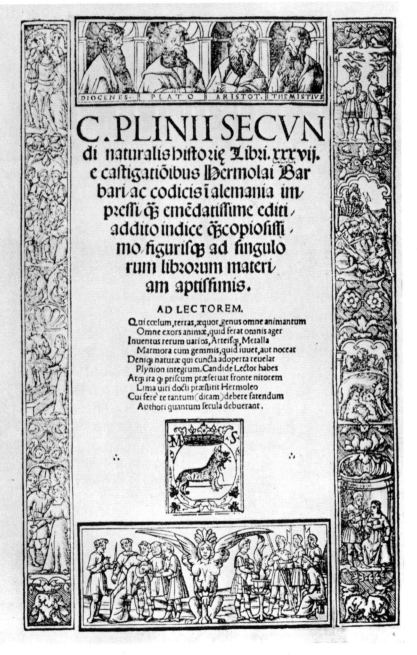

FIG. 7. Title-page of Pliny, *Historia Naturalis*, Venice, 1525
This edition contained the *Castigationes* of Hermolaus Barbarus

Another humanist attacked by Leonicenus is Gentile da Foligno for his description of the duodenum and of the bile duct. The second edition shows a remarkable improvement on the first. The attack on Leonicenus must have spurred him to more attentive and courageous critical work; in this edition and in the following we find him very cautious in his manner but decided in his opinion.

This edition of 1509 contains a letter of Hieronymus Menochius, a physician who staunchly supported the judgment of Leonicenus. The fourth book is dedicated to Franciscus Tottus of Lucca, who also wrote a strong defence of his teacher, which is published in the same book.

Among the supporters we should mention a physician of the Leipzig school, Martin Pollich of Mellerstadt, who published a *Defensio Leoniceniana* (Magdeburg, 1499). Besides this, many other physicians entered the field in the second phase of the controversy, in which, as we have seen, the criticism was no longer limited to philological discussion, but dealt also with many important anatomical and physiological questions. Not only Pliny but many other famous authors now came under fire.

On still another occasion Leonicenus was concerned with Pliny. In 1509 a book by Stephanus Guilliretus, *C. Plinii Secundi Medicinae libri quinque*, was published in Rome. It was the first printed edition of the so-called 'Plinian medicine', sometimes erroneously attributed, following a suggestion of the historian Paolo Giovio, to Plinius Valerianus. Of this Plinian or pseudo-Plinian medicine different manuscripts exist. They are evidently the work of some compilers of the third or fourth century A.D., who collected portions of Pliny's book and added some chapters from the works of others. The first edition, as we have said, was published in Rome in 1509. In 1516 another book appeared with a somewhat different title, *Aureum Opus, Integerrimi Philosophi et Medici, C. Plinii Secundi ad medellam non parum utile*. This book was published in Bologna by a well-known printer, Hyeronymus de Benedictis, who had published Galen's works with a commentary by Leonicenus. This new edition of the 'Plinian medicine' differs greatly from the edition of 1509, and also from the later Basle edition of 1528. It is very little known, and it appears to have been published simultaneously by Benedictus Geraldus in Padua, since his name is on the colophon of one of the two copies in the British Museum. Kristeller knows of only three copies. A copy of this rare book is in the library of the New York Academy of Medicine. This volume includes a 'psuedo-Plinian medicine' printed, as the publisher states, from a very old manuscript, and also a reprint of the work on syphilis by Leonicenus, which we will mention later. It may appear strange that Leonicenus, who had been such a careful student of Pliny's genuine work, should have agreed to his book on syphilis being published along with a spurious book by Pliny which had never been accepted by the scholars, and by a printer with whom he was certainly on the best of terms. This arrangement encourages the reader to assume that, when Leonicenus speaks, in the preface to his book on syphilis, of his having corrected the mistakes of Pliny, he is referring to this work of Pliny, which is found in the same volume. This erroneous opinion is strengthened by the fact that on the first page of the book Leonicenus is referred to as the interpreter 'of both' (*ambobus*)—that is, of both the 'pseudo-Pliny' and of the book on syphilis by Juan de Almenar, which precedes his in the same volume.

The vast activity of Leonicenus in other fields of medical literature is directly connected with his first work. He appeared to students and doctors as a courageous fighter, as a man who was able to present the great medical classics in a new light; in fact, with these flattering words, Erasmus of Rotterdam praised his activity. The attack on Pliny had put Leonicenus in the spot light at a time when Ferrara was the centre of literary studies, and prominent teachers and students from all parts made the school famous in the world of learning.

III

The book on syphilis by Leonicenus (*De Epidemia, quam vulgo Morbum Gallicum vocant*), published in a beautiful edition by Aldus Manutius in Venice in June 1497, appeared two months later in another edition in Milan and in the year 1499 in Leipzig. It is evident that the book became at once extremely popular. It is not unimportant in the controversy regarding Pliny. The book is dedicated to Giovanni Francesco della Mirandola, and in the letter of dedication Leonicenus resurrects again the Pliny controversy. He mentions that G. F. della Mirandola had found many errors in Pliny, and then adds:

> We want to mention this to the malicious and shameless people who, guided by hatred, utter calumnies against those who have found errors in Pliny—in silence they approve—which they could not find themselves. I refer also to those who like sheep always follow others, and rely only on the judgement of others. These looked at first with favour on our writings, but we are hoping more to enjoy the applause of honest and learned people and especially your approval.

The book on syphilis marks another step in the activity of Leonicenus as a critic of classical works. He says that the book had its origin in an academic disputation in Ferrara, and the academic element is emphasized throughout. Charles Singer made an exhaustive study of it in his edition of Sudhoff's *Earliest Printed Literature on Syphilis* (Florence, 1925), in which the book by Leonicenus is reproduced in facsimile. Singer correctly observes that the work is largely made up of criticisms of Avicenna and of his commentators. There are endless discussions of the pathological errors of the great Arabian. The ancients were not forgotten, and the shortcomings of Pliny are again soundly criticized.

The book has to be considered chiefly as an attack on astrology and the contemporary attribution of the origin of epidemics to unfavourable positions of the stars. Syphilis is believed to be a punishment for sins committed, or to be due to corruption of the air. The clinical observations are neither exact nor exhaustive, and the contagiousness of syphilis by contact is denied. The treatment of syphilis by unctions is prescribed, and much of the book is devoted to the possible identification of it with other diseases described by the classical writers. Leonicenus asserts that syphilis is not a new disease, but gives no evidence in support of his assertions. His book cannot therefore be quoted to prove the existence of the disease in Europe before Columbus. The book immediately became popular, was reprinted again in Venice

PLATE XVIII

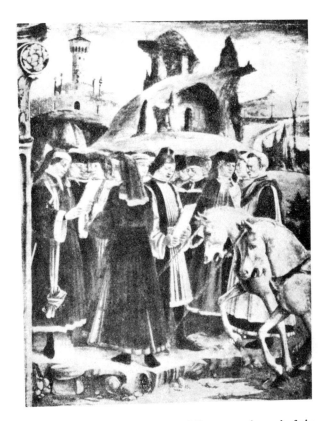

Fig. 8. Doctors at the School of Ferrara at the end of the fifteenth century (Fresco in the Palazzo Schifanoia in Ferrara)

(Patavinus et Ruffinelli, 1535) and in Basle (1532), and in a ponderous work compiled by Aloysius Luisinus, printed by Jordanus Zilettus in Venice in 1566–7. In this work all writings on the *Morbus Gallicus* written 'by all doctors of all nations' are diligently collected. It may be interesting to note that in the second edition (Milan) the passage on Pliny in the preface was omitted, and it was omitted also in the third edition published in Leipzig. In the edition of 1516 the preface is again slightly changed.

This work caused Leonicenus to suffer many attacks. A. de Scanaroli published at Bologna in 1498 a defence of the opinion of Leonicenus against an attack by Natalis Montesaurus, made in a work (Verona, 1498) which I have been unable to trace. In this defence Scanaroli asserted that the disease is not an infection and not necessarily connected with sexual intercourse: he maintained that it occurs also in virgins and old persons.

Another defence against the critics of his teacher was published in 1519 by a Roman pupil of Leonicenus under the title *Medici romani discipuli antisophisia* (Bologna, de Benedictis, 1519).

IV

The first commentary of Leonicenus on the *Aphorisms* of Hippocrates appeared in Venice in 1502, and was later published at Ferrara in 1509, at Venice in 1538 and at Paris in 1530. It caused such strong opposition that Leonicenus published in the same year an apology against his accuser, *Contra suorum translationum detractores apologia* (Ferrara, Maciochio, 1509). He asserted that some of the errors laid at his door were due to the printer and to the fact that he had used poor manuscripts. Berengar da Carpi and Thomas Leonicenus, who was professor of philosophy at Padua and died in 1531, joined the enemies of Leonicenus. The 'indignation and malediction' which he said were aroused first by his comments were very violent; but they belonged to the same class of literary controversies which were frequent among humanists. The *literati* and not the physicians began the criticisms of his editions of medical authors.

The first edition of Galen, with the comments of Leonicenus, showed diligent search for the best manuscripts. Leonicenus was entrusted with this work by the City of Ferrara, for which he was granted 400 Ferrara liras. It was published in Paris by Henricus Stephanus in 1514, but very soon polemics against Leonicenus began again. In 1522 he republished in Venice (Pentius de Leuco) a violent attack against his adversaries with the title *Contra obtrectatores apologia;* this was republished later in Basle by Cratander in 1532. Later Cratander published the commentary of Leonicenus on Galen's *Ars medicinalis.* This had many editions: in Venice by the Giunta Press in 1514, in Paris in 1528 and 1530, and again in Venice by De Tortis in 1538.

Summarizing the critical activity of Leonicenus which starts from his work on the errors in Pliny, we may say that it is a remarkable landmark in the history of humanism in a time of transition between the Middle Ages and the Renaissance, between scholasticism and experimental science. Leonicenus was among the first who criticized the texts of the ancients but not their ideas. We must remember, however, that even forty years later Vesalius also proceeded very cautiously in advance of Galen and always tried to attribute to copyists a part of Galen's errors. He was himself later a victim of the Galenists. From the criticism of the texts, which had its origin in the School of Ferrara, there arose criticism of the scholastic doctrines themselves.

V

The first real objective criticism of the scholastic writers began in Ferrara with Antonio Musa Brasavola, the successor of Leonicenus in the Ferrara chair.

Antonio Musa Brasavola, born in 1500, was one of the most famous teachers at the Medical School of Ferrara. He became the physician of Francis I of France, who bestowed upon him the name of Musa, the great physician of Augustus, to honour him for having sustained publicly in Paris a thesis, *De quolibet scibili*. The discussion lasted for three days and the vast erudition of Brasavola caused general admiration.

Brasavola represented in a most obvious way the transition from scholastic erudition to experimental observation. He was an excellent botanist and persuaded the Duke Hercules II of Este to send boats to the Greek islands in order to collect rare plants. He was the originator of the splendid botanical garden at the Belvedere. There was at this time a great passion for botanical research in Ferrara, where no less than five botanical gardens existed, and scholars came from abroad in order to visit them. It was in Ferrara that the English botanist Falconer began his herbal. In 1536 Brasavola's book *Examen omnium simplicium quorum usus est in publicis officinis* was printed in Rome. It is in the form of dialogues between a physician, a herbalist, and an old pharmacist. The work defends the use of traditional empirical remedies, while the author maintains that no remedy can be valuable until it is tested by personal experience. In fact, we know that Brasavola carried out a great number of experiments on dogs and other animals, and on prisoners with the permission of the Duke. He gives exhaustive descriptions of experiments concerning the use of different purgatives, of diuretic remedies, of narcotics and other remedies, and he shows his exact observation of the effects. He was an outstanding clinician who first described exactly the consequences of lesions in different parts of the brain, and he related loss of memory, speech, and the other faculties to the site and gravity of the lesion. His observation on the symptoms and course of plague are excellent.

Brasavola was a pupil of Leonicenus, whose chair he occupied. While he always spoke of his master with great reverence, he introduced original experimental research in medicine. He was considered in his own time, and also in the judgement of later clinicians, as the first to initiate at Ferrara the new trend towards experimental research. At the same period an outstanding piece of work was carried out by Antonio Canano, the most remarkable of the pre-Vesalian anatomists.

Up to the end of the seventeenth century the popularity of Leonicenus held sway. His books were often published and quoted after his death; his work on syphilis was republished by Boerhaave in 1728. The violent attacks against his person and his books prove how deeply imbued the scholars were at that time with scholastic thinking and blind acceptance of the classical texts. It is clear that no little courage was required to make even a superficial correction of some mistake. In fact, the apologies and justifications never ended, so that re-reading these old books we get the impression that sometimes even Leonicenus felt guilty. The conclusion which we may draw from the study of this famous controversy and its origins and consequences may lead us to believe that in the development of medical thought the episode itself did not have the immediate importance which had been attributed to it by some historians. However, the influence of Leonicenus and his school was certainly remarkable and his earliest criticism of the ancient authors played an important role in the history of medicine.

The School of Ferrara shows very clearly the evolution of medical thought at the end of the fifteenth century and at the beginning of the Renaissance. In this evolution the City of Ferrara played a remarkable part. It was there that from all over Europe great scientists and writers—Pietro Bembo and Erasmus, Ariosto, Copernicus and Paracelsus, Barbarus and Linacre—sought and found facilities for continuing their studies under the auspices of the ruling house, until the time when Renée of France was the animating genius of the group of persecuted Calvinists who found refuge at her court, and Rabelais drew from his sojourn inspiration for his work. This evolution began with the humanistic school of Guarino, of Benzi, of Savonarola. Leonicenus is its leading representative and we are able to follow it in his work. Finally, with Musa Brasavola and Canano, the greatest of the pre-Vesalian anatomists, the school made an important contribution to the Renaissance of science. The controversy on Pliny is therefore an important event in the evolution of scientific thought.[1]

---

[1] The literature dealing with the controversy on Pliny is vast. All medical historians, and especially the older historians such as Haeser, Sprengel and De Renzi, have dealt with it and have emphasized the importance of the work of Leonicenus. See also an exhaustive chapter on the subject by Lynn Thorndike in his excellent book, *A history of magic and experimental science.* New York, Columbia University Press, vol. iv, 1934, pp. 593–610, which has a rich bibliography.

The reproductions of pages from books in this essay are made from copies in the New York Academy of Medicine.

LA RÉFORME ET LE PROGRÈS DES SCIENCES EN BELGIQUE AU XVIe SIÈCLE

par

JEAN PELSENEER

L'AUTEUR de ces lignes s'est efforcé d'acquérir quelque teinture de l'histoire de la pensée scientifique et de l'histoire des sciences physiques et mathématiques, mais il ne fait aucune difficulté pour reconnaître que l'histoire de la médecine et de la biologie constitue un domaine où il s'avoue particulièrement incompétent. S'il se risque à l'aborder dans la première partie de cette brève contribution, que l'on veuille bien songer que son excuse est double : il n'a pas voulu se dérober à l'honneur qui lui était proposé de rendre hommage à un éminent historien des sciences; il n'a rien à refuser non plus à un représentant d'une nation grâce à qui il est de nouveau un homme libre.

I

Dans une note récente,[1] intitulée « L'origine protestante de la science moderne », nous avons cru pouvoir établir que la science moderne est née de la Réforme. Sans entrer dans une justification psychologique détaillée, nous avons montré, par deux exemples de caractère statistique, que le protestantisme avait joué un rôle déterminant au point de vue scientifique au cours de la période 1521–1600. En effet, que l'on considère le progrès des sciences en Belgique ou en Europe au cours de cette période, on constate, dans l'un et l'autre cas, que les mentions de travaux dus aux hommes de science acquis à la Réforme, l'emportent nettement sur le nombre de publications dues aux savants demeurés fidèles au catholicisme, l'avantage allant jusqu'à atteindre, pour certaines décades, la proportion de 6 à 1 en faveur des premiers.

Nous nous proposons aujourd'hui d'établir tout d'abord que l'histoire de la médecine en Belgique au XVIe siècle fournit une troisième preuve à l'appui de notre thèse selon laquelle les idées religieuses nouvelles ont joué un rôle primordial dans la genèse de la science moderne.

Rappelons quelques nombres que nous avons publiés en 1941, dans notre note intitulée « Aspect statistique du progrès des sciences en Belgique à travers les siècles »,[2] basée sur le dépouillement des vingt-sept tomes de la *Biographie Nationale publiée par l'Académie royale de Belgique* (1866–1938). Voici, pour différentes époques, le nombre de personnages figurant dans ce vaste dictionnaire biographique — il en comporte quelque 10,000 au total — et qui cultivèrent les sciences naturelles et la médecine, y compris la médecine vétérinaire, la pharmacie, etc. :[3]

$$1500 : 1$$
$$1525 : 22$$
$$1550 : 42$$
$$1575 : 39$$
$$1600 : 16$$

[1] *Lychnos*, 1946–7, pp. 246–8.

[2] *Académie royale de Belgique, Bulletin de la Classe des Sciences*, 5e série, t. XXVII, 1941, pp. 269–76; 1 pl.

[3] *ibid.*, p. 273.

Dans aucun des quatre autres domaines d'activité intellectuelle que nous avons également pris en considération dans le dépouillement en question (y compris le domaine des sciences physiques et mathématiques), l'accroissement du nombre de personnages n'est aussi brusque[4]. Or, Alphonse de Candolle, dans son enquête statistique,[5] a noté l'importance singulière du protestantisme, par rapport au catholicisme, au point de vue du progrès des sciences et tout particulièrement des sciences naturelles. Il y a là une présomption sérieuse que la Réforme est susceptible d'expliquer le démarrage soudain et rapide que connaissent les sciences médicales et naturelles en Belgique à partir de l'époque 1525.

Nous avions cru tout d'abord que la publication suivante — *Ministère de l'Instruction publique. Bibliothèque royale de Belgique. Histoire des sciences en Belgique jusqu'à la fin du XVIIIᵉ siècle. Exposition*[6] — pourrait servir de base à notre nouvelle investigation; ceci impliquant le postulat que nous identifions littérature scientifique et progrès scientifique. Mais ce catalogue est, en réalité, loin d'être systématique : c'est ainsi qu'aucune contribution de Charles de l'Escluse n'y apparait; en outre, il ne s'en tient pas à des contributions strictement scientifiques. Sa consultation nous permet cependant de consigner deux remarques. Abstraction faite des auteurs de langues grecque et arabe, toutes les mentions qu'on y trouve de traductions publiées durant la période 1521–1600 sont, sans exception, relatives à des oeuvres dues à des auteurs protestants ou traduites par des protestants. D'autre part, il est intéressant de noter que c'est à Bâle que Vésale fit paraître la plupart de ses ouvrages, notamment les deux éditions de sa *Fabrica*.

Force nous a été de recourir à une publication plus que centenaire, celle de Broeckx,[7] pour obtenir la seule vue d'ensemble quelque peu détaillée — encore qu'étrangement sommaire au regard des exigences de l'historiographie actuelle — que l'on possède jusqu'à présent sur l'état des sciences médicales en Belgique au XVIᵉ siècle. La lecture de Broeckx nous a permis d'établir, pour le XVIᵉ siècle, une liste de 45 médecins. Utilisant ensuite la *Biographie Nationale* et accessoirement le *Dictionnaire historique* d'Eloy,[8] nous constatons que, abstraction faite de 3 médecins dont il est impossible, dans l'état présent de la documentation, de préciser la confession, 24 médecins mentionnés par Broeckx se rattachent plus ou moins ouvertement aux idées réformées; 18 seulement appartiennent sans équivoque au catholicisme. Résultat remarquable, si l'on songe que le seul centre scientifique du pays, l'université catholique de Louvain, entendait demeurer une citadelle de l'orthodoxie et que, d'autre part, la proportion de la population protestante n'avait jamais été considérable.[9]

[4] *ibid.*

[5] *Histoire des sciences et des savants depuis deux siècles*, 2e édn., Genève, 1885.

[6] 1 vol., Bruxelles, 1938.

[7] C. Broeckx, *Essai sur l'histoire de la médecine belge avant le XIXᵉ siècle*, Gand, 1837.

[8] N. F. J. Eloy, *Dictionnaire historique de la médecine ancienne et moderne*, 4 tomes, Mons, 1778.

[9] Selon Pirenne, jusqu'au milieu du XVIᵉ siècle, avant l'abdication de Charles–Quint (1555), « dans toutes les provinces, la très grande majorité des habitants restait fidèle au catholicisme » (H. Pirenne, *Hist. de Belg.*, 3e édn., t. III, 1923, p. 372). D'après le même auteur, on n'a « que des indications bien incomplètes... qui ne permettent point d'établir avec quelque approximation le chiffre des protestants qui quittèrent le pays » vers 1585. « On l'a porté sans preuves suffisantes à plus de 100.000 personnes, et cette évaluation est d'autant moins admissible qu'un nombre considérable d'émigrés rentrèrent en Belgique durant les dernières années du XVIᵉ siècle. Mais si l'exode ne semble point avoir été très important en quantité, il le fut, en revanche, en qualité » (*ibid.*, 3e édn., Brux., t. IV, 1927, p. 340). Ajoutons qu'au XXe siècle, la population protestante de la Belgique est estimée à moins de 0,8 0/0 de la population totale.

Il faut souligner en outre que la valeur scientifique moyenne des premiers est nettement supérieure à celle des seconds; c'est ainsi qu'il n'y a généralement pas de protestants parmi les auteurs d'almanachs à tendances astrologiques.[10] La liste dressée d'après Broeckx ne représente que la moitié environ du nombre de médecins figurant dans la *Biographie Nationale*. Parmi ceux dont on ne trouve la mention que dans ce dernier recueil et qui sont ignorés de Broeckx, les protestants ne manquent pas, tel Samuel Quickelbergs (1529-67), dont l'ouverture d'esprit, l'activité, la soif d'instruction sont caractéristiques.

Le protestantisme — du moins à ses débuts qui seuls nous intéressent ici — c'est l'esprit de recherche, la liberté dans la ferveur. La Réforme, en élevant un groupe de citoyens au-dessus de la masse, n'aurait-elle fait que catalyser le développement de la science moderne naissante, ce rôle, méconnu jusqu'à présent, mériterait d'être systématiquement mis en lumière, à la fois dans les différentes branches des sciences et au sein des nations qui ont été témoins de cette naissance.

II

Dans cette seconde partie de la présente note consacrée au sujet de la signification de la Réforme pour la genèse et les premiers développements de la science moderne, nous voudrions indiquer succinctement quelques aspects et conséquences de l'influence du protestantisme au point de vue de l'histoire des sciences physiques et mathématiques en Belgique au XVIe siècle. Ce sera, on va le voir, une quatrième démonstration de notre thèse.

Rappelons les nombres que nous a fourni le dépouillement de la *Biographie Nationale*; il s'agit, pour différentes époques, des savants ayant cultivé les sciences physiques et mathématiques, ainsi que des cartographes et ingénieurs, dans la mesure où ils ont apporté des contributions originales à ces sciences:[11]

1500 : 1
1525 : 4
1550 : 9
1575 : 20
1600 : 14

Ces nombres seuls suffisent déjà à attester une corrélation entre la culture des sciences et les fortunes diverses du courant intellectuel constitué par les idées religieuses nouvelles. Dans quelle mesure celles-ci ont-elles déclenché le mouvement de pensée d'où est née la science moderne? Il est difficile d'apporter des preuves formelles sur ce point important, mais des remarques significatives peuvent être faites.

Toujours en minorité, les protestants furent cependant une élite. Si nous étudions la biographie des 43 mathématiciens, physiciens et astronomes que mentionne la *Biographie Nationale* pour les trois époques 1550, 1575 et 1600, nous constatons que, mis à part trois personnages sur qui les données font défaut, les protestants sont à égalité avec les catholiques;[12] plusieurs de ceux-ci d'ailleurs connurent des ennuis graves (Taisnier, par exemple, fut mis à l'*Index*). Mais cette division en deux groupes numériquement bien équilibrés,

[10] Rappelons que Calvin écrivit en français un *Traité ou avertissement contre l'astrologie* (1549).

[11] *op. cit.* (2), p. 273.

[12] Un seul protestant, Bert (1565-1629) (*Biogr. Nat.*, t. II, 1868, col. 292-8), s'est converti au catholicisme.

correspond en réalité à une répartition des savants en deux classes nettement caractérisées.

Les savants catholiques représentent ce qu'on peut appeler l'école de Louvain. C'est parmi eux que figurent les arpenteurs, les maîtres d'école, les comptables, les poètes-mathématiciens; nombreux sont ceux qui sacrifient à la chiromancie et à l'astrologie. Leurs travaux, généralement insignifiants au point de vue scientifique, sont souvent demeurés manuscrits; ce sont avant tout des auteurs d'ouvrages élémentaires. Une exception, extrêmement brillante, empressons-nous de le reconnaître — Adrien Romain.

Les protestants, au contraire, surclassent les catholiques. C'est parmi eux que se rencontrent les savants dont la réputation est internationale. Leur activité gravite de préférence autour d'Anvers, comme l'avait déjà remarqué Quetelet : « Anvers, à cette époque, méritait sans aucun doute d'être considérée comme notre principale cité sous le rapport intellectuel ».[13] Cette supériorité des savants réformés est confirmée par les résultats d'une double enquête, que nous avons donnés dans notre note sur « L'origine protestante de la science moderne », et qui montrent, répétons-le, que, pour la période 1521–1600, les mentions de travaux dus aux hommes de science acquis à la Réforme l'emportent toujours en quantité, dans l'historiographie des sciences, sur celles relatives aux auteurs demeurés fidèles au catholicisme, l'avantage en faveur des premiers allant jusqu'à atteindre la proportion de 6 à 1 pour certaines décades.

Doués d'un esprit de progrès, fort instruits, les savants protestants écrivent avec prédilection en langue vulgaire, les catholiques s'en tenant de préférence au latin. Voici par exemple le protestant Pierre Heyns (1537–97),[14] dans la vie de qui les langues vulgaires jouèrent un grand rôle; il ne publia rien en latin. La biographie de son coreligionnaire Mulerius (1564–1630)[15] nous fournit un excellent exemple de l'étendue de la curiosité et du rôle des langues vulgaires chez un savant protestant de niveau moyen. Mais il est un parallèle tout à fait caractéristique à cet égard, celui qu'on peut établir entre deux mathématiciens contemporains d'un mérite comparable, le catholique Adrien Romain (1561–1615) et le protestant Simon Stevin (1548–1620). Si l'on fait exception pour des calendriers, prognostications et almanachs rédigés en allemand,[16] toutes les publications de Romain sont en latin. Chez Stevin au contraire un ouvrage seulement sur 13 a vu le jour dans cette dernière langue;[17] proportion insignifiante.

L'histoire des sciences physiques et mathématiques en Belgique au XVIIe siècle nous apporte des confirmations *a posteriori* de l'importance du protestantisme au point de vue de l'évolution de la science moderne.

C'est au triomphe de la Contre-Réforme que la Belgique doit de ne pas pouvoir s'enorgueillir de la plus brillante dynastie que compte, avec la famille Bach, l'histoire intellectuelle. Jacob Bernoulli, notable anversois, mort en

---

[13] Ad. Quetelet, *Hist. des sc. math. et phys. chez les Belges*, Bruxelles, 1864, p. 97.

[14] *Biogr. Nat.*, t. IX, 1886–7, col. 359–60.

[15] *ibid.*, t. XV, 1899, col. 343–7.

[16] N°s. 10, 17, 18, 21, 24, 25, 26, 28, 29, 34, 35, 36, 44, 45, dans la notice par Bosmans, in *Biogr. Nat.*, t. XIX, 1907, col. 848 et ss.

[17] D'après la notice par Bosmans, in *Biogr. Nat.*, t. XXIII, 1921–4, col. 887 et ss. Il s'agit des *Problematum Geometricorum… lib. V.*

1583, s'exila à Francfort-sur-le-Main; de Nicolas Bernoulli — qui alla s'établir à Bâle, où il fit souche et où il mourut assesseur à la Chambre des Comptes — et de Marguerite Schonaver naquirent notamment Jacques et Jean Bernoulli.

Dans une leçon sur « L'histoire des sciences physiques »,[18] nous avons récemment commenté les condamnations successives que dut souffrir le cartésianisme en Belgique dans la seconde moitié du XVIIe siècle.   Les censures de la faculté de théologie de Louvain datent de 1662; elles ont ainsi devancé la condamnation prononcée à Rome par la Congrégation de l'Index (1663).

Nous avons déjà signalé[19] qu'aux époques 1650 et 1675, 60 à 70 0/0 des mathématiciens, physiciens et astronomes dont s'occupe la *Biographie Nationale* appartenaient aux ordres religieux,[20] comme si les laïques eussent couru quelque danger à s'occuper de science.

Péril réel, ainsi qu'en témoignent les malheurs de Martin-Etienne Van Velden (1664–1724), que nous avons eu l'occasion de retracer brièvement.[21]   Ce professeur de l'Université de Louvain s'était avisé, quelques années après la publication des *Principia* de Newton (1687), de défendre le système de Copernic.

L'incidence du protestantisme sur l'évolution des sciences physiques et mathématiques, attestée par les faits que nous venons de noter et de rappeler, mérite d'autant plus de retenir l'attention que c'est cependant dans le domaine des sciences naturelles que cette influence, ainsi que l'a magistralement montré de Candolle, s'est le plus évidemment manifestée.   Les faits en question n'en sont que plus probants en faveur de notre thèse sur l'origine protestante de la science moderne.[22]

[18] *Université libre de Bruxelles. Notes et conférences*, 3 s.d., 1946, pp. 62-89.

[19] *op. cit.* (2), p. 276, note 2.

[20] Cf. H. Pirenne, *Hist. de Belg.*, 3e édn., Brux., t. IV, 1927, pp. 449 et 454.

[21] In *Biogr. Nat.*, t. XXVI, 1936-8, col. 562-7.

[22] Depuis la rédaction de la note ci-dessus, une contribution décisive a été apporté par Mr. Jacques Putman dans son profond article : 'De l'origine et de la fin de la science grecque et de l'origine de la science moderne.' *Archives internationals d'histoire des sciences*, 1949, t. II, pp. 444-51.

ASTRONOMICAL TEXT-BOOKS IN THE SIXTEENTH CENTURY

by

FRANCIS R. JOHNSON

HISTORIANS of science date the beginning of modern astronomy from the sixteenth century. Looking backward, with the perspective of four centuries of scientific progress to direct our view, we can see that the publication of Copernicus' *De revolutionibus* in 1543 was the decisive event initiating the subsequent series of hypotheses and discoveries which has radically altered man's conception of the structure of the universe. For us of the twentieth century to reverse the vista, however, and to put ourselves in the position of men of the sixteenth century, requires a difficult exercise of the historical imagination. Unless we can for the moment jettison all the scientific knowledge mankind has acquired during the past four hundred years, we will be inclined to expect evidence that Copernicus' heliocentric hypothesis had a discernible—if not a startlingly manifest—impact upon every student of astronomy throughout the last five decades of the century. It will seem to us that all open-minded contemporaries of Copernicus should certainly have abandoned other systems in favour of the superior heliocentric theory: that the text-books of astronomy, the surest guide to the changes in the teaching of the subject in the schools, should display a marked alteration soon after 1543.

Such expectations would actually be unwarranted. The evidence of the text-books would reveal that no text-book widely used in Europe in the sixteenth century expounded the Copernican theory, and few even mentioned it.[1] Faced with these facts, the modern scholar is likely, with understandable

[1] One text-book recorded in contemporary bibliographies, to judge from its title, may have expounded the Copernican theory, but I have been unable to discover any extant copy of the treatise. Lynn Thorndike, also, in his *History of magic and experimental science* (New York, vol. vi, 1941, p. 45), reports his failure to find any trace to-day of a copy of this book, or of another which later bibliographers record, but which I believe is a 'ghost' created by an erroneous listing of the first treatise.

The earliest notice of the book in question appears in the great bibliographical catalogue of the late sixteenth century, Israel Spach's *Nomenclator scriptorum philosophicorum* (Strassburg, 1598). On p. 363, under the section entitled 'De Motibus Coelestibus', Spach has the following entry: 'Alberti Loniceri Theoria motuum coelestium, referens doctrinam Copernici ad mobilitates Solis. Colon. 8^s. 8.' Nearly a century later, what is apparently the same book is recorded as follows in the compilation of Martinus Lipenius, *Bibliotheca realis universalis* (Frankfurt A.M., 1679-85): 'Ad. Loniceri Theoria motuum coelestium ad mentem Copernici. Colon. 8. 1583.' Jerome de Lalande, *Bibliographie astronomique* (Paris, 1803, p. 114) lists: '1583 Colon . . . Mart. Alb. Loniceri Theoria motuum coelestium juxtà hypothesim Copernici.' J. C. Houzeau and A. Lancaster, *Bibliographie générale de l'astronomie* (Brussels, 1887-9, no. 2756) give this entry: 'Lonicerus, M.A. Theoria motuum coelestium juxta hypothesim Copernici. 4$^°$, Coloniae, 1583', which is obviously derived from Lalande.

The record of this work by one Lonicerus (the first name varies in the different listings) can therefore be traced back to Spach in 1598. Though later listings give a title that would indicate the book expounded the Copernican system, the wording in Spach would lead one to believe that Lonicerus, like so many other astronomical writers of his day, accepted Copernicus' mathematical calculations but sought to reconcile them with the old hypothesis of an immobile earth and a revolving sun (see below, p. 298). Only an examination of a copy of Lonicerus' book, if one can ever be found, can settle the question.

Houzeau and Lancaster, No. 2723, also list: 'Leoninus, A.=Leeuwen, A. van. Theoria motuum coelestium secundum doctrinam Copernici. 8$^°$, Coloniae, 1578. 8$^°$, Coloniae, 1583.' Since no record of this work can be found in Spach, Lipenius, or the *Bibliotheca belgica* of Valerius Andreas (1623), I am certain that the entry in Houzeau and Lancaster must be an error due to confusion with Lonicerus' book.

annoyance, to blame intellectual obscurantism and religious bigotry for the slow acceptance of the heliocentric system by text-book writers and teachers of astronomy. Lynn Thorndike, in the sixth volume of his great *History of Magic and Experimental Science*, admirably summarizes both the facts and the indictment customarily put forward to explain them:

> Next to astrological predictions, elementary textbooks after the manner of the *Sphere* of Sacrobosco seem to have been the most frequent publication in the astronomical field in the sixteenth century. Apparently almost every university had at least one elementary astronomical text produced for local consumption during this period. Their authors seldom reached the theory of the planets, the intricacies of which they usually postponed to a future volume which never appeared. The intricacies of the Copernican theory likewise were eschewed by such writers as beyond the reach of the beginning students for whom they wrote. They commonly adhered strictly to the Ptolemaic system, both as customary and as presenting the heavens the way they looked to an observer on the earth. This dead weight of pedagogical tradition and inertia did far more to delay the spread and general acceptance of the Copernican hypothesis than any religious opposition to it. Galileo might have done better to write a systematic textbook than his provocative dialogues. Hardly a single elementary textbook was written on the Copernican basis. Usually a passing sentence or two was all the recognition given to it. After examination of such textbooks had given me this idea, I found my impression confirmed by Hortensius in the preface to his Latin translation of Blaeu's *Institutio astronomica* in 1668. He states that, if the Copernican theory had been graphically presented sooner, as it had been recently by Blaeu, it would not have been condemned as absurd before it had been seen how it saved the phenomena, and that more probably than any other system. But because Copernicus himself was 'too obscure in his writings to be understood by everyone,' and because the use of the Copernican sphere and hypothesis was not explained in a popular way by any astronomer, many condemned it as false without understanding it.[2]

While admitting the accuracy of the foregoing description of the content of sixteenth-century astronomical text-books, can one offer any defence for their writers to mitigate the severity of this wholesale indictment? Let us first examine more fully the implication of Professor Thorndike's charges, not neglecting to inquire whether the elementary scientific manuals of that period were any more culpable than similar works of the present day. After we have done this, we can proceed with greater assurance to a survey and classification of the multifarious types of astronomical text-books published between 1500 and 1600.

To begin with, we must remember that up to 1600 no new scientific evidence was forthcoming to strengthen the case for the heliocentric hypothesis as compared with the older geocentric theory. Worse still, systematic observation of the nova of 1572 rudely dashed the hopes, which Copernican adherents such as Thomas Digges had evoked, of discovering a proof of the Copernican theory by measuring the parallax of that star (that is, its difference in apparent direction from the earth when the earth is at diametrically opposite points in its orbit about the sun).[3] Since the sixteenth-century astronomers failed

---

[2] New York, vol. vi, 1941, pp. 6–7.

[3] For Digges's support of Copernicanism see Francis R. Johnson and Sanford V. Larkey, 'Thomas Digges, the Copernican System, and the Idea of the Infinity of the Universe in 1576', *The Huntington Library Bulletin*, 1934, No. 5 (April), pp. 69–117. This article reprints Digges's

to detect any parallax with the then existing instruments, Copernican supporters were forced to postulate an incredibly huge distance between the orbit of Saturn and the fixed stars.   To counter this objection to the heliocentric theory, they could only cite the equally implausible assumptions fundamental to the Ptolemaic system, and finally fall back on the principal argument that Copernicus had used.   Based upon the philosophical axiom that the simpler explanation of a group of related phenomena was necessarily the truer one, it emphasized the greater mathematical simplicity of the heliocentric system.

As far as scientific evidence went, however, there was, in the light of the then available knowledge, little to choose between Copernicus and Ptolemy. Each system had certain points in its favour, but each likewise contained certain apparent absurdities which its opponents flaunted before defenders embarrassed by their inability to make a satisfactory reply.   The soundest position, scientifically, for the writers of elementary astronomical text-books to take in the last half of the sixteenth century was one of suspended judgement, presenting the arguments on both sides, analysing their validity, and finally, though perhaps indicating a preference, stating that further evidence was necessary for determining which hypothesis was correct.   Under such circumstances, Tycho Brahe's compromise system, first proposed in 1588, was welcomed by many lesser astronomers because it incorporated the mathematical advantages of the Copernican hypothesis yet avoided the physical objections which condemned that hypothesis in the eyes of its opponents.   Tycho retained the central, motionless earth of the Ptolemaic system, but made the sun the centre of all the other planetary orbits except that of the moon.   Thus, whether the sun revolved about the earth, carrying with it all the supralunary planets, or the earth, with the moon, revolved about the sun, made no difference mathematically; one was concerned merely with two bodies whose *relative* motions were known.

The scientists partial to the Copernican hypothesis, previously unable to offer a physical explanation for the motions Copernicus assigned to the earth, first found notable encouragement in Gilbert's *De magnete* (1600).   In the sixth book of that treatise, Gilbert asserted that the earth was a magnet, and that the principles of magnetism accounted for the rotation of the earth. Later in the seventeenth century, the discoveries of Galileo and Kepler, and finally the mechanics of Newton swelled the tide of arguments in favour of the Copernican system until it became irresistible.   But before 1600— hard as it may be for us of the twentieth century to realize it—the weight of scientific evidence was evenly balanced between the two systems.   Though some might scornfully reject the Copernican theory for such unscientific reasons as religious prejudice or reluctance to consider new ideas, there was, nevertheless—and this cannot be too strongly emphasized—no compelling

supplement to his father's *Prognostication euerlastinge* (1576 and later eds.), in which he translates most of Book I of the *De revolutionibus,* and discusses Digges's earlier espousal of the Copernican theory in his treatise on the nova in Cassiopeia of 1572, his *Alae seu Scalae Mathematicae* (1573).   For a fuller discussion of the scientific position of the Copernican theory in the sixteenth century, and the increasing support it received among scientists after 1600 as experimental and observational evidence accumulated to support the arguments in its favour and weaken those of its opponents, see Francis R. Johnson, *Astronomical Thought in Renaissance England,* Baltimore, 1937, chap. iv, vii, and *passim.*

scientific evidence in its favour. Consequently, failure to espouse Copernicanism cannot be taken as an infallible sign of the 'dead weight of pedagogical tradition and inertia.'

Once we become historically aware of the scientific position of the Copernican theory in the sixteenth century, we must admit that the reasons that writers of astronomical text-books gave for failing to go into the intricacies of the heliocentric system might well be valid. So long as the principal argument in favour of that system was its greater mathematical simplicity, that argument could only be made clear to the advanced student who had already mastered the complex mathematics of the calculation of the movements and positions of the planets. The subject was out of place in an elementary text-book. Indeed, no introductory astronomical text-book of to-day gives a detailed treatment of the complexities of the calculations of planetary orbits.

There were, moreover, compelling pedagogical reasons for beginning the exposition of the movements of the planets with the *apparent* rather than with the *actual* motions. Inasmuch as the observer is located on the earth, this means starting with the hypothesis of a geocentric rather than a heliocentric universe. Furthermore, both the celestial globe and the armillary sphere constructed according to the Ptolemaic hypothesis were practical instruments, by means of which a sixteenth-century student could solve graphically many simple problems calling for the position in the heavens where the sun, the moon, or one of the planets would be found on a certain day in the year.[4] A sphere constructed according to the Copernican system, on the other hand, would be no more than an interesting toy. Therefore a sixteenth-century teacher, even though he was a supporter of Copernicus, would begin by explaining the apparent motions in terms of a geocentric system. To follow a different course would have been unsound pedagogy. For this assertion the best evidence is the action of Galileo himself. Although already, since 1597 at least, an ardent Copernican, Galileo, when he composed about 1604 an elementary treatise on the use of the sphere, based his exposition of that astronomical instrument on the necessary assumption that the earth—the location of the observer—was the centre of the stellar universe.[5]

If students to-day were first introduced to astronomy by being taught the *apparent* motions of celestial bodies according to a geocentric hypothesis, observation could reinforce theory at the early stages of learning. Instead their elementary instruction acquaints them with a theory which hinders rather than facilitates their making any practical use of daily observations of the motions of the stars and planets. To this fact, more than any other, did Augustus De Morgan attribute the low level of rudimentary astronomical knowledge among educated people of the nineteenth century when compared with their ancestors of the sixteenth and seventeenth centuries.[6]

Further vindication of the sixteenth-century text-book writers will emerge if one examines the treatment in present-day text-books of the most obvious

[4] For a history and description of these astronomical instruments see Edward Luther Stevenson, *Terrestrial and celestial globes*, 2 vols., New Haven, Conn., 1921, and F. Nolte, *Die Armillarsphäre*, Erlangen, 1922.

[5] *Le opere di Galileo Galilei*, ed. A. Favaro. Florence, vol. ii, 1891, pp. 203–55.

[6] *The globes, celestial and terrestrial*. London, 1845, pp. 1–2.

twentieth-century analogy to the Copernican theory—Einstein's theory of relativity. In one respect the analogy is imperfect. Within twenty years from his publication of the special theory of relativity in 1905, and ten years from his announcement of the general theory in 1915, the principal consequences of Einstein's hypothesis had been tested and received experimental confirmation in a variety of ways. Therefore Einstein's theory won rapid acceptance among scientists, whereas Copernicus had to wait more than a century before the majority of scientists became his firm supporters. In other respects, however, the analogy is manifest, though not always recognized by writers on the history of science. Both Copernicus and Einstein proposed hypotheses depending upon the most specialized mathematical knowledge of the age for their complete elucidation. Neither hypothesis is a proper subject for an elementary text-book. Just as no sixteenth-century manual of astronomy began by expounding the Copernican system, so no modern text-book for the first college course in physics commits the absurdity of beginning with an explanation of Einstein's theory of relativity.

In fact, the amount of space given to relativity in eighteen text-books being widely used in the United States in the year 1943 (the four-hundredth anniversary of the publication of the *De revolutionibus*) corresponds almost exactly to the space given to the Copernican theory in the astronomical text-books current in the late sixteenth century.[7] Seven of these books make no mention whatever of Einstein's theory of relativity; three make a brief allusion to it in passing. The remaining eight, although stating that a full discussion of relativity is beyond the scope of an elementary course in physics, devote from one to three pages, at or near the end, to an exposition of the basic postulates of the theory and their physical implications.

[7] The group of eighteen text-books that I checked consisted of the sample copies supplied by publishers to my colleague Professor Paul Kirkpatrick, chairman of the Department of Physics at Stanford University, with the hope that the book might be chosen as the required text-book for the introductory course in physics. The following books were in the group:
(1) Newton Henry Black, *An introductory course in college physics*. New York, Macmillan, 1941.
(2) H. G. Heil and W. H. Bennett, *Fundamental principles of physics*. New York, Prentice-Hall, 1938.
(3) H. A. Perkins, *College physics*. New York, Prentice-Hall, 1941.
(4) Randall, Williams, and Colby, *General college physics*. Revised ed. New York, Harpers, 1937.
(5) A. W. Smith, *Elements of physics*. 4th ed. New York, McGraw-Hill, 1938.
(6) S. R. Williams, *Foundations of college physics*. Boston, Ginn & Co., 1937.
(7) W. Weniger, *Fundamentals of college physics*. New York, American Book Co., 1940.
(8) H. Howe, *Introduction to physics*. New York, McGraw-Hill, 1942.
(9) H. D. Smyth and C. W. Ufford, *Matter, motion, and electricity*. New York, McGraw-Hill, 1939.
(10) L. W. Taylor, *Fundamental physics*. Boston, Houghton-Mifflin, 1943.
(11) A. W. Duff, and others, *Physics*. 8th ed. Philadelphia, Blakiston, 1937.
(12) A. W. Duff and M. Masius, *College physics*. New York, Longmans, 1941.
(13) J. A. Eldridge, *College physics*. 2nd ed. New York, John Wiley & Sons, 1940.
(14) A. L. Foley, *College physics*. 3rd ed. Philadelphia, Blakiston, 1941.
(15) E. Hausmann and E. P. Slack, *Physics*. New York, D. Van Nostrand, 1935.
(16) A. L. Kimball and P. I. Wold, *A college text-book of physics*. 5th ed. New York, Holt, 1939.
(17) F. L. Robeson, *Physics*. New York, Macmillan, 1943.
(18) F. A. Saunders, *A survey of physics for college students*. Revised ed. New York, Holt, 1936.
The first seven of the text-books listed do not mention Einstein's theory of relativity; Nos. 8, 9 and 10 give it a brief notice in passing; Nos. 11 to 18 inclusive devote two or three pages to a short exposition of the fundamental principles of relativity.

If elementary text-books in the 1940's consider relativity of such mathematical complexity that, at most, they merely describe it briefly and defer fuller treatment to more advanced treatises, we are certainly not justified in expecting astronomical text-books before 1600 to expound in great detail the Copernican theory, especially when the heliocentric hypothesis had as yet failed to receive any sort of experimental or observational confirmation.

Once we look upon the sixteenth-century manuals of astronomy through lenses undistorted by unwarranted expectations, our principal objective need no longer be a search for evidence of the writer's attitude toward the Copernican theory.[8] Instead we can examine them objectively as records of the state of scientifically accepted astronomical knowledge, noting the fidelity with which they expound the latest doctrines of the time within the broad framework of the geocentric system which we loosely term 'Ptolemaic'. Thus we can analyse their relative merits more accurately and make some discerning and helpful classifications of the many types of text-books whereby the students of that day acquired a familiarity with the elements of astronomy.

As a starting point for surveying the hundreds of astronomical text-books published during the sixteenth century, the first basic classification to suggest itself is one according to the scope of the volume—the quantity and degree of difficulty of the information set forth. In this way we could make a rough division between the short introductory manuals, the more comprehensive and advanced text-books, and the specialized treatises addressed to mature students already expert in astronomy. The last group, which would include such works as Ptolemy's *Almagest*, Purbach's *Theoricae novae planetarum*, and, of course, Copernicus' *De revolutionibus*, can scarcely be called text-books, for they actually belong to a different category. If we omit this group, the plan upon which the text-book is arranged becomes a more revealing basis of initial classification than a division according to degree of difficulty. This basis, furthermore, would have a special advantage: it would emphasize the dominance of one supremely popular manual, Joannes de Sacrobosco's *Sphaera mundi*, in determining the order in which the subject matter of astronomy was presented to the students of the sixteenth—and also of the seventeenth—century.

The fame of John Holywood, the thirteenth-century writer whose name was Latinized as Joannes de Sacrobosco, rests on the little handbook of astronomy that he composed about 1225. His *Sphaera* became by all odds the most popular elementary text-book on the subject throughout Western Europe for over four hundred years. No other text-book save Euclid's on geometry has had a longer period of supremacy.

The book is a short treatise, requiring no more than twenty-four quarto pages in the first printed edition (Ferrara, 1472). Yet even from the century of its composition it established its dominance as the basic introductory manual for students of astronomy, so that other works going more deeply into certain phases of the subject took the form of commentaries on Sacrobosco's *Sphaera*. Faber Stapulensis, Michael Scot, and Cecco d'Ascoli

---

[8] Lynn Thorndike, *op. cit.* (1), pp. 3–66, gives an excellent survey of the post-Copernican text-books of astronomy from the point of view of their allusions to Copernicus.

were the most noted writers of the early commentaries that appeared in the printed editions of the late fifteenth and early sixteenth centuries. The later sixteenth-century editions customarily interspersed the text of Sacrobosco with more or less extensive scholia by the editor, who made use, in turn, of earlier commentaries. Thus the changing ideas and controversies in astronomical theory were presented in the annotations.

The doctrine set forth in any given Renaissance edition of Sacrobosco, therefore, would be the sum of the original text plus the editor's commentary. Consequently, a summary of Sacrobosco's treatise will serve to give us the plan of organization and the common denominator of the teachings to be found in the majority of the sixteenth-century text-books of astronomy.

The *Sphaera* is divided into four chapters. The first deals with the definition of a sphere, the structure of the universe, its division into the elementary and the aetherial regions, the number and order of the celestial spheres, and proofs of the spherical form of the heavens, and of the shape, position, and size of the earth. In short, it presents the fundamentals of astronomical theory, and, since the topics treated were to be the subjects of later modification and controversy, we shall return to examine its teachings in greater detail.

The second book is concerned with the practical matters of astronomical co-ordinates. It defines and explains the various circles of the celestial sphere: the equinoctial circle; the zodiac; the two colures; the meridian and the horizon; the minor circles (that is, the two tropic and the two polar circles); and finally, the five zones into which these minor circles divide the sphere. Here the doctrine set forth is, in all major details, the same as in text-books to-day. The third chapter deals with the rising and setting of the signs of the zodiac and of the constellations, the causes of the unequal lengths of days and nights, and concludes with the division of the earth into seven climates. The fourth chapter—the shortest of all—gives a rather sketchy explanation of the circles (equant, deferent, and epicycle) whereby the motions of the planets are represented, defines the elements of the planetary orbits, mentions the direct and retrograde motions of the planets, and concludes with explanations of the causes of eclipses. This is the weakest section of the book, for the complexities of the 'theorics of the planets' are too great to be elucidated in so brief a space.

Let us now return to the first chapter and summarize it more fully, so that the later additions and modifications of Sacrobosco can be more sharply distinguished.

The chapter begins by citing and explaining the geometrical definitions of a sphere, and then states that the spheres dealt with in astronomy are divided in two ways: 'secundum substantiam', and 'secundum accidens.' The division according to 'substantia' is into the nine celestial spheres: the *primum mobile*; the sphere of fixed stars, or firmament; and the seven planetary spheres, of which that of Saturn is greatest and that of the moon the least. The division according to 'accidens' gives the right sphere (that in which the equinoctial circle is at right angles with the horizon and would occur only when the observer was at the earth's equator), and the oblique sphere.

The next paragraph states that the frame (*machina*) of the universe is divided into two regions: the elementary and the aetherial. The elementary region comprises the earth, in the centre of the universe, surrounded by the three other elements in the order: water, air, and fire, the latter reaching to the sphere of the moon. This sublunary region is subject to continual alteration, whereas the aetherial region which encompasses it is immutable, a realm of changeless circular motion. The celestial spheres of this aetherial region are nine in number, beginning with that of the moon, and followed in order by those of Mercury, Venus, the Sun, Mars, Jupiter, Saturn, the Fixed Stars, and the highest heaven or ninth sphere. These celestial spheres have two motions: (1) the diurnal rotation from east to west of the ninth sphere about its axis, whose extremities are the poles of the world; and (2) the rotation of the eight inferior spheres from west to east about the poles of the zodiac, which are distant, according to Sacrobosco, 23° 33' from the poles of the ninth sphere. The diurnal motion of the ninth sphere drags the lower spheres with it. Their periods of rotation in the contrary direction are given as: Sphere of Fixed Stars, 36,000 years (or 1° in 100 years, the rate of precession of the equinoxes according to Ptolemy's calculations); Saturn, 30 years; Jupiter, 12 years; Mars, 2 years; the Sun, 365 days and about 6 hours; Venus and Mercury, the same as the Sun; the Moon, 27 days and 8 hours.

Sacrobosco then proceeds to give two proofs that the heavens move circularly, and three reasons for their being circular in form.[9] Next he takes up the question of the shape of the earth, and gives five proofs of the earth's sphericity.[10] He continues with these proofs that the earth is at the centre of the universe:

[9] Sacrobosco's proofs are: (1) The heavens revolve from east to west because: (a) stars always rise in the east and set in the west, while retaining the same position relative to one another; and (b) stars near the celestial pole (the pole of the ninth sphere or *primum mobile*) describe circles about the pole, while remaining always in the same relative positions.

(2) The heavens are spherical in form for these three reasons: (a) *Similitudo*, that is, the physical world should be similar to the archetypal world, in which there is neither beginning nor end; therefore the sphere, to which one cannot assign a beginning nor end, is the most appropriate figure. (b) *Commoditas*, that is, since the circle has the greatest area of all isoperimetric figures, for the universe, which contains everything, the sphere is the most commodious form. (c) *Necessitas*, for if the heavens were of some form other than spherical, as pyramidal or cubical, two impossibilities would follow: either certain spaces in the corners would be occupied by a vacuum, which is contrary to nature, or these spaces would contain material bodies lacking a natural place, and these bodies would consequently shift about in these angular spaces as the heavens revolved. Furthermore, as Alfraganus says, if the heavens were flat, the sun and stars would appear larger, because nearer, when at the zenith than when rising or setting; yet actually they appear larger when near the horizon because of the effects of the atmosphere.

[10] The proofs are: (1) The stars rise and set earlier in regions to the east and later in regions to the west; for example, an eclipse of the moon that appears to us just after sunset will appear to an observer farther east some time after sunset, because the sun has set earlier there. This proves that the earth has a curved surface in an east-west direction. (2) The earth's curvature in a north-south direction may be demonstrated as follows: As an observer proceeds from north to south, stars which formerly were never above the horizon become visible and stars formerly visible drop below the horizon. Since this change in the elevation of the stars is directly proportional to the distance travelled, the earth's surface must be circular in this direction. (3) If the earth were flat from east to west, stars would rise at the same moment to an observer in the east as to one farther west; but this is manifestly contrary to fact. Also, if the earth were flat in a north-south direction, stars always visible in one locality would be always visible in a locality farther north or south. (4) That the water of this earth partakes of its curvature is proved by the fact that, as a ship sails from a port, an observer at the top of the mast can still see a mark on shore after it has disappeared below the horizon of an observer at the foot of the mast. (5) Water being a homogeneous body, the form of the whole would agree with the form of its parts. Water drops assume a globular form; therefore the mass of water seeks a spherical form.

1. To an observer on earth the apparent size of a star remains the same as it moves across the sky; hence its distance must remain the same.

2. If the earth were not in the centre, an observer on the side of the earth nearest the firmament would see less than half of the heavens, whereas one on the side farthest distant would see more than half. This is contrary to Ptolemy and all philosophers, who state that wherever a man may be, exactly half the heavens are above his horizon.

Sacrobosco here adds that this fact is likewise a proof that the earth is but a point in respect to the firmament, for if the earth had any appreciable magnitude compared to the eighth sphere, an observer on its surface would see less than half the heavens. Furthermore, Alfraganus says that the smallest visible star is greater than the earth. Therefore, since the star is no more than a point compared to the firmament, this would be even more true of the earth.

To prove the immobility of the earth, Sacrobosco cites its *gravitas*. This natural quality of the element earth causes it to seek the centre of the universe and there remain unless violently displaced. Should the earth move naturally, it must move toward the circumference of the universe, which we know is absurd. The first chapter then concludes by stating the size of the earth, giving its circumference, according to Eratosthenes and later writers, as 252,000 stadia, and describing how this figure was ascertained by measuring the length of one degree along a meridian.

The foregoing summary displays the underlying pattern of the usual elementary course in astronomy from the thirteenth century to the end of the sixteenth. With Sacrobosco as a text, the teacher could supplement the information epitomized therein by means of fuller explanations and illustrations, by adding to or revising the proofs of some of its propositions, and by annexing tables of the sizes of the stars and planets, their distances from the earth, and the ratios between deferent, epicycle, and eccentric of the various planetary orbits. Moreover, he could readily bring the text in line with new astronomical calculations and theories by explaining the reasons which impelled astronomers to abandon the older doctrines and adopt the new. Consequently, in the medieval manuscripts of the *Sphaera*, the commentary of an expositor usually accompanies Sacrobosco's text, either following it or being interspersed with it. The same practice was followed in the early printed editions. To find the bare text of the treatise separately printed is comparatively rare; most editions are differentiated by the name of the editor and the extensiveness of his commentary.

To record and to distinguish between the numerous editions of Sacrobosco's *Sphaera* published before 1600 is far beyond the scope or aim of this study. Indeed, after some time spent in tracking down and examining as many as possible of the hundreds of astronomical text-books of the sixteenth century,[11] I am convinced that anything approaching a complete census of the editions of Sacrobosco's treatise is impossible, for hitherto unnoted printings keep turning up all the time. Two statements, however, I can make with assurance. Before 1501 at least thirty different printed editions were issued. From 1501 to 1600 at least two hundred distinct editions, in Latin or in

---

[11] The research on which this study is based was done in 1942–3, when the writer was a fellow of the John Simon Guggenheim Memorial Foundation.

translation, came from the various presses throughout Europe; since there were probably many editions of which no copy has survived, the true figure may well be twice that number.[12]

Without attempting to mention all the text-books grounded on Sacrobosco, we can nevertheless indicate their nature and variety by describing very briefly some of the most important and widely used volumes. If we also do the same for the principal text-books that followed a different plan of presentation, the result will be a faithful portrait of the astronomical knowledge received by the sixteenth-century student. From this we can then discern which ideas he would consider matters of universal agreement, beyond dispute, and which he would find debatable, with highly respected authorities arrayed on either side. Furthermore, by dividing the period into three sections and noting shifts in the types of text-books most popular, we may be able to draw some inferences concerning the trends of astronomical education during the course of the century.

Sacrobosco, writing in the early thirteenth century, based his manual chiefly upon the work of the ninth-century Arabian astronomer Alfraganus. He follows Alfraganus in accepting Ptolemy's figure for the rate of precession of the equinoxes ($1°$ in 100 years) and in making no reference whatever to the theory of trepidation; that is, the notion that the rate of precession was variable. To Thâbit ben Kourrah, a generation younger than Alfraganus, later writers gave the credit for the discovery of trepidation. The Arab astronomer Albategnius, a contemporary of Thâbit, after comparing his observations of the stellar positions with those of Ptolemy, had computed the rate of precession to be $1°$ in 66 years. Although Albategnius considered the discrepancy between his value and Ptolemy's to be due to inaccuracies in the observations of Ptolemy's predecessors, Thâbit accepted both values and elaborated the theory of trepidation to explain this imaginary variation in the rate of precession. Thâbit's works may not have been known to Sacrobosco, but the scholars in Spain who compiled the Alfonsine tables about the year 1256—two or three decades after Sacrobosco wrote his treatise —were thoroughly conversant with all the astronomical writings of the Arab and Jewish world, both those that had been translated into Latin and those still in the Semitic languages. They accepted the notion of trepidation, added a tenth sphere to the previous nine so as to portray that imaginary phenomenon, and based their calculations on a period of 49,000 years for the cycle of precession and 7,000 years for the cycle of trepidation.

Within a few decades, therefore, after Sacrobosco wrote his *Sphaera*, a teacher using his manual would feel obliged to point out that the most recent astronomical opinion favoured ten spheres instead of nine, in order to account for the motion of trepidation, which had been unknown to Sacrobosco. The 'trepidation talked' of Milton's *Paradise Lost*[13] had thus been a subject of debate in the astronomical text-books of Europe for over 400 years. Every student knew that it was a fundamental point upon which reputable authorities disagreed.

[12] Allan H. Gilbert, in 'Milton's textbook of astronomy', *Pub. Mod. Language Assoc.* 1923, xxxviii, 297, states that there are at least seventy Latin editions before 1647, but his estimate is much too low.

[13] iii. 483.

In the early days of printing the text of the *Sphaera* was usually accompanied by extensive commentaries by one or more authors, or by other astronomical works which carried the subject further than Sacrobosco's introductory manual. Three such collections stand out in importance; each first appeared before 1500 but continued to be reprinted during the first thirty years of the sixteenth century. The earliest of these evolved from the edition published in Venice in 1478, which added the *Theorica planetarum* of Gerard of Cremona (twelfth century) to Sacrobosco. In the Bologna edition of 1480 (Hain-Copinger No. 14109) Georg Purbach's *Theoricae novae planetarum* was also included. In the 1482 and later editions the publishers, realizing that Gerard's treatise was out of date, substituted a criticism of it by Regiomontanus but retained Purbach's work as the most recent comprehensive exposition of the planetary motions. The collection, in this final form, was published at least six times before 1500, and had at least four more editions in the sixteenth century.[14]

A second popular collection included the fourteenth-century commentary of Cecco d'Ascoli (predominantly astrological) and the fifteenth-century commentaries of Franciscus Capuanus de Manfredonia and Faber Stapulensis (Jacques Le Fèvre d'Étaples). Frequently added were Purbach's *Theoricae* and Capuanus' commentary on that work. The earliest edition I have seen is that of 1499; Houzeau and Lancaster (No. 1642) record an earlier edition printed at Basel in 1485, but this seems to be an error. During the first decades of the sixteenth century this was the most frequently printed collection. Eight editions, some of them containing additional astronomical works, are recorded.[15] Both Capuanus and Faber Stapulensis accepted trepidation and explained the reasons for postulating ten moving spheres instead of nine.

A third collection that was popular included the commentary of Pedro Cirvelo and the questions on Sacrobosco of Pierre d'Ailly. Houzeau and Lancaster (No. 1643) record the date of the earliest edition as 1498. I have seen the editions of 1508, 1515, and 1526; the first two were printed in Paris and the last at Alcala.

Besides these collections, there were editions with extensive commentaries by only one writer. In France, in the early sixteenth century, by far the most popular was that by Faber Stapulensis, which published Faber's commentary sometimes separately and sometimes interspersed with the text. Houzeau and Lancaster (No. 2289) list twenty editions between 1500 and 1559; only three of these, however, were later than 1534.

The two most scholarly, fully annotated editions first composed and issued during the three opening decades of the sixteenth century came from Poland. One was by John of Glogau, professor of philosophy at the University of Cracow when Copernicus was a student there. His *Introductium compendiosum in tractatum Spere materialis . . . Joannis de Sacrobusto* was published at Cracow in 1506 and 1513, and again at Strassburg in 1518. The other edition emanating from the teachers at the University of Cracow was the *Sphericum opusculum cum lucido & familiari expositione per Matthaeum Shamotulieñ*, issued in 1522.

[14] Hain, Nos. 14110 to 14114 and Copinger No. 5208; the later editions, Venice 1501, 1513 and 1515, and Paris, about 1515.

[15] Venice, 1514, 1518, 1519, 1531; Basel, 1523 and 1551; Paris, 1515; Cologne, 1516.

One other extensively annotated edition achieved wide circulation at the beginning of the century, that by Wenceslaus Faber of Budweis. The earliest copy I have seen is that printed at Cologne in 1515, but the text indicates that the original date of composition was shortly after 1491. Houzeau and Lancaster (No. 1644) list the first edition as about 1495, and note other editions in 1498, 1500, 1501, 1503, and 1508. From the catalogues of the British Museum and the Bibliothèque Nationale two more editions, both of 1505, can be added.

Next to Sacrobosco in popularity, but trailing by many lengths, was Proclus' *Sphaera*, an even more elementary work. It saw many editions in the Latin translation of Thomas Linacre, and was also translated into French, Italian, and English. One of the most comprehensive and influential astronomical treatises of the first half of the century was based on it—Johann Stoeffler's *In Procli . . . Sphaeram mundi . . . commentarius*, published at Tübingen in 1534 and frequently referred to by later writers. Another original treatise, too advanced for a handy beginner's manual but often used by subsequent compilers of text-books, was the French physician and scientist Jean Fernel's *Cosmotheoria* (Paris, 1528). Fernel's measurements and calculations of the size of the earth were far more accurate than those set forth in any other contemporary work.

To complete the picture of the text-books from which students before 1530 might learn the elements of astronomy, the popular encyclopædia of Gregor Reisch, entitled *Margarita Philosophica*, should be included. Arranged in sections according to the seven liberal arts of the medieval curriculum, it had a book on astronomy which summed up the contents of Sacrobosco and of the fourteenth and fifteenth-century commentaries. It was twice printed before 1500, republished eight times between 1503 and 1535, and reissued after a lapse of almost half a century in 1583.[16]

Up to about 1530, as the preceding survey demonstrates, printers of astronomical text-books concentrated on issuing volumes designed to put into the hands of the student and scholar the sort of collections of treatises on astronomy that he had customarily found in the manuscript volumes of the preceding century. Yet already the tendency is noticeable toward smaller, less expensive text-books, with the notes and amplifications of a single author rather than a collection of commentaries and treatises. In the period between 1530 and 1570 the smaller text-book became the dominant type. Though older collections were occasionally reprinted, the wider popular market which the newer works commanded made printers turn increasingly to producing the cheaper manuals.

By far the best of these, though not the least expensive, was a work notable for the excellence of its diagrams. Written by Peter Apian and revised by Gemma Frisius, it was issued first in 1524 with the title *Cosmographicus liber*. It combined elementary astronomy and geography, and was entirely independent of Sacrobosco in text, yet came nearest to equalling him in popularity. The astronomy it expounded was conventional, embracing trepidation and the ten moving spheres which that theory necessitated.[17]

[16] See Houzeau and Lancaster, No. 2250.

[17] The diagram of the universe from Apian's *Cosmographia* is reproduced as Fig. 1. It is typical of the diagrams based on a system of ten moving spheres.

In later editions the title was changed to *Cosmographia*. Under this name the book was reprinted until the end of the century, although its greatest vogue was during the fifty years following its first publication. At least twenty-five

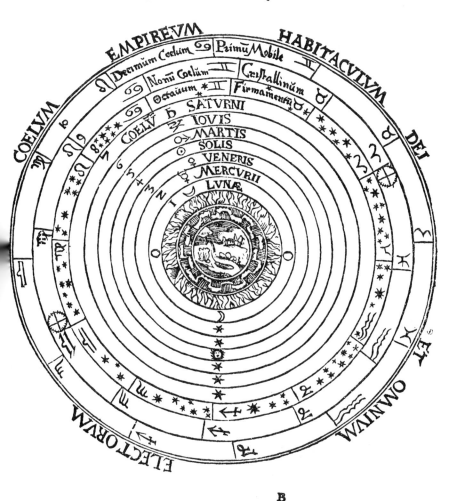

B

Fig. 1. Diagram of the Universe from Apian's *Cosmographia*.

different Latin editions appeared; moreover, an abridgment with the title *Cosmographia introductio*, first issued in 1529, was many times reprinted. Translations of the work into French, Spanish, and Flemish each had several editions.

Not so widely used as an elementary text-book except in France and England, but of great intrinsic importance, was another original astronomical work, *De mundi sphaera sive cosmographia*, written by Oronce Finé, Regius Professor of Mathematics at the Collège de France. It was first printed in 1542 in two editions, the octavo being a slightly abridged version of the folio, with many of the illustrations omitted. Editions in quarto appeared in 1551 and 1555, and a French translation in 1551. The chief distinction of the *De mundi sphaera* is its proclaiming unequivocally that eight spheres are sufficient to account for all the stellar motions. Finé states that neither

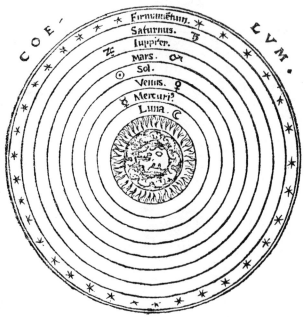

Fig. 2. Diagram of the Universe from Finé's *De mundi sphaera*.

the presence of stars, nor any other convincing reason, forces us to imagine any moving orb above the eighth sphere, or firmament.[18] Therefore, in his diagram of the universe, he is content with eight stellar spheres (see Fig. 2).

The sixteenth-century source for the astronomical system that refused to postulate any moving sphere which, being void of visible stellar bodies, could not be observed by man was a little treatise by Augustinus Ricius, *De motu octavae sphaerae*. First published at Trino in 1513, it was issued again at Paris in 1521, edited by Oronce Finé. Ricius, after reviewing the history of astronomical theories concerning the motions of the eighth sphere and the measurements of the rate of precession, concludes by denying the existence of trepidation and therefore casting aside the ninth or crystalline sphere, and by rejecting as unnecessary a separate sphere as a *primum mobile*.

[18] *De mundi sphaera* (1542), fo. 3ʳ of the folio edition.

Instead, he allots the uniform movement of precession to the eighth sphere, but accounts for the diurnal rotation of the heavens by having the entire assemblage of eight spheres turned about as a unit, by a separate 'intelligence', once every twenty-four hours.

After Finé, adopting the ideas of Ricius, published his text-book supporting a system with only eight moving spheres, students could not fail to recognize, as some treatises before and many afterwards proclaimed, that the evidence for any spheres beyond that of the fixed stars was doubtful. Although the majority of writers during the rest of the century accepted trepidation with its ten spheres, many rejected it and were content with Sacrobosco's nine, while some of the more empirically sceptical followed Ricius and Finé in rejecting more than eight.[19] In fact, toward the end of the century, because they wished to adopt the mathematical calculations of Copernicus without sanctioning his hypothesis of the triple motion of the earth, many astronomers added an eleventh moving sphere. Copernicus, assuming the conflicting observations of his predecessors to be accurate, included two imaginary phenomena to his system—trepidation and the notion that the obliquity of the ecliptic was subject to a cyclic variation between 23° 52' and 23° 28'. To explain these, he assigned a wobbling motion to the earth's axis. The non-Copernicans, accepting the supposed variation in the obliquity of the ecliptic on Copernicus' authority, portrayed it by means of an additional sphere.[20]

The period between 1530 and 1570, besides being characterized by the less expensive astronomical text-book, was the period of original manuals rather than elaborate commentaries on Sacrobosco. Among these original text-books, besides those of Apian and Finé, which we have already mentioned, the following were the most important and widely used. I have indicated for each work the approximate number of sixteenth-century editions, based on the listings in Houzeau and Lancaster, supplemented by my own notes of copies I have seen or found recorded in the catalogues of the world's major libraries.

1. Gemma Frisius, *De principiis astronomiae et cosmographiae*, a text-book similar to Apian's *Cosmographia*, to which Gemma Frisius had contributed, but containing a few more details in the astronomical sections. First published in 1530, the book was reprinted five times by 1578, and three editions of a French translation were issued between 1556 and 1582.

2. Franciscus Maurolycus, *Cosmographia*, an advanced rather than an elementary text-book, first printed at Venice in 1543. There were new editions in 1558, 1575, and 1590.

3. Alessandro Piccolomini, *De la sfera del mondo*, usually issued jointly with his *De le stelle fisse*, a book that was by far the most popular and best text-book in Italian. Between 1540, when the first edition was published at

---

[19] Robert Recorde, in his *Castle of Knowledge* (1556)—the first important astronomical work in English—favours eight spheres, although explaining why most writers portray ten (see pp. 10 and 278-9).

[20] The fullest mathematical exposition of the post-Copernican system with eleven moving spheres is found in Giovanni Antonio Magini's *Novae coelestium orbium theoricae congruentes cum observationibus N. Copernici*, Venice, 1589, although Clavius, in his commentary on Sacrobosco, and other astronomers had already, on the basis of Copernicus' work, expounded a system with eleven spheres.

Venice, and 1597 there were at least twelve editions, besides two editions of a French translation by J. Goupyl.

4. Cornelius Valerius, *De sphaera et primis astronomiae rudimenta*, a small conventional handbook which enjoyed a great popularity, especially in the Low Countries. Eleven editions are recorded between 1558 and 1596.

5. Caspar Peucer, *Elementa doctrinae de circulis coelestibus et primo motu,* which, although it mentions Copernicus and his system with respect and adopts some of his figures, rejects the motion of the earth and portrays a system of nine moving spheres, following Ptolemy, Alfraganus and Sacrobosco. Thus, in agreement with most of the books emanating from the University of Wittenberg, it ignores the theory of trepidation. Between 1551 and 1587, seven editions, at least, of this work were printed at Wittenberg.

During the middle decades of the sixteenth century Wittenberg was, in fact, the chief centre for the publication of cheap octavo handbooks of astronomy. More often reprinted than any other was a little book which merely presented Sacrobosco's text, with a preface by Melanchthon eulogizing the practical value of astronomy. It helped set the fashion, in editions of Sacrobosco's *Sphaera*, for small manuals with a minimum of commentary. The earliest edition listed is dated 1531, and at least twenty-eight editions were issued at Wittenberg and elsewhere in Europe by 1578.

Two other small manuals, following the general order of Sacrobosco's but arranged in the form of question and answer, were produced at Wittenberg during the same decades. I give the date of the earliest edition in each case, but both were reprinted several times. The first was Sebastian Theodoric's *Novae quaestiones sphaerae* (1564); the other, Thomas Blebel's *De sphaera* (1576–7). None of the Wittenberg manuals except Peucer's was distinguished for scientific merit; they rejected trepidation because of Ptolemy's authority rather than for any scientific reasons.

Of a slightly higher order was the edition of Sacrobosco's text with the rather cursory annotations of Elie Vinet. First published in Paris about 1550, it became the most popular inexpensive handbook in France, being reprinted at least fifteen times before the end of the century. In 1564 Vinet's scholia were combined with notes by Francesco Giuntini to produce another edition of Sacrobosco that achieved considerable vogue. It was issued at least thirteen times from presses in Lyons, Paris, Antwerp, and Cologne; with notes by other scholars added, it continued to be republished well into the seventeenth century.

During the last thirty years of the sixteenth century, the relatively inexpensive manuals of astronomy that we have been describing were frequently reprinted, but no new works of this type gained a widespread vogue in those three decades. On the contrary, this was the era of what might well be termed comprehensive 'variorum' editions of Sacrobosco's *Sphaera*, in which the compiler subjoined to almost every sentence of that thirteenth-century writer's text several pages of commentary reviewing the divergent views put forward by various astronomers. Thus his book became an encyclopædia of astronomical knowledge and speculation. The first work of this sort was Erasmus Schreckenfuchs' *Commentaria in sphaeram*

Joannis de Sacrobusto, a folio of over 300 pages printed at Basel in 1569. In 1577 an equally comprehensive treatise was composed by Francesco Giuntini and printed at Lyons in two thick octavo volumes entitled: *Fr. Iunctini . . . commentaria in sphaeram Ioannis de Sacro Bosco.* Reissued in 1578, this commentary was in 1581 included in the folio edition of a collection of Giuntini's works having the title *Speculum astrologiae*—a collection which was published a second time in 1583.

Neither Schreckenfuchs' nor Giuntini's encyclopædic commentaries achieved the success of Christopher Clavius' *In sphaeram Ioannis de Sacrobosco commentarius.* First issued in Rome in 1570, this thick quarto volume, running to some 500 pages, became the principal advanced text-book of astronomy throughout Western Europe for the next three-quarters of a century. Nine editions had appeared by 1600, and there were at least as many more after that date.[21]

The only text-book produced in the late sixteenth century which rivalled that of Clavius was Michael Maestlin's *Epitome astronomiae,* published at Heidelberg in 1582.[22] The author avowedly followed Sacrobosco in his order of arrangement but did not, like Schreckenfuchs, Giuntini, and Clavius, present his material as a commentary on Sacrobosco. All four of these writers set forth and amplify the basic data in Sacrobosco, often adding further proofs of the earth's sphericity, of the insignificant size of the earth with respect to the firmament, and the like. Although Maestlin alone was favourable rather than averse to the Copernican system, he was content, after mentioning it, to present the Alfonsine system of ten spheres. Clavius and Giuntini review the arguments of Ricius and Finé for a system comprising only eight moving spheres, of Copernicus for an explanation of the stellar motions by a triple motion of the earth, of other astronomers for nine, or ten, moving spheres. Clavius finally favours eleven moving spheres in order to represent Copernicus' notion of the cyclical variation in the obliquity of the ecliptic. Giuntini's vote is cast for ten.

This trio of works by Clavius, Giuntini, and Maestlin constitute the most up-to-date and best among the widely used astronomical text-books at the close of the sixteenth century. At its opening the typical text-book had been made up of Sacrobosco's text plus either some more advanced treatises or a collection of commentaries by fourteenth- or fifteenth-century writers. The middle decades witnessed the wider dissemination of elementary astronomical instruction, which gave rise to the vogue of the less costly manual, whether it be an original text-book or an edition of Sacrobosco supplemented by a minimum of commentary. The closing decades turned once again to the comprehensive work that brought together in a single volume the divergent ideas of various writers, both ancient and modern. Hence the welcome given to the encyclopædic text-books of Giuntini, Clavius, and Maestlin.

Throughout the entire period, however, the one point of difference among astronomers that would be most strongly impressed upon any student was

[21] The sixteenth-century editions were: Rome, 1570, 1575, 1581, 1585; Venice, 1591, 1596; Lyons, 1593, 1594, 1600. I have used the 1581 edition.
[22] Other editions before 1600 were published at Tübingen in 1588, 1593, 1597 and 1598.

not the conflict between the Ptolemaic and the Copernican theories. On the contrary, it was the debate over the number of motions of the eighth sphere or firmament, and consequently the number of moving spheres beyond the firmament that must be postulated to account for these motions. Above all, it centred upon the acceptance or rejection of the supposed phenomenon of trepidation. A majority of astronomers accepted it, and Copernicus was among their number. Indeed, Copernicus was often cited as an authority by his contemporaries, who adopted his figures for the period of trepidation, even when they scornfully discarded his method of explaining it by assigning a third motion to the earth.[23]

[23] After this essay was written Professor Lynn Thorndike published *The 'Sphere' of Sacrobosco and its commentators*, Chicago, 1949. The volume prints a Latin text and an English translation of Sacrobosco's *Sphere*, and also a text and translation of three early commentaries: those by Robertus Anglicus, Cecco d'Ascoli, and that ascribed to Michael Scot. The reader may consult this book for fuller details concerning the contents, date of composition, and sources of Sacrobosco's popular handbook of astronomy.

NAUTICAL SCIENCE AND THE RENAISSANCE*

by

ARMANDO CORTESÃO

Middle Ages to Renaissance

MAN'S mentality emerged from the Middle Ages as if it had been a chrysalis for some ten centuries. Greek culture and the universalism of Imperial Rome had been superseded by the œcumenical Roman Church, which in turn had to give place to the universality of knowledge of the Renaissance. Scholasticism, with its sterile dislike of experimental investigation, had by the end of the fourteenth century been succeeded by an ardent thirst for rational proof. The interests of man's mind were gradually transferred from the misty domains of dialectical analysis to the observation of nature and constructive thinking which, with the revival of learning, led to the experimental philosophy and synthesis of modern times.

The crystallization and cleavage of amorphous feudal Europe, more or less ruled by the Popes, into well defined nationalities and languages, the gradual development of the science of navigation, and the invention of the printing press were the main factors which, through that cosmopolitan enlightenment of the Renaissance, led to the foundation of Western Civilization. If printing was the most wonderful and powerful agency for the expansion, spreading and popularization of knowledge, the technique of navigation on the high seas was the master-key which opened all the doors of the unknown world to the curiosity and needs of a Europe just awakening from its medieval lethargy.

Until almost the end of the fifteenth century Europe was practically isolated from the rest of the world: to the west, the legendary vast expanse of the ocean; to the south, that huge dark continent; to the east, the fabulously rich and strange countries of which so little was known; northward, the frigid wastes closed the circle of the unknown. Any medieval world-map, of which there are many extant, bears witness to that. Some information came from North Africa, and the countries of the Eastern Mediterranean maintained commercial contacts with the East; some European travellers had even gone as far as China, but the knowledge they had brought back was very limited, scanty, often wrapped in marvel and legend, and scarcely spread. Such a scholar as Pierre d'Ailly simply ignores Marco Polo and other more recent great travellers in the famous *Imago Mundi* (*c.* 1410); he does not even mention his own countryman Jean de Bethencourt, who had gone to the Canary Islands in 1402. In his cosmographical and geographical divagation, Dante had also ignored his contemporary Marco Polo, and does not seem to have believed in the habitability of the southern hemisphere and the antipodes. D'Ailly was still too much imbued with Aristotelian physical theory and, though in his next book—*Cosmographiae*

* This essay, originally written for this book, was published, without illustrations, in *Archives Internationales d'Histoire des Sciences*, 1949, 2s., ii, 1075–92, and is reprinted with some amendments by the author. [Editor.]

tractatus duo (*c.* 1414)—he acknowledges Ptolemy's *Geography*, which had recently been translated into Latin, his advance in the trend of thought just dawning is not the greater. Although some scholars, such as the German Albertus Magnus and the English Roger Bacon, braving Ptolemy (the *Almagest* had been translated into Latin in 1175) and ecclesiastical authorities, had since the thirteenth century decided—with the support of Aristotle—in favour of the habitability of the earth south of the Equator, many fifteenth century writers still believed that it was uninhabitable, and Ptolemy's notion of an enclosed Indian Ocean was also almost generally accepted during the whole of that century and part of the next; as a matter of fact it was not definitely dispelled before the eighteenth century!

To know the world in which he lives has always been one of the main desires of man's intellectual curiosity. Besides, economic and political circumstances in the late Middle Ages had made the expansion of Europe quite imperative. Positive geography had thus to become one of the most eventful factors in the new social structure which was developing. The veil of mystery and legend that had covered all the world around Europe was lifted only after the ships, enabled to navigate the high seas far from sight of the coast-lines, could cross the Atlantic and reach the Far East. This was accomplished gradually, in a series of steps which remained known as 'The Great Age of Discovery'.

The first condition of high sea navigation with any measure of security is the possibility of finding the ship's position with practical accuracy and at reasonable intervals. Out of sight of known land, the only way for the ship to find its position is by determining the latitude of the place in which it is at a given moment; and this cannot be done properly but by means of astronomical observations at sea, i.e. calculating the meridian altitude of some heavenly body. Nautical astronomy is, then, the basis of distant seas navigation, and its discovery and development is the foundation of modern geographical science. The Portuguese were the designers and founders of nautical science in the fifteenth century, and until the first quarter of the sixteenth century they were unrivalled by any other people in its development and progress.[1] From other people they received, however, the scientific preparation which constituted the background of their performance. Their merit lay above all in the fact that they gave a practical application to a branch of scientific knowledge that so far had been used for speculative purposes only, thus solving a problem on the solution of which depended the progress of mankind. With the foundation of nautical science—a first step only in the great age of discovery of which they were the leading

---

[1] This has been demonstrated (among other Portuguese scholars such as Luciano Pereira da Silva, Jaime Cortesão and Gago Coutinho) by Joaquim Bensaúde, *L'astronomie nautique au Portugal à l'époque des grandes découvertes*, Bern, 1912, and subsequent works, and acknowledged by all leading authorities.
'It was the Portuguese who originated and developed the means of making and delineating discoveries. . . . Thus was a fairly correct system of navigation over distant seas established.' (Sir Clement R. Markham, *The history of the gradual development of the groundwork of geographical science*, London, 1915.)
'Nowadays it is widely accepted that the Portuguese were the founders of nautical science.' (G. H. T. Kimble, *Esmeraldo*, 1937, and *Geography in the Middle Ages*, 1938.)
See also : Edgar Prestage, *The Portuguese pioneers*, 1933, and E. G. R. Taylor, *The English debt to Portuguese nautical science in the Middle Ages*, London, 1938.

artisans—the Portuguese came to play a leading role in the Renaissance. They were indeed the performers of a plan, imposed by the economic and political necessity of European expansion, which had been in gestation since the thirteenth century.

Now, how did this situation originate in Europe, and how did this small people, of little more than a million souls at the beginning of the fifteenth century, come to solve it? What was their technique of navigation, how did it develop and from what scientific background did its roots spring? The importance of this subject of Portuguese navigation and discoveries can be gathered from the enormous literature it has brought about among Portuguese as well as foreign writers, in the past and the present. Among British writers alone are Major, Bethune, Alderley, Yule, Danvers, Beazley, Whiteway, Ferguson, Ravenstein, Markham, Prestage, Dames, Taylor, Boxer, Rey, Crone, Kimble, Welch, Axelson and Blake, to mention only a few of the more noteworthy.

Gold and Spices

In the Europe of the late Middle Ages aromatic spices such as cloves, mace, nutmeg, cinnamon, ginger, and above all pepper, had become so important that they were often used as currency and to pay taxes, as well as for seasoning. Until the first half of the fifteenth century spices came from the East to Europe via the Red Sea and Egypt or Syria, whence they went to southern and western Europe through Venice and Genoa, and to eastern Europe through Constantinople. So Europe became steadily more dependent on the levantine intermediaries. The development of international commerce, especially that of spices, was one of the main reasons for the scarcity of gold then felt in Europe. It was known that North Africa was one of the main sources of the gold coming into Europe, and since the beginning of the fourteenth century the Genoese had tried to find out the routes by which the caravans brought it to some south-Mediterranean ports, of which Ceuta was one of the most important. Some pepper also came from the north-west coast of Africa. The Portuguese took Ceuta from the Moors in 1415, and three years later initiated a series of systematic explorations down the west coast of Africa. This was the first great step in the maritime enterprise which culminated in the arrival of a Portuguese fleet in India in 1498. Although it was said that the attack upon Ceuta was moved by the spirit of chivalry of the King's sons, who wanted to be knighted in combat against the traditional enemies of the Christian faith, and that Prince Henry, called the Navigator, in charge of the maritime expeditions, was inspired above all by his religious zeal, contemporary evidence shows that the real motive behind all these early undertakings and ventures was chiefly economic and political. It has also been said that Prince Henry conceived, from an early date, the plan of reaching India by sea; but this is a doubtful point.

The Portuguese had been active at sea since the twelfth century. Their ships went as far as the Levant, Normandy and England and they had established commercial factories at Bruges; in 1226 alone over one hundred safe conducts were given to Portuguese merchants in England. In 1335 they discovered the Canaries. In the last decades of the fourteenth century Lisbon had become the greatest port of call between the Mediterranean and Western Europe, thriving on shipping and merchandise of all sorts and origins. The conditions in which the second Portuguese dynasty (1385–1580) began, with a king chosen or elected by the people, and his marriage to an English princess, contributed powerfully to the dynamism which characterized the new ruling generation. The Portuguese were in the splendour of their sturdy virility, and as every people in ample contact with the sea, they always craved for liberty, adventure and wider horizons. At the beginning of the fifteenth century, then, Portugal could well feel the pulse of Europe, and her situation in the extreme south-west of the continent, facing the vast ocean, may explain why these people, in spite of their small numbers and limited resources, but who had reached their majority, were naturally called upon to accomplish an historical mission of world importance. Europe was then on the prongs of an intellectual, social and economic crisis which was to attain its climax a few decades later. One century earlier the Catalan mystic Ramon Lull (c. 1235–1315) had already suggested the circumnavigation of Africa in order to reach the East. There were people who believed or suspected that Africa was surrounded by sea, and it is only natural that, coupled with the purpose of getting the African gold, the idea arose of going directly to fetch the oriental spices in ships. But if such an idea did not occur immediately to Prince Henry and his advisers, who were well abreast of the latest geographical developments, it did not take long to become the chief aim in a well thought out, systematic, scientific and sustained national plan. Henry the Navigator may have been moved by the spirit of chivalry in his youth, and he certainly was always imbued with religious fervour; but after the earlier years of his career he was, above all, the administrator of an economic enterprise of national magnitude and international consequence.

Modern capitalism was born in 1447, when Genoa adopted the gold standard. The scarcity of gold became more than ever wide-spread all over Europe, and the need of procuring it paramount. Then, in 1453, the Turks took Constantinople, and subsequently conquered Asia Minor and the Balkans, which deeply affected the prosperity of Venice and Genoa, chiefly the latter. The importance and demands of Egypt, as exclusive commercial intermediary between East and West, only became greater. Arab pirates from the north-African ports grew still more daring and infested the Mediterranean to such an extent that navigation in those waters was practically at their mercy. The economic difficulties, resulting from the increased price of gold and cost of spices, were only aggravated by the new order of international relations kindled by the end of the Hundred Years' War, also in 1453. On the other hand, the Roman Church, long alarmed by the Turkish menace, especially after the fall of Constantinople, tried to rally the European powers against the danger of the Ottoman invasion of Europe, and several appeals were made to Portugal. This was the situation in the middle of the fifteenth century—a most momentous period in history. If it were possible to reach the Indian Ocean by sea, to bring the precious spices and other riches directly from the East, and there to attack the Moslem power in the rear (as Lull and the Venetian geographer and traveller Marino Sanuto had already proposed more than a century before), the European problem would be eased, or even solved, as indeed it was later at least in part, when the Renaissance entered into its splendour.

In the last ten years before his death in 1460, Prince Henry had sent several emissaries to Egypt and Abyssinia, not only to gather information but also with the design, it seems, of obtaining the support of Prester John, to whom legend had lent fabulous power, as a Christian ally against Islam. There is no doubt that the idea of reaching the East by sea was then rife and, though the full plan developed and matured only after the Prince's death, much progress had already been made in its preparatory phases. By 1460 the Portuguese ships had already rediscovered Madeira and the Azores archipelagos, and reached as far south as Sierra Leone and perhaps Cape Palmas, if not farther. And above all the Portuguese sailors had begun to learn how to navigate on the high seas.

The greatest figure in the whole of Portuguese history, and the real organizer of the master plan of the circumnavigation of Africa, was King John II, born in 1455. Though he began his reign only in 1481, Afonso V, his father, had already handed over to him in 1474 all matters concerning navigation and discoveries. By this time the Cape Verde Islands had been discovered (1462), João de Santarém and Pedro Escobar had crossed the Equator and reached Annobon Island (1471), and Lopo Gonçalves had pushed on to Cape Lopez (1473). Maritime activity was carried on more eagerly than ever, especially after Prince John became John II in 1481. In 1482–4 Diogo Cão continued the exploration along the coast of Africa, visiting the mouth of the Congo River and reaching Saint Mary's Cape (13° 26' S.). In his second voyage of 1485–6 Cão reached Sierra Bay (21° 48' S.), just north of the Cape of Good Hope. Then, in 1487–8 Bartolomeu Dias rounded the Cape of Good Hope and reached the Great Fish River—at the doorway to the Indian Ocean. This much is known officially.

The plan was in full swing, but Dias' voyage was only a part of it. In 1485 (?) John II sent two emissaries, António de Lisboa and Pedro de Montarroio, by land to the East, but they were unable to go beyond Jerusalem. It was essential, however, to find out whence the spices came, to know something about the south-east coast of Africa, and to gather positive information concerning Prester John. Thus, a new attempt was made with Pedro da Covilhã and Afonso de Paiva in 1487. The two travellers reached Aden together, via Cairo, and then parted. It seems that Paiva sailed towards Abyssinia, and it is only known that he died in the venture. Covilha went to Cannanore and Calicut, returning to Aden via Goa and Ormuz, whence he went to Sofala, thus learning of the Arab navigations to Madagascar and beyond, and then returned to Cairo at the end of 1490 or beginning of 1491. There he met two men who had come from Portugal and were searching for him. He knew then of Paiva's death and decided to go to Abyssinia himself; but first he wrote an account of his mission to the king and sent him a map he had brought from Portugal, on which he had put the names of many places about which he had enquired and learned, chiefly the Moluccas and Banda Islands where the cloves, nutmeg and mace came from.

As a result of Dias' navigation to the southern coast of Africa and Covilhã's voyage along the other coast as far as Sofala, John II had got the last piece of information he needed for the great expedition to India, and he also knew where the coveted spices were to be found. There is no doubt to-day that he knew as well of the existence of a vast continent to the west, running from high northern to high southern latitudes; Diogo de Teive had been in American waters in 1452, since when the Portuguese had never ceased to reconnoitre westwards in the greatest secrecy. There are even reasons to suppose that Columbus, whose life has always been involved in a veil of mystery so thick that it could never be satisfactorily lifted, was a secret agent in the service of the cunning king of Portugal.[2] His mission was, it seems, to distract the attention of the Spanish kings from the Portuguese plan of reaching the East by sea, convincing them that it would be easier to reach the Far East by way of the West. The Portuguese, then incomparably more advanced in nautical science and geographical knowledge than the Spaniards, knew quite well that the way to Cathay and India was much longer and more difficult westwards, and that not far away in that direction there was a vast land which could pretty well absorb their dangerous competitors' attentions.

Columbus, a man whose nationality is even yet a subject of passionate discussion, discovered America officially in 1492. However, the nautical science which enabled him to go there was Portuguese and his exploit fitted perfectly in the transcendent plan of John II. This plan was a masterpiece and it had been organized scientifically, technically, and politically to the last detail. But the great King could not see its climax. He died in 1495, when the final expedition to India was being prepared. Vasco da Gama's fleet sailed from Lisbon in July 1497, arrived at Calicut ten months later and returned in 1499. A few years later Afonso de Albuquerque practically destroyed the Moslem power in the East and took Malacca in 1511; the Portuguese reached Banda and the Moluccas in 1512, China in 1513 and Japan in 1542. Before the middle of the sixteenth century they had discovered and established themselves, to a greater or lesser extent, in the Atlantic Islands, Africa, Brazil, Abyssinia, India, Malasia, China and Japan.

There were only about a million and a half inhabitants in Portugal at the beginning of that century, and this small number was reduced nearly to a million and a quarter in less than a hundred years and, before rising again, the number went down nearly to the million mark in the seventeenth century. They had contributed manfully to the foundation of a new era in the history of mankind—but at a heavy price. The great enterprise of unveiling the unknown world was initiated by Prince Henry but finally organized by John II—a giant whose place in world history has not yet been fully acknowledged. One is known as the 'Navigator'; the other, who was then called 'El hombre' by Queen Isabella of Castile, remains in Portuguese history as the 'Perfect Prince'.

[2] See A. Cortesão, *Cartografia e cartógrafos Portugueses dos séculos XV e XVI*. Lisbon, 1935, vol. i, pp. 187-248; and *idem*, 'The Mystery of Columbus', *Contemporary Review*, 1937, March.

PLATE XIX

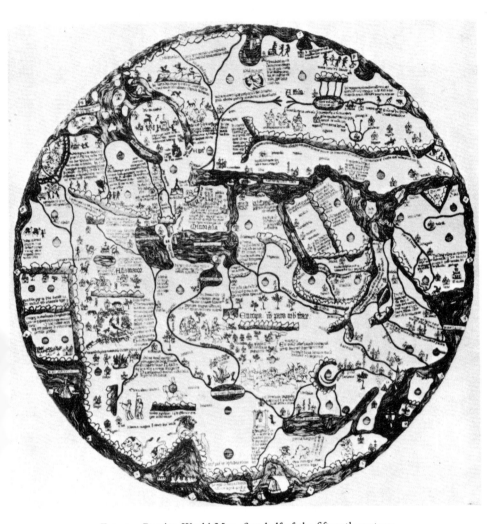

Fig. I. Borgian World Map, first half of the fifteenth century

The south is at the top of the map, which shows Europe still surrounded by mystery and legend. In Ethiopia, guarded by dragons and other fabulous animals, are the Golden Mountains with the inscription: 'Hic sunt môtes aurei in quibus sunt deserta maxima et ab infinites serpentibus habitata.' Near the north-west coast of Africa is the River of Gold with the inscription: ' Fluvius aureus hic habet VIII leucas latitudine '

PLATE XX

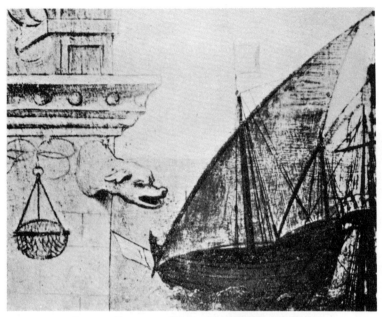

FIG. 2.   Two-masted Caravel with lateen sails only
(From a contemporary Portuguese drawing by the ' Master of St. Auta ')

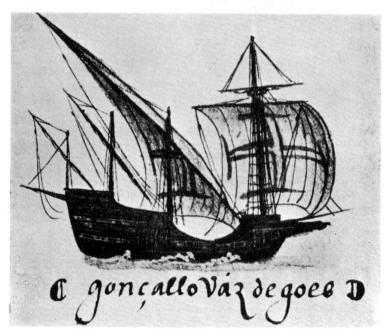

FIG. 3.   Four-masted Caravel with square sail at foremast
(From a contemporary Portuguese manuscript of *Livro das Armadas*)

The Birth of Nautical Science

The practical application of the magnetic needle to navigation, and the elaboration and development of the navigation chart were, so to say, the first steps towards the Medieval Renaissance in geographical science. Although in ancient Greece it was already known that the lodestone attracted iron, and the Chinese used some magnetic apparatus for polar direction in the second century of the Christian era, it seems that in the West such knowledge dates from not earlier than the eleventh century. There is evidence that from that time the polarized needle was used by European mariners and that the Italians were most probably the originators of the early form of the modern compass-box. The gradual improvement and popularizing of the magnetic needle was followed by the development of the first accurate maps or compass-charts of the Mediterranean and Black Sea made by Italians and Catalans. The *Carta Pisana* of *c.* 1300 is the earliest of these charts extant, and Vesconte's map of 1311 the first one dated; but no doubt many others were made before this, and by that time they had already become more or less standardized. These charts represent a great progress, if we consider that their proportion between the length and width of the Mediterranean is incomparably more correct than in the Ptolemaic maps. It seems, however, that such charts were rather for study, information or even decorative purposes, the sailors preferring the real *portolani* or rutters, of which there were many good ones, for actual navigation. The Pole Star and the magnetic needle were good enough for orientation in the confined waters of the Mediterranean and along the western coast of Europe. Even when by accident or design some navigator was drawn westwards, far from sight of the European coasts, he was always sure of finding land once he returned eastwards. This was the case with the unknown discoverers and rediscoverers of Madeira and the Azores Islands, which appear on several maps of the second half of the fourteenth century, though the first known voyages thither, by the Portuguese, date respectively from 1423 and 1427. However, in 1291 two Genoese galleys had already gone to the Canaries, and many other expeditions followed, both Genoese and Portuguese; it was perhaps during one of these voyages that Madeira and the Azores were discovered for the first time.

Arab geographers had spread the legend that beyond Cape Bojador (26° 6' N.) there was the Sea of Darkness and that torrid zone which would turn black any man who dared to penetrate into it. When the Portuguese doubled Cape Bojador in 1435 and reached Garnet Bay (24° 51' N.) they not only dispelled a centuries-old legend of terror but opened a new age in the history of navigation. In the following years their ships never ceased to push farther south using the prevailing north-east winds; but the round sails of the small boats they used were not easy to trim to sail near the wind, that is, with the side wind, on the return voyage. So they built the caravel, a vessel of fifty tons and upwards, of small draft and with lateen sails, very suitable for exploring the coasts and for running before the wind. Caravels, the first of which appeared no later than 1436, were soon exclusively used by the Portuguese along the coast of Africa. This type of ship gave them superiority and great advantage. Bartolomeu Dias' voyage round the Cape of Good Hope in 1487–8 was still made with four caravels of two or three masts and only lateen sails. Their size was then increased to 150 and 200 tons, for longer or trans-oceanic voyages, with three or four masts, the foremast having one or two round sails. Columbus' three ships on his famous voyage of 1492 were three-masted caravels of this type.

The Portuguese soon discovered, especially after rounding Cape Bojador, that the return voyage was much easier when they sailed westwards with the favourable winds and currents, far out on the high sea, and that there was a belt with a high percentage of calms between the Canaries and Azores parallels; but north of the latter islands, after passing the eastern fringe of the Sargasso Sea, they met another belt of prevailing west winds and currents which would take them to the coast of Portugal. There is evidence that ever since 1424 they had made a systematic study of these prevailing winds and currents, and the voyage through the high sea became a regular practice before 1446 and was known as the *Volta da Mina* (Return from Elmina) or *Volta do Sargasso*. With this came the necessity of devising some accurate and practical means of finding the ship's position on the high seas. At first, and for many years to come, the navigation was by dead reckoning, i.e. the ship's position was estimated from the distance run and the course steered by the compass. Though the sailors' experience could sometimes bring amazing accuracy to the process, the inefficient reckoning of the distance run and of the corrections for currents, leeway, etc., showed that something better had to be found. Hence arose the idea of determining the astronomical latitude on board ship, by adaptation of the process used on shore.

To find latitudes, i.e. our position on the earth's surface in relation to the poles and to the Equator, has always been relatively easy by observing the course of the Sun or stars. Eratosthenes' calculation of the circumference of the Earth in the third century B.C., by difference of latitudes between two points in Egypt, is a classical example. In this case the zenithal passage of the Sun on the day of the summer solstice at noon was simply observed at one of the points by the absence of shadow at the bottom of a well, and at the other the Alexandrine used an instrument resembling a sun-dial; but the use of the astrolabe was more than a century old. Through the Arabs the use of the astrolabe came down to the Middle Ages, the Moslems being interested in astronomical matters, not only out of scientific curiosity but also for religious purposes, in order to determine accurately the direction of Mecca. It was the Arabs, indeed, who transmitted Ptolemaic geography to the Christian Occident. They also used astronomical observations for astrology, and it was specially for this purpose that it passed into Spain and Portugal mainly through the Jews. But there is no reason to assert, as some have done, that any goniometric instrument was used to determine latitudes at sea before the second quarter of the fifteenth century—certainly not in Europe. It is true that when Vasco da Gama arrived in the Indian Ocean he found that the Arab pilots could determine the astronomical latitude at sea by means of a rudimentary apparatus of their own; but the process was inferior to that used by the Portuguese; we do not know when it began, and it never spread to Europe.

PLATE XXI

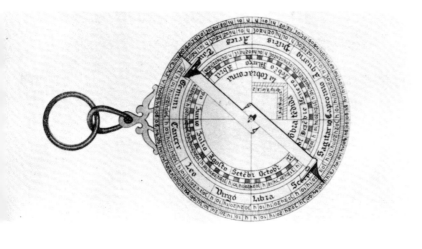

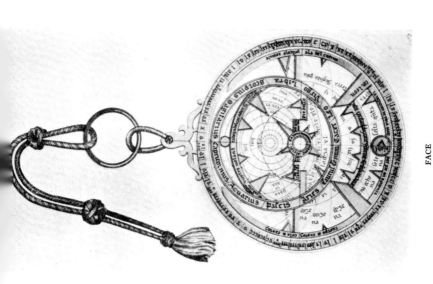

BACK

FACE

FIG. 4. Thirteenth-century Astrolabe of King Alphonso X. From the *Libros del Saber de Astronomia del Rey D. Alfonso de Castilla*, edited by M. Rico y Sinobas, Madrid, 1863–7, vol. ii

This complicated medieval instrument was used mainly for astrology.

King Alphonso X of Castille (1252–84), *El Sabio*, ordered a number of learned men assembled in Toledo to write the famous *Libros del saber de astronomia*, a vast work in which are contained all the contemporary astronomical knowledge and detailed instructions for the making of astrolabes and quadrants. It is believed that he gave a copy of the precious book to his grandson, King Denis of Portugal (1261–1325), a learned monarch who founded the University of Lisbon in 1290. That astronomical knowledge developed in Portugal at an early date is shown by the *Tabulae astronomicae*, a codex with 55 parchment leaves written in Portuguese and Latin at Coimbra in the first half of the fourteenth century, extant in the Biblioteca Nacional of Madrid. King John I shows some astronomical knowledge in his *Livro da Montaria*, and his son, King Duarte (1391–1438), wrote another book, *Leal Conselheiro*, two chapters of which are devoted to the calculation of the hour by the Guard in Ursa Minor. It has also been asserted that Prince Henry the Navigator wrote a book called 'Secret of the Secrets of Astrology', now lost, and he also established a chair of mathematics and astronomy at the University of Lisbon in 1431. There is other evidence that the Portuguese were well abreast of contemporary astronomical knowledge when Prince Henry engaged in his service the Catalan cartographer Jafuda Cresques, who came to Portugal between 1420 and 1427. He was the son of Abraham Cresques, author of the famous Catalan map of the world, 1375–81, which he probably helped to draw. This remarkable man's knowledge of cosmography, cartography and instrument making must have had considerable influence in the preparatory phase of Portuguese nautical science.

In view of the new demands brought about by high sea navigation, more and more a regular feature in the discoveries, and familiarity with astronomical matters, the idea of using the astrolabe and quadrant for determining latitude at sea came naturally to the mind of Prince Henry's cosmographers and navigators. Of the many applications of the astrolabe only one was essential for navigation, i.e. to determine the height of heavenly bodies. So the first thing to do was to simplify the astrological astrolabe and quadrant, and enlarge their size in order to get a better division of the graduated circle. The date at which the first Portuguese experiment with astronomical navigation began has been the subject of discussion among Portuguese scholars, but most probably it was during the second quarter of the fifteenth century. The first recorded actual observation of astronomical latitudes at sea with the quadrant was during a voyage to the coasts of Guinea in 1462, though there are references to similar observations with astrolabe and quadrant in 1451 and 1455. The first recorded use of the nautical astrolabe was during a voyage to Elmina in 1481. There is no evidence of the cross-staff being used by the Portuguese before the sixteenth century. At first the latitude was deduced from the height of the Pole Star, but as the observers drew near to the Equator it was necessary to find a method of calculating it by the height of the Sun at noon, which needed the preparation of tables of declination plain enough for the use of the mariners. This problem was solved by John II's Junta of astronomers, who once more had to adapt the precepts of the *Libros del saber de astronomia* to the new circumstances. The chief scientist in the Junta was Master José Vizinho, a disciple of Abraham Zacuto, professor of astronomy at Salamanca, who in 1473–8 had composed in Hebrew an *Almanach perpetuum*. This was probably used by Vizinho, when he was sent to Guinea in 1485 in order to practise the new method on board ship. Zacuto went to Portugal in 1492

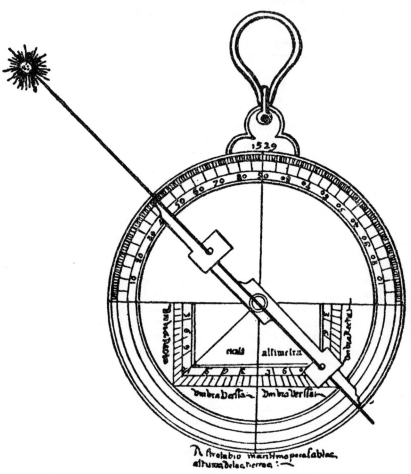

Fig. 5. SIMPLIFIED ASTROLABE OF THE PORTUGUESE MARINERS

As represented on Diogo Ribeiro's World Map of 1529 (Rome). The instrument was in fact still further simplified by the suppression of the altimetric scale of shadows seen in the lower half of this picture.

as royal astronomer, and his *Almanach* was translated by Vizinho and published in Leiria in 1496. As Zacuto's Tables were too complicated for the sailors' needs, they were simplified and compiled, with other data, in a practical manual known as *Rule of the astrolabe and of the quadrant*. These

Rules or *Regimentos*, though often copied by hand, were soon printed. The earliest known is the so-called (because the only copy extant was found in a Munich library) *Regimento de Munich*. Though this copy is not dated it was printed in Lisbon perhaps in 1509, and it seems that its earliest edition dates from 1495. The *Regimento* is divided into two parts. Part I contains: (1) Detailed instructions for calculating the latitude from the Sun's meridian altitude, with 17 examples according to whether the observer is north or south of the Equator or on the Equator; (2) rules for finding the latitude by measuring the height of the Pole Star; (3) list of the latitudes of 60 different points on the sea coasts, north of the Equator (the next edition known, the *Regimento de Evora* of 1517 (?), gives the latitudes of 193 points north and south of the Equator); (4) rule for plotting the ship's track; (5) calendar and tables of Sun's declination for twelve months. Part II contains only a Portuguese translation of the thirteenth-century English cosmographer Sacrobosco's *Tractatus de sphaera*. Later editions show considerable improvements in the rules and tables, and such additions as rules for the tides and determining the hour by the Pole Star and Guards.

These *Regimentos* soon found their way into Spain, either in works such as Martin Fernandez de Enciso's *Suma de geographia*, published for the first time in 1519, or were originally written in Spanish by Portuguese, such as Francisco Faleiro's *Tratado del esphera y del arte del marear*, published in 1535. In the words of Professor E. G. R. Taylor, 'Enciso appears simply to have translated into Castilian an example written early in 1518 by one Andreas Pires, a Portuguese pilot who, like Magellan and Ruy Faleiro, had transferred his services to Spain'.[3] Enciso also used largely the *Regimento de Munich*. Other similar Spanish books which appeared later, such as Pedro de Medina's *Arte de navegar* (1545) and Martin Cortés' *Breve compendio de la sphera y de la arte de navegar* (1551), are largely based on Portuguese works. It was mainly through Spanish books that Portuguese nautical science passed to the Dutch, English, French and Italians. The earliest of such English works is Roger Barlow's *Brief summe of geographie* written in 1540–1, which 'embodies an almost word for word translation of the volume which was prepared by Enciso in 1518'.[4] Next came Jean Rotz's *Boke of ydrography* (1542) which 'also closely follows the early Portuguese model'.[5] Thomé Cano, a Spanish pilot, wrote in his *Arte para fabricar, fortificar y apareiar naos de guerra y mercantes*, published in Seville, 1611: 'Spaniards, French, English and Dutch owe what they know to the Portuguese, who taught them how to navigate on the high seas and in distant regions: to them not only Spain but the whole of Europe owes the application of the astrolabe, which the ancient always used in order to know the movement of the stars, to the use and art of navigation—such a great invention as its consequences show.'[6] And the famous Fray Bartolomé de Las Casas had already asserted in the *Historia de las Indias*, which he wrote in its final form from 1552 to 1561: 'Certainly the Portuguese were the first who found and

[3] *A brief summe of geographie by Roger Barlow*. Ed. E. G. R. Taylor, 1932, p. xv

[4] *ibid.*, p. xi.

[5] *ibid.*, p. 185.

[6] fo. 5v, 6.

used this manner of navigating; and from them we Spaniards took it—do not deprive them of their deserts, but let us rather thank them.'[7] This might well be read by some who, even to-day, still try to deprive small Portugal of her due as the founder of modern nautical science.

Climax

Portuguese nautical science reached its climax in the first half of the sixteenth century, and among its many exponents three outstanding names must be mentioned: Duarte Pacheco, João de Castro and Pedro Nunes. Wide is the range of their contributions to nautical science, such as Pacheco's first scientific study of tides, Castro's research on magnetic declination, and Nunes' mathematical attainments, to mention only a few of the most remarkable. In the Introduction to his translation of Pacheco's *Esmeraldo*, Kimble refers to 'his almost unique geographical and nautical knowledge'. C. R. Boxer says that 'the works of Castro form a veritable landmark in the history of nautical science, and as regards Portuguese *Roteiros*, the standard they set was never surpassed . . . . those works on navigation and sailing directions which served as guides and models to the early English and Dutch navigators, who were destined to deprive their Lusitanian predecessors of their hard-won inheritance, and were the origin of the magnificent English *Pilots* series of the present'.[8]

There is ample evidence that cartography developed *pari passu* with Portuguese navigation. Azurara, Prince Henry's chronicler, refers to the detailed 'navigation charts which the Infant caused to be prepared' of the newly discovered coasts. In Beazley and Prestage's words, 'this passage shows in the clearest manner that the first hydrographical maps of the west coast of Africa, beyond Bojador, were made by the Portuguese, and that these maps were adopted and copied by the cosmographers of the whole of Europe'.[9] Of the many Portuguese fifteenth-century maps, often referred to in documents and chronicles, none is known to exist to-day. Some of them were used for the making of foreign maps, such as those of Bianco (1448), Fra Mauro (1457), Benincasa (1467, etc.), Toscanelli (1474), Soligo (*c.* 1475), Martellus (*c.* 1492), Behaim's globe (1492), map of *c.* 1471 in Modena, Egerton MS. 73, etc. With observed latitudes recorded on the charts, these acquired special geographical value, and after the navigations had gone beyond the Equator the degrees of longitude had the same size, and the north-south rhumb lines were perpendicular to the Equator, i.e. true meridians. Such a chart has been rightly called *carta plana quadrada* (square plate chart). This is specially noticeable when it took the form of a planisphere, such as the so-called Cantino map of 1502, which is actually drawn upon the equidistant cylindrical projection of a sphere. As the newly named coasts were delineated according to positions determined by dead reckoning and corrected by observed latitudes, magnetic declination had not been studied and distant longitudes were most inaccurate, the distribution of lands over such maps was often far from reality, and its representation

---

[7] lib. i, cap. 27.

[8] C. R. Boxer, 'Portuguese Roteiros, 1500–1700'. *Mariners' Mirror*, 1934, xx, 172–6.

[9] Azurara's *Chronicle*. Hakluyt Soc. ed., p. 345.

PLATE XXII

FIG. 6.   First page of the Portuguese translation of J. de Sacrobosco, *De Sphaera*

This treatise constituted the second part of the earliest known printed copy (? 1509) of the *Regimentos* or Nautical Rules.   The first edition was probably published *c.* 1495

,did not actually correspond to a cylindrical projection. The unknown nature of the declination (it was only in 1538 that Castro came to the conclusion :that 'magnetic deviation has no connexion with differences of meridian') brought the misplacement in latitude of distant coasts, even when the chart had a scale of geographical latitudes. This led some cartographers to add another small scale indicating the true geographical latitudes off Newfoundland, a region then specially visited by the Portuguese. There are still at least eighteen specimens of such charts extant; the first one is that of Pedro Reinel of c. 1504, and the last that of Denis de Rotis, dated as late as 1674.[10]

Pedro Nunes was the first to draw attention to the fact that cartography not rigorously scientific was worthless for accurate navigation. Perhaps the most remarkable of his contributions to nautical science was to recognize, and publish in 1537, that when a ship follows a fixed course it does not describe a straight line but a curve which cuts successive meridians at the same angle, i.e. a loxodrome. This could not be traced as a line on a square plate chart, except when the rhumb followed was dead north-south or east-west. His definition of the loxodrome is classical: 'The rhumbs are not circles, but irregular curves which go on forming with every meridian we pass equal angles as on the chart; and if we went straight towards the sun, under the arch which is a part of the greater circle, at every hour and moment we should be changing the course.' Nunes presented this question for the first time in the *Tratado em defensam da carta de marear* contained in his book *Tratado da sphera*, published in 1537, and later on dealt more scientifically with the problem, teaching how to trace the curve, in another of his books, *De arte atque ratione navigandi*, published at Basle in 1566. This is perhaps the most important work on nautical science ever written before his death. The keen mathematician described the nature of the loxodromic curve—a peculiar double spiral rising from the Equator to the poles without ever reaching them—but did not give the practical solution of the problem in its application to cartography. Such glory was reserved for the Flemish cosmographer Mercator, with the famous projection, graphically used for the first time in his map of 1569, which initiated a new era in nautical science. Mercator's projection was studied and improved by the Cambridge mathematician, Edward Wright, in his *Certaine Errors in Navigation detected and corrected* (1599). In another book, *De Crepusculis*, published in 1542, Nunes presented his invention of the *nonius*, for reading the exact divisions on a scale, eighty-nine years before Vernier. Great was the repercussion of Nunes' works. The famous English mathematician John Dee, says Professor Taylor, 'had formed a close friendship with his great Portuguese contemporary Pedro Nunes, and throughout his career as a mathematical adviser to a long succession of English explorers he is found to be applying the principle laid down in Nunes' important works upon nautical science'.[11]

During the first three centuries of distant seas navigation the sailors had no means of determining longitudes accurately; their instruments for observing eclipses were too rudimentary and chronometers were unknown.

[10] Personal communication from my friend Commander D. Gernez, who has given much attention to this problem.

[11] E. G. R. Taylor, *The English debt to Portuguese nautical science*, p. 8.

But even so, Duarte Pacheco calculated the length of the degree at eighteen leagues (106,560 metres), that is, with an error of 4 per cent only. At the Treaty of Tordesillas signed in 1494, which divided the world into a Portuguese and a Spanish hemisphere, one of the Portuguese delegates, Pacheco, demanded that the meridian of partition should run 370 leagues westwards of the Cape Verde Islands. Thus they made sure that a great part of the coast of Brazil—of the existence of which they already knew and which they needed as place of call for rounding the south of Africa on the voyage to the Indian Ocean—would remain within their zone, and that the coveted Spice Islands—of which they also had fairly precise information after Covilhã's voyage to India in 1488—would fall inside it by five degrees. This may show what surprisingly good results could be reached by the method of combining, repeatedly, differences of latitudes with the ship's true course derived from observations of the Polaris, Southern Cross and even the Sun for determining the longitude.

The rise of navigation to its present position of almost an exact science may fairly be dated from the invention of Mercator's projection, and from the English invention of the sextant in 1731 and of the chronometer in 1735; but its foundation was the fifteenth- and sixteenth-century nautical science of the Portuguese who, in their turn, derived theirs from the navigational experience and astronomical knowledge of the Mediterranean peoples. The great maritime enterprise was achieved through successive geographical steps in the transition from the Middle Ages to the Renaissance, the six foremost of which were the doubling of Cape Bojador in 1435, the crossing of the Equator in 1471, the rounding of the Cape of Good Hope in 1487, the officially accepted discovery of America in 1492, the arrival of a European fleet in India in 1498, and the discovery of the Straits of Magellan in 1520 followed by the first voyage across the Pacific. The discovery of the rest of the world became then a matter of course; modern geography was born. In less than a century cosmographers and seafarers had endowed mankind with new and wider horizons; the sea became the great route of the world; spices, gold, precious stones and other riches from remote countries began arriving more easily, or for the first time, in Europe; economic and intellectual intercourse between far away continents and peoples developed gradually into the internationalism which is now leading to the World Federation of Nations in, let us hope, a not very distant future.

Columbus went to America, Gama to India and Magellan to the Western Pacific thanks to the newly created nautical science—the key that opened one of the universal gates of the Renaissance.

FROM MEDIEVAL HERBALISM TO THE BIRTH OF
MODERN BOTANY*

by

AGNES ARBER

FROM the earliest times plants must, through sheer necessity, have compelled the interest of man, because of their usefulness in providing both food and protection. The incidental discovery that herbs had various effects in curing or mitigating the ills the flesh is heir to, must also date from the remote past. This discovery was, indeed, of the first importance in promoting plant study, for any herb, even those that had no other obvious use, might prove to be of medicinal value; thus the need to recognize those that, on trial, had proved effective, resulted in the gradual building up of a body of botanical knowledge. In the Middle Ages, although the accepted religious picture of the Universe, as limited in space and time, had an inhibiting influence upon scientific study in general, the Church fortunately never discouraged a knowledge of the herbs used in the arts of healing.[1] For Western Europe this knowledge found its record in a long series of herbal manuscripts, of which the sources date largely from the classical period. To Professor Charles Singer we owe an illuminating study of these works.[2] They continued to be copied and recopied by hand up to the time of the invention of printing, when some of them started a revived career in printed form. At the beginning of the sixteenth century there was thus in existence a considerable corpus of writings representing a tradition dating back to the Greek physician Dioscorides, who lived in the first century of the Christian era. These writings were, it is true, limited in scope, but they bore within themselves many of the seeds of that vast development in the systematic knowledge of the flowering plants which took place in the sixteenth and seventeenth centuries.

Side by side with the study of medicinal herbs through the literature, acquaintance with them was being kept alive continuously on the less sophisticated plane of folk medicine. The chief repositories of this kind of knowledge seem to have been country-women,[3] who handed down their lore from mother to daughter, and to them the learned sometimes express their debt. At the end of the thirteenth century Simon Corda of Genoa acknowledged that he was taught the Greek names of plants and their virtues by an old wife of Crete.[4] More than two hundred years later, Otto Brunfels alludes in his herbal to *vetulas expertissimas*,[5] 'highly expert old women', while Euricius Cordus, writing soon after Brunfels, says that he had in his

---

* In preparing this essay, use has been made of a lecture given on 29 January 1944, for the History of Science Lectures Committee of the University of Cambridge.

[1] Charles Singer, *A short history of science.* Oxford, 1941, pp. 154–5.

[2] *idem*, 'The herbal in antiquity'. *Journ. Hellenic Studies*, 1927, xlvii, 1–52.

[3] T. A. Sprague, 'The herbal of Otto Brunfels'. *Journ. Linn. Soc. Lond., Bot.*, 1928, xlviii, 79–124; cf. p. 82.

[4] Lynn Thorndike, *The Herbal of Rufinus.* Chicago, 1946 ; cf. p. xiii.

[5] Otto Brunfels, *Herbarum vivae eicones.* Argentorati, apud Joannem Schottum, 1530–6, vol. iii, p. 13.

time learned from the lowliest women and husbandmen (*cum a vilissimis nonnunquam mulierculis et colonis didicerim*);[6] while Anton Schneeberger, a Polish botanist, declared in 1557 that he 'was not ashamed to be the pupil of an old peasant woman'.[7] In England this folk medicine tradition was carried on into relatively modern times. Sir Joseph Banks, when he was at Eton in the mid-eighteenth century, was seized with a desire to know some botany, and the plan he adopted was to pay herb-women to teach him, giving them sixpence for every specimen they brought to him.[8] Somewhat later in the same century, Goethe was learning his plants from the herb-gatherers in the Thuringian forest.

Until well into the sixteenth century, such botanical information as was generally current in England can have been transmitted only by word of mouth, for the reason that herbal manuscripts were uncommon and inaccessible to the unlearned, while there were no printed books in existence from which simples could be identified. It was not until 1526 that the first British book with a series of plant pictures was published; this was *The grete herball*,[9] a translation of a French treatise, *Le grand Herbier*.[10] That it should have been Englished may seem surprising, since in those days Latin was the recognized medium for anything of a learned character; but it has recently been shown that, in the period from 1500 to 1640, a much higher proportion of scientific works appeared in the vernacular in this country than in any other, with the possible exception of Italy.[11] Moreover, in the case of *The grete herball*, there was every reason for using the mother tongue, since the purpose of the book was wholly practical, and it aimed at giving information about herbal remedies to a large, unlearned public. We are specially told that the work is arranged on a systematic plan, so that the 'herbes and trees in this booke comprehendyd [are] everyche of them chaptred by hymselfe, and in every chapter dyvers clauses wherin is shewed dyvers maner of medycynes in one herbe comprehended which ought to be notyfyed and marked for the helth of man'. When the modern reader observes how many herbs are each credited with the cure, not of one type of illness, but of complaints of all sorts, he cannot but wonder whether most of the remedies had any validity at all, except in so far as they introduced a fresh vegetable element into the people's diet, which must in those days have been generally deficient in this regard, especially in winter. A proportion of the herbal remedies named have survived, however, into our present pharmacopœia. The compiler of *The grete herball* noted that 'the iuce of the leves of wilowe is good to delay the heate in fevers yf it be dronken'; if he could return now, and see the extent to which drugs based on salicylic acid are used for this purpose, he would feel that his statement had been confirmed to an extent of which he could scarcely have dreamed.

[6] Euricius Cordus, *Botanologicon*. Coloniae, apud Joannem Gymnicum, 1534, pp. 26–7.

[7] B. Hryniewiecki, 'Anton Schneeberger (1530–81) ein Schüler Konrad Gesners in Polen'. *Veröffentlichungen des Geobot. Institutes Rübel in Zürich*, Heft 13, 1938, 64 pp.

[8] Sir J. Barrow, *Sketches of the Royal Society*. London, 1849, pp. 12–13.

[9] *The grete herball*. Southwark, Peter Treveris, 1526.

[10] Cf. A. Arber, *Herbals, their origin and evolution*. 2nd edition. Cambridge, 1938, pp. 26–8, 44–50.

[11] F. R. Johnson, *Astronomical Thought in Renaissance England*. Baltimore, 1937, p. 3.

The grete herball, though its actual date of publication is in the sixteenth century, illustrates the way in which medieval modes of thought lingered on into this period. Making no pretensions to originality, it is avowedly compiled from the works of ancient writers, such as Avicenna, Platearius, Albertus Magnus, and Bartholomew the Englishman, who themselves drew their information ultimately from classical sources. The book contains a large number of woodcuts, derived from continental illustrations of the previous century. Fig. 1, which represents the henbane, is one of the better examples, but not many of them are such as to enable the most ingenious student to identify the plant. Besides the conventional character of the pictures, another feature of the book, which must have been baffling to the enquiring reader, is the discordance which not infrequently occurs between figures and text.

𝕮𝖉𝖊 𝕵𝖚𝖘𝖖𝖚𝖎𝖆𝖒𝖔.𝕳𝖊𝖓𝖇𝖆𝖓𝖊.𝕮.𝕮𝕮.𝖗𝖑𝖎𝖎.

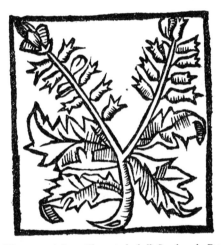

Fig. 1. Henbane (*Hyoscyamus*) from *The grete herball*. Southwark, Peter Treveris, 1526.

Occasionally economy is effected by using the same woodcut for more than one plant. The date palm, for instance, is illustrated by a picture which is recognizable though diagrammatic, so that it is disappointing to find this appearing again as the tamarind. Another woodcut does duty both for the cherry and for the deadly nightshade (*Atropa Belladonna* L.), but it is not probable that this led to fatalities, since the drawing does not bear the slightest resemblance to either plant. The account of 'Calendula', or 'Ruddes', undoubtedly relates to the marigold, for we are told that 'Maydens make garland of it when they go to feestes and brydeales', but it is associated with a figure which is distinctly a wallflower, and not a marigold at all. Discrepancy between text and illustrations occurs, in fact, so often that one can only suppose that, in those days of lack of picture books, the printer felt that his duty was done when plenty of decorations had been supplied, and that their relevance to the text was a matter of little moment.

In *The grete herball* there is not much attempt at a description of each plant, but sometimes an indication of its character is given. A word may be said, for instance, about shape and colour of fruit structures; corn-cockle 'hath blacke sedes tryangled or syded', while the seed of gromwell is 'clere and whyte shynynge and therfore it is called grayne of ye sonne'. In general, however, such description as is vouchsafed almost limited to comparison with other plants. For example, 'Lupulus is an herbe that groweth on hedges and rampeth in maner of an herbe called bryony or whyte vyne and is called hoppes, ye leves therof be lyke nettles, and hath sharpe savour and tarte'. One of the most adequate descriptions is that of *Polygonatum*. We are told that 'Sigillum sancte Marye, or Sigillum Salamonis is al one herbe that is called Salamon's seale or our ladies seale. It groweth in derke shadowy places and in forestes and hath leves lyke [Polygonum] and lytell smal whyte floures, and bereth reed sedes on a rowe two and two one as another in ordre and hath a whyte knotty rote as kneholme or fragon [butcher's broom]'. In most cases, however, description is almost completely neglected. Such an account as 'Borage is an herbe y^t hath rugh leves and is named bourage', seems to be regarded as sufficient. The cornflower, again, is discriminated merely as 'an evyll wede y^t groweth in the wheate', while ceterach is still more simply distinguished as 'an herbe so named'.

It was obviously essential for collectors of medicinal herbs to know where to look for their plants, and this need is met in *The grete herball* by a certain amount of information about habitats. 'Polypodi', for instance, is described as 'a wede moche lyke to ferne, and groweth on walles, stones, and upon okes'. About the homes of exotics the writer is pardonably vague, and 'beyond the sea' evidently passed as an exact enough localization. 'Aloes', then famous for the perfume derived from it, is described as 'a wood . . . founde in a flode of hye Babylone nygh wherby renneth a ryver of Paradyse terrestre'. This may seem a fantastic account, but it was long before it was improved upon, for the origin of aloes remained an incompletely solved problem, even in comparatively recent times.[12] It is perhaps possible that references to Babylon in *The grete herball* were not intended to be taken literally, but were merely a graceful way of indicating that the writer had no idea whence the plant came. Cassia wood is another example; we learn that it is 'the barke of a lytell tree that groweth towards the ende of babylon'. The traditional children's game 'How many miles to Babylon?' suggests that the word had associations hinting at something remote from the prosaic factual world. It is hardly surprising that *The grete herball* should fail to be specific about the provenance of foreign vegetable drugs, when we remember how belatedly they have sometimes been traced to the plant producing them. We have just mentioned the instance of aloes; kostus, also, was a well-known perfume from the time of Dioscorides or earlier, but its botanical source (*Sausurrea Lappa* A. B. Clarke, Compositae) was not discovered until the middle of the nineteenth century.[13]

The impression one gains from turning over the pages of *The grete herball*— taken as representative of the popular aspect of medical botany in its overlap

[12] Lign-aloes, calambac, calambour, or eagle-wood, is now known to be derived from *Aquilaria Agallocha* Roxb. (Thymeleaceae.)

[13] T. A. Sprague, 'Early Herbals'. *Pharm. Journ.*, 1937, cxxxix, 515–8.

from the medieval into the Renaissance period—is that this type of study had advanced very little since the days of Dioscorides, some 1500 years earlier, for both text and illustrations were derived from classical sources, and had, on the whole, altered only in the direction of degradation through continued copying from generation to generation. Moreover, there seemed to be no reason why this imitative process, having gone on for so long, should not have continued indefinitely; but, happily, a fresh impulse arose in the sixteenth century. It was not, however, the herbalists themselves who in the first place breathed this new spirit into their subject, but the artists who were summoned to collaborate with them. This is exemplified in the work of Otto Brunfels, a German botanist who produced a Latin herbal in 1530, the *Herbarum vivae eicones*.[14] The text, though it revealed great learning and had much more botanical content than the group to which *The grete herball* belongs, showed no definite advance on the classics, being frankly a compilation from Dioscorides, Apuleius Platonicus, and other writers. It was the Italian botanists of the fifteenth and the beginning of the sixteenth centuries who had been the pioneers in translating and commenting on the earlier authorities, and it was through their interpretative work that Brunfels gained his information. It appears that Brunfels was himself perfectly satisfied to depend entirely on classical sources; he does not show the smallest inclination to describe in his own words even the most familiar plants. As an example we may take his account of the water-lilies. The white water-lily, he says, 'has broad leaves emerging somewhat above the water, solid, firm, leathery, strongly scented. Sometimes, however, they are also under water, many arising from one root. Flower white like a lily, having a yellow centre. The flower, after it has shed, is round, and similar in its roundness to an apple or to the head of a poppy, and of a dark colour. Root [rhizome] large, rough, knotted like some kind of club'. Of the yellow water-lily he writes: 'It springs forth like the first; the root, however, is paler and rough. It has shining yellow flowers like a rose. It also bears from the root, as it were, the tails of dormice.' On comparing this description with that given by Dioscorides,[15] one finds that Brunfels took over the earlier account almost word for word. The only point original to him seems to be the similitude suggested between the adventitious roots of the yellow water-lily and the tails of dormice—an apt touch.

On plant nomenclature and classification[16] such ideas as one can gather from Brunfels are unimpressive. He did not attach importance to choosing one Latin name and sticking to it; for instance, he calls the various buttercups indifferently *Pes Corvinus*, *Coronopus*, or *Galli Crus*—all three names being suggested by the resemblance of the leaf to the foot of a bird. Of species in the modern sense he had no clear conception. To him a species simply meant a 'kind', and he sometimes included plants which are now allotted to different families under what, in modern parlance, is one generic name. He distinguished, for example, three Scrophularias—*major*, *media*, and

---

[14] *idem*, *op. cit.* (3). Much use has been made of this memoir in the following account of Brunfels' herbal.

[15] Dioscorides, *The Greek Herbal of Dioscorides . . . Englished by John Goodyer*, 1655. Ed. by R. T. Gunther. Oxford, 1934, bk. iii, 148–9, pp. 377–8.

[16] Sprague, *op. cit.* (3), pp. 84–5.

minor—but these are the plants of which the Linnean names are *Scrophularia nodosa* (fig-wort); *Sedum Telephium* (orpine) ; and *Ranunculus Ficaria* (lesser celandine).

H Y O S C Y A M V S

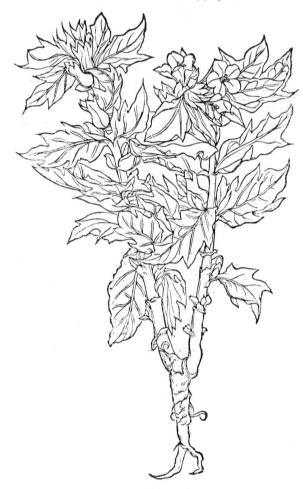

Bylſam kraut.

Fig. 2. Henbane (*Hyoscyamus*) from Otto Brunfels, *Herbarum vivae cicones.*
Strasbourg, 1530–6.

The significance of Brunfels' herbal in the history of botany is not, indeed, to be looked for in the text, but in the illustrations, which are superbly drawn though with no sacrifice of realism to artistry. Fig. 2 is an example, but justice could not be done to their quality without reproducing them all, and on the original scale. The drawings were not Brunfels' own work. Either he himself or his publisher called in an extremely gifted artist, Hans Weiditz, who was made responsible for the figures. The introduction of Weiditz to collaborate in the preparation of the herbal had unforeseen consequences; he seems to have soon assumed the upper hand, with results that have been welcomed by posterity, but were evidently disconcerting to Brunfels himself. Brunfels regarded the classical names of herbs as the *real* names, and he had intended to relegate to a mere appendix those plants which could not claim to have been sponsored by antiquity, and were so luckless as to possess vernacular names alone. He called these poor things *herbae nudae*,[17] forlorn or destitute herbs. His neat plan for thus separating the sheep from the goats was, however, dislocated, because Weiditz and his assistants insisted on drawing what they chose when they chose, and their choice sometimes fell upon these botanical outcasts; so that—with the printer waiting for copy— Brunfels was faced with the inclusion of pictures of upstart plants, unknown to the ancients, which he had had no intention of honouring in this way. For this unfortunate situation he apologizes in connexion with the pasque-flower (*Anemone Pulsatilla* L.) and the ladies' smock (*Cardamine pratensis* L.), neither of which had previously received scientific recognition. He would, no doubt, have been startled if he could have known that these two woodcuts, which he admitted so grudgingly, would be accorded an outstanding place in the history of plant delineation, both because of their own admirable quality, and as being the original type pictures of two Linnean species.[18] On account of its realistic illustrations, which belong to a different world from the symbolic decorations of *The grete herball*, Brunfels' work is the first in which it is possible to identify a high proportion of the species enumerated. This herbal may thus be regarded as in some respects the starting point of modern systematic botany.[19] Of the 258 species and varieties dealt with in the *Herbarum vivae eicones*, rather more than four-fifths were already known to classical and medieval writers, while the remaining 47 species were new to science when they were published by Brunfels.[20] There is a clear line of descent from Brunfels, through Gaspard Bauhin, to Linnaeus, and thence to twentieth-century systematics, for Linnaeus as a rule cites Bauhin's *Pinax* of 1623 as his earliest authority, while Bauhin himself generally refers back to Brunfels.[21]

As we have seen, Brunfels' text was essentially classical and medieval, and was not itself rejuvenated by the illustrations associated with it. But it was these illustrations which had a searching influence upon contemporary and later herbalists, opening their eyes to features of form and structure hitherto disregarded. We can trace this effect in the work of the two great German botanists who immediately succeeded Brunfels—Leonhart Fuchs and Jerome Bock. In Fuchs' case the influence was specially direct, for it concerned his pictures rather than his text. In 1542 he produced a magnificent herbal, *De historia stirpium*;[22] its figures owed much to Weiditz's woodcuts, which

---

[17] 'nudas herbas, quarum tantum nomina germanica nobis cognita sunt, praeterea nihil' (*Herbarum vivae eicones, op. cit.* (5), 1530, vol. i, p. 217).

[18] Sprague, *op. cit.* (3), p. 90.

[19] *ibid.*, p. 79.   [20] *ibid.*, p. 113.   [21] *ibid.*, p. 89.

[22] Leonhart Fuchs, *De historia stirpium*. Basileae, in officina Isingriniana, 1542. For an authoritative study of this herbal, see T. A. Sprague and E. Nelmes, 'The Herbal of Leonhart Fuchs', *Journ. Linn. Soc. Lond., Bot.*, 1931, xlviii, 545–642.

had shown the way to combine full botanical content with artistic excellence. His picture of henbane is reproduced here as Fig. 3. The three illustrations of this plant which are reproduced in this essay will enable the reader to

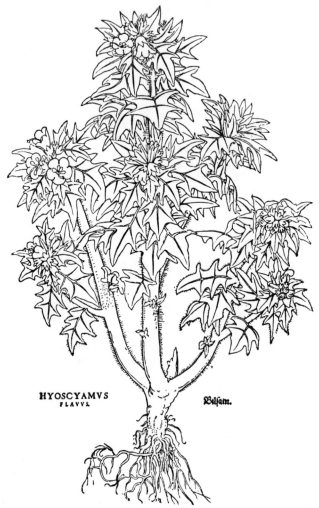

HYOSCYAMVS
FLAVVS.   Bilfam.

Fig. 3. Henbane (*Hyoscyamus flavus*) from Leonhart Fuchs, *De Historia stirpium.*
Basle, 1542, fo. 833.

compare the stylized medievalism of *The grete herball* with the 'back to nature' tendency of work that originated in the sixteenth century.

So far as the text[23] was concerned, Fuchs' herbal was based essentially upon Dioscorides. Like Brunfels he was a medical man, and his interest

[23] Cf. *ibid., p.* 553.

was concentrated primarily upon the improvement of the German pharma-copœia. He aimed at reaching correct identifications of the plants whose virtues were detailed not only by Dioscorides, but also by Galen, and other early authorities. Struggling towards this end, he, like Brunfels, suffered from one severe handicap—the failure to realize how vastly different the Mediterranean flora, described by the classical writers, actually was from the plant world north of the Alps which he himself knew.

We may sum up the contributions of Brunfels and Fuchs by saying that, while their text to some extent clarified and increased the existing knowledge of plants, it was their illustrations which opened a new era in botany. What their artists saw with their own eyes, and conveyed in their drawings, constituted a more complete impression of plant nature than the limited and imitative accounts which these two writers gave in words.

In 1539, that is to say between the appearance of Brunfels' herbal and that of Fuchs, Jerome Bock (Hieronymus Tragus) produced a botanical work which, as regards its text, showed more originality than the other two. Bock tells us[24] that 'Otto Brunfels of pious memory', urged him 'to put the vast work in order and to communicate it to our Germany'. Patriotism was evidently a powerful factor in inducing Bock to submit to so much labour; he says that nothing could delight him more than that his results should be of use to 'our most beloved country'. It was consistent with this attitude that, unlike Brunfels and Fuchs, he chose to write in German. By his expressive and masterly use of his own native tongue, he painted word pictures of the plants which he handled, pictures which share the vivid and first-hand quality of Weiditz's drawings. It has been suggested that the special excellence of Bock's descriptions was the result of a compensatory effort to make up for his inability to pay for illustrations for the first edition of his herbal. It seems more likely, however, that it was in reality due to an inherent instinct for observing plant life, and a natural gift for finding fit words in which to clothe his impressions. We have previously quoted Brunfels' account of the water-lilies, which showed very little advance on Dioscorides. Bock progressed much further, especially in paying considerable attention to the flower. He described the buds of the white Nymphaea as 'certain oblong heads, almost like ripe almonds, enclosed in purplish-green leaves'. From each of these buds is produced in June, 'a white lily or rose of many leaves crowded together, so that one flower verily appears to consist of twenty-eight leaves, or sometimes fewer. These leaves, considered individually, resemble in form a thumb or the leaf of a houseleek'. So definite an attempt to give an idea both of the number and shape of the perianth members in a flower of this type was, at that time, something new. The nature of the stamens and radiating stigmas in the centre of the flower was of course mysterious to Bock, but he suggests their appearance by describing them as 'something saffron-coloured, not very different from a figure of the sun'. He notes the smoothness and spongy texture of the leaf-stalk, and the absence of scent and taste in the rhizome. Passing to the yellow water-lily, he mentions the resemblance of its buds to those of the marsh marigold (*Caltha palustris* L.).[25]

[24] Jerome Bock, *De stirpium*. Argentorati, 1552. Preface, cap. xiii. (Throughout this account of Bock's work, I have used this Latin version of his herbal.)
[25] *ibid.*, ii, cap. xlviii, pp. 695–6.

Brunfels, though he was the first to record the pasque-flower (*Anemone Pulsatilla* L.) gives no description of it because it was unknown to the ancients. Bock, on the other hand, instead of being inhibited by the absence of any previous account upon which he could draw, gives out of his own head a good description[26] of this 'unknown herb', which he says the herb-women call dinner bell or cow bell. The plant in its vegetating state he likens to fennel, and its black and hairy root to that of the Christmas rose. He adds that it flowers in March, and that in May the flower comes to an end in a smooth, hoary, hairy head, which he says 'may be compared, not infelicitously, to a rudiment of a hedgehog'. He likens the individual threads to hogs' bristles, but recognizes their seed nature; he notes that the stalk, which bears the head, may be nine inches long. He has observed in his garden that the hot biting taste of the plant keeps it safe from the attacks of animals. On the evidence of its pungent taste, he decides that it is a kind of ranunculus—an idea which shows real insight into relationships.

This description of the pasque-flower brings out one of the best characteristics of Bock's work—namely that his conceptions were dynamic rather than merely static. When he described a plant, his ideal evidently was to give a concise account of the life-history, rather than to limit attention to the flowering epoch—a phase to which systematic descriptions are still too often confined. The stress which Bock lays on the developmental sequence from season to season of the year comes out conspicuously in what he says of the lesser celandine (*Ranunculus Ficaria* L.).[27] His description of the leaves and root is adapted from Dioscorides,[28] but his account of the flower and of the life-history is his own. He explains that the plant appears about the end of February, on moist hills, in vineyards, and in certain meadows, and is rendered conspicuous by its green hue. Like arum and the orchis kind, it comes to life afresh every year, with new roots, leaves, and flower. A slender stalk shoots up, bearing a very beautiful yellow bloom, which clearly represents a little star, and recalls that of ranunculus. Withering in the month of May, it dies away, letting fall its leaves and flowers, the rootlets meanwhile lying hid in the earth until the beginning of February in the following year.

It will not give a just idea of Bock's position in the history of botany if we recall only those parts of his work in which he was relatively advanced; so, as a counterpoise to the sound observations already quoted, we may consider his theories about the origin of the wild orchids[29] of the German countryside, with which he was familiar. He notes that, when the flower has fallen, certain small pods appear, filled with fine dust. He does not recognize this dust as their seeds, but this is scarcely surprising; even with the advantage of a microscope, the minute embryo, with its fantastically exaggerated envelope, does not in the least recall a seed of the ordinary type. Having then decided that orchids have no seed, Bock sought about for their means of propagation, and thought that he had discerned it. Influenced no doubt by the curious animal-like form of the flowers in some members of the group, he was

---

[26] *ibid.*, i, cap. cxxxvii, pp. 413–4.
[27] *ibid.*, i, cap. xxv, p. 112.
[28] Dioscorides, *op. cit.* (15), ii, 212, p. 227.
[29] Bock, *op. cit.* (24), ii, cap. lxxxii, pp. 783–5.

prepared to find that they sprang from an alien source, and he suggests in all seriousness that they are the offspring of thrushes and blackbirds. The bird's-nest orchid (*Neottia Nidus-avis* L.) he regards somewhat differently; it seems to him a monstrosity, and he propounds the theory that it takes its origin from putrefaction. That views of this kind should have been held by so intelligent a man as Bock, is an indication of the existence of a dark background of superstitious beliefs; it helps one to realize how difficult it must have been in the sixteenth century to achieve a fully scientific approach to natural history, when the general atmosphere was charged with a credulity that recognized no impossibilities.

We noticed that Bock's fervour for his fatherland was potent in inciting him to make his herbal. The same fervour is clearly apparent in his account of sweet root, or liquorice, the Mediterranean *Glycyrrhiza glabra* L.[30] He indites a paean in praise of 'this most excellent and most noble plant', saying that, 'just as other nations proclaim and extol sugar, so Germany can glory in liquorice'; and he notes that a certain region in Bavaria could supply enough of this product for the whole of Germany. The woodcut which Bock gives includes, as well as the picture of the plant, a coil of the long, dark, pliable sticks of liquorice, which are still familiar to us in the twentieth century. He is also moved to reward the plant's dedication to the service of the state by decorating it with a cartouche of the two-headed eagle of the Holy Roman Empire.

Among contemporary botanists rather younger than the three Fathers of Botany, another German, Valerius Cordus, has special claims to remembrance; but as he died in 1544, before he was thirty, as a result of the hardships of an Italian journey, and as his botanical work was not published in his own time, he is too often overlooked. Cordus was not the only herbalist whose life was sacrificed to plant hunting in Italy in those days. The British botanist William Turner recorded in 1568 that a certain Gerhardus de Wijck was 'so earnest a sercher of simpels [medicinal herbs] when he was in Italy, that he went into the mount Appennine wyth manye other, to finde out simplesse, wherof he onelye wyth two or thre other escaped death, for all the other dyed ether in there yorneye or shortely after that they came home '.[31]

Cordus left in manuscript an *Historia plantarum*[32] written about 1540, which was published posthumously in 1561. It is his ability to give identifiable diagnoses that is his chief distinction. When one considers descriptions of plants by early botanists, there is a temptation to judge them as if they were inferior specimens of twentieth-century descriptions, whereas they are really something of rather a different kind. Dr. Sprague, who has specialized in identifying plants from Cordus' *Historia*, finds that this is best done by setting his accounts side by side with good modern *figures* of the plants concerned, rather than with the corresponding *descriptions*. This can only mean that the artist takes a view of the plant which is less limited by contemporaneity than that of the botanist, who describes it technically on

[30] *ibid.*, ii, cap. cl, pp. 934–7.

[31] William Turner, *The first and seconde partes of the Herbal of William Turner . . . with the Third parte, lately gathered.* Collen (A. Birckman), 1568, p. 6.

[32] See T. A. and M. S. Sprague, 'The Herbal of Valerius Cordus'. *Journ. Linn. Soc., Lond., Bot.*, 1939, lii, 1–113. (Abstract in *Proc. Linn. Soc.*, Lond., 1936–7, Session 149, 156–8.)

some preconceived scheme; and that the artist thus includes features in his drawing which are omitted in modern descriptions, but which may find a place in a sixteenth-century account. A modern diagnosis emphasizes only such characteristics as seem, in our particular period, to be of importance, and generally those only which can be recognized in dried material, special significance being attributed to the structure of the flower. A sixteenth-century account, on the other hand, diverges from this in several points. It tends, for instance, to stress comparisons with unrelated plants; but a more important difference is that it lays the general emphasis on another set of characters from those to which we turn to-day. Considerable notice is taken of the vegetative habit and of the root, and also of features detectable by senses other than sight. For instance, Cordus, in describing a kind of goat's-beard, says that the root, 'when cut, . . . yields a copious supply of greyish-white latex, which, when worked with the fingers or tongue, becomes like bird-lime, and can be drawn out into a long string, and when dried becomes red and by degrees black; the whole herb is sweet to the taste, and the latex actively astringent but without smell'.[33]   Odour and taste were studied intensively because of their real or supposed value in indicating medicinal properties, and they often revealed good diagnostic characters which have been lost to sight in modern botany. For example, it has been pointed out by Sprague that one of the meadow rues[34] described by Cordus can be identified as *Thalictrum flavum* L., because he describes the rhizome as yellow internally, and indicates that the leaves are intermediate in form between the lower leaves of coriander and those of rue (two genera quite unrelated to *Thalictrum*), while the whole plant has a bitter and somewhat acrid taste. These details, though taken together they do in fact serve for recognition, would not be emphasized in a modern description. In the same way, another of his species is known to have been *Thalictrum angustifolium* L., because he mentions that its flower has a strong smell, recalling that of the elder. So little attention is paid to-day to odour and taste, that systematists no longer feel it their duty to estimate them comparatively from the evidence of their own senses. The seventeenth century, however, took a different view. In 1682 Nehemiah Grew[35] analysed all plant tastes into ten basic elements, which he considered might be present in graded strengths, and in various combinations, and might lead altogether to 1,800 recognizable 'variations of taste'. This may seem to us now fantastic, but no doubt perception in such matters increases with careful cultivation; and when Grew spoke of the 'Green Pods' of a certain species of clematis as being hot in the tenth degree, we may take it that he at least conveyed a somewhat more definite idea to his own generation than he does to ours.

Though we may have fallen below the standards of earlier days in the discrimination of tastes and smells, it sometimes seems as if the reverse were true where colour is concerned; but this is probably in part a misleading impression due to changes in the use of names for different hues.[36]   For

[33] *ibid.*, p. 30.
[34] *ibid.*, pp. 25–6.
[35] Nehemiah Grew, *The anatomy of plants.* London, 1682, pp. 279–82.
[36] Sprague, *op. cit.* (3), p. 87.

instance, 'brown' in English and 'braun' in German were applied in the sixteenth century to flowers which we would now call mauve, purple, or pinkish. In *The grete herball* one of the small crane's-bills is described as having a 'browne' flower (chap. ccclxi), while Brunfels calls the purple comfrey 'brown', and Fuchs uses the same adjective for the fox-glove, though translating it into Latin as *purpureus*. *Niger* and *candidus*, again, are also words that sometimes cause confusion, since they did not always mean black and white, but sometimes merely dark and pale.

The few German botanists we have named, who flourished in the first half of the sixteenth century, and their great Italian contemporary, Pierandrea Mattioli—whose work, though it is of the first importance, must here be left untouched—were succeeded, in the latter part of the sixteenth century by a galaxy of herbalists, scattered over most of the countries of Europe, who collectively assembled a vast corpus of information, which as time went on became more and more unwieldy and overwhelming. At first there had been no idea of any rigid system of nomenclature. The naming depended largely on the herbalist's personal fancies; for example, various authors, from Brunfels onwards, had given at least seven different names to the hoary plantain, the *Plantago media* of Linnaeus.[37] The muddle was increased by the fact that the names sometimes took the inconvenient form of whole descriptive phrases; but gradually, out of the welter of confusion, an approach was made towards the binominal system, which Linnaeus was destined to crystallize in the eighteenth century.

The most convincing indication of the increase in the mass of material available between the early sixteenth and early seventeenth centuries is given by a comparison of Brunfels' herbal with Gaspard Bauhin's *Pinax theatri botanici* of 1623.[38] Brunfels includes less than 260 species, whereas Bauhin deals with about 6,000. As an index of the momentum attained after another two centuries, we may recall that a single systematist, A. P. de Candolle, in the early nineteenth century himself described more than 6,000 *new* species— that is to say, more than the total number which had become known between the beginning of scientific botany in Greece and the days of Bauhin.[39] Bauhin's *Pinax* (or chart) was a successful effort at sorting out plant names, and bringing order into the crowd of unco-ordinated facts that had gradually accumulated. In thinking of the history of plant nomenclature and classification, we have to remind ourselves that no one actually *perceives* anything but individual plants. The idea of a species is a mental abstraction from the direct knowledge of individuals, while the idea of a genus is a further abstraction from the idea of species. Bauhin sharply differentiated genera and species, giving names to genera, but without descriptions, while distinguishing species by diagnostic phrases. Tournefort made a further advance at the end of the seventeenth century, since he treated genera as being themselves entities susceptible of description.[40]

---

[37] M. L. Green, 'History of plant nomenclature'. *Kew Bull.*, 1927, 403–15.

[38] Sprague, *op. cit.* (3), p. 79.

[39] A. L. P. de Candolle, 'La vie et les écrits de Sir William Hooker'. *Bibliothèque Universelle*, Genève, 1886, xxv, 44–62. (Especially see p. 59.)

[40] Green, *op. cit.* (37).

Though the earlier writers often tacitly recognized genera, in the modern sense, as units, the way in which they grouped these genera was as a rule merely a matter of convenience. *The grete herball*, and even Fuchs' herbal, were alphabetical in plan, and though Bock objected to this scheme, and definitely aimed at setting like plants side by side, he achieved this only within narrow limits. Throughout the sixteenth century the prevailing tendency was to group together those plants which did the same sort of service or disservice to man; for instance, herbs which would heal wounds, herbs suitable for garlands, and poisonous herbs, might each form a group. It is true that the herbalists in this way occasionally builded better than they knew, for, in associating plants which had special scents or special medicinal qualities, they sometimes unconsciously grouped them according to valid chemical criteria; but this was an exceptional happening. It was only in the most gradual way that botany ceased to be distorted by man's egoism, and plants began to be thought of as creatures with their own lives and relationships, which were independent of human needs and whims. Even when the idea had arisen of classifying plants according to their own nature, and not merely to provide man with a utility key to the vegetable creation, the question as to which of their characteristics were basic for taxonomy still remained open. The sixteenth-century herbalists did not face this question explicitly, and, so far as they attained to a natural classification, they reached it through an intuitive feeling for affinity, which they did not attempt to rationalize. This instinctive process reached its highest point in Mathias de l'Obel, a botanist of the Low Countries who lived long in England. He succeeded, chiefly on leaf characters, in segregating at least partially the groups that we now call dicotyledons and monocotyledons. Unlike most of the herbalists of his period he had a profound and almost mystical sense of the underlying meaning of classification, which he thought should reveal a certain universal order.[41] Possibly he had in mind the Great Chain of Being,[42] passing without discontinuity from inanimate objects through all the forms of life, and culminating in creatures transcending man. This conception played a great part in medieval and Renaissance thought, and it is surprising that the herbalists on the whole showed little obvious trace of its influence.

If we regard the sixteenth century as a time of instinctive groping after plant relationships, we may correspondingly look upon the seventeenth century as the period in which a number of possible criteria for classification were tested in their application. The various schemes which were then propounded all suffered alike from a certain narrowness, because they depended upon the idiosyncrasies of their authors, who selected individual features at choice and used them as if they were universal clues to relationship. Rivinus,[43] for instance, was obsessed by the corolla, while Morison[44] stressed the characters of the fruit and seed. Both Morison and Ray were too much influenced by the habit distinction between trees, shrubs, and herbs. Ray's system is held to be the best devised in the latter part of the seventeenth

[41] Mathias de L'Obel and Petrus Pena, *Stirpium adversaria nova*. London, 1570. See preface.
[42] See A. O. Lovejoy, *The Great Chain of Being*. Harvard, 1934.
[43] A. Q. Rivinus, *Introductio generalis in rem herbariam*. Lipsiae, 1690–9.
[44] On Morison, see S. H. Vines and G. C. Druce, *The Morisonian Herbarium*. Oxford, 1914.

century. He invented the terms dicotyledon and monocotyledon, and separated these groups on seedling structure more effectively than de l'Obel had done on leaf characters. Ten years ago, in a biography by Dr. Raven,[45] full justice was done to Ray for the first time. This book contains a complete study of Ray's work on plants, and is helpful in including extensive translations from his Latin, which—though in itself of admirable quality— has hitherto acted as a barrier between him and the average botanist.

The progress of systematic botany, throughout the period which we are considering, showed a steadier progress than that of most scientific subjects. Though the seventeenth century was a revolutionary time in the non-biological sciences—since the overthrow of Aristotelian physics changed men's attitude to the universe as a whole—botany, being modestly concerned with our one planet alone, remained unaffected. Even in the last decade of the seventeenth century, Camerarius, whom we shall consider later, quotes Aristotle respectfully, though he thinks it necessary to apologize for doing so. So far as classification is concerned, the influence of the Aristotelian school showed itself chiefly in the long survival of the division into trees, shrubs, and herbs. However, as time went on, it became more and more apparent that the detailed structure of the flower and fruit, which the ancient writers had understood but little, furnished clues to classification which could be followed more readily than those derived from the vegetative system; but in taxonomics full use could not be made of floral structure, until the nature of the stamens, and their function in relation to the carpels, had been elucidated. Before considering how this was brought about, we must turn to certain other developments which preceded the discovery of sex in plants.

From the classic days of Greece, a great botanical treatise representing the teachings of Theophrastus, Aristotle's successor, had been handed down. This treatise, which dealt with the plant on broad general lines, influenced the theoretical botany of the Renaissance much as the *Materia medica* of Dioscorides dominated it on the medical side. Now and then these two influences interpenetrated; Brunfels, for instance, in his herbal, which is essentially Dioscoridean, introduces as an appendix some of the work of Theophrastus on the parts of plants. The share of botany in the seventeenth-century revolt against the Aristotelian tradition mainly resolved itself into a call for the replacement of book knowledge by direct observation; this was obviously a sound plea, but the insistence on it, as though it were something new, was manifestly unjust to the Aristotelian school. Both Aristotle and Theophrastus were admirable observers, and they never claimed that their work should be treated as final. The harm had been done, not by their own teachings, but by unintelligent and slavish repetitions, which had fossilized their dicta into a body of dogma which it was treasonable to question. Those who approached the teachings of the classical school in the right way, seeking from them suggestions for their own thought rather than a ready-made creed, continued to find in them intellectual wealth. Aristotle, Theophrastus, and their successors had been deeply impressed by the analogy traceable between animals and plants. This, like most analogies, was a two-edged weapon, and its uncritical use in some ways did harm to botany, since it led to plants

[45] C. E. Raven, *John Ray Naturalist.* Cambridge, 1942.

being fitted forcibly into an alien scheme derived from a prior knowledge of animals. In opening up new fields of research, however, the comparison was a fruitful one, especially since it led Marcello Malpighi in Italy, and Nehemiah Grew in England, to embark in the latter half of the seventeenth century upon the study of the internal structure of plants, with the aid of the newly-invented microscope. Though they were both indebted to the Aristotelian analogy, they approached it from different angles. Grew[46] thought that, since the bodies of animals and of plants were both 'the *Contrivances* of the same *Wisdom*', he might search hopefully in the field of plant structure for discoveries similar to those which had already been made among animals. Malpighi, on the other hand, tells us that in the enthusiasm of youth he chose the higher animals for anatomical study. The grave difficulties he encountered suggested to him that he might get help through a comparison with simpler forms of life, so he turned to insects. Here, not unnaturally, he again found special difficulties; so he decided to proceed to plants, as a still lower and simpler level of creation. No doubt the clues to animal structure that he hoped to find among plants must have eluded him, but incidentally he laid the foundations of a new science. It is impossible to give any adequate idea of the work of Malpighi and Grew in a few words, so it must be left untouched. We will only say that anyone who turns over their great folios must stand amazed at the amount of anatomical detail which they discovered and portrayed, considering that there was no previous knowledge whatever upon which they could build. An unaccountable feature in the history of botany is that, after the time of Malpighi and Grew, plant anatomy remained virtually stationary for about a hundred and fifty years. There is no obvious reason why it should not have advanced steadily after so favourable a beginning, but in actual fact it failed to do so.

Grew was just as much concerned with general morphology, and with ideas about function, as he was with what is commonly called plant anatomy. He dealt in detail, for instance, with the structure of flowers. When he first became interested in the subject, he was at a disadvantage because the nature of the stamens was unknown. It is true that from early days plants had sometimes been distinguished as male and female, but this distinction was metaphorical only. Brunfels, for instance, in the case of colour varieties, calls the plant with the stronger colour the male.[47] That the scarlet pimpernel is male, and the blue, female, is a statement which is found in Dioscorides, and is repeated by Brunfels, who also called the purple-red dead-nettle (*Lamium maculatum* L.) male, and the white dead-nettle (*Lamium album* L.) female. Fuchs also sometimes uses these terms, but with him they scarcely mean more than calling two varieties α and β.[48] When Grew wrote his first book in 1672, a full century after Fuchs' death, though the problem of the function of the stamens was no longer ignored, it was still unsolved. Grew saw that the beauty of the stamens was agreeable to man, and that they might be useful in helping him to tell one plant from another. While it was also clear that they had a part to play in connexion with insect life, he felt

---

[46] Grew, *op. cit.* (35), preface.

[47] See Sprague, *op. cit.* (3), p. 87.

[48] Sprague and Nelmes, *op. cit.* (22), p. 552.

that explanations of this type were incomplete; and he thought that the stamens must also have some meaning, still undeciphered, in the plant's own economy. A few years later he had reached the right conclusion, and in his *Anatomy of Plants* of 1682[49] he definitely adopted the view that the androecium (or 'attire', as he calls it) 'doth serve, as the *Male*, for the *Generation* of the *Seed*'. This view, he says, Sir Thomas Millington had suggested to him in conversation, but apparently after he had already reached it on his own account. Millington,[50] though well known in other fields, does not, except through this one reference, figure in the history of botany; he just flashes across the scene, secures immortality with a single remark, and vanishes again.

Grew made no attempt to *prove* the male nature of the stamens. It was reserved for a German botanist, R. J. Camerarius, to do so in 1694 in a little work called *De sexu plantarum epistola*,[51] produced when he was twenty-nine. As literature it has none of the merits of Grew's writings. It is cumbrous and ill-arranged, and its Latinity has been described as barbarous; but its quality transcends these defects, and it has come to be recognized as one of the minor classics of botany. It was written in the midst of the distresses of war. In construction it is unlike a modern treatise, since.it takes the form of an epistle addressed by Camerarius to one of his friends. In the seventeenth century men of science were in the habit of communicating their results to one another by letters, which passed from hand to hand, or were read at meetings of societies, and which to a great extent took the place of the journals and offprints upon which we rely to-day. Camerarius' memoir dates itself, not only by its epistolary form, but also by the fact that a didactic ode, written by an admirer, is appended to it; in this poem the thesis of *De sexu plantarum* is expounded with lyrical fervour through twenty-six stanzas. The writer has no easy task, since Camerarius does not talk only about lilies and roses, but largely about inconspicuous unisexual flowers, such as those of hops and hemp, spinach and dogs'-mercury, which are less amenable to poetic diction. However, the bard faces the problem boldly, singing of 'The spinach oft in kitchens used', and so on.

De sexu plantarum is somewhat confusing as a piece of presentation; and one has to pick out the main thread of the argument from among the items of a learned historical account of all that had been written previously on the subject. Camerarius begins by drawing attention to the fact, long known, that in some species certain individual plants are sterile; while others are fertile; and he cites the principal theory current in his time—namely, that flowers of the sterile kind are borne by plants which in cultivation have been neglected. He shows, however, that this explanation will not hold, partly because there is persistence in the sex character of each individual stock, and partly because, both in the wild state and also in gardens, plants of both sexes may be found growing freely intermingled. So it cannot be the

---

[49] Grew, *op. cit.* (35), p. 171.

[50] Millington belonged to Trinity College, Cambridge, but migrated to Oxford, where he became Sedleian Professor of Natural Philosophy; he was eventually President of the Royal College of Physicians. Grew's description of him as 'Savilian' Professor is a slip.

[51] For a translation see M. Möbius, *R. J. Camerarius. Über das Geschlecht der Pflanzen* (*De sexu plantarum epistola*). Ostwald's Klassiker der Exakten Wissenschaften, Leipzig, No. 105.

environment that is responsible. He then considered how he could arrive at some less unsatisfactory hypothesis through experimental work. He chose two species in which the same individual bears both sterile and fertile flowers—*Ricinus communis* L., the castor oil plant, and *Zea Mays* L., maize. From a plant of ricinus he cut away the buds of the sterile flowers before the unfolding of the stamens, and found that when he did so, he never got fully developed seeds. In a plant of maize, also, from which he had cut away the sterile tassel, he found that he obtained two cobs without seeds. In diœcious plants, again, he got similar results; he discovered that a mulberry tree, which occupied a solitary station, bore seeds which contained no embryos, and that a plant of dogs'-mercury with ovaries, which was quite cut off from the neighbourhood of other plants, produced seeds which would not germinate. From these and other observations of the same type he concluded that plant reproduction is comparable with that of animals, and that it demands the presence of stamens; he qualifies this conclusion, however, by expressly excluding spontaneous generation and vegetative propagation through buds. He laments that he does not know exactly how the pollen fertilizes the ovule. 'It would be greatly to be wished', he writes, 'that we should learn from those who, through their optical instruments, have more than lynx-eyes, what the granules of the anther contain, how far they penetrate the female apparatus, whether they arrive uninjured at the place where the seed is receptive, and what, when they burst, comes out of them.' This consummation was still far off, for it was not until 1846—more than a hundred and fifty years later—that Amici[52] established the main facts of the process with any exactness, while the fate of the second male nucleus was not determined for another half-century.[53] Just as anatomy made no advance for a very long period after Malpighi and Grew, so the knowledge of the function of the parts of the flower went through a similar phase of marking time; indeed, until well into the nineteenth century many botanists remained sceptical about the existence of sex in plants. The lingering influence of Aristotle's dicta may have been responsible for this, since he was reputed to have denied the existence of sexuality in plants. This denial was not, however, so categorical as it was sometimes made to appear, for he qualified it by saying that 'even in plants we find in the same kind some trees which bear fruit and others which, while bearing none themselves, yet contribute to the ripening of the fruits of those which do'; and he names the fig as an instance.[54]

Camerarius was not merely a man who made a remarkable discovery on observational and experimental grounds; we have to remember him for something more fundamental—his unalloyed intellectual integrity. He put forward his theory, not as a barrister whose business it is to make the best of his case, but as a seeker after truth, who lays as much stress upon the evidence against his thesis as on that which is in its favour. He writes, in terms which remind one of Francis Bacon, that the mind is wont to dwell upon what

[52] G. Amici, 'Sulla fecondazione delle Orchidee'. *Giorn. Bot. Ital.*, 1846, ii, 237–48; translated in *Ann. d. Sci. nat.*, 3s., bot., 1847, 193–205.

[53] On this discovery see P. Maheshwari, *An introduction to the embryology of Angiosperms.* New York, 1950, pp. 18–21.

[54] Aristotle, *De generatione animalium*, i. 1; 715[b]. (*Works*, vol. v, translation by Arthur Platt. Oxford, 1910.)

suits it, and only reluctantly allows itself to turn to the consideration of those things which are irreconcilable with a cherished opinion. He sees the consequences of this tendency so clearly that he takes a firm stand against it in his own case, and he concludes his memoir with a detailed account of the difficulties with which his views are confronted. To begin with, he cites lycopodium and equisetum—in which he mistook the spores for pollen-grains—as plants which have stamens, but no female organ. This idea was not unreasonable, given the state of ignorance of the time. He recognized, indeed, that both these genera belonged to the category of plants of which the origin and mode of reproduction were still obscure. He then passed on to examples among the angiosperms, in which the female bears fruit without the help of the male. 'This is another thing', he says, 'which does not fit in with my view.' In the maize plant with its male inflorescence removed, which he discussed earlier in his memoir, though two of the cobs produced no seed, a third cob gave eleven fertile seeds, and thus, as he writes, 'broke through the law of the absolute necessity for male pollen'. He knows that he removed the staminal head with great care, and he does not think that there were other maize plants which could be responsible, since there were none in the near neighbourhood. In this matter, however, he was probably mistaken, through not realizing the distance to which maize-pollen might be conveyed; according to modern work,[55] it may travel a quarter of a mile in a high wind. In the hemp (cannabis) also Camerarius found a certain discordance between the facts and his own theory. He transferred three young female plants from field to garden, and though there was no male anywhere near, they produced a number of seeds. He tried again, this time starting with seeds, and keeping the pot in a place remote from other hemp plants. He happened to get three male and three female individuals. He cut down the three males before the stamens were developed, and anxiously awaited the fate of the others. Again he got some fertile seeds in addition to abortive ones. Probably the explanation was that some of the flowers were hermaphrodite, and not unisexual, a possibility of which he was not aware. This seems to be the more likely since he notes that it was the first flowers which bore seeds; for it is a well-known fact that early flowers in an inflorescence tend to be hypertrophied, and may show the development of parts which remain latent in the succeeding flowers. Whether this was so or not, the important point is that he frankly confesses himself baffled, and does not try in the least to belittle such facts as might seem to invalidate his theory. Moreover, he expresses the intention of experimenting further, and of trying to detect any errors which may lurk in his earlier observations. In all respects his thesis was worked out according to the strictest tenets of the new experimental philosophy. As the author of *De sexu plantarum*, Camerarius deserves indeed to be remembered side by side with his older contemporaries, Malpighi and Grew. These two workers had a wider sweep of genius than Camerarius, and Grew, individually, had a gift of insight, and a capacity for making literature out of scientific material, to which the other two did not attain. But their qualities were complementary, and it is jointly to these three physicians—an Italian, an Englishman, and a German—that the honour

[55] P. Weatherwax, *The story of the maize plant.* Chicago, 1923, p. 128.

belongs of having initiated modern scientific botany.   The subject, as they visualized it, formed a world of experience on a wholly different plane from the tissue of medieval lore preserved in *The grete herball*, which was the starting point of the present study.

THE HISTORY OF ALBRECHT DÜRER'S RHINOCEROS IN ZOOLOGICAL LITERATURE

by

F. J. COLE

ALBRECHT DÜRER'S well-known and justly admired woodcut of the Indian Gomda[1] was drawn and cut in 1515. It was for over two centuries accepted as a trustworthy representation of the rhinoceros, and it figures so often and in so many disguises in early zoological works that a history of its 'deambulations' is worth attempting.[2] Before doing so, however, it is material to summarize briefly what was known of the animal in classical times.[3] The references in the Bible to the 'unicorn' are too vague to admit of satisfactory identification, and indeed probably do not refer to the rhinoceros; but Aristotle is more definite in the *Historia animalium* and in the *De partibus animalium*, where he states, it is true at second hand, that the 'Indian ass' has a single horn and a non-cloven hoof. This may possibly be a reference to the Indian rhinoceros in spite of the fact that the species has three sufficiently distinct toes, albeit less obvious than in other Ungulates. Strabo the geographer (*c.* 64 B.C.–A.D. 21) is the first to give us a recognizable description of a rhinoceros with one horn, based on a single individual which he claims to have seen. He refers, at second hand, to its combats with the elephant—a tale which is widely repeated in the writings of the Middle Ages and in some later works. Strabo uses the word rhinoceros or nose-horn, ῥινό-κερως. He mentions the plicae of the skin, and hence his example was of the Indian species.

The mosaic pavement of the Temple of Fortune at Praeneste, now Palestrina, which was constructed probably between 80 B.C. and A.D. 200,[4] illustrates scenes on the Nile, and includes a figure of a rhinoceros with *two* nasal horns, which hence must have been the African species, *R. bicornis*, and so fits into the scene.[5] Another Roman mosaic discovered in a garden at Perugia includes an undoubted figure of the African rhinoceros, but the disproportion in length between the two horns is somewhat exaggerated[6] (Fig. 1). According to Pliny, an Indian rhinoceros made its first appearance

---

[1] This is the Hindu equivalent of rhinoceros adopted by Dürer himself. Other variants are: Ganda, Genda, Gainda, Gomela, Gonda, Gainra.

[2] I ought to explain that I have not specifically searched the literature for Dürer material, but have used only such examples as have been accidentally encountered during many years when engaged in other historical studies. A complete list has therefore still to be compiled. See the bibliography, arranged alphabetically by authors, for detailed references to the works cited in these footnotes. Except for Fig. 2, all the illustrations are from copies of works in my own library. For the excellent photographs I am indebted to Mr. F. C. Padley.

[3] For further details consult the works of Oken (1838), Camper (1782), Klein (1751), Buffon (1754), Shaw (1800), and the early encyclopaedists.

[4] Marucchi (1904) and Hinks (1933) put the date of this mosaic at about the time of Hadrian, and the former suggests that it may have been inspired by Aelian, who was a native of Praeneste. The rhinoceros figured here has three digits in the foot, and not one as in the horse.

[5] Athenaeus quotes Callixenus of Rhodes (? third century B.C.) as his authority for the statement that an Ethiopian rhinoceros took part in Ptolemy's parade, which was held in the third century B.C. No horn or horns are mentioned, and hence it is not certain that this was the two-horned African rhinoceros.

[6] Cf. Guardabassi (1877).

in Rome during the games organized by Pompey the Great on his return to Italy (?61 B.C.), and Suetonius mentions that the Emperor Augustus (63 B.C.–A.D. 14) exhibited a rhinoceros in Rome, which has been interpreted as a contradiction of Pliny, but may refer to another occasion. Domitian (A.D. 52–96)[7] also brought a rhinoceros to Rome, and the interest so aroused was responsible for the references to the animal in the epigrams of the poet Martial (c. A.D. 40–104)[8] and for the minting of two Roman coins representing the two-horned rhinoceros, in one of which the animal is facing right and in the other left. A rhinoceros was again shown in Rome in the reign of Antoninus Pius (A.D. 86–161), but on the fall of the Roman Empire living examples did not appear in Western Europe until the sixteenth century, when the original of Dürer's figure arrived in Lisbon from India in 1515.

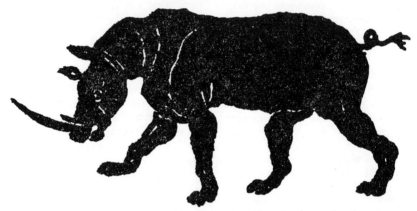

Fig. 1. The two-horned African rhinoceros as figured in a Roman mosaic at Perugia.

Martial's observations on the rhinoceros have been frequently discussed by learned editors. What he *says* is that the rhinoceros 'tossed a heavy bear with his double horn', which can refer only to the two-horned African species. This attribution is confirmed by the Domitian coins and the testimony of Pausanias (second century A.D.), whose 'Ethiopian bulls called rhinoceroses' have one horn at the end of the nose and behind it another but smaller one.[9] Owing to ignorance or scepticism of such a species, various modern commentators have attempted to explain away Martial's 'double horn', and the text has been emended by the substitution of 'urus' for 'ursus', which transfers the two horns to the victim, and even to the tossing of two bears with a single horn. In the latter case, however, we are assured that the bears would not have been tossed simultaneously. Another solution was suggested by Scaliger, who welcomed the publication of Dürer's woodcut as a sufficient confirmation of Martial's species.

    An interesting reference to the rhinoceros in the Middle Ages occurs in a Latin hymn to Saint Paul by Abelard, written in the first half of the

[7] Cf. Mattingly (1930).

[8] Cf. Martialis, *De spectaculis*, xxii.

[9] The Ethiopian rhinoceros was re-described by the geographer Cosmas (*fl.* A.D. 535–47).

PLATE XXIII

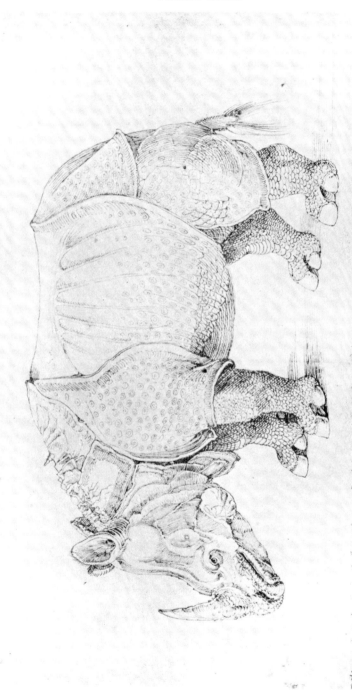

FIG. 2.   Albrecht Dürer's drawing of the Indian rhinoceros.   (British Museum, Department of Prints
and Drawings.   Reproduced by permission)
The date '153' in the legend is an error for '1513'

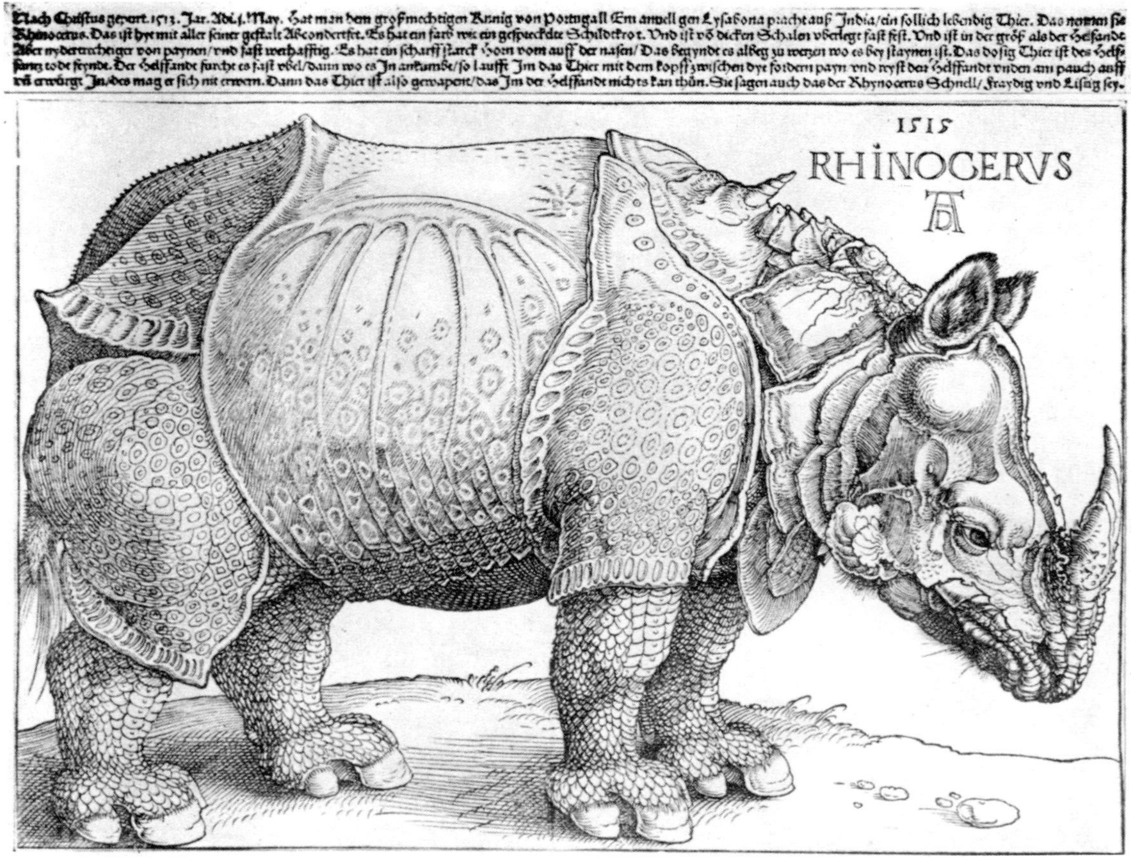

PLATE XXIV

FIG. 3. Dürer's woodcut. From an impression of the very rare first state in the author's possession

... the woodcut itself is correctly dated '1515'

twelfth century.[10] The verse runs:

Ut rinoceros est indomitus,
Quem ad aratrum ligans Dominus,
Glebas vallium frangit protinus.

Saint Paul is unrestrained and untiring, even as the rhinoceros, when his hand has been put to the plough.

The story of Dürer's rhinoceros was first told by Giovio[11] in 1555, and recently da Costa[12] and Campbell Dodgson[13] have added considerably to what was previously known. It is only necessary here to summarize very briefly the more important facts. The specimen, an Indian rhinoceros, *R. unicornis*, was presented by the Sultan of Guzerat to the Portuguese Mission in India in 1514, and it arrived at Lisbon on 20 May 1515. It was sketched and briefly described by a Portuguese artist, and this was the document[14] which later reached Dürer at Nürnberg, and provided the basis and stimulus for his famous drawing[15] and woodcut of 1515. Da Costa considers that the drawing was the work of the Portuguese artist, but on all grounds the Dürer attribution is unassailable. The rhinoceros itself left Lisbon in December 1515 and reached Marseilles in January 1516, on its way to Rome as a present to Pope Leo X. The ship sailed at the end of January, but in February a storm overwhelmed the vessel in the Gulf of Genoa and it was lost with all on board. The corpse of the rhinoceros, however, was washed ashore, and, after being stuffed, was dispatched to the Pope. Dürer's drawing was made in 1515, and impressions of the woodcut were published in the same year. The date on the drawing, viz. '153' (for '1513'), and in the inscription of the early states of the woodcut, is an error. The drawing (Fig. 2) became the property of the English physician Sir Hans Sloane, whose collections were purchased by the nation in 1754, and are now in the British Museum. Dürer himself had never seen a rhinoceros, living or dead, when his drawing was made.[16] Nevertheless, it envisages the distinctive congruity of the animal better than later ones executed from the life. It should be noted that a woodcut of a rhinoceros, also dated 1515, by Hans Burgkmair is known only from a single impression in Vienna. This appears to be relatable to the Portuguese sketch, but has none of Dürer's embellishments; and it may well be that the first valid representation of the animal which has come down to us was swamped by the rapid success of Dürer's print.

It is surprising that of all the authors who reproduced Dürer's figure Gesner[17] is the only one who acknowledges the obligation. Some of them

[10] *v.* under Abelard in bibliography. (Sir Eric Maclagan kindly drew my attention to this passage.)

[11] *v.* Giovio (1555).

[12] *v.* Da Costa (1937).

[13] *v.* Dodgson (1903, 1938).

[14] The document has since been lost, but an Italian translation has survived.

[15] The original sketch plays no part in the present story, since it was obviously unknown to the numerous plagiarists of the woodcut.

[16] The edition of Dürer's woodcut issued by Hondius, *c.* 1620, includes the erroneous statement that a living rhinoceros was sent by the King of Portugal to Germany, where Dürer made a sketch of it from the life.

[17] *v.* Gesner (1551 and 1553).

comment on the woodcut in a way which strongly suggests that they had seen it. The learned Bochart,[18] however, refers to Dürer as a distinguished artist who had in 1515 'accurately' drawn an Indian rhinoceros which was at the time alive in Portugal. The dorsal horn, he correctly says, is known only from that drawing. Bochart was not convinced of the existence of a rhinoceros with two *nasal* horns, although he was familiar with the classical references to such a species. If something can be said in extenuation of Dürer's imposing coat of armour, which after all is only an artistic elaboration of the plicae of the skin, it must be conceded that the small dorsal spiral horn is entirely and gratuitously fictitious. What induced him to introduce this quaint and not unpleasing feature? He had presumably heard of a two-horned rhinoceros, but in his own time and for long after there was no convincing evidence of the occurrence of a species with two *nasal* horns. On the contrary, much dubiety existed as to its reality. The Portuguese sketch showed only one, and Dürer, perhaps anxious that his figure should not be found wanting in so striking a feature, ventured to invent an inconspicuous second horn on the withers, where it might easily have escaped the notice of his predecessors. In this connexion it should be borne in mind that the two-horned African rhinoceros does not appear in modern zoological literature until 1661, when it was described and figured by Estienne de Flacourt,[19] who saw the animal in South Africa on his way home from Madagascar. The rhinoceros does not occur in Madagascar itself. Dürer therefore would not have at his disposal a contemporary description or figure of the two-horned species.

A comparison of Dürer's drawing in the British Museum with the first state of the woodcut (Fig. 3) reveals some noteworthy differences.[20] The most important is that in the woodcut the body is relatively shorter and heavier, and hence less natural. It is difficult to escape the conclusion that a deficiency in width of the block compared with its height was the factor that determined the ungainly proportions of the woodcut. Thus the horn actually touches the border-line of the block and there is not sufficient room for the whole of the tail, although it is pressed closer to the body. In the woodcut the dorsal horn becomes more prominent, hairs are added to the chin and neck, the shading at the edges of the plicae of the skin is converted into an ornamental pattern, and the median dorsal projection behind the ears is omitted. In both drawing and woodcut the toes are too distinct, but their number is correct.

The first author to copy Dürer's figure was Gesner (1551).[21] As already mentioned, the woodcut, and not the drawing, is the only source known to the plagiarists.[22] Gesner's figure (Fig. 4) has been accurately reduced so as not to disturb the proportions of the parts, and it is a faithful copy of the original, no attempt being made to improve upon it or to add to Dürer's

[18] *v.* Bochart (1663).

[19] *v.* Flacourt (1661). It may be necessary to alter the date of the first appearance to 1658, when the first edition of this work was published. I have not seen this edition.

[20] According to A. M. Hind, Dürer did not cut the blocks himself, but duplicated his drawings on the wood and left the cutting to a craftsman.

[21] *v.* Gesner (1551).

[22] Edward Wotton, in his *De differentiis animalium,* 1552 (colophon dated 1551), was evidently not acquainted with Dürer's woodcut.

PLATE XXV

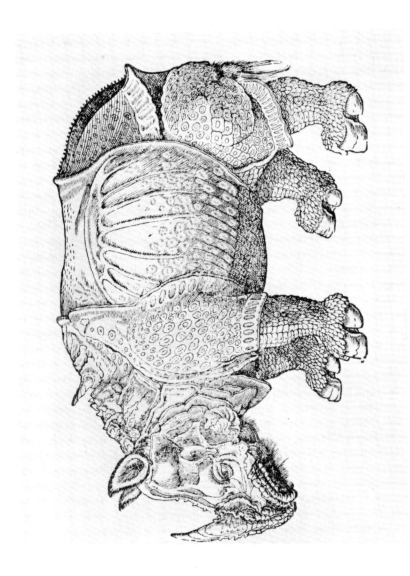

FIG. 4.   Copy in reverse of Dürer's woodcut

Gesner, 1551.

embellishments. The second horn is perhaps slightly less prominent. The origin of the figure is acknowledged, and its merit and popularity are referred to in terms of great admiration. No other author admits his debt to Dürer, nor can their failure to do so be ascribed, at least in many cases, to ignorance of the original. Gesner was aware of the references to a two-horned rhinoceros in classical literature, and he may even have assumed that Dürer's figure was the animal there referred to, notwithstanding that the second horn was not on the nose.

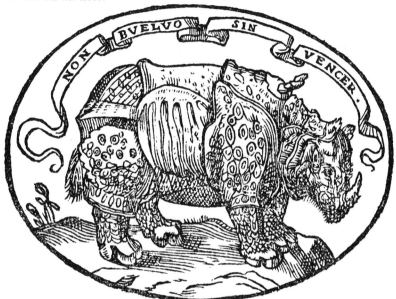

Fig. 5. Giovio's emblematic figure of Gomda, (?) 1556.   Enlarged.
Reproduced from the 1574 edition.

In a posthumous work on decorative devices or emblems with appropriate mottoes (?1556), Giovio[23] includes a reduced figure of Dürer's Gomda as the symbol of unconquerable might (Fig. 5). This was the accepted view of the animal, and is expressed by almost all the early writers. Bishop Giovio's version is an ungainly distortion of the original, in which the ears are too small and the dorsal horn is exaggerated until it is as large as the nasal horn. In the unillustrated first edition (1555) Giovio provides the first account of the fatal voyage of the Lisbon rhinoceros, which doubtless explains his knowledge of Dürer's figure and its appearance in the Dialogo.   In the following year (1556) Valerianus,[24] inspired by Martial's epigram, introduced a figure of Dürer's rhinoceros tossing a bear—apparently with its ears (Fig. 6). The analogous figure by Camerarius (1595) is much more realistic. Valerianus' emblematical woodcut at first suggests a comparison with that of Giovio, but there are points of difference which indicate that it is based

[23] v. Giovio (1555 and 1574). Cf. Redgrave, Trans. Bib. Soc., 1910, xi, 39–58. The first edition of the work of 1555 has no illustrations. I do not know in which edition the figure of the rhinoceros appeared, but it must have been before 1574, possibly in 1556.

[24] v. Valerianus (1556).

directly on Dürer, who, however, is not mentioned. Valerianus was familiar with the coins of Domitian embodying the two-horned African rhinoceros, but he distinguishes between this species and the Indian rhinoceros sent to Portugal, which, he says, 'has the second and smaller horn farther back, as all who saw the animal agreed'. This is obviously a reference to Dürer's figure, which is thus regarded as a reliable drawing of the Indian species.

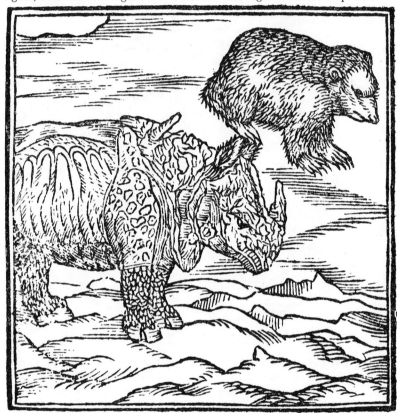

Fig. 6. Valerianus, 1556.   Dürer's rhinoceros tosses a bear.

Paré's woodcut of 1573 (Fig. 7) is a shapeless caricature of Dürer's Gomda.[25] It appeared in many editions of Paré's works. In 1579 he used also Thevet's figure of a combat between the rhinoceros and the elephant.[26] He used both figures again in his *Discours . . . De la Mvmie* (1582). (Johnson, in his translation of Paré's works (1634), copied Gesner's figure in addition.) Paré credits Pausanias with the statement that the second horn is very small, sharply pointed and situated high up on the shoulder. This is Dürer but not Pausanias.

Thevet[27] (1575) was the first to introduce major divergences from Dürer's Gomda, and his figure (Fig. 8) was used not only by Paré but also by Valentin in 1704. Thevet is credited with having seen a rhinoceros in Cairo in 1554,

[25] *v.* Paré (1573).   [26] *v.* Paré (1579).   [27] *v.* Thevet (1575).

Figure du Rhinoceros armé de toutes pieces.

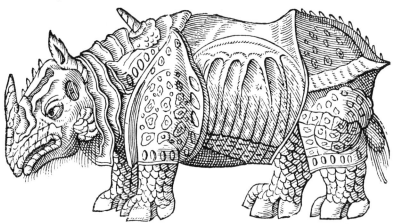

Fig. 7. Ambroise Paré's woodcut, first used in 1573, reproduced from his
Discours . . . De la Mvmie, 1582.

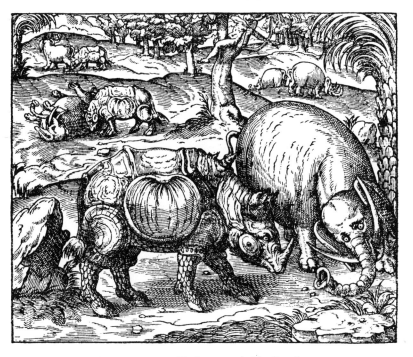

Fig. 8. Thevet, 1575. Elephants attacked by Gomda.

but nevertheless he describes scales in the skin like those of a crocodile. Dürer's second horn is increased almost to the size of the first, the appearance of external armour plating is much exaggerated, and the three toes of the foot are replaced by a cloven hoof like that of an ox. The old story of the rhinoceros attacking the elephant is repeated and illustrated. A drawing (or picture) of a rhinoceros was executed by Marcus Gheeraerts the Elder (Gerardus

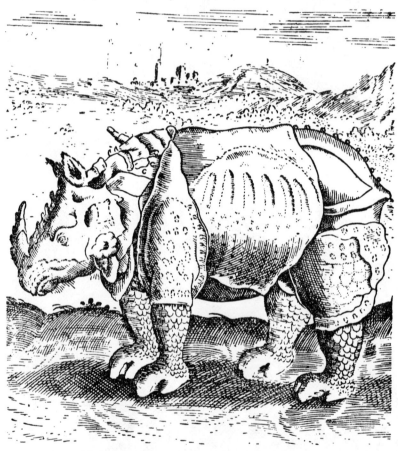

Fig. 9. Marcus Gheeraerts the Elder, 1583 [enlarged].

Brugensis) in 1583,[28] and was published by C. J. Vischer about 1630 in an oblong atlas of animal types without text (Fig. 9). It is based on Dürer, and its crude departures from the original are chiefly those arising from a lack of skill on the part of the engraver. The tail is omitted. Also, the head of an Indian rhinoceros appears in the engraved title-page of this work.

Very attractive miniature etchings by Hans Sibmacher of two rhinoceroses, one of which is tossing a bear (Fig. 10), were published in 1595 by Camerarius

[28] v. Gheeraerts (c. 1630).

the younger,[29] who acknowledges that the source of his information is an accurate drawing *received from Spain*.   If the figures are not too accurate, they are at least based on nature, and, apart from Burgkmair's print, they are the first representations of the Indian rhinoceros in modern literature of which this can be said.   There is no suggestion of Dürer's influence in them, nor does Camerarius mention his name, but he is familiar with Dürer's Gomda, which he identifies with Martial's two-horned species.   He wrongly criticizes Martial for an abuse of the privilege of poetic licence, since, he says, the second horn is

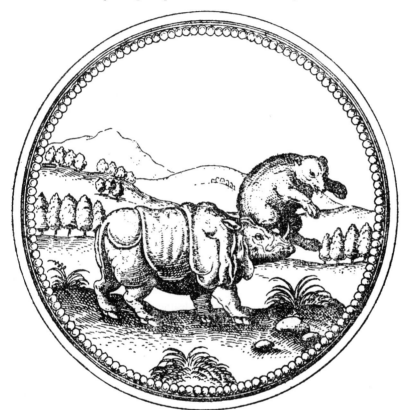

Fig. 10. Camerarius, 1595 [enlarged].   Not based on Dürer.

only a tuberosity on the back and not a true horn.   This is clearly a reference to Dürer's second horn, from which it seems that he shared the prevailing ignorance of the existence of the African two-horned rhinoceros, which figures on Roman coinage in the first century, is unmistakably described by Pausanias in the second century, and in his own time was figured by Agustín[30] in 1587. Camerarius, it is true, mentions Pausanias, but says nothing of his reference to the two horns.

[29] *v.* Camerarius (1595).
[30] *v.* Agustín (1587).

Topsell's figure (1607)[31] is a woodcut, and is a remarkably close copy of Gesner's figure. He admits that he has never seen the animal, but believes that Gesner's figure was taken from the life in Lisbon before many witnesses. Eucherius is quoted as stating that the rhinoceros has two horns on its nose, which Topsell says is 'utterly false', in spite of the fact that Martial 'seems to express' the same thing. He concludes that Pausanias' second horn *is the dorsal horn of Dürer*, and hence he has no knowledge of the African species.

The first modern attempt to figure in detail the two-horned African rhinoceros is the *Asinus cornutus* of Aldrovandus[32] (Fig. 11), published in 1616, and copied with modifications by Jonston, Kircher and Scheuchzer.

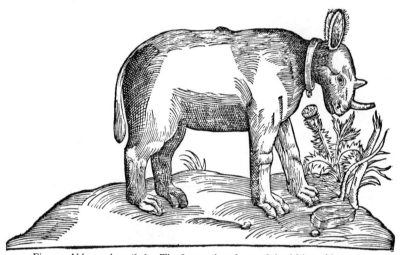

Fig. 11. Aldrovandus, 1616. The first modern figure of the African rhinoceros.

It is a tame young animal provided with a leather collar, and the species is said to occur in India, Scythia and Africa; but Aldrovandus disclaims that he speaks from personal knowledge and cannot therefore vouch for what he has heard. This doubtless explains the asinine bias. The source of his information may have been the German traveller Samuel Kiechel (1563–1619) although he admits indebtedness to Camerarius. In Johnston's copy[33] the proportions and strength of the parts are so transformed that the figure is less like a rhinoceros than ever. His object may have been to make it look more like an ass, and in this he succeeds.

The armorial bearings of the Society of Apothecaries,[34] dating from 1617, are remarkable in having a crest which is a greatly reduced and simplified version of Dürer's Gomda (Fig. 12). In spite of these modifications, however, the relationship is beyond question, if only in virtue of the ribs and dorsal horn, which latter is greatly increased in relative size so as to be almost as large as the spiralized nasal horn. The figure of a rhinoceros occurs in the coats of arms of many English families subsequent to the fifteenth century, but

[31] *v.* Topsell (1607).   [32] *v.* Aldrovandus (1616).
[33] *v.* Jonston (1650).   [34] *v.* Dickinson (1929).

all such examples portray the single-horned Asiatic species without trace of the Dürer convention. The coat of arms of the Apothecaries was the work of William Camden (1551–1623), antiquary and historian. The suggestion that he introduced the rhinoceros as a foil to the unicorns ignores the fact that its horn was then important in the pharmacopœia. Its inclusion was thus justified on medical grounds. The validity of Dürer's drawing had not so far been challenged; it is thus strange that his well-known figure, more

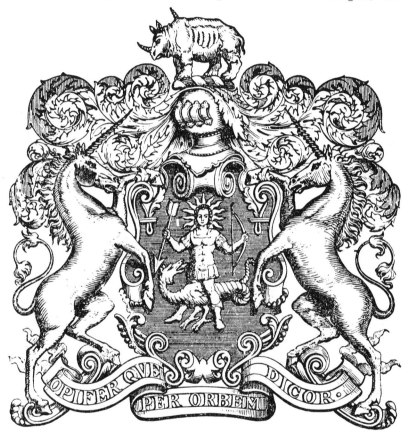

Fig. 12. Armorial bearings of the Society of Apothecaries, 1617. The only appearance of Gomda in heraldry.

artistic and accurate than its competitors, should have been preferred only once. I have discovered that the book-plate of Peter Butcher, of Ipswich, plagiarized the arms of the Apothecaries. The book is not dated, but below the arms is written, 'Peter Butcher, his book, MDCCXXIII'. The Society's archives contain no reference to Butcher.

Aldrovandus never saw a rhinoceros, but he was familiar with Dürer's print, and his later figure[35] of 1621 is based on Gesner's version, of which it is a

[35] v. Aldrovandus (1621).

full-sized fairly close copy, except that the dorsal horn is slightly less prominent.[36] Parkinson[37] (1640) has preferred to imitate Camerarius rather than Dürer, except that his rhinoceros is engaged in a more peaceful and amiable diversion than in tossing a bear (Fig. 13).

Jonston's copperplate (Fig. 14) of 1650,[38] which was copied by C. Bartholin in 1678, and by Scheuchzer, without the tail, in 1732, is a reduced copy of Dürer's woodcut; but the reduction has accurately preserved the proportions of the original, and the superior perspective obtainable by the use of a metal plate larger than the subject has resulted in a less ponderous

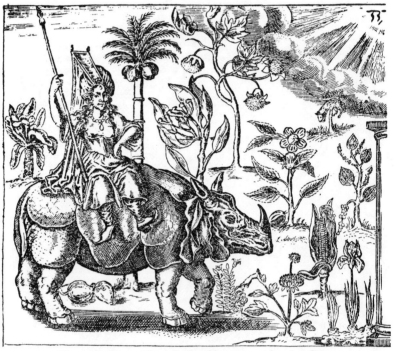

Fig. 13. Parkinson, 1640. Indian rhinoceros, not based on Dürer.

rhinoceros than Dürer gives us.[39] In 1650 G. G. Rossi published, in an oblong atlas without text, figures of animals stated to have been drawn and engraved by Antonio Tempesta (d. 1630).[40] Tempesta's rhinoceros (Fig. 15) is also based on Dürer's woodcut, and he was probably familiar with Paré's figure of 1573. Dürer's animal is accurately reduced to one-half, but the accuracy applies only to the outline. The decision to retain the size of the detail whilst reducing the area it occupies has resulted in falsifying the general appearance of the animal as drawn by Dürer.

[36] Klein quotes Catelanus (*q.v.* 1625) as accepting Dürer's figure, but I have not seen this work.
[37] *v.* Parkinson (1640).   [38] *v.* note (33).
[39] The *Theatrum universale omnium animalium.* Amsterdam, 1718, nominally by Hendrik Ruysch (1663–1727), is only a later issue of Jonston with a cancel-title, and hence may be relegated to the limbo of pirated works.   [40] *v.* Tempesta (1650).

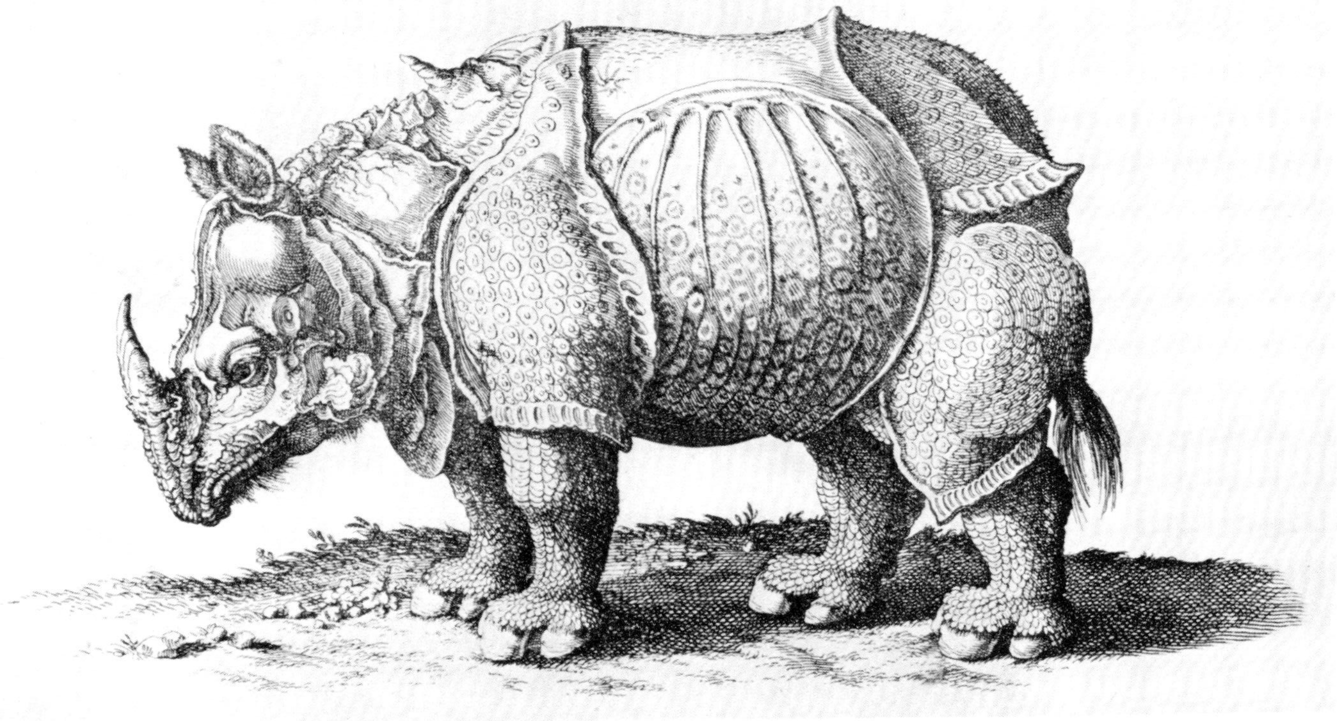

PLATE XXVI

RHINOCEROS. *Hornnaſe* Rʰᵢₙₒᶜᵉʳ

FIG. 14. **Jonston**, 1650. The first detailed and competent metal engraving of Gomda

PLATE XXVII

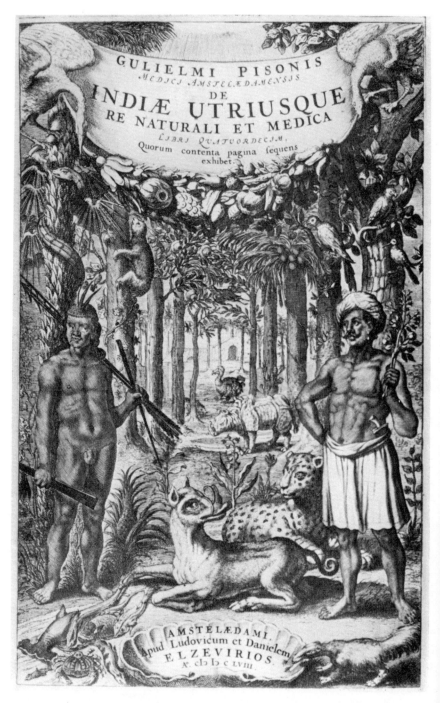

Fig. 16.   Engraved title-page of the second edition of Piso's work on the East Indies, 1658, in which Gomda is accompanied by the Dodo, the Babirusa and other valid species

The second edition of Piso's work on the East Indies (1658) includes a contribution by Bontius,[41] and an engraved title-page not present in the first edition (Fig. 16). Bontius has personally observed large numbers of the Indian rhinoceros, and he rejects Dürer's dorsal horn, armour plating and decorations, without, however, mentioning his name. The separate dermal plates, he says, correctly, are simply continuous folds of the skin. His own figure, which was supplied by Piso, is very poor, especially as regards the head and feet, the latter seeming to be provided with claws. It has, however, some importance as one of the first attempts to draw the animal from the life. The imposing engraved title of this work includes three interesting figures—the babirusa, the dodo and Dürer's Gomda, and it is the only work in which a rhinoceros taken from the life appears together with the creation of Albrecht Dürer.

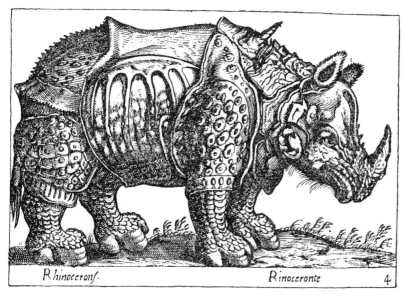

R *hinoceronſ.*   R *inoceronte*   4

Fig. 15. Tempesta, 1650. Engraving, derived from Dürer, but not comparable with Jonston's published in the same year.

The second figure of the African two-horned rhinoceros to appear in modern times was published by de Flacourt[42] in 1661. He encountered the animal in South Africa on his way home from his investigations in Madagascar. The figure is very small and crude, with no traces of Dürer influence, but there can be no question of its identity. In Kircher's highly imaginative work on Noah's Ark (1675)[43] we find among the fortunate occupants of that capacious vessel two species of rhinoceros—one a woodcut copy of Jonston's travesty of the *Asinus cornutus* of Aldrovandus, and the other a greatly reduced and deplorable caricature of Dürer's Gomda (Fig. 17). The latter appears again

---

[41] *v.* Bontius (1658).   [42] *v.* Flacourt (1661).   [43] *v.* Kircher (1675).

alongside some of his aquatic refugees, and the place assigned to him in the Ark has in adjacent cubicles the elephant and the bear—the traditional foes of the rhinoceros. We may congratulate Noah, therefore, in refusing to countenance the tales which celebrate the mutual encounters of these formidable monsters.

In the second edition of Thomas Bartholin's work on the Unicorn, edited and extended by his son Caspar (1678),[44] we find a greatly reduced but competent etching of Jonston's version of Gomda, without any noteworthy modifications. The Jonston source is acknowledged, but Dürer's name is not mentioned. Bartholin is aware of the existence of a species with two nasal horns and gives figures of them removed from the body. Grew[45] (1681) is one of the numerous authors who, in ignorance of the two-horned African rhinoceros, interpret references to such a species in terms of Dürer's figure.

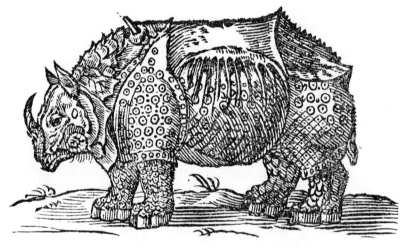

Fig. 17. Kircher, 1675. Gomda enters Noah's Ark.

A reviewer of Tachard's voyage into Siam (1686),[46] writing in the *Philosophical Transactions*, remarks: 'I know not by what mistake he makes the *Rhinocerote* a two-horned animal.' Nevertheless, Tachard evidently saw the detached double nasal horns of *R. sumatrensis*, but not the animal itself, or he would not have figured Dürer's Gomda basking in the forests of Siam (Fig. 18).

Valentin's figure of 1704 is copied without acknowledgment from Thevet, but in his second volume (1714)[47] he produces three variants of Dürer, although one of them lacks the dorsal horn (Fig. 19). They differ from all previous figures which I have seen and there is no mention of them in the text. Gomda thus appears to have relatives, and Valentin's discovery of three new species must be recorded and duly accredited to their industrious

[44] v. Bartholin (1678).
[45] v. Grew (1681).
[46] v. Tachard (1686).
[47] v. Valentini (1704, 1714).

PLATE XXVIII

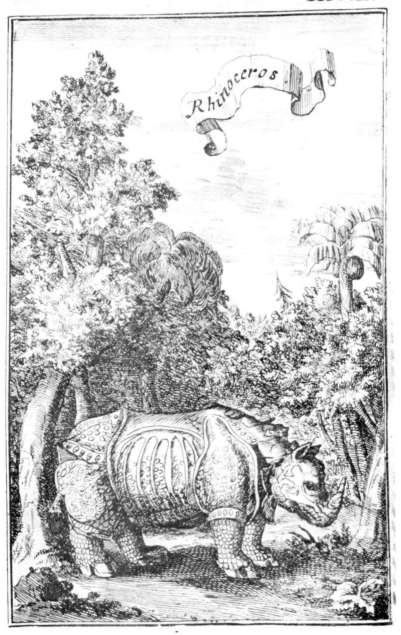

FIG. 18. Tachard, 1686. Gomda in the forests of Siam

PLATE XXIX

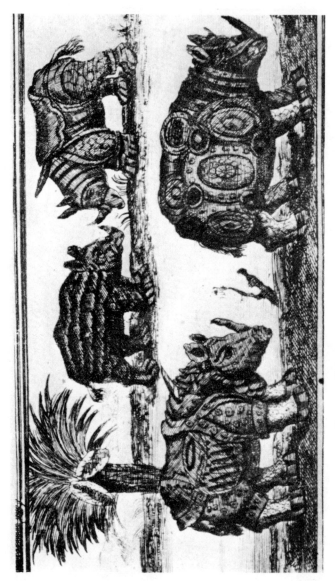

Fig. 19. Valentini, 1714. Three new species of Gonua

inventor.[48]   Chardin[49] (1711) saw living rhinoceros many times, and his figure was based 'very exactly' on a captive example and owes nothing to Dürer.   Yet it is an indifferent and lifeless caricature, and is actually less suggestive of the species than Gomda, despite the extravagances of the latter.   Hartenfels[50] (1715) revives the old story of the combat between the elephant and Gomda, who resembles some of his predecessors without being a close copy of any one of them (Fig. 20).   Here, however, the elephant is the aggressor and his onslaught is awaited by a calm and even contemplative victim.

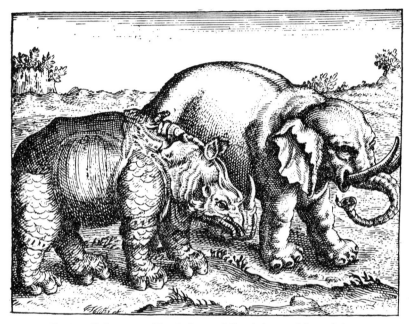

Fig. 21.   Kolbe, 1719.   The elephant and Gomda in peaceful association.

Kolbe[51] (1719) accurately describes the African rhinoceros from his own observations, and bluntly criticizes previous descriptions of the animal, which, he says, embody little truth or agreement.   And yet his figure (Fig. 21) is a gross perversion of Dürer's Gomda, with its limbs covered with large fish-like scales.   Such a flagrant violation of the obligations of veracity would call for severe condemnation were it not for the fact that Kolbe must be acquitted of responsibility for the figure, which was introduced by an anxious but misguided publisher intent on alleviating the dullness of the text. Scheuchzer,[52] in his work on the Natural History of the Bible (1731–5),

[48] It is difficult to believe that these figures are original, but if they are not their source is still to be discovered.

[49] v. Chardin (1711).

[50] v. Petri ab Hartenfels (1715).

[51] v. Kolbe (1731).

[52] v. Scheuchzer (1731–5).

reproduces Jonston's modified copy of the *Asinus cornutus* of Aldrovandus (1616), which has the additional defect of still further exaggerating the asinine, at the expense of the rhinocerine features of an original already sufficiently transmuted. This author also introduces five versions of Dürer's Gomda. In the first (1731) the second horn is shown on the back but not as a spiral, thus resembling the nasal horn. In the second a male and female are included in the procession entering Noah's Ark. The third (1732) is an artistic copy of Jonston's in picturesque surroundings (Fig. 22), but the engraver has not left himself room for the tail. The fourth is clearly a variant of Dürer, but I have been unable to trace its source, which, as in the other cases, is not given. The fifth (1733) illustrates only a part of the animal, and then not in detail. It represents the reasonable alarm of the Psalmist when attacked by lions, wolves and Dürer's rhinoceros.

Carwitham's unsatisfactory but original figure of a rhinoceros[53] (published 1739) is based on the specimen exhibited in London in 1685; but Parsons's drawings[54] of immature individuals of the Indian species which reached England in 1739 and 1741 are better and more natural, and were intended to correct the embellishments of Dürer. They are, however, unsatisfactory in detail, and their failure to focus more successfully the attributes of the living animal is an unconscious tribute to the intuition of the great painter who never saw the animal he was drawing. It is interesting to note that Parsons's second specimen was the animal seen and figured by Albinus[55] in 1742, and his sketches were introduced into the background of two of the Albinus plates of the skeleton and muscles of the human body (1747). They are somewhat impressionist in character, as befits their adventitious role in the plates, but more life-like than any previously published. The author excuses the instrusion of this irrelevant monster in a work on human anatomy on the ground that the species is rare, and provides a more agreeable perspective than a fictitious landscape.

It is difficult to understand why Hill,[56] the critic of the *Philosophical Transactions* in 1751, should ignore in 1752 Parsons's figures of 1743 in the same publication, and perpetuate the tradition that Dürer's Gomda was a valid picture of the rhinoceros. His version is Jonston's, without, however, the dorsal horn and with some modification of the head. Edwards's figure (1758),[57] drawn 'from the life' in 1752, is a passably good representation of an immature Indian rhinoceros with no suggestion of Dürer. He refers to a species with two horns, but he is not certain whether such specimens are true species or only 'accidental sports of nature'. Even Klein[58] and Buffon,[59] writing in 1751 and 1764, are still doubtful whether the one- and two-horned rhinoceroses are distinct species or merely varieties, and Klein and Valmont de Bomare[60] (1769) suggest that the male sex only has the small second horn on the back at the right shoulder, which is obviously Dürer's dorsal horn. To complete this comedy of errors J. Bruce,[61] the African explorer (1790), who

[53] *v.* Carwitham (1739).   [54] *v.* Parsons (1743 and 1766).
[55] *v.* Albinus (1747).   [56] *v.* Hill (1752).
[57] *v.* Edwards (1758).   [58] *v.* Klein (1751).
[59] *v.* Buffon (1764).   [60] *v.* Valmont de Bomare (1769).
[61] *v.* Bruce (1790).

PLATE XXX

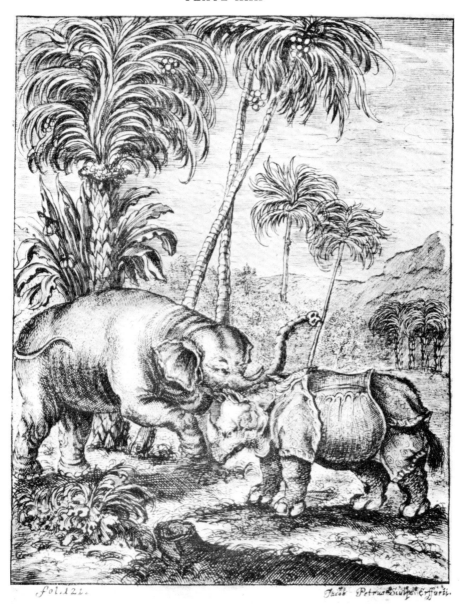

fol.121.   *Jacob Petrus Sculpsit Erffurti.*

FIG. 20. Hartenfels, 1715. The elephant turns on Gomda

PLATE XXXI

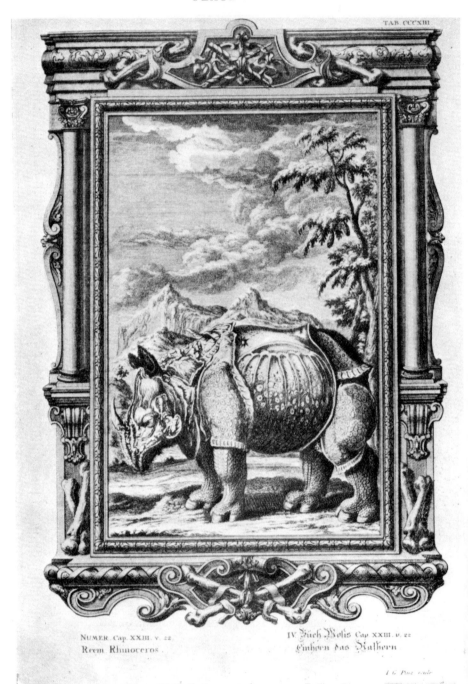

TAB. CCCXIII.

NUMER. Cap. XXIII. v. 22.
Reem Rhinoceros.

IV Buch Mosis Cap. XXIII. v. 22
Einhorn das Nashorn

J. G. Pinz. sculp.

FIG. 22. Scheuchzer, 1732. Gomda enriches the fauna of the Old Testament

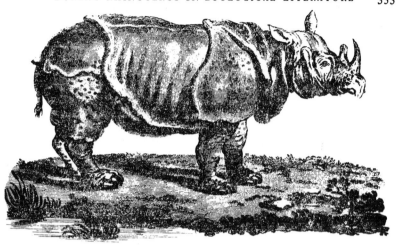

Rhinoceros of Africa

Fig. 23. Bruce, 1790. An Indo-African ghost.

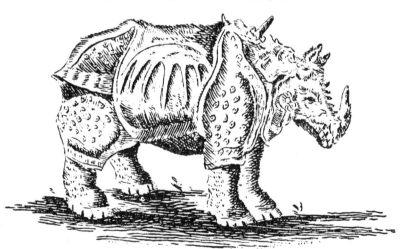

A RHINOCEROS

Fig. 24. Boreman, 1769. The last appearance of Gomda on the stage.

claims to have been thoroughly familiar with the appearance of the African rhinoceros, believes that the single-horned Asiatic species occurs also in Africa—a lapse which perhaps explains, but does not excuse, his own figure of the African species (Fig. 23). Dürer's woodcut, he says, 'was wonderfully ill executed in all its parts, and was the origin of all the monstrous forms under which that animal has been painted ever since, in all parts of the world'. Bruce asserts that his drawing 'is the first that has been published with two horns, it is designed from the life, and is an African'. All this from the man who appropriated Buffon's figure of the *Indian* rhinoceros of 1764, adorned it with a second nasal horn, and thereby produced a hybrid which ranks with Dürer's Gomda as one of the simulacra of zoological literature.[62] He even testifies to the occurrence of traces of a third horn, and quotes native hunters as saying that they 'frequently see rhinoceroses with three horns grown', but ' only upon the male'. Labat[63] (1732), who travelled in Ethiopia, believed that the rhinoceros there had three horns, one on the nose, a second on the forehead and a third on the back. And so Dürer's dorsal horn, so far the prerogative of the Indian rhinoceros, now adorns the shoulders of its African relative.

Gomda's fate was by this time sealed. Attacked as he was on all sides, he is still to be found fighting hopefully for his life in unexpected and humble places. He has now a senile and weather-beaten appearance. His attempt to compensate for the loss of his tail by a parade of extra toes fails to divert the attentions of the doomster, and he finally expires (Fig. 24)—not in a magnificent and learned folio with hand-coloured plates, but in an unremembered, shabby compilation by a hack writer to which the author did not even put his name.[64] For over 250 years Gomda was in constant demand, he travelled over the whole world, and, especially in his younger days, he foregathered with the very aristocracy of natural history, albeit not always recognized for what he was. And even now that his active life is spent, and he has been laid aside among the bibliographical curiosities of his period, he still lives in the memories of the well-affected; and if you wish to possess his image as he was when he was born, you will need to thrust your hand deep into your pocket.

Peace be with thine ashes Albrecht Dürer, great artist and creator of the olympian rhinoceros.

BIBLIOGRAPHY

ABELARD, P. (1079–1142). Cf. J. P. MIGNE, *Petri Abaelardi Abbatis Rugensis opera omnia*. Paris, 1885, no. lxvii, col. 1806. 4to.

AGUSTÍN, ANTONIO [AUGUSTINUS]. *Dialogos de medallas.* Tarragona, 1587. 4to.

ALBINUS, B. S. (1697–1770). *Tabulae sceleti et musculorum corporis humani.* Lugd. Bat. et Leidae, 1747. Fol.

ALDROVANDUS, U. (1522–1605). *De quadrupedibus solidipedibus.* Bononiae, 1616. Fol.

—— *Quadrupedum omnium bisulcorum historia.* Bononiae, 1621. Fol.

BARTHOLIN, T., Sen. (1616–1680). *De unicornu.* Second edition. Amstelaedami, 1678. 12mo.

BOCHART, S. (1599–1667). *Hierozoicon, . . . de animalibus S. Scripturae.* London, 1663. Fol.

---

[62] Bruce's figure is reproduced in the 1807 edition of Boreman.

[63] *v.* Labat (1732).

[64] *v.* under Boreman (1769). The author of this work was Thomas Boreman, a bookseller of whom little is known.

BONTIUS, J. (1598–1631). In G. PISO (1611–1678), *De Indiae utriusque re naturali et medica*. Amstelaedami, 1658. Fol.

[BOREMAN, T.] *A description of three hundred animals*. Tenth edition. London, 1769. 12mo.

BRUCE, J. (1730–1794). *Travels to discover the sources of the Nile*. 5 vols. Edinburgh, 1790. 4to.

BUFFON, COMTE DE (1707–1788). *Histoire naturelle*. Paris. Vol. xi, 1754 (*sic* 1764). 4to.

CAMERARIUS, J., Jun. [KAMMERMEISTER] (1534–1598). *Symbolorum et emblematum ex animalibus quadrupedibus desumtorum centuria altera*. Norimberg, 1595. 4to.

CAMPER, P. (1772–1789). *Natuurkundige verhandelingen . . . over den Rhinoceros met den Dubbelen Horen*. Amsterdam, 1782. 4to.

CARWITHAM, J. *Various kinds of floor decorations*. London, 1739. 8vo.

CATELANUS, L. *Von der natur . . . des Einhorns*. Franckfurt am Mayn, 1625. 8vo.

CHARDIN, J. (1643–1713). *Voyages en Perse, et autres lieux de l'Orient*. Amsterdam, 1711. 12mo.

DA COSTA, A. F. *Deambulations of the Rhinoceros (Ganda) of Muzafar, King of Cambaia, from 1514 to 1516*. (Portuguese Republic Colonial Office. Division of Publications.) Lisbon, 1937. 8vo.

DICKINSON, T. V. 'The armorial bearings of the Worshipful Society of Apothecaries.' *Proc. Roy. Soc. Med.*, 1929, xxiii (Sect. Hist. Med.), 11.

DODGSON, CAMPBELL, *Catalogue of Early German and Flemish woodcuts preserved in the . . . British Museum*. London. Vol. i, 1903, p. 307. 8vo.

—— 'The Story of Dürer's Ganda.' In H. A. FOWLER, *The romance of fine prints*. (Kansas City Print Society.) Kansas, 1938. 8vo.

EDWARDS, G. (1694–1773). *Gleanings of natural history*. London, 1758, pt. i. 4to.

DE FLACOURT, E. (1607–1660). *Histoire de la grande Isle Madagascar*. Paris, 1661. 4to.

GESNER, C. (1516–1565). *De quadrupedibus viviparis*. Tiguri, 1551. Fol.

—— *Icones animalium quadrupedum viviparorum*. Tiguri, 1553. Fol.

GHEERAERTS, MARCUS, Sen. [GERARDUS]. *Animalium. Quadrupedum. Omnis. Generis. Verae. et. Artificiosissimae. Delineationes, pictore Marco Gerardo Brugense. A° 1583*. [Amsterdam, *c.* 1630] Obl. 4to. No text, 21 Pls.

GIOVIO, P. [JOVIUS] (1483–1552). *Dialogo dell'imprese militari et amorose*. Roma, 1555, 1574, and other editions. 8vo.

GREW, N. (1641–1712). *Musaeum Regalis Societatis*. London, 1681. Fol.

GUARDABASSI, M. *Not. scavi antic. Accad. Lincei*. Roma, ann. 1877, p. 6. 4to.

HILL, J. (1716–1775). *An history of animals*. London, 1752. Fol.

HINKS, R. P. *Catalogue of the Greek, Etruscan and Roman paintings and mosaics in the British Museum*. London, 1933, p. xlix. (The Nilotic pavement at Palestrina dates from the Hadrianic period.)

JONSTON, J. (1603–1675). *Historia naturalis de quadrupetibus*. Francofurti ad Moenum, 1650. Fol.

KIRCHER, A. (1602–1680). *Arca Noë*. Amstelodami, 1675. Fol.

KLEIN, J. T. (1685–1759). *Quadrupedum dispositio brevisque historia naturalis*. Lipsiae, 1751. 4to.

KOLBE, P. (1675–1726). *The natural history of the Cape*. London, 1731. 8vo. (First edition in German, Nürnberg, 1719, fol.)

LABAT, J. B. (1663–1738). *Relation historique de l'Ethiopie Occidentale*. Paris. Vol. i, 1732. 8vo.

MARTIALIS, MARCUS VALERIUS (*c.* A.D. 40–104). *De spectaculis liber*. xxii, 'De rhinocerote'.

MARUCCHI, O., *Bull. Comm. Archeol. Roma*, 1904, xxxii, 258. (For Palestrina mosaic.)

MATTINGLY, H. *Coins of the Roman Empire in the British Museum.* London. Vol. ii, 1930. 8vo.

OKEN, L. (1779–1851). *Allgemeine Naturgeschichte für alle Stände.* Stuttgart. Vol. vii, 1838, p. 1187. 8vo.

PARÉ, A. (1510–1590). *Deux livres de chirurgie . . . 2. Des monstres tant terrestres que marines, avec leurs portrais.* Paris, 1573. 8vo.

—— *Les œuvres.* Paris, 1579. Fol.

—— *Discours . . . Asçauoir, de la mvmie, de la licorne.* Paris, 1582. 4to.

—— *The workes of that famous chirurgion, Ambrose Parey.* Trans. T. Johnson. London, 1634. Fol.

PARKINSON, J. (1567–1650). *Theatrum botanicum.* London, 1640. Fol.

PARSONS, J. (1705–1770). 'The natural history of the rhinoceros.' *Phil. Trans. Roy. Soc.*, 1743, xlii, 523–41.

—— 'On the double horns of the rhinoceros.' *Phil. Trans. Roy. Soc.*, 1766, lvi, 32–4.

PETRI AB HARTENFELS, G. C. (1633–1718). *Elephantographia curiosa.* Erfordiae, 1715. 4to.

SCHEUCHZER, J. J. (1672–1733). *Physica sacra.* Augustae Vindelicorum et Ulmae, 1731–5. Fol.

SHAW, G. (1751–1813). *General zoology.* London, 1800. Vol. i, pt. i, p. 201. 8vo.

[TACHARD, G.] (*c.* 1650–1712). *Voyage de Siam des Peres Jesuits.* Paris, 1686. 4to.

TEMPESTA, A. (1555–1630). *Nova raccolta de li animali piu curiosi del mondo disegnati et intagliati da Antonio Tempesta.* Roma, G. G. Rossi, 1650. Obl. 4to.

THEVET, A. (1502–1590). *La cosmographie universelle.* Paris, 1575. Fol.

TOPSELL, E. (*c.* 1570–*c.* 1638). *The historie of foure-footed beastes.* London, 1607. Fol.

VALENTINI, M. B. (1657–1729). *Museum Museorum.* Franckfurt am Mayn, 1704, 1714. Fol.

VALERIANUS, J. PIERIUS [VALERIANO BOLZANI, G. P.] (1477–1558). *Hieroglyphica.* Basileae, 1556. Fol.

VALMONT DE BOMARE, J. C. (1731–1807). *Dictionnaire raisonné universel d'histoire naturelle.* Yverdon. Vol. x, 1769, p. 30. 8vo.

THE MEDICAL CURRICULUM OF THE UNIVERSITIES OF EUROPE IN THE SIXTEENTH CENTURY

WITH SPECIAL REFERENCE TO THE ARABIST TRADITION

by

DONALD CAMPBELL

THE intimate contact of the Arabians and Latins in Sicily and the Iberian Peninsula in the seventh century, and the subsequent formation of the school of translators in Toledo, led to a vast number of Arabic translations of works on Graeco-Arabian Medicine reaching the Latin West. Scholars at that time possessed of necessity a generous combination of intellectual curiosity and physical vigour; any less well equipped would have fallen by the wayside. All Europe up to the thirteenth century, with the exception of parts of Italy, was in a state of barbarism, the original Greek manuscripts had not reached the West, and the practice of medicine was a degraded occupation which was subject to the penalties of the Draconic Code.

During this period Islam displayed a conspicuous activity, and though the Muslims destroyed much of the 'heretical' literature of the second Great Library of Alexandria, they rescued much of Greek Medicine through Byzantium and the Nestorian cloisters. Some of the Greek works would have been completely lost had it not been for the translating zeal of the Arabians. For example, the tenth to the fifteenth books of Galen's *De anatomicis administrationibus* survive only in the Arabic.

The period of translation in the Iberian Peninsula did not come to a close until A.D. 1285, which marks the death of the Sicilian Ibn Faradj. This was followed by the scholastic period, when the Arabic teaching was transmitted by the 'mystics' and then by the 'systematizers'. The medieval scholastic was not a specialist; he sought to be an encyclopaedist and to elaborate 'a complete scheme of things' with an unreasoning reverence for the wisdom of antiquity. By the thirteenth century we enter the second post-Arabian period of medicine and science, when the teaching was systematized by the 'transmuters', and accepted by the 'scholastics'. The Latin manuscripts which bear on the teaching in the sixteenth century will be discussed later.

The University of Seville was devoted to the study of Arabic, and its geographical position led to its being called upon to transmit the Arabic culture of the Western Caliphate to Latin Europe. By the sixteenth century there were sixteen universities in Spain alone, though the Spaniards made no appreciable contribution to the spread of learning.

The term *universitas*, until the latter part of the fourteenth century, was applied to the scholastic guilds within the *studia generalia*, and as the Middle Ages progressed, the distinction between the two was lost. Peripatetic students appointed their own teachers and founded universities, among which were Oxford and Cambridge; though in this connexion it should be stated that the scholar of the Middle Ages was usually a man of mature age who had already made his mark—not necessarily a good one—in some walk of life.

It was a common practice for both professors and students to migrate yearly from one university to another, and an appreciable number of them could be described as able-bodied vagabonds, who combined the study of medicine and philosophy with a life of adventure.

In this way of life they had the example of Algazirah (d. 1004), a medical practitioner of Kairawān, a portion of whose work was translated into Latin by Constantine the African. Algazirah is credited with a work entitled a *Guide to the Poor*, and at the same time enjoyed a reputation as a buccaneer of mean parts. Constantine's versions of this and other works were used in Europe long after the time of Gerard of Cremona, of whom more later.

The sixteenth century saw the foundation of a number of new universities, for example, Leyden (1575), Edinburgh (1582), and Dublin (1593), in all of which the students elected their rectors—amid a hail of missiles—and determined the courses of study. The actual curriculum consisted in the main of disputations in which professors and students took part; this custom became the foundation of the system of dissertations and theses presented before graduation at the universities.

In order to appreciate the methods of study at the European universities in the sixteenth century, it will be necessary to examine in some detail the extant Arabic manuscripts, and the 'Latino-barbari' versions of these documents.

In the course of this disquisition we shall show concrete examples of the results of transliteration from the Arabic manuscripts, and the effect of these 'new' words on the minds of the Schoolmen of the Middle Ages. It will be necessary to examine the relevant Latin translations in detail, and to note the dates of the findings of the original Greek manuscripts, in order to elucidate our point. It will also be necessary to refer briefly to the growth and development of Arabism prior to the century under review.

The scholasticism of medieval times was a main outcome of the Arabic teaching inseminated in the Iberian Peninsula. The School of Montpellier was a famous Arabist centre, and at a time when the medical library of Paris was limited to under a score of books, Montpellier had all the Latin translations, from the Arabic manuscripts, by Constantine and Gerard of Cremona. A tabulation of Constantine's works is to be found in the writings of Petrus Diaconus of Montecassino.[1] The order of Gerard's translations of the principal medical works was : (i) The ten books of the *Liber ad Almansorem* by Rhazes; (ii) the three surgical tracts of Albucasis; and (iii) the fourth book of Avicenna's *Canon*, of which the fourth and fifth chapters deal with surgery. Gerard of Cremona—not to be confused with Gerard of Sabbionetta, who succeeded him—translated into Latin some seventy Arabic works. Gerard had great faith in his own translations, but despite this, the versions of Constantine were used in Europe long after Gerard had done his work. Gerard died at Toledo in 1187, at the age of seventy-three years.

Among the far-reaching results of the Arabic contacts that have survived we might mention the introduction of Arabic numerals, the voluminous pharmacopœias, and the use of such words as syrup, elixir, alcohol, cypher, and many others. This was due to the fact that the translators were unable to find Latin equivalents, and they therefore transliterated the Arabic words.

[1] F. Puccinotti, *Storia della medicina*. 3 vols. Livorno, 1850–66. Vol. ii, p. 304.

Among other interesting words brought over to Europe were admiral, amber, sofa, and tabby. Though these examples are not strictly essential for our purpose, they denote a widespread tendency to the expansion of our language.

The *Antidotarium* (*parvum*) of Nicholas Præpositus, of which several editions exist,[2] contains the foundation of our modern apothecary's weights and measures, i.e., 20 grains = 1 scruple, and 3 scruples = 1 drachm. This work contains the Arabic formula for the 'soporific sponge', which was used to produce anaesthesia.

Owing to the lack of direct contact between the Latin Europe of the Dark Age and the Greek centre of Byzantium, the Greek language became a diminishing quantity. In the time of Roger Bacon (1214–94) Greek was a spoken and written language in southern Italy, and by the year 1360 we have the authority of Petrarch for the statement that there were scarcely ten men of learning in Italy who were acquainted with it. In this connexion it is significant that the bulk of the extant Greek manuscripts are later than the Latin renderings from the Arabic sources.

The medical writings of the thirteenth and fourteenth centuries consisted of compilations, commentaries, and concordances, most of which were based on the Latin translations of Arabic works available at Toledo. During these two centuries the medical system of Europe became a hopeless tangle of superstition, ignorance, and bigotry. The pre-Renaissance period was one during which Arabic teaching assumed a dominant position in Europe. It was not until 1543 that the modern works of Vesalius and Copernicus rekindled that intellectual independence which gradually brought to a close the Arabist tradition. This influence continued in the intellectual life of the scholastics up to the end of the sixteenth century, and we find that the medical curriculum of the universities of Europe demanded a knowledge of Avicenna's *Canon*, Galen's *Ars parva*, the *Aphorisms* of Hippocrates, and the *Materia medica* of Dioscorides.

Avicenna (d. 1037) was born in the province of Bokhara. Among the hundred books he is credited with, the most important was *Al-Qānūn fi't-Tibb* —which was known to the Latin West as *Canon*. Avicenna presents us with the doctrines of Galen and Hippocrates modified by the system of Aristotle, together with illustrative material from later writers. He surpassed both Aristotle and Galen in dialectical subtlety, and his train of reasoning appealed to the scholastics when passages that were obscure or unintelligible were considered sublime. On the other hand we find that Avenzoar (d. *c.* 1199), who performed tracheotomy and operated for renal calculi, described the *Canon* as waste paper; and Arnald da Villanova (d. 1312) referred to Avicenna as a professional scribbler whose misrepresentations of Galen stupified European physicians.

The *Canon*, which was the final codification of Graeco-Arabic Medicine, remained until 1650 the standard text-book in the Universities of Montpellier and Louvain. This work contains about a million words and is subdivided into five books and numerous major and minor sections. The first two books are concerned with physiology and hygiene, and are based on Aristotle and Galen. The third and fourth books deal with treatment, while the fifth is on

---

[2] e.g., Venice, 1471, 1497, 1532.

materia medica. A great number of manuscripts are extant. This work was translated by the two Gerards of Cremona. A beautiful Arabic edition, founded on the Florentine manuscript, was published in Rome in 1593.[3] The principal Latin editions are those published at Milan in 1473,[4] at Padua in 1476 and 1479,[5] and at Venice in 1482, 1486 and 1500.[6] The fifteenth century saw the appearance of *Maximus Codex totius scientiae medicinae*, which consisted of a mass of commentaries on the *Canon*.[7]

In common with other Arabic works which were translated into medieval Latin at Toledo and elsewhere, the *Canon* never did convey a true conception of Arabian Medicine to the Latin West. This is well illustrated in the Latin translation,[8] where the Arabic *al-ʿIshq* (love) is rendered as *De ilixi* with *Alhasch* as a variant. The first part of the third book of the Latin version is entitled *Sermo universalis de soda;* the Arabic *ṣudāʿ* means 'a splitting headache'. It will thus be seen to what controversial depths the medieval scholastics must have gone, with their fondness for dialectical subtlety, in their disputations and commentaries on elixir, soda, love and a splitting headache.

Anatomy was closed to Avicenna owing to his religious beliefs. He is said to have obtained his anatomical material from Rhazes (d. 926), who was one of the most original of the Arabic writers. Avicenna was translated into Greek.[9]

Galen's *Ars parva* (τέχνη ἰατρική) was translated into Arabic from the Syriac by Johannitius the Nestorian, and by Gerard of Cremona from Arabic into Latin. Constantine the African, who ended his days at Montecassino, also translated this work from the Arabic into Latin. The basis of the teaching in European universities was in the last resort the rendering of Johannitius, whose full name was Ḥunayn ibn-Isḥāq. He was the Erasmus of the Arabic Renaissance and was known to the Latin West as Hunayn, Onan, and Humainus. The Arabic translators led by him reviewed the works of Galen as a whole; this is evidenced by the Arabic manuscript at Stamboul.[10] Greek, Hebrew, and Latin manuscripts of the *Ars parva* are known.

This work is not to be confused with Galen's *Methodi medendi* (θεραπευτικῆς μεθόδου βιβλία ιδ'), i.e., *Megatechne*, of which Greek, Arabic, and Latin manuscripts are known. Of the Latin manuscripts there are eight in Oxford and four in Cambridge. There is an illuminated copy, presented to King Henry VIII, in the British Museum. For a full list of the Arabic manuscripts and Latin translations of the *Megatechne* my work on Arabian Medicine should be consulted.[11]

[3] [Libri v Canonis Medicinae. Arabic text]. Rome, Medicea, 1593.

[4] *Canon*. Lib. i–v. Milan, Philipp de Lavagna, 1473.

[5] *Canon*. Lib. i–v. Padua, J. Herbort, 1476 and 1479.

[6] *Canon*. Lib. i–v. Venice, Pt. Maufer and Nic. de Contengo, 1482; P. Maufer et soc., 1486; Simon Papiensis, 1500.

[7] *Maximus Codex totius scientiae medicinae*. 5 vols. Venice, Philipp. Pinzi, 1523. The commentaries are by Averroës, Dinus, Gentilis, Thaddaeus of Florence, Ugo, and others.

[8] *Canon*. Venice, Junta, 1544, fo. 208 *b*.

[9] Paris MSS. 2256, 2260, 2307–9.

[10] MS. Aya Sophia 3631.

[11] Campbell, *Arabian Medicine and its Influence on the Middle Ages* 2 vols. London, 1926. Vol. i, p. 26 and vol. ii, pp. 89–94.

Galen's *Ars parva* is the same work as *Ars medica*, and was known under several alternative titles, such as *Tegni*, *Microtegni*, *Microtegnon*, and *Techne*. Latin translations were published at Vienna in 1496, 1521, 1523, and 1527.

Numerous manuscripts were issued under the name of Haly Eben Rodan or Rodoham, without the mention of Gerard's name. The exception to this sin of omission is a manuscript in the British Museum.[12] Seven of Haly's commentaries are in the Bodleian and other Oxford libraries.[13] In Cambridge there are three Latin translations incorporating Haly's commentaries.[14]

The Caesarian Collection published in 1534 at Strasbourg contains the following: *Isagoge s. introductio Johannitius in artem parvam Galeni de medicina speculata*. The *Isagoge* was the Arabised version of Galen's *Ars parva* (or *Ars medica*), and a complete list of the Latin translations that were extant until the year 1939 has been published.[15] There are eleven in Cambridge and sixteen in Oxford. Of the thirty-seven other copies of this work in the British Museum, one was by Octavius the Scot who published it in Venice in 1498;[16] this translation begins 'Turisani monaco plus microtegni galieni'. Another is entitled 'Galieni . . . micro Tegni', and is based on the translation of Gerard of Cremona and issued together with Haly's commentaries.[17] There are no Arabic manuscripts of this work extant. A complete English translation of the *Isagoge* is given by Withington.[18]

A collection of Latin works, which includes Galen's *Ars medica*, came to be known as *Isagogici libri*.[15] This collection is included in the 1550 Lyons edition of Galen's works under the heading 'Elenchus librorum Galeni omnium qui in hoc opere continentur'.[19]

The presence of these Arabised works, and the fact that Europeans produced writings under Arabic pseudonyms, resulted in the Arabist tradition attaining a supremacy that was not seriously challenged until the fifth decade of the sixteenth century. In that decade the Arabist tradition was positively arraigned by the publication at Venice in 1547 of the Aldine Collection of *Medici antiqui*[20] and of the Estienne Collection of *Medicae artis principes*.[21] But the influence of the Arabist tradition continued until the period 1769–74, when the Haller Collection entitled *Artis medicae principes* was first published. It included references to the *Surgery* of Albucasis and to the *Liber de variolis et morbillis* of Rhazes. It will be noted that the former is illustrated, and that

---

[12] Brit. Mus. MS. I.B. 21384.

[13] The following are the press-marks of these seven Oxford MSS.: (i) Coll. Omn. Animar. 71; s.xiv. in fo. 113. (ii) Bodley 2303; s.—. (iii) Coll. St. Joh. Bapt. 10; s.xiii. fo. 99. (iv) Coll. Novi 170; s.xiv. fo. 17. (v) Merton 220; s.xiv. fo. 110. (vi) Merton 221; s.xiv. fo. 161. (vii) Univ. 89.

[14] The following are the press-marks of these three Cambridge MSS.: (i) Cantabr. Coll. Caii 59; s.xiv. fo. 251. (ii) St. Petri 14. s.xiv. fo. 101. (iii) Univ. J. i. II. 5; s.xiv. fo. 17–24.

[15] The list given in my *Arabian Medicine, op. cit.* (11), vol. ii, pp. 19–31 was still correct in 1939.

[16] Brit. Mus. MS. I.B. 22976.

[17] Brit. Mus. MS. I.B. 21384.

[18] E. T. Withington, *Medical history from the earliest times*. London, 1894, App. iv, pp. 386–96.

[19] For a list of these works, see *Arabian Medicine, op. cit.* (11), vol. ii, pp. 194–5.

[20] *Medici antiqui omnes, qui latinis literis diversorum morborum genera et remedia persecuti sunt.* Venice, 1547.

[21] *Medicae artis principes post Hippocratem et Galenum. Graeci Latinitate donati.* Excudebat H. Stephanus. 2 vols. Francfort, 1567.

the latter is a lucid account which may be read in an English translation,[22] and which is almost modern in its presentation of clinical detail.

The effect of the three surgical tracts of Albucasis on Latin Europe was that, while it tended to remove surgery from the hands of travelling mountebanks, it retarded its natural development, and the fictive anatomy of the Arabians took the place of human dissections. The teaching of Albucasis led to the extensive use of the actual cautery and meddlesome surgery in western Europe.

Galen's anatomical work, in terms of modern thought, may be looked upon as a first-hand study of comparative anatomy, though his conclusions and those of his followers were erroneous. It is stated that his work on practical anatomy was based on dissections of the barbary ape, the tailed monkey, and other animals such as the baboon, bear, and pig. Withington published an illuminating paper on Galen's Anatomy, and this should be consulted.[23]

It should be recorded that Galen's exhortations to original research were omitted by Oribasius and the great Arab writers. This grave injustice had disastrous results on medical education. The observation that 'a dog looks up to man, a cat looks down on man, and the pig gives man a level stare', might well have been first made in the 'dark age of anatomy', that is, up to the time of the dissectors Leonardo da Bertapaglia (d. 1460) and Leonardo da Vinci (d. 1519).

The *Operum Galeni* of 1550 contains a section on the anatomy of the pig (*De anatomia porci*).[24] This pseudo-Galenic work had a wide influence in the teaching centres of the Latin West.

An edition of a work by Galen was issued in 1622. This was the *Ars parva* or *Galeni Ars Medicinalis argumentis . . . locupletata e J. Thuilo.*[25] The date is significant; Galen was undoubtedly still an important authority in the early part of the seventeenth century.

The *Aphorisms* of Hippocrates were widely produced in Arabic translation, and until 1939 there were three Arabic manuscripts in Algiers, five in Berlin, two in Cairo,[26] one in Cambridge, four in Florence, six in Gotha, three in Leyden, eleven in Paris, two in Rome, nineteen in Stamboul, one in Vienna, two in the British Museum, and five in Oxford.[27]

The Arabic version of the *Aphorisms* in Cambridge[28] has the customary Arabic commentary. Most of the Latin translations of this Arabised work were published together with Galen's *Tegni*. The ubiquitous Haly in 1479 issued a Latin version 'cum commentario Galeni ex arab latine verso a Constantine Africano monacho'; this edition also contains Galen's *Microtechnon* (or *Ars parva*). A Latin edition in the British Museum[29] published

---

[22] Rhazes, *A treatise on the small-pox and measles.* Trans. W. A. Greenhill. London, Sydenham Soc., 1848.

[23] E. T. Withington, *Proc. Third Internat. Congr. Hist. Med.* Antwerp, 1923, pp. 96–100.

[24] *Operum Galeni.* Lyons, 1550, cap. i.

[25] Brit. Mus.: 12mo, 740a. 17 (1); 16mo, 544a. 34(2).

[26] Bibl. Khediviale 7663; 7666.

[27] Bodl. 533; 544; 608; 614; 627.

[28] Bibl. Univ. 1386; s.xii–xiv, No. 6.

[29] Brit. Mus. 539 i. 14(1–3).

in 1498 contains 'Espositio Ugonis Senensis super libros Tegni' and 'Espositio Ugonis . . . super aphorismos Hippocratis'. The text is interpolated.

The *Materia medica* of Dioscorides was widely used. It was the standard work on the subject in the period of Arabic dominance among the scholars in the West, and maintained its lead until the sixteenth century, when a knowledge of its contents would justify a scholar in claiming recognition in the subject.[30]

The Arabised teaching of Dioscorides was incorporated in the *Operum Galeni* (Lyons, 1550); volume iii, folio 297 mentions Dioscorides and some three hundred and fifty remedies and their substitutes ('De substitutis medicinis'). Among the remedies that appear to have survived until recent times, Zingibere and Pyrethrum may be mentioned. The substitutes are Succo papaveris—Mandragorae fructus; Refina pini—Terebinthi; Hyaenae adipe—Vulpis adeps; and Pipere albo—Nigri duplum. Among the other items in the armanentum of the physician of the sixteenth century, this work mentions Nardus indica, Lotus herba, and Ricini oleum, all of which indicate an Eastern origin. Cap. ccl (vol. iv), which is on Ginger, contains the following: 'Inuentur maxime in Troglodytis et Arabiae partibus.' Cap. cclx contains the following: 'Syrum nascitur in Africa, et in India optimum tamen habetur Arabum . . .'; and cap. cclxxvii reads: 'Thus, lacryma est arboris, quae in Arabia, et in India nascitur, quae Graece . . . dicitur. Quod ergo de Arabiae arbore manat, candidus est; quod de India . . . Expl. in nullo possit reprobus inueniri.'

John of Gaddesden (d. 1361), court physician to King Edward II, who is said to have been the original of Chaucer's Doctor of Physick, wrote his *Rosa Anglica* while at Merton College, Oxford. In this work he quotes from the Arabists Bernard de Gordon and Henry de Mondeville. Fifty-seven years later, the Arabist surgeon Guy de Chauliac condemns the work as containing 'the fables of Hispanus (Pope John), Gilbert, and Theodoric'. It was published at Pavia in 1492 and 1517; at Venice in 1502; and at Augsburg in 1595. This work was also translated into Gaelic; one of these Gaelic manuscripts, dating from about the mid-fifteenth century, was published with an English translation for the Irish Text Society in 1930.

John Arderne, another Englishman, in his *De arte phisicali et de cirurgia* (1412), mentions the work of Rhazes, Serapion and Avicenna. An English translation by Sir D'Arcy Power was published in 1922.[31]

---

[30] The following is a comprehensive list of the *De materia medica* of Dioscorides in Arabic manuscripts:
Bologna: Bonon. Marrigli 424.
Escurial: Scorial. 845.
Leyden: Bibl. acad. 1301.
London: Brit. Mus., Supp. MS. 1785 (Lib. iii, iv).
Madrid: Matri. bibl. nac. 125 (Gg. 147); 233 (Gg. 257).
Oxford: Bodl. 573. This manuscript, presented by the widow of the late Sir William Osler, is a splendid specimen of Arabic writing. Its special value lies in its coloured pictures of plants. It was translated in 1239 (probably in Spain) by Stephanus ibn Masail, and copied by Al-Hasan ibn Muhammad al-Nasāwi.
Paris: Parisin. 2849; 2850 (fragments).
Stamboul: Aya Sofia 3702; 3603; 3704 (illustrated).
[31] Publications of the Wellcome Historical Medical Museum, o.s. No. 3. London, 1922. (The translation was from a transcript, made by Eric Millar, of the facsimile of the Stockholm MS. which is in the Wellcome Museum.)

No judgement on the variety and range of Arabian Medicine would be permissible without the mention of such works as the pseudo-Galenic *De incantione, adjuratione et suspensione*, Latin manuscripts of which are in Rome,[32] and at Munich.[33] The following quotation from the *Operum Galeni* explains itself: 'Inscr. Cl. Galeno Adscriptus Liber de Incantione, Adjuratione, & Suspensione. Est autem inter Constantini Africani opera excusus. . . Libri de incantione, & amuletis, quem inter Constantini Africani opera legimus.'[34]

Medicine between the twelfth and seventeenth centuries, as will be seen by the Arabic manuscripts and Latin translations described above, was largely based on Avicenna, Rhazes, Albucasis, Avenzoar, and Averroës. The New Pharmacy found its roots in Serapion (Senior and Junior). The latter wrote *Liber de medicamentis simplicibus*, which was based on Galen and Dioscorides. There are no Arabic manuscripts of this work extant. Among the Latin translations was *Liber Serapionis aggregatus in medicinis simplicibus, translat. Simonis Januensis interprete, Abraham Judaeo Tortuosiensi de arabico in latinum* (Milan, 1473). Other Latin versions of this Arabic work were those published at Venice in 1479 and 1552, and at Strasbourg in 1531.

Aben-Guefit, or Ebn Wafedal Lachmi of the Arabians, wrote a work on 'simples' based on Dioscorides and Galen; a Latin translation by Gerard of Cremona was printed later and issued as supplements to the *Opera* of Mesuë, and published together with the work of the Arabic writer Alkindus at Strasbourg in 1531. Another Arabic writer who drew on Dioscorides was Ebn Albe'thar; a Latin translation of his writings, *Liber magnae collectionis simplicia medicamentorum et ciborum continens*, is a compendium of materia medica and dietetics; it is the fullest work on the subject in Arabian Medicine. Versions in Latin were published at Venice (1593), Paris (1602), and Cremona (1758). With Ebn Albe'thar we come to the last of the Arabians whose work influenced the medical curriculum of the Latin West.

Medicine and Philosophy were linked in the Middle Ages, and Averroës, to whom reference has been made earlier, was a friend of Avenzoar the great Arabian clinician; his system of Aristotle was derived from the Arabic translations, as he knew no Greek. The doctrines he propounded exercised an important influence in Latin Europe in the sixteenth century. When the Jews were expelled from Spain they took with them the Averroistic interpretation of Aristotle to southern France and Italy.

The principal work of Averroës was *Kitab-al-Kullyat*, transliterated in the Latin West as *Colliget*. It was translated by Bonacosa at Padua in 1255, and a Latin translation was published at Venice in 1482. The Latin edition published at Strasbourg in 1531 also contains the work of Rhazes, Serapion Junior, and Avenzoar.

Leonardo da Vinci (d. 1519) used the medieval Arabic anatomical nomenclature, e.g., *meri* for oesophagus, *siphac* for peritoneum, and *myrach* for stomach.

With the dawn of modern times, when the experimenters and anatomists began to publish their findings, we observe that the Arabist tradition in

---

[32] MS. Vatic. 2378.
[33] MS. Apogr. libri Venetiis a.1503 editi.
[34] *Opera Galeni*. Lyons, 1550, vol. iii, fo. 1497.

Europe began to fade. The direct appeal to Nature for her secrets, and the fundamentally modern works of Vesalius and Copernicus, published in 1543, saw the final overthrow of the *Arabistae*. The recovery of the Greek texts in the sixteenth century increased the heat of the intellectual battle between the Arabists and Hellenists. These disputations were joined by the experimenters, who agreed with neither. Among these were Achillini (d. 1512); Paracelsus (d. 1541); Servetus (d. 1553); Fallopius (d. 1562); Eustachius (d. 1574); Varolius (d. 1575); Ingrassias (d. 1580); Arantius (d. 1619); Fabricius ab Aquapendente (d. 1619); and William Harvey, who was a pupil of Fabricius.

The spirit of enquiry and criticism that broke the authority of the Medieval Church was the same spirit that was directed against the 'medical pope', Galen, and his servile and subtle followers, the Arabists. The impulse arising in the fifteenth century gathered momentum in the sixteenth, but the great expansion of knowledge was not fully apprehended at first. The early effort of the forward-looking scholars was sternly opposed by the matured Arabists whose only opponents hitherto were the Hellenists. Experiment and observation eventually brought the fictive anatomy of the Arabians into a state of ridicule. While the sixteenth century still saw the *Arabistae* in positions of influence in the universities, the final signal of the breakdown of Arabised Greek Medicine was the rediscovery of the *De medicina* of Celsus and other classical writings in the previous century.

Here, we would note that Pomponazzi (1462–1525), who was a doctor of medicine of Padua University, wrote *De immortalitate animae*. This work gave rise to a great controversy which heralded the Renaissance.

Paracelsus, who demonstrated his contempt for the Arabists by publicly burning the works of Galen and Avicenna, showed great originality in his description of a 'natural balsam' (the plastic lymph of Harvey). 'Paracelctic Medicine' was assailed by the Royal College of Physicians. Among the English writers, Francis Anthony (1550–1623) showed a decided Arabist leaning in his reliance on Arnald da Villanova and Raymond Lull, and did not quote Paracelsus.

The intellectual conflict in the last decade of the fifteenth century and during the first half of the sixteenth led to the replacement of the Arabist versions of the Greek texts in Latin garb by the Latin translations from the original Greek texts.

Despite the discovery of the original Greek texts in 1443, we find that a publication such as the *Collectio Chirurgia Veneta* (Venice, 1497) begins as follows: 'Guidonis de Cauliaco chirurgia parva, Albucasis Chirurgia, Jesu Haly et Canamusali de oculis. . . . Leon. Bertapalia recollectae super IV canonis Avicennae.' Other editions of this work were issued in Venice in 1498, 1499, 1513, 1519, and 1546 (Giunta).

Guy de Chauliac (d. 1368) was surnamed 'The Restorer' because his works re-introduced Arabic terms; he made free use of the anatomical nomenclature of Galen and Avicenna, and his writings show the frequent use of such medieval Arabic terms as *meri, sumen* or *sumac, myrach, siphac,* and *zirbus.* The vigour of Guy's work led to his influence on surgery extending to the sixteenth century and later.

Guy's Arabic-scholastic surgery was printed in fifty-two editions in Europe during the fifteenth and sixteenth centuries, and despite the schools of anatomy in Bologna and Padua, the Arabist tradition maintained its dominant position. Guy's *Chirurgia magna*, which was written in 1363, was a popular and most important vade-mecum even after the sixteenth century. In this work he refers to Avicenna, Rhazes, and Albucasis and presents us with a treatise on anatomy and chapters on materia medica and therapeutics. This work is representative of medical science during the High Scholastic Period. It may be noted that Guy does not mention Celsus. Four manuscripts contain diagrams of surgical instruments. Guy was the most eminent exponent of the Arabised Galen and Albucasis.

Arnald da Villanova's *Opera omnia* were published at Lyons in 1532. The work *Breviarum practicae* has been ascribed to Arnald; the third book is on gynaecology and begins thus: 'In this book I propose, with God's help, to consider the diseases peculiar to women, and, since women are for the most part poisonous creatures, I shall proceed to treat of the bites of venomous beasts.'

Gynaecology and obstetrics in the sixteenth century are well illustrated in *Collectio gynaeciorum* published at Basle in 1566 and 1586. The second book commences: 'Ex Albucasis libro secundo . . . affectus mulierum.' Another edition of this work was published in 1597 at Strasbourg. These and other works illustrate the fact that in the last decade of the sixteenth century Arabist tradition survived in the centres of learning. There is no sharp line of demarcation between the eclipse of Arabism and the rise of the Modern Age.

At Oxford University the medical curriculum included the *Tegni* of Galen, the *Antidotarium* of Nicholas of Salerno, and the *Aphorisms* of Hippocrates. The course of study extended from six to eight years. Leipzig required a knowledge of Avicenna's *Canon*, Galen's *Ars parva*, and the *Nonus Almansoris* of Rhazes. The last was the ninth book of the *al-Kitābu-l-Manṣūrī* of Rhazes which was dedictated to al-Manṣūr, the prince of Khurāsān; the Latin translation of this work was entitled the *Liber ad Almansorem*. The sources used by Rhazes for the first book were Hippocrates, Galen and Oribasius; the second book comes from Hippocrates, Galen, Oribasius, Aëtius, and Paul of Aegina, and contains chapters on 'slave buying'; the third book is from the same Greek sources and is concerned with dietetics; the fourth book is based on Galen and is on personal hygiene; the fifth is on dermatology; the sixth, which is also from Greek authors, is on 'diet for travellers'; the seventh is on surgery, and is taken from Hippocrates, Paul of Aegina (Book vi), the *Synopsis* of Oribasius (Book vii), and Aëtius (Books xiv and xv); the eighth book is on toxicology. The ninth book is devoted to a consideration of diseases of the body from 'top to toe'. Rhazes derived his material for this book from the *De morbis* of Hippocrates, the *De locis affectis*, *Methodi medendi*, and *De compositione medicamentorum secundum locos* of Galen, Aëtius (Books vi–xii), Oribasius (Books viii and ix) and Paul of Aegina (Books iii and iv). The *Nonus Almansoris* was famous throughout the Middle Ages, and was the subject of numerous commentaries. It formed a part of the regular medical curriculum of the University of Tübingen. The tenth and last book of this famous descriptive treatise is on fevers, and is based on Hippocrates, the *De crisibus, De differentiis febrium, Methodi medendi* (Books iv–x) of Galen, Aëtius (Book v), and Paul of Aegina (Book vi). The ten volumes of this work by Rhazes demonstrate the carrying over of Greek Medicine to the Arabians, and the Latin translations (published at Milan in 1481, at Venice in 1497, at Lyons in 1510, and at Basle in 1544) are evidence of the esteem in which it was held by the universities in the sixteenth century. The ninth book, together with commentaries, was published separately at Venice in 1483, 1490, 1493, and 1497, and at Padua in 1480.

The medical curriculum at Vienna (1520) and at Frankfort-on-the-Oder (1588) included the *Canon* and the ninth book of the *Liber ad Almansorem*.

The demand for Latin versions of the Arabic works of Avicenna, Averroës, and Serapion in particular, was supplied in a very generous manner by Andreas Alphagus Belluensis (d. 1520). Andreas, like his predecessors labouring under a weight of contentious commentary, made correct translations from the Arabic texts of Avicenna's *Canon*, his *Aphorismi de anima*, and a number of his other works; he also translated Serapion's *Practica*.

All the universities in the Latin West demanded a knowledge of the Arabised versions of the Greek works, and the *Arabistae* were undoubtedly the most influential of the learned members of society throughout the sixteenth century.

It was not until the seventeenth century that the gathering forces of the experimenters and sceptics dissipated the miasma of incantations, amulets, and 'blind belief' that characterized the medieval mind. Arabian Medicine and Science had outlived their usefulness.

The assertion that Arabian Medicine had its appeal in its culinary and sexual content will not bear investigation. An examination of any one of the standard works accepted by the universities of the sixteenth century, such as the *Liber ad Almansorem* of Rhazes, reveals a spirit of wide enquiry and a desire to alleviate, if not cure, human suffering.

The *Arabistae* have not been vanquished completely. Our numerals, our system of weights and measures, our language, our pharmacopœias, and the fact that medicine was raised from the grade of a discreditable business to the status of a dignified calling, are due to the Arabians whose intellectual activities permeated Europe in its Dark Age.

SOME VESALIAN STUDIES *

by

HERNANI MONTEIRO

I. *The Woodcut Portrait of Vesalius and the Editions of the 'Fabrica'*

IN 1912 Belgium had decided, on the initiative of Professor Paul Heger, to commemorate in a fitting manner the quatercentenary of the birth of Andreas Vesalius. The celebration was to have been held in Brussels, the city of his birth, in December 1914. A 'Liber Memorialis' was to contain studies by various authorities on different aspects of Vesalius as man and scientist.

The war held up this tribute to the distinguished anatomist. But M. H. Spielmann, the contributor to the memorial volume who had been entrusted with the section on the portraiture of Vesalius, completed his first draft and then continued to extend his work. In 1925 it was published in London by the Wellcome Historical Museum with the title, *The Iconography of Andreas Vesalius*. This fine work deals exhaustively with its subject, and contains full critical descriptions of all the known portraits of Vesalius, whether in the form of paintings or prints, or in sculptured busts or reliefs on medals.

The fourth chapter of this work deals with engravings, and opens with a list of portraits in the various editions of the *Fabrica*. With reference to the wood-cut portrait of Vesalius designed by Jan van Calcar,[1] which bears the date 1542, and which was published in the 1543 edition of the *Fabrica* and in the *Epitome*, Spielmann notes that it also appeared in the German edition of 1543, in the *Epistola . . . Radicis Chynæ* (1546), and also in the second (1555) edition of the *Fabrica* which, like the first, was published at Basle by Oporinus. In a foot-note this explanation is given: 'It is easy to distinguish to which book each of the three different impressions of this Woodcut belongs, when found apart from the volume. Above the portrait in each case appears the printed name, ANDREÆ VESALII. In the first edition (1543) the space occupied by these words is $3\frac{7}{8}$ in. (9·8 cm.) wide; in the second edition (1555) it is $3\frac{3}{16}$ in. (8·1 cm.) wide; and in the *Epistola . . . Chynæ* it is $3\frac{1}{2}$ in. (8·[9] cm.) wide'. And immediately after these words are added: 'It is to be noted that in the impressions of 1546 and 1555 the block has suffered damage at the top left corner, and can be so recognized.'[2] And in another note, on the portrait and engraving of the second edition of the *Fabrica*, Spielmann says: 'Professor Roth was in error in supposing that the block used in 1555 is not the same as that of 1543. This first error entails a second—the claiming as evidence the presence of the mark over the right eyebrow (the *Muttermal* = birth-mark, or wart) as "confirmation" that the mark is an element of the true portraiture! The fact is that this so-called

---

* Translation kindly supplied by Mr. A. C. Hawkins, Director of the British Institute, Oporto.
[1] C. Singer, *Journ. Anat.*, 1943, lxxvii, 261–5. Singer considers the head only of Vesalius to be the work of an artist of merit, Calcar or another.
[2] Spielmann, *Iconography*, p. 121.

PLATE XXXII

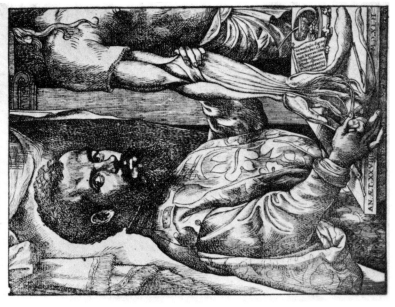

Fig. 2. Portrait of Vesalius in the *Fabrica*, 1555
(From the copy in the Library of the Instituto de
Anatomia, Lisbon)

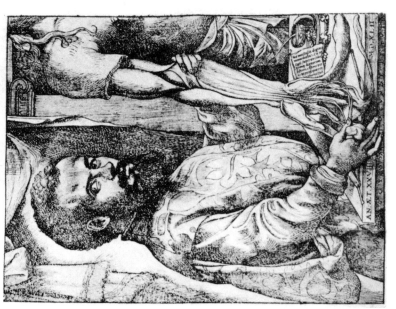

Fig. 1. Portrait of Vesalius in the *Fabrica*, 1543
(From the copy in the Oporto Municipal Library)

PLATE XXXIII

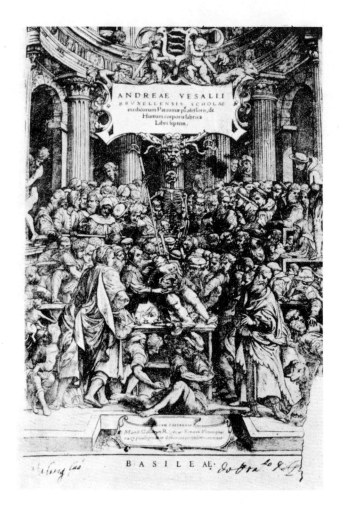

FIG. 3. Title-page of the *Fabrica*, 1543
(From the copy in the Oporto Municipal Library)

"repetition" is not repetition at all, but a simple case of the reprinting of the same woodblock.'[3]

Since the war of 1914–18 deprived the medical world of the chance to celebrate the fourth centenary of the birth of Vesalius, I suggested in 1938,[4] four centuries after the publication of his *Tabulae anatomicae*, that the opportunity should not be lost of celebrating in 1943 the quatercentenary of the publication of his *Fabrica*. A fortunate date when one comes to think of it, inasmuch as nearly all the best results of the scientific researches of Vesalius are as it were enshrined—as Charles Singer points out[5]—in that book, to the publication of which he owes his title of Father of Anatomy : 'Vesalius and his great work *On the fabric of the human body* are one. Without the book he would be but a ghost.'

But in 1939 a new war broke out and spread over almost the whole of Europe, and Belgium once again found herself unable to stage a solemn tribute to the memory of the great anatomist.[6] Far from the struggle, Spain, Portugal and Argentina did so.[7] America—involved in the conflict, it is true, but outside her own territory—likewise organized a number of ceremonies.[8] And yet,

[3] *ibid.*

[4] H. Monteiro, *Bruxelles-Medical*, 1938, xix, 205, 242.

[5] C. Singer, *The evolution of anatomy*. London, 1925, p. 115.

[6] Nevertheless, in Belgium the date was commemorated in Brussels (see *Bruxelles-Médical*, Sept. 1944 : special number) by the Académie Royale de Médicine at its meeting on 26 June 1943, during which Professor G. Laboucq gave an address and read an unpublished translation of the preface to the *Fabrica*. In addition, the hitherto unpublished biography of Vesalius, written in 1933 by Professor Léon Frédéricq, was issued in the *Mémoires de la Société Royale des Sciences de Liège* (1942, 4s., vi).

[7] In Spain I gave a lecture in the Faculty of Medicine of Santiago de Compostela, on 16 May 1942, on the historiated capitals in the *Fabrica*. In October 1943 at my suggestion as President of the Sociedade Anatómica Portuguesa there was held in the same university an Anatomical Congress in honour of Vesalius, at which this society and the Sociedade Anatómica Luso-Hispano-Americana met together (the latter under the presidency of Professor Henrique de Vilhena). In passing it may be mentioned that on 10 June a scenario for a film about Vesalius was published in the Madrid review *Fantasia*.

In Portugal, in commemoration of that date, I made two communications to the Academia das Ciências on the initial capitals (2 July and 22 October 1942) and gave two lectures in the Faculty of Medicine in Oporto (18 March and 13 May 1943). In March and April of 1943 this Faculty organized a series of lectures as a tribute to the memory of the Flemish anatomist. See the following :

Hernani Monteiro, 'Comentarios às Estampas do Tratado de André Vesálio *De humani corporis fabrica*, Bâle, 1543'. *Arq. de Anat. e Antropol.*, 1942–3, xxii, 161–200. The Italian translation of the sonnets connected with the prints may be found in the same journal, 1945, xxiii, 529–59.

idem, 'As letras capitulares de Tratado de Anatomia de Vesálio *De humani corporis fabrica*, Bâle, 1543'. *ibid.*, 1942–3, xxii, 433–76.

idem, 'André Vesálio. No quarto centenário da publicação da *Fabrica*'. *ibid.*, 1944, xxiii, 15–53; and *Jornal do Médico*, 1943, iii, Nos. 62–3.

idem, 'Três anatómicos célebres da Renascença italiana : Leonardo da Vinci, Berengario da Carpi e André Vesálio'. *Arq. de Anat. e Antropol.*, 1943–5, xxiii, 135–40; and *Jornal do Médico*, 1943, iii, Nos. 62–3.

idem, Address given at the opening session of the Anatomical Congress of Santiago de Compostela in October 1943. *Arq. de Anat. e Antropol.*, 1943–5, xxiii, 135–46 and *Jornal do Médico*, 1943, iii, Nos. 62–3.

idem, 'Iconografia de liçoes e Trabalhos anatómicos antes de Vesálio'. *Arq. de Anat. e Antropol.*, 1943–5, xxiii, 273–90.

In the Sociedade Argentina de la História de la Medicina in Buenos Ayres, the date was commemorated in July 1943 by a series of lectures dealing with various aspects of the life and work of Vesalius.

[8] Particulars of the celebrations held in the United States in honour of Vesalius may be found in the editorial written by Henry Sigerist to introduce the special number (December 1943) of the *Bulletin of the History of Medicine*, which was entirely devoted to the Flemish anatomist. See also the December number (1943) of *The Yale Journal of Biology and Medicine* (vol. xvi,

much was done to mark the date by the publication in that year 1943 of Harvey Cushing's posthumous work, *A Bio-Bibliography of Andreas Vesalius*, which constitutes, in the just words of Sigerist, 'the iron foundation for all research on Vesalius'.

That fine work of Cushing opens with the celebrated portrait of Vesalius, without an indication of the book from which it was reproduced. The caption runs as follows: 'ANDREAS VESALIUS. The well-known contemporary portrait of Vesalius which appeared in the *Fabrica* of 1543, the *Epitome* of 1543, and the China-root Epistle of 1546. Although still fresh in 1546 (and in 1555), the block had been chipped in the upper left corner. This is the only authentic portrayal of Vesalius.' From this and from the flaw in the upper left corner of the woodcut it seems safe to conclude that the portrait was reproduced from the 1546 work. And it also seems safe to conclude that Cushing—or Professor Fulton, who, with the assistance of Dr. W. W. Francis, so devotedly undertook the posthumous publication of his book—thought, just as Spielmann had already said, that the defect in the wood-block only appears in the impressions of 1546 and 1555.

In Portuguese public libraries I saw two copies of the first (1543) edition of the *Fabrica* : one in the Oporto Municipal Library (originally in the possession of the Congregação do Oratório), and one in the Academia das Ciências in Lisbon (originally in the library of the Convento de Jesus in Lisbon).

There is a copy of the second edition of 1555 in the Library of the Instituto de Anatomia in Lisbon, which was left to the Escola Médico-Cirúrgica by Dr. Simão José Fernandes.[9]

pp. 105–50). It contains the speeches made in the Historical Library of Yale University Medical School in the session of 30 October 1943. In the offprint, a copy of which I received from Professor John Fulton, there is also a description of the Vesalius exhibition held in the Yale Medical Library.

In England the date was commemorated by Drs. Charles Singer and Ashworth Underwood. From the former we have : 'To Vesalius on the Fourth Centenary of his *De Humani Corporis Fabrica*', *Journ. Anat.*, 1943, lxxvii, 261–5; 'A New World', *Times Lit. Supp.*, June 1943; 'Two Forerunners. Our debt to Copernicus and Vesalius. The Passing of Medieval Science', *Times Lit. Supp.*, 29 May 1943; 'Vesalius the Man', *Brit. Med. Journ.*, 1944, ii, 407. And from the latter : 'The *Fabrica* of Andreas Vesalius. A Quatercentenary Tribute', *Brit. Med. Journ.*, 1943, i, 795.

In Palestine Professor Sh. E. Franco, of the Hebrew University of Jerusalem, is preparing a work on Vesalius. In a local periodical he has already published a note on the relations between the anatomist and the Jews : 'Andreas Vesalius and the Jews', *Journ. Palestine Jewish Med. Assoc.*, 15 June 1945, xxviii, No. 12.

[9] There is a copy of the 1568 edition in the library at Evora, originally in the library of the Convent of the Congregação do Oratório at Estremoz.

Of the edition of 1604 a copy is in the care of the Faculty of Medicine at Oporto; and of the 1725 edition (*Opera omnia*) there is a copy in the Instituto de Anatomia of Coimbra (which belonged at one time to the Convent of Santa Cruz there), another in the Biblioteca Nacional in Lisbon (from the Library of the Cistercian Convent at Alcobaça), and yet another in the Academia das Ciências in Lisbon. This copy, as may be read in a manuscript note, came from the library of Casimiro da Costa Caetano. I may add, from information which I owe to Dr. Silva Carvalho, that Casimiro da Costa was born in Oporto, studied philosophy, Greek and medicine in Paris and took his degree at Leyden. In 1767 he defended his thesis *De stadio medico*. Thereafter he studied at hospitals in London and Edinburgh and came, in 1769, to qualify at Coimbra University in order to establish himself in practice in Lisbon.

I have also seen two very well preserved copies (two volumes each) of the 16vo. edition of 1552 (Lyons) : one in the library at Evora, the other in the Biblioteca Nacional in Lisbon (originally in the Carthusian foundation at Evora, according to the MS. note which appears in both volumes : 'Liber Carthusiae scalae coeli dono datus ab Illmo. et Rmo. Inno. Patre D. Theotonio a Bragança Archiepiscopo Eborĕn, fundatore et dotatore eiusdem domus').

The library of the Faculty of Medicine at Oporto also owns copy No. 529 of the *Icones anatomicae* (New York and Munich, 1934–5).

Now, in the copy of the *editio princeps* (1543) of the *Fabrica* in the Oporto Municipal Library,[10] the print of the Vesalius portrait (inserted facing sig. A[1] = page 1) shows the defect referred to in the top left corner, as may be seen from an examination of Fig. 1.[11]

That the print, even if loose, did in fact belong to a copy of the edition of 1543 is shown by the space occupied by the name of Vesalius printed above the portrait. One has only to compare it with the print of the 1555 edition of the *Fabrica*, in the copy belonging to the library of the Instituto de Anatomia in Lisbon.

It is thus clear that, contrary to what Spielmann supposed, the flaw in the top left corner of the engraving does not give sufficient grounds for the assertion that a portrait of Vesalius belongs to one of the works printed in 1546 or 1555. The fact that the copy of the *editio princeps* of the *Fabrica* in the Oporto Municipal Library already exhibits the flaw in question proves that the wood-block was damaged not after but during the printing of the work in 1543. And it also proves, in confirmation of Spielmann's statement and contrary to what Roth thought, that a new block of the portrait was not made for the 1555 edition of the *Fabrica*, but that the same 1543 wood-block was used.

By reason of two wars Europe, and Belgium in particular, could not celebrate, as was its wish, either the quatercentenary of the birth of Vesalius or the publication of his outstanding treatise. May Sigerist's hope be realized with the commemoration, in 1964, of the fourth centenary of his death 'in a pacified, rejuvenated and joyful world'.

II. *The Title-page of the 'Fabrica'—A Lesson in Anatomy*

In 1942 I published, in the *Arquivo de Anatomia e Antropologia*, some comments on the woodcuts of the *Fabrica*. I referred also to the ornate title-page, in which the artist lets his imagination run riot in a sumptuous setting for the great master's lecture. And in my interpretation of this print I recorded my verdict against the symbolism which some attribute to it. This lavish anatomical theatre never existed. Let us overlook the natural phantasy of Calcar—and perhaps of Vesalius as well, for one may be sure that the whole of the artist's work was carried out according to the anatomist's instructions; and let us discount the magnificence of the hall, decorated with rich and elaborately worked columns and also the position of the figures dictated by the balance of the composition as a whole. Then it does not seem to me that the interpretation requires recourse to complicated symbolism.

Though we do not know whether Vesalius or Calcar suggested the idea for the design, it is evident that one or other, or both, wished to represent the new method of studying and teaching anatomy, and, moreover, in a rather exaggerated fashion. They did not therefore follow the dissection scenes as illustrated in some of the older books. In these the professor is seen reading the text aloud from his high chair. The demonstrator carries out the crude dissection; while the ostensor—who is not always shown in these illustrations—

[10] In this copy, bound in leather, the unpaginated half-sheet *m*3 is present and intact with his eight anatomical figures (Type 1 of Huntingdon).

[11] The portrait of Vesalius is missing from the copy belonging to the Academia das Ciências in Lisbon, the page having been torn out.

indicates the parts to which the professor refers in the course of his reading. In the print Vesalius is not seated in the professor's chair. He stands by the body among the students and performs the dissection himself. He uses no book, but speaks from his own knowledge. The students help him when necessary, and the menial demonstrator is relegated to a subordinate position. In the dedication of the *Fabrica* to Charles V he describes his method. There he states that in his work at Louvain, Padua, Bologna, and Pisa he had tried to free himself from the yoke of masters and schools, and was striving to demonstrate Man on Man himself.

In the fine title-page of the *Fabrica* which we are discussing, the body is of the highest importance; for Vesalius set out to study and teach anatomy not merely, as hitherto, almost solely through animal dissection, repeating and commenting upon the words of Galen, but by dissection of the human subject. But in addition the upright skeleton is very evident. When we remember how troublesome it was to secure human bones for anatomical studies and how skilled Vesalius was in the preparation and mounting of skeletons, and further how difficult it was in those days to obtain subjects, we can well understand why a central position was reserved in the composition for the skeleton; in this way the importance of the study of osteology was emphasized.

It may be noted that in the *Fabrica* the initial letter O of Books I and III represents the preparation of the bones by boiling; in the letter C can be seen a stage in the complicated preparation of a natural skeleton by the old method of maceration, while in the letter P reference is made to the process employed by Vesalius for mounting skeletons.

The naked man (he was dressed in the edition of 1555), who appears on the left of the title-page supporting himself on a column, may very well represent the model used by the master for his demonstrations of surface anatomy, although artistically stylized in his total nudity, or he may be nothing but a figment of the artist's imagination. We must bear in mind, as both Roth and Singer have pointed out, that Vesalius was vitally interested in living anatomy.

As for the monkey and the dog which appear in the right and left foreground of the print, I consider their presence there to be very appropriate, for what Vesalius wished to demonstrate in some of his courses and in his famous book was that Galen's school was based on animal and not human dissection. To this end he clearly had to devote himself to studies in comparative anatomy, for which dogs and monkeys were indispensable, and he even dissected goats (this animal duly figures in the frontispiece of the 1555 edition), sheep, oxen and cats. This he had seen done by Sylvius, his master in Paris. In the work published in 1555 Vesalius quotes observations on those and other animals such as the pig, horse, and lion.[12]

On the other hand, it is also well to remember that Vesalius—incontestably the reformer of anatomical studies, by his efforts to base the knowledge of Man on the observation of Man himself and not merely on that of animals—had very few human subjects at his disposal for complete and careful dissection.

Vesalius used animals freely for his dissections, even though they were difficult to obtain, and he also used them for vivisection. In the last chapter of

---

[12] Singer, *op. cit.* (6), p. 145.

the *Fabrica* he discusses the vivisection of pigs, dogs and cats. Despite the fact that his anatomy is essentially human—which constitutes its claim to immortality—in some instances in the *Fabrica* the parts described are those of animals and not of man. These parts Calcar drew in some of the figures of the bones and muscles.

Vesalius himself wrote in chapter xix of Book V of the *Fabrica* (p. 547): 'and then, in the sight of all, I dissected a man and a dog and, when opportunity offered, a monkey, calling attention diligently to all things which are described by me.'

At the beginning of his public demonstrations he used to refer briefly to the anatomy of the various organs, using a dissected dog or sheep for their demonstration. Only afterwards did he demonstrate on a human subject. He finished with some vivisections; and in order that this should be made clear, at the bottom of the title-page of the second (1555) edition of the *Fabrica*, which was printed during the lifetime and under the direction of Vesalius, we can see the board with the ring, the holes and the ropes for fastening the animals.

When dealing in his demonstrations with the age and sex differences in the joints, he used the bones of various animals as well as those of man. For demonstrating the placenta, he used the uterus of a goat or a sheep. As the eye-ball in the human subject was often in an early state of decomposition, he always dissected the eyes of oxen, and in the capital letter R the enucleation of the eye of the ox is shown.

In the capital letter Q (as for example at the beginning of the dedication and of Book V) there is shown the vivisection of the pregnant sow, which Vesalius describes in detail in chapter xix of Book VII: 'De vivisectione nonnulla.'[13] The dog figures in four of the historiated initials: in the T, both in the larger woodcut with which one of the books begins and in the smaller initial capitals in several chapters, and also in the S and the Q (smaller picture). In the latter a Caesarean operation is being carried out on a bitch.

This emphasis on the dog clearly shows that it was not a mere symbol of an archaic anatomy,[14] but that this animal was much used in anatomical studies.

If, for Vesalius, the monkey, the dog and other animals were springs in which he had to slake his thirst for knowledge, driven as he was to do so by the difficulty of obtaining human subjects, it is not to be wondered at that they figure at the threshold of his work, and I do not think it necessary to invent lofty symbolism in order to explain their presence there.

These views I expressed some years ago, and further reflection strengthens my opinion. I note with satisfaction that both Singer and Underwood hold the same views as I do regarding this famous title-page. As Singer has written: 'Much symbolism has been discovered in it and all or nearly all, in my opinion, unnecessary, misplaced and mistaken.'

---

[13] Shows the beginning of the work—the cutting of the skin of the neck to uncover the recurrent nerves—and not the opening of the trachea, as is indicated in the legend to Fig. 65 ('The trachea is being opened') on p. 118 of Charles Singer's fine work *The evolution of anatomy*, London, 1925. Only in the last phase, with the work far advanced after the opening up of the abdomino-pelvic viscera, and the opening of the thorax and of the pleural cavity, did the operator open the trachea to introduce air into the lungs through a reed inserted in the orifice, in order to prevent the death of the animal by asphyxiation.

[14] See Spielmann, *op. cit.* (3).

VESALIUS AND THE GALENISTS

by

M. F. ASHLEY MONTAGU

IT is a remarkable fact that the two books which are conventionally agreed upon by scholars as marking the end of the Middle Ages and the birth of the new spirit of science were published within one week of each other. The first by the Polish canon Nicholaus Copernicus (1473–1543), *De revolutionibus orbium coelestium*, published at Nürnberg on 25 May 1543, when the author was seventy years of age; the second by the Flemish-born physician and anatomist, Andreas Vesalius (1514–64), *De humani corporis fabrica*, published at Basle on 1 June 1543, when the author was but twenty-eight years of age. (It was possibly a pardonable confusion of these facts which accounts for a certain medical student's malappropriate definition of anatomy as 'the study of celestial bodies'!)

The achievement of Copernicus was much greater than that of Vesalius and considerably more original, yet interestingly enough his book was much more in the tradition of an earlier period than was that of Vesalius. The work by Copernicus had been eagerly awaited for many years, and when at long last it made its appearance it was well received. But not nearly as well nor as widely acclaimed as was the book by the young Professor of Anatomy at Padua.

The *Fabrica* of Vesalius, an achievement on a somewhat lower intellectual plane than that of Copernicus, represents the culmination of a tendency which was already well developed in the first half of the sixteenth century. The achievement of Vesalius was to give that tendency its clearest and most complete expression in his book. And it was at once accepted for what it was, not so much as representing a break with the Galenical tradition, as has so frequently been stated, but rather as an advance upon it.

It has been the custom to represent the *Fabrica* as having made a complete break with the old traditional anatomy,[1] and to portray the Galenists as the bad violent men, 'head-pieces stuffed with straw,' while Vesalius is almost invariably painted as the heroic young genius whom the plodding, leaden Galenists, barking like the dogs of St. Ernulphus, were resolved to destroy.

In the case of Copernicus the Church is cast in the role of villain. In the case of Vesalius it has always been the Galenists, with a bit of Church thrown in to provide the right *décor*. There is no truth in the first legend, and very little in the second. I should like to do something towards restoring a truer perspective to the facts than has thus far been attempted. A great deal has been taken out of context which should never have been removed in the first place. These excerpts need to be restored and viewed in relation to the terms and the times to which they properly belong.

Let us now briefly engage ourselves with the life of the principal character in our story.

---

[1] How untrue this is Charles Singer has recently shown in an interesting article, 'Some Galenic and animal sources of Vesalius.' *Journ. Hist. Med. and Allied Sci.*, 1946, i, 6–24.

Andreas Vesalius was born at Brussels, the metropolis of Brabant, on the last day of December 1514. His father, of the same name, was court physician to Charles V. His mother, Isabelle Crabbe, seems, so far as the biographers are concerned, chiefly remarkable for the fact that she was of English ancestry. Vesalius came from a family which had already produced five generations of physicians, and as the great eighteenth-century anatomists Boerhaave and Albinus say, 'sprung from such a stock, born of such parents, he felt impelled not to suffer himself to fall away from the ancient virtue of his fathers'.[2] The young Vesalius was sent to the military college at Louvain where, among other things, he acquired an excellent knowledge of Latin and Greek, and under the influence of his teacher Guinterius Andernacus developed a burning enthusiasm for the natural sciences. At school he was already depopulating the fauna of his region by dissecting mice, dormice, moles, cats and dogs. And with the aid of the anatomically-inclined Guinterius he succeeded in obtaining a human skeleton by robbing a gibbet.

From school he proceeded to Montpellier, returning on several occasions to continue his studies at Louvain. Meanwhile Guinterius had given up Greek for the teaching of anatomy at Paris, where another erstwhile teacher of classics at Amiens was now the most celebrated lecturer on anatomy in Europe, Jacobus Sylvius, which is but the Latin for the French Jacques Dubois, and as Charles Kingsley Englished or rather Scotched it, 'alias Jock o' the Wood'.[3]

At the age of eighteen Vesalius proceeded to Paris in order to study medicine under these two men, among others, but more particularly under Sylvius. Here, a devoted pupil, he remained for three years.

Whatever may have been the origin of the anatomical interest shown by Sylvius and Guinterius, the easiest way to systematize that interest was to begin with the study of the standard texts, and then, with their aid, proceed to the dissection of a human body or that of a monkey, a pig or a bear, each of them in turn, if possible. Since the standard texts of the day were all Galenical, it is scarcely surprising that they read them and became confirmed Galenists. They could hardly have done otherwise, for the Pergamean Galen (A.D. 130–200) had a reputation of 1300 years to lean upon, not alone as a great anatomist but as a master of every branch of medicine and biology. And it must certainly be the judgement of every unbiased student of the history of science that that reputation was well deserved. There were some who found Galen dull. In Rabelais' copy of the Greek Galen is written in a bold hand, 'This Galen is an uncommon dull fellow, a dud, a lump of lead'. The truth is, however, that most students of Galen found him rewarding and interesting enough to devote a good many of their student and later years to the study of his writings. His discussion of the systems of the human body are truly remarkable achievements, and he is sufficiently accurate to make it easy to gloss over his errors.

---

[2] Hermann Boerhaave and Bernhard Siegfried Albinus, 'The Life and Works of Andreas Vesalius'. (Translated by Benjamin Farrington from the Preface to their edition of the works of Vesalius, *Opera omnia anatomica et chirurgica*. Lugd. Bat., 1725. *Trans. Roy. Soc. South Africa*, 1930, xix, 49–78; passage quoted on p. 54.)

[3] Charles Kingsley, 'Andreas Vesalius'. In *Health and Education*. London, 1887, pp. 385–411.

If one did not pay too much attention to detail, and one could hardly do so under the conditions prevailing during the dissection of an unpreserved, uninjected, putrefying body which it was possible to keep for no longer than three days, Galen would do very well, especially if one read him in the editions of the learned commentators, who had frequently 'becommentated' him with such a wealth of matter, that fewer words of Galen's than of the commentator's were to be found upon each page. There was no anatomy superior to Galen's, and under such circumstances the best men could hardly be other than Galenists—which is what Sylvius, Guinterius and Vesalius were.

It is necessary to insist upon these points in view of the uncritically costive attitude of many modern writers towards any medieval figure who was a follower of Galen. Such writers are themselves guilty of the very sins for which they condemn the Galenists, namely, the uncritical repetition of what has most often been said before them, and a lack of acquaintance with the first-hand sources. It is easy to repeat what others have said; it is somewhat less easy to discover the truth for oneself.

With the defects and virtues of his classical scholarship to support him, and the experience and tradition of anatomy into which he had grown, Sylvius was book-learned and competent in the subject to a degree which earned for him the reputation of being the greatest anatomist in Europe. As one of his pupils, Loys Vassé, wrote in 1540: 'From everywhere flocked to him Germans, English, Spaniards, Italians and others of all nations who all agreed that the like of this admirable and almost divine man was not to be found in the whole of Europe.'[4] Allowing for the ease with which such blossoms bloomed in the verbal springs of the Middle Ages, such a eulogy from an old student suggests that there was more in Sylvius than those of a later age would allow who see in him nothing more than a pretentious, fee-hungry, old dunce. In spite of Sylvius' alleged personal unconcern with dissection, Vesalius none the less always entertained a considerable respect for him.

When, in 1533, Vesalius had gone to Paris to study under Sylvius, the latter had been in that town but a few years, having returned from Montpellier, where at the age of fifty-three he had been granted a bachelor's degree on 28 June 1531.

These bare facts require some elaboration; and since we shall be concerned with the encounter of Vesalius with what might properly be called 'Galenitis' rather than Galenism through the person of Sylvius, let us inquire what manner of man Sylvius was.

Born in 1478 in the little village of Louvilly, near Amiens, he was the seventh of fifteen children, eleven boys and four girls. His father was a poor weaver. An older brother, François, became the principal of the college of Tournay, near Paris, and succeeded in entering his brother in that institution. Here young Sylvius exhibited an extraordinary talent for languages, and in the course of several years acquired a thorough knowledge of Latin, Greek, and Hebrew. A French grammar written by him remained for many years a classic. He wrote tolerably good verse, excelled in mathematics, invented machines for transportation by water, and in good time developed an intense

---

[4] LeRoy Crummer and J. B. de C. M. Saunders, 'The Anatomical Compendium of Loys Vassé (1540)'. *Ann. Med. Hist.*, 1939, 3s., i, 351–69.

interest in the structure of the human body through the careful perusal of the works of Hippocrates and Galen. From passages in his works it would appear that he took advantage of every chance that came his way to examine bodies: a mason killed by a fall from a roof, a woman dying in childbed, and so on. He was deeply interested in pharmacy, and is said to have travelled to distant cities in order to learn new pharmaceutical methods. His poverty was such that he was unable to defray the very appreciable expense of obtaining a medical degree; 'but his erudition in medical matters was so well known that there gathered about him a considerable number of pupils, and he was so successful that the Faculty of Medicine at Paris forbade him to teach, as it interfered with the regular schools.'[5]

It was at this time that he betook himself to Montpellier where, as we have said, he obtained his bachelor's degree in 1531. When, therefore, he returned to Paris it was as a teacher with an already established reputation in that city. His classes are said to have numbered as many as 400 to 500 students. It was surely not simply Sylvius' reading of the Gospel of Galen which attracted such a vast throng. We know that he did not read particularly well, that his voice was rather harsh and grating, and that his personality, to say the least, was not excessively appealing. We may be sure that he had something to say worth hearing.

With respect to dissection this was distinctly not a task customarily performed by the professor, but by demonstrators specially employed for the purpose. It should be pointed out here that this pattern of teaching anatomy has survived to the present day. The professor will give a course of lectures, or perhaps a few introductory lectures, while the junior members of the department supervise the dissection. If Sylvius ever learned very much about the human body from dissection, the surest way to forget it for all practical purposes was to teach in the *ex cathedra* style which was the custom of his day. But all this does not imply that what Vesalius asserted of Sylvius was true, namely, that he was averse to dissection, for in his little *Introduction to Anatomy* Sylvius says:

'I would have you look carefully and recognize by eye when you are attending dissections or when you see anyone else who may be better supplied with instruments than yourself. For my judgment is that it is much better that you should learn the manner of cutting by eye and touch than by reading and listening. For reading alone never taught anyone how to sail a ship, to lead an army, nor to compound a medicine, which is done rather by the use of one's own sight and the training of one's own hands. . . .

'You would do well to dissect the bodies of those who have died of some disease in order that, by recognizing the cause of the malady, you may treat others wisely. Do not dissect only the bodies of men, but also those of monkeys and other animals similar in many respects to man. Yet I will recommend that at first you should work only upon human bodies, thus you will obtain a profound knowledge of the different parts of man which you can apply in dissecting other animals. . . .

'Now many do not like at first to view the dissection of man and cannot endure it without great disturbance of mind. Notwithstanding this, they

---

[5] Frank Baker, 'The Two Sylviuses. An historical study'. *Bull. Johns Hopkins Hosp.*, 1909, xx 329–39; passage quoted on p. 330.

ought, if they can, to accustom themselves from the very beginning to look diligently at the body of man while it is being dissected, and then to perform the dissection with their own hands. For this simple manner of learning is the shortest, most certain, and easiest to retain.'[6]

These, surely, are not the words of a man with small experience of the dissection of the human body, nor are they, clearly, those of a man who was averse to dissection. The truth is that Sylvius is known to have given a fair number of practical demonstrations on the human body to many of his classes, to the admiration of all those present, including Vesalius.

Among other subjects in which his fame as a teacher was justly deserved was materia medica. Here, as in anatomy, he placed great emphasis on observation and practical work. Long before the establishment of botanical gardens Sylvius was growing medicinal plants, both indigenous and foreign, in the garden of his house just outside Paris, so that his students might learn in the shortest and easiest way, by inspection and observation, the principal characters of these plants.

Study of the works of Sylvius reveals the fact that he had at least as good a knowledge of anatomy as any man of his time, that he made a fair number of dissections of the human body; but it is clear that what he saw he saw, for the most part, through the eyes of Galen. Nevertheless, he did make an important and lasting advance upon Galen's terminology. The muscles of the arms and legs, for example, Galen had distinguished by numbers, a notation which was followed by all other authors, including, later, Vesalius. The nomenclature we use to-day is, for the most part, where he named the muscles, Galen's, and where he did not, that of Sylvius but not of Vesalius. Sylvius performed the same service for the vessels, and it is due to the fact that he did not do so for the nerves that we still call them by number to-day.[7] But perhaps his chief anatomical distinction is the fact that he distinguished voluntary from involuntary muscle, and described their differences.

Vesalius' judgement of his contemporaries has always been accepted at its face value. Sylvius was no giant, but neither was he a pygmy. He appears to have been a rather austere, avaricious, ill-tempered person, not the perfect preceptor but a teacher from whom one could learn about as much as there was to be learned from the best of the day. Vesalius later disclaimed learning anatomy from him. But as Baker has said: 'Vesalius was in the habit of making derogatory remarks about his preceptors that do not bear close scrutiny. It is incredible that he should have stayed with Sylvius for three years if he had had no opportunity to learn anything while with him. The generally received opinion that Vesalius sprang like Minerva from the head of Jove, armed cap-à-pie, and broke the record of all previous ages by dissecting the human body for the first time, does not bear critical examination. Without wishing to detract in any way from his well-merited fame, it seems quite

[6] Jacobus Sylvius, *Opera medica*. Genevae, 1635, p. 127. The translation is by Frank Baker, *op. cit.* (5).

[7] Sylvius did not give his name or any other to certain structures commonly referred to him, but which belong rather to an anatomist of the seventeenth century with whom he is often confused, namely, François de le Boë (1614–1672), professor of practical medicine at Leyden, who was also known by his Latin cognomen as Sylvius. It was Franciscus and not Jacobus who gave the really first adequate anatomical description of the brain and sinuses of the dura mater, and it is after Franciscus that the fissure of Sylvius is named, as is also the aqueduct, which was, in fact discovered long before either Sylvius was born.

certain that he must have been indebted to his master for a good deal, and that the foundations of the *Fabrica* were laid in Sylvius's laboratory.'[8]

Late in 1536, in the midst of the tumult of the approaching war between France and the Empire, bound by every tie of loyalty to the Emperor Charles V, Vesalius hurriedly returned to Louvain, without taking his doctor's degree, although he had fulfilled all the requirements. Less than a year later (6 December 1537) the Senate of Venice had appointed Vesalius, at the age of twenty-two, State Professor of Anatomy. At Padua Vesalius read the anatomical books of Galen three times to his students before he convinced himself that Galen's descriptions frequently failed to agree with his own observations on the human body. In 1538 Vesalius is still almost wholly a follower of Galen, as his *Tabulae Sex* show. Indeed, up to this time 'he used to extol Galen as the second leader of medicine after Hippocrates, as the first and foremost exponent, the coryphaeus, of dissection, a rare marvel of nature and a great admirer of nature, and the author of all good things'.[9]

Meanwhile, as his dissections proceeded Vesalius accumulated so many corrections to Galen that together they formed a fairly large volume. By 1539 he had resolved to write his own anatomy, 'if', as he tells us in *The Blood letting Letter* published in that year, 'the opportunity of bodies offers, and Joannes Stephanus [Van Calcar], outstanding artist of our age, does not refuse his services'.[10]

The Bloodletting Letter, which represented the entrance of Vesalius into a heatedly discussed controversy, namely, as to where best to bleed, contains some very definite but very diffidently, even deferentially, made corrections to Galen's description of the veins. Thus, he writes: 'For this opinion of mine on venesection in pleurisy, conceived by no one previously, I might strive to extract from the statement of Hippocrates in the second book of *The Regimen in Acute Diseases* except it too pointedly contradicts the authority of Galen, which I am afraid of disputing almost no less than if in our very sacred religion I were secretly to doubt the immortality of the soul.'[11]

In spite of such protestations of loyalty, the defection of Vesalius from the Galenical description of the character of certain veins was obvious.

Vesalius appears to have been perfectly aware of the thinness of the ice over which he was skating, and was, in fact, at some pains to avoid situations in which there lay a possibility of giving offence to the more vellum-bound Galenists. Thus, when the great Giunta edition of Galen's works was being planned, an edition in which the most learned scholars of the day were to participate, Vesalius was invited by Montanus to re-edit the large section *De anatomicis administrationibus* earlier translated by Guintherius. He at first declined for fear of giving offence to his former teacher. He was, however, finally prevailed upon. As Augustinus Gadaldinus, the reviser of the final proofs, tells us in his preface to the volume: 'It was he who contributed

[8] Frank Baker, *op. cit.* (5), p. 331.
[9] Boerhaave and Albinus, *op. cit.* (2), Farrington's trans. of Preface, p. 62.
[10] 'Andreas Vesalius Bruxellensis: The Bloodletting Letter of 1539.' Translated by J. B. de C. M. Saunders and Charles D. O'Malley. In *Studies and Essays in the History of Science and Learning offered in homage to George Sarton on the occasion of his Sixtieth Birthday.* Ed. by M. F. Ashley Montagu. New York, 1946, pp. 3–74; passage quoted on p. 74.
[11] *ibid.*, pp. 66–7.

the books on the dissection of veins, arteries and nerves, with corrections in many places. Persuaded finally by the entreaties and arguments of ourselves and others, to the effect that he would be doing great harm should he let the fear of giving offence to his teacher Andernach—a fear which obsessed him— deprive others of so much that was useful, he also improved the books on dissection to such an extent as almost to make them new.'[12]

In this work on the bones Vesalius made many corrections in Galen's text, but except, possibly, for some verbal rumblings from Paris and other places, the work was favourably received. This sort of encouragement served but to re-enforce Vesalius in his determination to proceed with his anatomical treatise, all the more so since the talents of an exceptionally distinguished artist, who evidently had no mean knowledge of the human body himself, had become available to him.

The two years from 1540 to July 1542 Vesalius spent working at a feverish pace on his great book. The *Fabrica* when published in June 1543 contained a total of 663 folio pages including the 278 magnificent woodcuts and numerous decorative woodcut initials. This remarkable *tour de force* represented the most original work on the human body published since Galen's writings were first given to the world.

The name of Galen must continue to be honoured and revered as one of the greatest discoverers and systematizers in the history of biology. Galen was, of course, not himself a Galenist in the pejorative sense of that term. He was first and foremost an observer and discoverer of nature. Where he erred was in his tendency to extrapolate, to transfer without checking, his findings on one animal to the structure of a totally different one. Thus, the details of many structures observed by Galen in pigs, monkeys, and other animals are by him described as normal structures in man. Human bodies were not easily available to Galen, and so between wounded gladiators, monkeys, bears and pigs, he did what he could. But unlike most Galenists he was not one to obtain 'base authority from other's books,' but deep-searched nature 'with saucy looks'. Indeed, Galen would have been the first to welcome the work of Vesalius. And, in truth, most of Galen's followers and admirers joyfully welcomed Vesalius' book from the day of its appearance. They were quite willing to accept the Galen corrections made by Vesalius even when Vesalius was wrong and Galen right. It is sufficient to mention the names, among these, of Fallopius, Aeccius, von Veltwiyck, Roelants, Gesner, Cornarius, Fuchs, Henerus, and Paré. There was no battle for the acceptance of the new anatomy and the new method of observation: both were accepted at once. Who could help but be overwhelmed by this glorious work? Alas, the sort of people we should expect. At first, the ungenerous and the poor in spirit, persons who, like Sylvius, had been planning an anatomy of their own, and had now had all the underpinning knocked away from under them by this unfledged usurper of their authority. For what, indeed, should a bold and impetuous upstart of twenty-eight years be doing writing such books challenging thus not alone their own but also Galen's authority? There is a point beyond which impetuosity becomes madness. And this is, in fact, what Sylvius did say of Vesalius.

[12] *Galeni omnia opera.* Venetiis, vol. i, 1541. Quoted from Harvey Cushing, *A bio-bibliography of Andreas Vesalius.* New York, 1943, p. 64.

Then there were those who were biliously jealous, the choleric and dyspeptic, the avowed and unavowed enemies and detractors. Under the cloak of strict adherence to the evangel of Galen, to which the generations and Time had given the imprimatur of unchallengable truth, these combined forces became that skulking of bigots whom it has been the custom to identify as 'the Galenists'. But the point it is highly desirable to establish is that they were not Galenists, but bigots, and that most of them were so not because they were the children of their time, but because, for purely personal reasons, they didn't like Vesalius, and the reason why they were going to tell—even though it wasn't the true one.

There has, in the past, been a strong tendency to romanticize Vesalius and to represent him as something of a martyr who was eventually hounded to death by 'the Galenists', those phlogistonists of anatomy, who resented the attack upon their doctrine, and who

> Carved in their groove,
> By apostolic knocks
> Proceeded to prove
> Their doctrine orthodox

by anatomizing Vesalius in barbed words. The ingredients, indeed, are all there for the purposes of the writer of romantic history[13] or the occasional medical essayist. The serious student appraising the facts views the evidence somewhat differently, and, I think, more justly. He sees that the few stupid attacks, which were made upon Vesalius a fair number of years after the publication of the *Fabrica* by those who disliked him personally, have been dissociated from particular persons and generalized for the age in which Vesalius lived. The notion which it has been sought to convey is that the Middle Ages were in spirit antipathetic to Vesalius' way of thinking—reliance upon observation rather than upon authority; that his *Fabrica* came upon the last phase of those Ages as a bolt from the blue; that the *Fabrica* represented a clean break with the existing tradition of anatomical knowledge and teaching; and that for all these 'obvious' reasons, as well as his alleged bumptiousness, the opposition to Vesalius and his work was great. This conventionalized story does not agree with the facts. As Lynn Thorndike has recently indicated,[14] the movement among anatomists of the first half of the sixteenth century was, in general, definitely oriented in the direction of greater reliance upon observation and rejection of Galen where he was in disagreement with the observed facts. Thus, Jacopo Berengario da Carpi (*c.* 1470–1530), professor of surgery at Pavia and Bologna, dissected over a hundred human bodies, and was the first to introduce anatomical figures into an anatomical text. In his popular commentary upon the medieval handbook of Mundinus, published in 1521,[15] and which as late as 1664 was translated into English,[16] he decries the habit of

---

[13] See, for example, Charles Kingsley's wholly delightful but thoroughly euhemeristic piece, *op. cit.* (3).

[14] Lynn Thorndike, *A history of magic and experimental science.* New York, vol. v, 1941, pp. 498–531.

[15] *Carpi commentaria cum amplissimis additionibus super anatomia Mundini una cum textu eiusdem in pristinum et verum nitorem redacto.* Bononia, 1521.

[16] Μικροκοσμογραφια *or, a description of the body of man; being a practical anatomy, shewing the manner of anatomizing from part to part. . . . Done into English by H. Jackson.* London, 1664.

anatomical writers who follow authorities like cattle and warns the reader not to be deceived 'by some of our moderns who involve anatomy with authorities and not with observation'. He says also that he always accepts Galen's views except where observation is at discord with them.[17] In keeping with the humanist tradition of the age Carpi's textual criticisms were minute and extensive. Fallopius not unjustly called him the first restorer of anatomy. A careful study of his work serves to show to what an appreciable extent a man like Carpi paved the way for Vesalius.

A work transitional between that of Carpi and that of Vesalius is represented by the *Liber introductorius anatomiae* of Nicolaus Massa (d. 1569), which was published at Venice in November 1536, and dedicated to Pope Paul III.[18] Massa criticizes the anatomists of his day for writing so much that is not essential to the science of dissection, for their sophistical arguments and distinctions which so befog the minds of youthful students that they fail to grasp anatomy itself (fo. 3v, 15v), 'moderns who know things only by name,' and who 'by trusting in the dicta and questions current in the schools have failed to observe' (fo. 10r). In his little volume Massa describes only what can be seen in a single dissection and is most essential in medicine; he omits all discussion of late medieval questions to which Carpi gave so much space, and insists upon the importance of frequent dissection as against disputations and the use of authorities. Furthermore, he provides the reader with a fair number of new observations based entirely upon his own dissections.

The books of both Carpi and Massa were widely read and approved, and there can be little doubt that Vesalius had read and been influenced by them. At any rate, these works clearly reflect the advancing new spirit of the age, and show beyond question that two of the most widely read immediate forerunners of Vesalius in anatomy were far from being blind followers of Galen, but that they were quite independent and critical in their judgement, and placed considerable stress upon the necessity of dissection and the importance of direct observation. In his *Fabrica* Vesalius simply continued in the spirit which was the best of his time, in the direction set by such men as Carpi and Massa. The age had been prepared and was ready for such a work. When it appeared it was welcomed as that complete presentation of the facts to which earlier introductory volumes, including one by Vesalius, had led the way. It was not a bolt from the blue, but a work which it had practically been expected that someone would write, and of a kind which several men, including Massa, had hoped to write. As for the alleged break with the Galenical tradition, this was in point of fact no more radical than was that of Carpi or Massa. Vesalius did on a grand scale what they had done on a small one. Being a young man of some means he was able to command the services of the best anatomical illustrator and of the best printers of his time to produce a folio volume which, even if the text had not been as good as it was, would have established itself instantly in the esteem of all students of medicine.

Though he often criticizes Galen, sometimes not altogether justly, the subject of anatomy is presented in seven books in the traditional Galenic order,

---

[17] Carpi, *op. cit.* (15), fo. 240r, 398r, fol. 412v.

[18] Nicolaus Massa, *Liber introductorius anatomiae sive dissectionis corporis humani nunc primum ab ipso auctore in lucem editus.* Venetiis, 1536, fo. 10r.

commencing with the bones, thence proceeding to the ligaments and muscles, and so on. Indeed, Vesalius is at pains to express his admiration for Galen, whom he calls 'after Hippocrates the prince of medicine', 'easily the foremost among the teachers of anatomy', and while correcting his errors he criticizes 'those who to-day call themselves Galenists but do not study anatomy and dissect as Galen did'.[19] The *Fabrica* actually reproduces many Galenical errors both in the text and in the illustrations, and reveals the shallowness of the knowledge possessed by Vesalius of certain obvious parts of the human body, and his reliance upon Galen.[20]

What would seem to be the almost deliberate neglect by Vesalius of any reference to contemporary anatomists who, like Carpi and Massa, were his immediate intellectual forerunners, and his rather over-aggressive preface in which he criticizes 'the supineness of the medical profession', and gives a somewhat critical picture of the state of medicine in his own day, undoubtedly annoyed some people and failed not to amuse others. Most agreed that its faults were few and its virtues many, that, in short, it was a splendid book. As Fallopius put it, what Carpi had begun Vesalius perfected.[21]

In his preface, without naming names, Vesalius made several pointed references which hit home hard. No one could fail to recognize Jacobus Sylvius as the object of these remarks.

Speaking of his attempt to restore anatomy to some degree of completeness Vesalius writes:

'But this effort could by no manner of means have succeeded, if, when I was studying medicine at Paris, I had not myself applied my hand to this business, but had acquiesced in the casual and superficial display to me and my fellow-students by certain barbers of a few organs at one or two public dissections. For in such a perfunctory manner was anatomy then treated in the place where we have lived to see medicine happily reborn ... except for eight muscles of the abdomen, disgracefully mangled and in the wrong order, no one (I speak the simple truth) ever demonstrated to me any single muscle, or any single bone, much less the network of nerves, veins and arteries.'[22]

Referring to his illustration, Vesalius writes:

'But there comes into my mind the judgment of certain men who vehemently condemn the practice of setting before the eyes of students, as we do with the parts of plants, delineations, be they never so accurate, of the parts of the human body.'[23]

Sylvius had a well-known prejudice against anatomical delineations, and especially inveighed against those of Carpi, saying that they could 'at best, only serve to gratify the eyes of silly women'.[24]

[19] Andreas Vesalius, *De humani corporis fabrica*. Basileae, 1543, Bk. ii, fo. 58, fo. 234–40, 342 ff.

[20] See Singer, *op. cit.* (1).

[21] Gabriel Fallopius, *Observationes anatomicae*. Venetiis, 1561, fo. 25r.

[22] Benjamin Farrington (Translator), 'The Preface of Andreas Vesalius to *De Fabrica Corporis Humani* 1543'. *Proc. Roy. Soc. Med.*, 1932, xxv, 1357–66; passage quoted on p. 1361.

[23] *ibid.*, p. 1364.

[24] 'They can at best only serve to gratify the eyes of silly women (*mulierculis oculos pasturis*), to the true physician they must always be a hindrance, for it is his duty to view and handle the body as a whole and in all its parts, becoming acquainted with the substance, size, number, shape, situation and connections of each as far as the fingers can reach, not confining this examination to the surface, the only portion that can be represented in pictures.' 'Ordo et ordinis ratio in legendis Hippocratis et Galeni libris.' Sylvius, *op. cit* (6), fo. 5.

Finally, Vesalius delivers himself of the following gentle blast:

'Moreover I am aware [first] how little authority my efforts will carry by reason of my youth (I am still in my twenty-eighth year); and [secondly] how little, on account of the frequency with which I draw attention to the falsity of Galen's pronouncements, I shall be sheltered from the attacks of those who have not—as I have done in the schools of Italy—applied themselves earnestly to anatomy, and who, being now old men devoured by envy at the true discoveries of youths, will be ashamed, together with all the other sectaries of Galen, that they have been hitherto so purblind failing to notice what I now set forth, yet arrogating to themselves a mighty reputation in the art.'[25]

Whether or not Vesalius had Sylvius in mind when he penned those words, it is hardly a precarious conjecture to suppose that Sylvius felt himself greviously offended; but apart from adversely criticizing in his classes the contributions to anatomy made by Vesalius, he held his peace. The picture generally conveyed is quite otherwise, Sylvius being cast in the role of mephitic leader of those who 'almost immediately' after the publication of the *Fabrica* rushed to the attack upon it and its author.[26] That 'almost immediately' lasted eight years, Sylvius publishing nothing till 1551, being provoked partially into doing so by the publication of the details of a private correspondence between them which Vesalius had initiated. This publication represented a rather long letter replying to certain queries of Joachim Roelants concerning the china root. The original epistle is dated 13 June 1546, and it was published late in 1546.[27]

Here Vesalius reveals that some time after the publication of the *Fabrica* he had written Sylvius with the greatest respect and deference, saying that if there were any comments in his books on anatomy which had displeased Sylvius, he, Vesalius, hoped that Sylvius would tell him what they were. To which Sylvius made answer at length to the effect that he could not believe that Galen was in error, and that friendship between himself and Vesalius was possible only if the latter made a complete retraction of his criticisms, which, he added, were probably due to his youth and too long association with the Italians. Upon which Vesalius replied that he could not oblige, since age and experience had served but to confirm his views.

'Many persons are hostile to me', he writes, 'because in my writings I seem to hold in contempt the authority of Galen, the prince of physicians and preceptor of us all, because I do not agree indiscriminately with all his opinions, and especially because I have demonstrated that some errors are discernible in his books. Surely scant justice to me and to our studies and indeed to our times! . . . I would rather have counted in this class any one than Jacobus Sylvius, an ornament to the physicians of our age; but, from the letter sent by your son, in which he disclosed that he had read my books, he proved very decidedly that he *does* belong to this group. So now you can

[25] Farrington, *op. cit.* (22), p. 1364.

[26] See, for example, the excellent lecture by Arturo Castiglioni, 'The Attack of Franciscus Puteus on Andreas Vesalius and the Defence by Gabriel Cuneus', delivered at the 400th Anniversary Celebration of the *De humani corporis fabrica*, *Yale Journ. Biol. and Med.*, 1943, xvi, 150; reprinted by The Historical Library, Yale University School of Medicine, 1943, p. 35.

[27] Cushing, *op. cit.* (12), p. 163.

easily deduce what ground I covered in my letter to him which I sent on to you from Nimwegen so that your son could deliver it to Sylvius.'[28]

It is a thousand pities that a copy of this letter has not survived, but we may well guess its contents, and we may be sure that Sylvius thoroughly disapproved of them.

In 1551, when Sylvius was seventy-two years of age, he published a broadside aimed against Vesalius entitled *Depulsio Vesani cuiusdam calumniarum in Hippocratis et Galeni rem anatomicam* (The Refutation of the Calumnies of Vesanus). The punning change of Vesalius into Vesanus (madman) was, as Kingsley has said, 'but a fair and gentle stroke for a polemic, in days in which those who could not kill their enemies with steel and powder, held themselves justified in doing so, if possible, by vituperation, calumny, and every engine of moral torture'.[29]

The absurdly fantastic arguments which Sylvius brought forward to show that Galen had indeed dissected and described the human body, and not that of monkeys, as Vesalius had asserted, convinced nobody, but they made a great many people laugh—at Sylvius.

When, twenty years after the publication of the *Fabrica* the sycophantic Franciscus Puteus published a scurrilous attack upon Vesalius,[30] one of the persons Puteus called upon to testify to the soundness of his criticism was Gabriel Cuneus. Cuneus, who was professor of anatomy at Pavia from 1554 to 1574, at once made it thoroughly and unequivocally clear that he was on the side of Vesalius. His reply to Puteus, published in 1564, was crushing and definitive, and put an end to the last of the detractors of Vesalius.[31]

Obviously, a number of people were jealous of the achievement of Vesalius and hostile towards him on that account, and some, too, because his self-conceit rubbed them the wrong way. In several cases, as for example, certain physicians of the Emperor Charles, elderly colleagues of Vesalius, an attempt was made to injure his standing with the king. The resentment, however, was a personal one, directed against the objectionable youth and imperiousness of its object. It was not a school of thought which through its followers was hostile to Vesalius, but frustrated persons who seized upon his criticism of Galen as a peg upon which to hang their abuse of the critic. Vesalius was himself a Galenist, and apart from a few bigots, the Galenists were with Vesalius from the first. In the past the personal enmity of a comparatively few men has been made to appear as if it were the reflection of the spirit of the times, the Middle Ages, in the person of the Galenists against the Renaissance in the person of Vesalius.

I have attempted to indicate that this view is not correct.

[28] *Epistola rationem modumque propinandi radicis Chynae decocti.* Basileae, 1546. See Cushing, *op. cit.* (12), p. 162.

[29] Kingsley, *op. cit.* (3).

[30] Franciscus Puteus, *Apologia in anatome pro Galeno, contra Andream Vesalium Bruxellensem.* Venetiis, 1562.

[31] Gabriel Cuneus, *Apologiae Francisci Putei pro Galeno in anatome, examen.* Venetiis, 1564.

ANDREAS VESALIUS IMPERIAL PHYSICIAN

by

CHARLES DONALD O'MALLEY and J. B. de C. M. SAUNDERS

IF the publication of the *De humani corporis fabrica* in June of the year 1543 marks the end of the achievement of Andreas Vesalius in the history of science, August of the same year sees him emerge as Imperial physician— an appointment which, by the standards of the time, could only be regarded as the complement to a distinguished career. The period during which Vesalius served at court, though relatively unimportant, is none the less of intense interest. Much of it is obscure, and the sources few and rare, yet one may glean here and there a few details, which have not as yet been utilized, to add to our knowledge of the man in his professional capacity.

As Charles Singer has remarked, after the publication of his epochal work, anatomy thenceforth becomes Vesalian, while Vesalius himself passes into the background. Many and various have been the conjectures put forward to explain what to modern eyes seems almost a mysterious withdrawal from academic life, in the fullness of his youth and on the threshold of a still more brilliant future. It has been suggested that he hoped to find, in an appointment at the court of the most powerful monarch in Europe, protection from the persecution of enemies who had become enraged at his new ideas and criticisms of the sacrosanct Galen. But, as we shall attempt to show, he had committed his services to the Emperor Charles V many months before any such opposition had developed. It may have been that his rifling of tombs in search of anatomical material, or the thoroughness of his dissections, transgressing the limits which custom imposed as desecration of the body, or even his dangerous excursions into biblical exegesis, had led him to decide upon a discreet withdrawal and the quest for a patron who might protect him against ecclesiastical wrath. It is possible that the great expense of illustrations and publication of the *Fabrica* determined him to search for a more lucrative position. All these may have some substance, but a simpler and more compelling explanation may be found in his own views on the ideal physician.

In the preface to the *Fabrica* Vesalius clearly shows his kinship with the peculiar aesthetic and philosophical views of the then current theory of humanism, and had expressed himself on the essential unity of the art of medicine, of which anatomy was but the foundation. He was fully aware, almost jealously aware, of the importance of his anatomical knowledge for an understanding especially of surgical lesions, 'in whose cure we behold the appointed place of the true and highest power of medicine'.[1] He recognized that he had made his mark and established recognition in the preliminaries which would gain him preferment and position in the most distinguished post-graduate school of the day, where he hoped to reach his goal as a physician. How high were these hopes may be measured by the disappointment he expressed at his failure to put his ideas into practice after scarcely two years of service with the Emperor. 'You yourself', he says writing to his friend Joachim

---

[1] *De humani corporis fabrica.* Basileae, 1543, Preface ; *Epistola rationem modumque propinandi radicis chynae.* Basileae, 1546, p. 39.

Roelants of Mechlin, 'are thoroughly aware of how greatly I was obstructed when I first came to court, not only in my study of anatomy—that subject which in our age has fallen into complete decay—but also in every enterprise I undertook with my medical students'.[2] The ideal of Vesalius was the complete physician which he could only attain by the practice of medicine. It is true he might have elected to do so at Padua or Pisa, but he had strong ties with the court of Charles V through the long and faithful service of his father as Imperial apothecary.

Vesalius had spent at least four years of hard work and a considerable sum of money on the preparation of the *Fabrica*. From his letter to Oporinus we know that the woodcuts and final instructions to the printer were ready for dispatch by 24 August 1542, and now he must impatiently wait on the typographers. Sometime early in 1543 Vesalius crossed the Alps to Basel to be on hand for the arduous task of proof reading, until at length the colophon marked the triumph of completion. Here he remained to enjoy a well-earned rest, and on 3 August served as godfather to a son of his old friend, Robert Winter, the Basel publisher.[3] Although the colophon of the *Fabrica* is dated June 1543, the work itself was apparently not ready for distribution until August. A letter (2 August) of Johannes Gast, a Basel friend of Vesalius, referring to a copy of the *Fabrica* sent to Heinrich Bullinger, the celebrated theologian of Zürich, suggests that the book had just been placed on sale.[4] Therefore it was perhaps the binder, as well as social obligations, which delayed Vesalius during the month of July.

At the earliest, on 4 August, Vesalius set forth for Speyer where the Emperor was then staying,[5] and it was presumably there that he presented to Charles V a copy of the *Fabrica*—the same copy, so it would appear, which remained in the university library at Louvain until its destruction during the invasion of Belgium in 1914. It was, we believe, at this time that he sought and obtained his appointment at the court and not in 1544, as Roth and many others hold.

The dedication of the *Fabrica* to Charles V is dated 1 August 1542. It is possible that Vesalius at that time had already decided to seek the Imperial service. The ground had long been prepared for such a move. His father as Imperial apothecary was in a position to smooth the pathway for him, and we know that the elder Vesalius had presented his son's *Tabulae* to the Emperor in 1538.[6] Furthermore, it is evident from the *China Root Letter* that a general impression existed at Padua that he would not return after publication of his books. Whatever the procedure may have been, Vesalius was accepted and performed his first service to the Emperor, as he tells us,[7] in the short campaign of September 1543 against the Duke of Cleves, a rebel vassal of Charles and an ally of Francis I.

The latter part of the year 1543 and the first half of 1544 were relatively

[2] *Epistola, op. cit.* (1), p. 40.

[3] M. Roth, *Andreas Vesalius Bruxellensis.* Berlin, 1892, p. 129.

[4] Gerhard Wolf-Heidegger, 'Über Vesals Aufenthalt in Basel im Jahre 1547'. *Gesnerus,* 1945, ii, 207.

[5] *ibid., loc. cit.* (4).

[6] *Fabrica,* 1543, fo.*4r; *Epistola docens venam axillarem dextri cubiti in dolore laterali secandam.* Basileae, 1539, p. 6; cf. Roth, *op. cit.* (3), p. 60.

[7] *op. cit.* (2), p. 176.

peaceful, since the fourth Franco-Imperial war was not to break out until the summer. Therefore the services of Vesalius do not appear to have been required, at least in a military capacity, and he was free to return to Italy and wind up his affairs there. It was therefore embarrassing for Columbus, who had assumed that his absence would become permanent, when his master, whom in the meanwhile he had been criticizing before the students, reappeared in December to hold another dissection. 'He thought that after the publication of my books I would not return to Italy, or (as you know) compare my writings with what I observed in bodies, in public dissections at Padua and Pisa.'[8]   Needless to say, Columbus remained conspicuous by his absence at this time.

Several months had now elapsed since Vesalius' book had been published and the presentation made to the Emperor—enough time to receive the first letters telling him of its reception by those at court and elsewhere. So unfavourable were these early criticisms that in a rage of disappointment he burned the manuscripts of his notes and works under preparation—an act which he was greatly to regret.[9]

From Padua, Vesalius travelled onward to Bologna with 'our Tronus, (who at that time was a travelling companion of his). Here he stayed with Albus who escorted him to the schools in which a dissection was being performed. Then, in the name of all the large group which had assembled, Buccaferreus asked Vesalius to oblige the students by dissecting something and speaking about it'. Vesalius chose to discuss the venous system; a fitting topic in the light of his newly acquired status, and one of great therapeutic importance, on which he had made his first original contribution in the *Venesection Letter* of 1539. Two bodies were available, and he proceeded to carry out a partial dissection of the vena cava and its branches before the large audience of Bolognese and others who had been attracted from the outside by the fame of the anatomist. The discussion turned into a wordy debate between the Galenists and Aristotelians on the origin of the veins and the source of the blood, and the meeting continued far into the night and was ended only by the discomfort of the cold. Wearied and bored by the fruitless philosophic turn in the discussion which he knew would likely last for days, Vesalius escaped, and setting out at dawn, proceeded on his way to Pisa, which he reached on 22 January 1544. As the dissection at Bologna was to have continued on the next day, his audience thought that they had been treated with scant courtesy by his precipitate departure and were not slow to express their extreme displeasure.[10]

The Duke of Tuscany, Cosimo de' Medici, had invited Vesalius to conduct an anatomy at the newly re-established and reorganized University of Pisa, and had offered him a permanent position, which the anatomist was compelled to decline since he had already committed his services to the Emperor. Nevertheless, dissection material was floated down the Arno to Pisa, and the course continued until the onset of the lenten season brought it to a close.[11]

[8] *ibid.*, p. 136.   [9] *ibid.*, p. 196 [for 195].
[10] Franciscus Puteus, *Apologia in anatome pro Galeno, contra Andream Vesalium.* Venetiis, 1562, fo. 116ᵛ ff.
[11] Andrea Corsini, *Andrea Vesalio nello studio di Pisa.* Siena, 1915.

It was therefore toward the end of February that Vesalius departed for Florence and thence to rejoin the Emperor, who was once more gathering his forces for a new campaign and would have need of the young physician.

It was apparently with some regret that Vesalius left Pisa, which under the control of Cosimo was exceedingly sympathetic to the new anatomy. The Duke fully appreciated the ability of Vesalius, as is indicated by his efforts, despite Imperial competition, to gain the anatomist's services on a permanent basis, and by the fact that when the position was finally offered to Columbus, it was at a salary some 200 ducats smaller than that offered to Vesalius. Indeed, Columbus seems to have been a third choice, since Leonhardt Fuchs had already been considered for the post.[12]

Vesalius had now gone northwards to participate in the war against the French which began in the summer of 1544, and it is in this war that we obtain the first clear picture of Vesalius as the Imperial physician. In the course of military operations the forces of Charles V besieged the town of Saint-Dizier, and during the siege René of Nassau, Prince of Orange-Châlon, and one of the Emperor's closest friends, lost his life on 15 July. On the fourteenth of the month the young prince accompanied by Don Fernando de Gonzaga, Captain-General of the armies, had proceeded to the inspection of the trenches and gun emplacements preparatory to an assault planned for the next day. While sitting in the same place from which Don Fernando had arisen a little before, he was struck in the right shoulder by a ball from a falconet. He was carried immediately to the Emperor's lodgings, where, to the great grief of Charles, he died around six in the evening of the following day. 'I examined the viscera of the Prince of Orange, the Lord of Halvin and several others whose bodies, wounded by the fiery bombs, had to be removed from our army, I know not whither', says Vesalius.[13]

It was not until the following year that the famous treatise disproving the ancient contention that wounds by fire-arms were poisonous was published by Ambroise Paré. The autopsy on the body of the prince may have been to determine the cause of death, but its chief purpose was to allow of embalming, a duty which devolved upon the physicians. We turn to Paré, who was in the opposing forces of France at Saint-Dizier and Landresi, for an account of the technique employed, and here we are informed of the special difficulties encountered in the preservation of the bodies of kings and princes.

For thus the body being over and above washed in strong vinegar, or Lye, shull be kept a long time, if so be that a great dissolving heat do not bear sway, or if it be not put in a hot and moist place. And this condition of time and place is the cause why the dead bodies of Princes and Kings, though embalmed with Art and cost, within the space of six or seven dayes, in which they are kept to be shewed to the people after their embalming, do cast forth so greivous a sent, that none can endure it; so that they are forced to be put in a leaden Coffin. For the air which encompasseth them groweth so hot by reason of the multitude of people flowing to the spectacle, and the burning of the lights night and day, that the small portion of the native heat which remaineth being dissipated, they easily putrifie, especially when as they are not first moistened and macerated in the liquor of aromatic things,

---

[12] Andrea Corsini, 'Nuovi documenti riguardanti Andrea Vesalio e Realdo Colombo nello studio pisano'. *Riv. d. storia crit. d. sci. med. nat.* Faenza, 1918, ix, 507–12.

[13] *op. cit.* (2), p. 176.

as the *Aegyptians* antiently used to do, steeping them in brine 70 dayes, as I formerly told you out of *Herodotus*.[14]

According to the report of Daza Chacon, the Spanish physician and associate of Vesalius, it was during the same campaign that Vesalius performed a clumsy amputation at the elbow upon a certain Captain Solis. Remarking upon the difficulties of disarticulation at this joint in the presence of gangrene, Daza Chacon wrote:

> ... the joint of the elbow, which is the most difficult to cut of the whole body because notwithstanding that Vesalius was very skilled in dissection and did it better than anyone else of his time, it happened in the year 1544, when the army of His Majesty the Emperor Charles was near Saint Dizier, that a Captain Solis wished him to amputate his arm (as was necessary) at the elbow, and although he laboured a great while, he was never able to do so, and we had to amputate four fingers' breadth above.[15]

Paré is reputed to have been the first to reintroduce the procedure of disarticulation of the elbow in 1538.[16] Almost all early surgeons comment on the difficulties encountered in this operation, which seems to have been due to the mistake of regarding the tip of the olecranon as the level of the joint. Considering the great anatomical knowledge of Vesalius, especially of the bones, one can hardly credit the Spanish surgeon's statement; but Vesalius at this stage in his career was admittedly a tyro in the art of surgery.

The war came to an end with the Peace of Crespy in September 1544. Sometime in the winter of 1543–4 the father of our Vesalius had died, leaving to his son a considerable inheritance, which included the family residence in Brussels. Upon his return from the campaign, and no doubt relying upon his inheritance and an assured position at court, Vesalius immediately (September 1544) ventured into matrimony with Anne van Hamme, daughter of a respectable bourgeois family in comfortable circumstances.[17] No longer is our physician to be the irresponsible grave robber and argumentative investigator. Two years later he writes: 'As if, too, youth, unrestrained by a wife, children, and every domestic responsibility, and free to enjoy the most delightful intimacies and friendships, were not the age by far most fit for treating anatomical matters'.[18]

His Imperial master Charles had returned to the Netherlands, and we hear of the Emperor being carried in January 1545 from Ghent to Brussels in a litter because of the disabling effects of gout,[19] incidentally his eleventh attack of

---

[14] Ambroise Paré, *Workes*. London, 1634, lib. xxviii, p. 749.

[15] Dionisio Daza Chacon, *Practica y teorica de cirugia en romance y en latin*. Madrid, 1678, vol. i, p. 181.

[16] Paré, *op. cit.* (14), lib. xii, c. xxv, p. 325.

[17] Alphonse Wauters, 'Quelques mots sur André Vésale', *Mém. d. l'Acad. roy. de Belgique*, 1897, lv, 26; M. H. Spielmann, *The iconography of Andreas Vesalius*. London, 1925, pp. 65–6.

[18] *op. cit.* (2), p. 194.

[19] Max Fisch, 'Vesalius in the English state papers', *Bull. Med. Lib. Assoc.*, 1945, xxxiii, 232. The Emperor was supposed, we believe euphemistically, to have suffered from gout. The term used by Vesalius is *morbus articularis* which, although translated in contemporary English as gout, was applied to any rheumatic or arthritic condition or bone pain in the region of the joints. True gout with the formation of tophi had been recognized since the time of Rufus of Ephesus, but it was not until Thomas Sydenham published his masterpiece, *Tractus de podagra et hydrope*, in 1683, that there was any clear clinical differentiation of gout from rheumatic disorders. In view of Charles V's extraordinary eating habits, he may have been suffering from true gout, but it would be unwise to accept the condition categorically as gout. Although Vesalius nowhere

the malady.[20] Vesalius had by this time grown sufficiently in professional stature, so that he was employed about the Imperial person for the first time, but only in a subsidiary capacity.

Charles was a difficult patient, and his eating habits the despair of his physicians. He relished highly spiced foods, and so exotic was his appetite that Monfaletto, the grand master of the kitchens, was always at his wit's end to supply something new. 'From the mass to the mess' had become a proverb at the court. In addition, he surrounded himself with quacks to whom he lent a willing ear. Impressed by high praises for the newly introduced remedy called the China root, a variety of sarsaparilla, 'he took the decoction by his own wish, rather than on the advice of Master Cornelius [van Baersdorp, first physician]'.[21] The drug had been introduced in 1535, but had rapidly fallen into disrepute. But now, owing to the imprimatur of the Emperor, it had once more surged into popularity. Vesalius had had previous experience with the remedy in Italy while visiting the sick as a student under the tutelage of the famous physician, Giovanni Battista della Monte (Montanus). This had rendered him extremely dubious of its efficacy; but the new remedy was now the fashion, and we find Vesalius called in to administer a decoction to Jean de Hennin, Count of Bossu and Paron de Reckheim, the Emperor's childhood friend and favourite, to Ludovic Sances, stated to be the viceroy of Sicily, and to many of their friends.[22] Vesalius was now more dubious than ever of the value of the much-praised panacea. 'No very powerful argument for the commendation of the China can be drawn from the case of the Emperor, since he used it for only fifteen days, with varied regimen, and with the method of administration frequently changed, principally at his own caprice.'[23] Indeed, in the following year, 1546, Vesalius wrote in no uncertain terms of the uselessness of the vaunted remedy in his letter on the China root, which carries in its title the phrase 'which was recently employed by . . . the Emperor'.

About this time while in Brussels, possibly during the winter of 1544-5, Vesalius and his Spanish colleague, Daza Chacon, treated a case of osteomyelitis of the lower end of the femur. We believe that this is one of the earliest recorded instances of deliberate operation for the treatment of this condition. The case is recorded by the latter physician thus:

> In the year '45 in Brussels, in company with the Doctor Vesalius, in regard to a Flemish knight who was called Busquen and was of the chamber of the Emperor Charles, our lord. He had a very severe pain in the inner part of the right thigh and three months of the most severe illness. And because of the most grave and continuous pain, he neither ate nor slept. He had been bled and purged many times, and given the China and sarsaparilla; yet all this did not help. We came to him to open the place where the pain was, although there was no sign of any obstruction; and we drew off from him a quantity of matter, slightly whitish, which as it came

specifically states that the Emperor had the French disease, nevertheless his discussion of the illness is in accordance with the use of the China root and guaiac for the treatment of syphilis, and both of these remedies were employed on the Emperor. In addition, the pains from which Charles suffered were chiefly around the shoulder and the tibiae; highly suggestive of the fleeting pains of syphilitic periostitis.

[20] Alfred Morel–Fatio, *Mémoires de Charles-Quint, texte portugais et traduction française*. Paris, 1913, p. 255.

[21] *op. cit.* (2), p. 12.

[22] *ibid.*, p. 17.

[23] *ibid.*, p. 18.

forth instantly the sick man commenced to rest, to eat and to sleep; and the outcome
was so successful that where he had been almost consumed, now in a short time
(as he was a youth) he was restored to his existence in full health.[24]

March 1545 was marked by the opening of the Diet of Worms, prompted by
the religious troubles in Germany.   However, Charles, first delayed by his gout,
and then travelling from Brussels to Anvers and thence by the Rhine to
Worms, did not reach that city until 16 May.[25]   We can do no more than assume
that Vesalius was with the Emperor at Worms.   Nevertheless, it is interesting
to note that it was while Charles was in that city that he received the news of the
birth (8 July) of a grandson, the prince Don Carlos,[26] who was later to be the
patient in the most important case of Vesalius.

The Diet closed in August, and Charles returned to the Netherlands by way
of the Rhine to Louvain and thence to Brussels.   From Brussels he continued
to Bruges and so to Bar-le-Duc, where he was delayed by another flare up of the
gout.   Finally he arrived in Utrecht for the meeting of the Order of the Golden
Fleece.   But once more his gout compelled him to extend his visit until better
health permitted him to continue his travels onwards toward Guelders.[27]

Although still tormented by his gout, Charles went on to Maestricht,
where in February 1546 he received information that the conference being held
at Ratisbon (Regensburg) was in danger of breaking up.   He therefore advised
the commissioners to prolong the meeting until he might arrive, and leaving
Maestricht, he travelled through Luxemburg to Speyer and eventually to
Ratisbon.[28]

Vesalius seems to have been with Charles in the Netherlands and to have
followed his passage of the country, but on the way to Ratisbon he was ordered
to remain at Nijmegen in order to attend Bernardino Navagerio, the Venetian
ambassador, who had fallen seriously ill.   Here he sat down to reply to a belated
letter, 'with its highly perturbed tone', which he had received from Jacobus
Sylvius, and in which Sylvius told of having read the *Fabrica* and discussed
certain offensive passages, which he desired Vesalius to withdraw if they were to
maintain their friendship.   Because of the opportunity of a messenger, Vesalius
answered him rather hastily and thus failed to make a copy of his reply.[29]
However, as soon as his patient was ready to travel, they completed the journey to
Ratisbon, and there Vesalius was able to give the purport of his reply to Sylvius
which makes up the greater bulk of his work known as the *China Root Letter*.
Here too, we find him called in to consult with the famous anatomist of Ferrara,
Joannes Baptista Canano, over the illness of Francesco d'Este—an occasion of
great significance, for in discussing the problems of venesection the matter of
the existence of venous valves was apparently brought up by Canano.[30]

In the Emperor's eyes Vesalius was constantly growing in professional
stature, and although he continued to repose the greatest confidence in his

[24] Daza Chacon, *op. cit.* (15), vol. i, p. 69.

[25] Morel–Fatio, *op. cit.* (20), p. 259.

[26] *ibid.*, p. 263.

[27] *ibid.*, p. 265.

[28] *ibid.*, pp. 267, 269.

[29] *op. cit.* (2), pp. 41–2.

[30] Andreas Vesalius, *Examen*: in the *Opera omnia*, ed. Boerhaave and Albinus. Leyden, 1725,
vol. ii, pp. 794–5.

protomedicus, Cornelius van Baersdorp,[31] he was desirous of having the young physician in attendance for a second opinion. In the meantime, Vesalius was gaining favourable attention abroad, and he was offered the post of court physician to the King of Denmark, an offer which he refused but suggested that the post might well be filled by his friendly correspondent, Jerome Cardan.[32]

The year 1547 marked the seemingly legendary meeting of Vesalius with the eminent botanist Leonhardt Fuchs[33] at about the time of the outbreak of the Schmalkald war, and the fact that Vesalius has been shown in attendance upon Charles at Heilbronn in December and January[34] tends to indicate his participation in the campaign.

In February Vesalius accompanied the Emperor to Ulm,[35] but in the beginning of March the physician took a brief trip to Basel, although for what purpose is uncertain. However, he left Basel by 25 March and was met on his return trip by an Imperial courier who hastened him to the Emperor, who needs must have his brilliant physician whenever he felt sufficiently indisposed to tire of irregular advice. A contemporary letter informs us that Vesalius had rejoined the Emperor in Nürnberg before 8 April.[36]

Vesalius was in attendance upon the Emperor during his sojourn in Augsburg from July 1547 to August 1548.[37] At this time Vesalius made what was perhaps his greatest contribution to the surgical art by the re-introduction of the classical operation for drainage of an empyema. With the passage of the years he obtained an extensive experience of the procedure, and his contribution was widely proclaimed by his contemporaries. The first record we possess of his operating for this condition is that given by Daza Chacon; in it the Spanish surgeon stresses unwarrantably his own importance and fails to mention, as may be gathered from the brilliant *consilium* of Vesalius (1562) on the subject,[38] that the ribs were counted from below. We can perhaps forgive the vanity of an old man writing in his senility.

In the year 1547 the Emperor's Majesty Charles being in Augsburg, I saw the most learned Vesalius open an empyema. Although he made anatomical sections almost miraculously (as I have seen many times), he was slow in surgery, and thus entrusted nearly all such to me. He opened this between the third and fourth [ribs], always keeping as far out as possible to protect the veins and arteries which go from side to side. The profusion of blood was great; although he penetrated the pleura, nothing came forth, except that which was extravenate, although great care was used. Therefore [the patient] died.[39]

In the fall of 1548 the Emperor returned to Brussels, and it was here that Vesalius made his dramatic prophecy of the imminent death of Maximilian of Egmont, Count of Buren, who fulfilled the prediction on 23 December.[40]

[31] The hypothesis that Narciso Vertunno (*Parthenopeus*, 1491–1551) remained Charles's protomedicus up to the time of his death has been disproved by Fausto Nicolini, 'New light on the Neapolitan physician Narciso Vertunno'. *Journ. Hist. Med. and Allied Sci.*, 1946, i, 335–7.

[32] Cardanus, *Opera omnia*. Lyon, 1663, vol. i, p. 23.

[33] Roth, *op. cit.* (3), p. 218.

[34] *ibid.*, p. 217.　　　　　　　　　[35] *ibid.*, p. 218.

[36] Wolf-Heidegger, *op. cit.* (4), pp. 209–11.

[37] Roth, *op. cit.* (3), p. 219.　　　　[38] *ibid.*, pp. 398–405.

[39] Daza Chacon, *op. cit.* (15), vol. ii, p. 232.

[40] Jacque-Auguste de Thou, *Histoire universelle*. London, 1734, vol. i, p. 364.

The accuracy of the prognosis created a great stir, but there were those who later became somewhat sceptical of the powers and motives of Vesalius in this direction. The Chancellor Granvelle, writing to the president of the privy council in 1558, says: 'M. de Lalaing se porte mieulx et ne crains pas beaucoup les jugemens de Vesalius sur ses malades, parce qu'il les déclare toujours d'arrivée mortelz, afin que s'ils meurent cela l'excuse, et s'ils vivent, qu'il aie faict miracle'.[41]

However, the ability of Vesalius was now receiving more than regal approval. In 1549 he was honoured *in absentia* at Basel through the dedication to him of the medical works of Alexander Benedictus,[42] and in a more material fashion by an increase of salary. From now on the Emperor seems to have had Vesalius and Cornelius van Baersdorp in general attendance upon him. In his capacity as court physician Vesalius cared for the most powerful figure at the court, the Cardinal Granvelle, who became ill in the summer of 1549 but died within the space of a year.[43] Granvelle was succeeded by his son, Antony Perrenot, Bishop of Arras and later, like his father, Cardinal Granvelle. Arras had been an old class-mate of Vesalius at Louvain and had been instrumental in obtaining the increase in salary. Vesalius had learned much at court. Writing to the famous schoolmaster, Jean Sturm, on the best method of addressing the potent Bishop of Arras, he reveals a practical diplomacy with which he is rarely credited:

Master Martinus has shown me your letter, and has most courteously and kindly delivered your good wishes. I am delighted that I continue to be so dear to you, and that you return my affection in such full measure. The day before yesterday I proffered my thanks to Arras for helping me to obtain from the Emperor an annual three hundred Rhenish florins above my regular stipend. At this same time I also told him that in your letter to me, you had asked to be commended to him; and he seemed to welcome my message with sincere feeling. Of course I do not know whether you write to him often: but if there is no need of writing, you will not, I believe, go far amiss if you write rather infrequently. On the other hand, I am sure he will be pleased to accept the dedication of books, and hence I urge this procedure on your part—although you should perhaps expect no notable recompense.

Praise him for his manifold skill in languages, in which, you will write, he is so thoroughly versed that he is at ease in addressing well-nigh all the nations of Europe and, in fact, seems to have been brought up in each of them; since, whenever he comes to discuss and to treat any matter with these nations . . . he adapts himself so well to its ways that he appears to have imbibed its customs along with its language. When you ascribe to him erudition in the various disciplines, particularly in law, mathematics, medicine, and natural philosophy, add that he also shows interest in the manual arts, namely in painting, sculpture, alchemy, and architecture: for it is amazing how greatly he excells in these arts, and how much he enjoys them, whenever he can snatch any time from his own very heavy duties; it is amazing too, what kindness he shows toward those who work with these arts. Mention the fact that he is the son of a very great man, who is to be counted most fortunate in that his five sons are all so equally adorned with virtues that it is difficult to determine which of them will show the greatest distinction in the fulfillment of his present activities. Express your wonder at a young man possessing judgment which is not

---

[41] Wauters, *op. cit.* (17), p. 27.

[42] Roth, *op. cit.* (3), p. 221.

[43] Fisch, *op. cit.* (19), p. 236.

rash or over-hasty, but fully mature and worthy of admiration by all. But points like this should come to your mind more readily than I can write them down. Yet be sure to add that you have no hesitation in writing rhetoric to so eloquent a man, and one who, Atlas-like, so sturdily supports his fatherland, etc. For the rest, my very best regards to you and please give my heartiest greetings to Master Guintherius. Brussels, 15 May.

If you will not laugh at me, I should beg you, in your preface to make incidental mention of your Vesalius, from whom, as from many others, you have heard the habits of Arras. For as boys we spent almost three years under the same teachers, and however many honours have been heaped upon him, I have always found him most affectionate towards me.

Yours devotedly,
And. Vesalius.[44]

In February 1553, the Emperor, then in Brussels, seems to have had a very bad attack of gout, so that it was said that he had prepared himself for possible death. Vesalius was in attendance as well as Charles's favourite protomedicus, Cornelius van Baersdorp, but the Emperor did not recover until well into the spring.[45] Charles finally arrived at his decision to abdicate in 1556, and upon retirement he gave Vesalius a life pension and permission to enter the service of the new ruler, Philip II.[46]

Not long after assuming his responsibilities under the new monarch, Vesalius was called upon in 1559 for consultation in the tragic case of Henry II of France. To celebrate the treaty of Cateau-Cambrésis ending the Franco-Spanish strife, and the double marriage of Henry's daughter to Philip II and the French king's sister to the Duke of Savoy, a passage of arms had been arranged to terminate the festivities. The French king participated in the jousts on the afternoon of 30 June. In running the last course he was wounded above the right eye by the broken lance of his opponent, Gabriel de Montgomery, Captain of the Scottish Guard. The wound proved fatal, and the unfortunate king died ten days later from injury of the brain by contrecoup.

The incident was widely mentioned by the chroniclers of the time, and from them we learn that four criminals were executed immediately to provide experimental material in order to determine the course of the splinters. The most outstanding of the French surgeons present was Ambroise Paré, to whom we are indebted for a brief but excellent account of the post-mortem findings.[47] Philip himself was at Brussels, the Duke of Alva serving as proxy at the wedding, and on hearing the news he promptly dispatched Vesalius to take charge of the case. Vesalius set off post-haste but did not arrive in Paris until 5 July, when it was too late to do more than pronounce a fatal outcome. Thus far the account of Daza Chacon has not been presented. This account does not differ materially from those previously mentioned, but it does provide some graphic details hitherto unknown. The Spanish surgeon writes:

[44] Roth, *op. cit.* (3), pp. 421–2.
[45] Fisch, *op. cit.* (19), pp. 238–40.
[46] Roth, *op. cit.* (3), pp. 241–2.
[47] Paré, *op. cit.* (14), lib. v, c. ix, p. 249. Paré, unlike other chroniclers of the event, writes that the wound was on the left side.

I wish to tell you this other story which it may please you to know; it is true, and I learned it from the most learned Vesalius and from others mentioned as present, and this was the case. When the King's Majesty Philip, our sire, the second of this name, was victor at St. Quentin, he made peace with Henry the Second, King of France, and in this they arranged marriages. King Henry (as was fitting) celebrated this peace and the marriage since these things were so important to him, and the more so since it concerned his daughter as the Queen of Spain. In the many celebrations which the king held, one day while jousting, he was wounded in the forehead in an encounter of lances. They immediately sent to the court of the King's Majesty, our sire, which at that time was in Flanders, for Doctor Vesalius. And a few days later, a surgeon who was with the court (he was at that time an Alcalde for lack of good men) negotiated with a court favourite that they should send him there, and it happened as he wished, for immediately they ordered him to leave by post. Having reached his destination, he saw the wound of the king, and it was decided to hold a consultation over the matter. There were many very distinguished physicians and surgeons, all very learned in Latin and Greek, and skilled in surgery. It is customary there that when the physicians gather to treat some sickness, especially in the case of a royal personage, they all sit down and the Chaplain, as we would say here Protomedicus, attends and orders whomever he thinks should give his opinions; and to honour Doctor Vesalius and his companion (if we may call him that), he left them to speak last. The French began to speak in that Latin they talk, and with very great facility, each one giving his opinion. The Chaplain ordered Vesalius to speak, and he left the Spaniard for the last because all had the greatest confidence (since he had been sent) that what he said would result in the health of the king. So Vesalius gave his opinion with that Latin and facility which I have seen in many consultations (which I have had with him) and treated of the essence of the wound, the signs and prognoses, and the treatment of it, which a good surgeon would be obliged to observe, and all with such wisdom that it was no wonder that all were very satisfied and admiring. At the conclusion, the Chaplain with much reverence and politeness said to the Spaniard that he should give his opinion. It is true and not a story, that those who told me about it said that the French, and even the lords who were present (as is customary in such cases) were waiting for what the surgeon would say, like the Carthaginians when Aeneas wished to speak to them from the throne. And the poor Spaniard, since the Latin he knew was very barbarous, and he did not know French, thought it well to begin to speak in his own language, as though the French had been in Portugal for a long time; and so in Spanish for a while, and for a while in the Latin which I have mentioned, he said things which were better left unsaid. This is not a joke but a fact. The French were in such a state that they did not know whether they saw it or whether they were dreaming it, because although they saw it, they could not believe it.[48]

Philip II was now to spend the rest of his life away from the Netherlands, and consequently Vesalius and his wife, completely breaking family ties with their native land, travelled in the king's retinue to Madrid. There Vesalius served the representatives of Flanders at the court, and on occasion members of the English diplomatic staff.[49]

In 1562 Vesalius participated in the celebrated case of the Infante, Don Carlos,[50] who had fallen down a flight of steps and had been thrown

[48] Daza Chacon, *op. cit.* (15), vol. i, pp. 174–5.

[49] Roth, *op. cit* (3), pp. 243–4; Fisch, *op. cit.* (19), pp. 246 ff.

[50] J. B. de C. M. Saunders, 'Vesalius and Don Carlos', in *Essays in biology in honor of Herbert M. Evans.* Berkeley, 1943, pp. 531–8.

against a door at their foot. The gossips had it that the spoilt and ill-tempered prince was chasing a serving maid whom he had terrified by his advances. The accident occurred on Sunday, 19 April, and at first the youth was attended by his personal physicians, Drs. Olivares and Vega, and later by Daza Chacon. Upon notification of the accident, Philip dispatched his protomedicus, Juan Gutierrez, a certain Portuguese doctor, and the royal surgeon, Pedro de Torres, to attend on the Infante.

Despite the multitude of attendants and the care with which the prince was treated, fear of erysipelas arose, and the indecision of the physicians, in the light of the rank of the patient, prompted them to dispatch a messenger to the king, who 'as soon as he heard the news, left Madrid on Friday, 1 May, before daylight and arrived at Alcalà before treatment time; the dressing was done in the presence of His Majesty and Doctor Andreas Vesalius, a very learned man'.[51]

Vesalius had accompanied the king to Alcalà, but being, as it were, an alien consultant who had been foisted upon the native physicians, his attendance seems to have promoted a certain amount of tension, which the arrogance of Vesalius would by no means lessen.

At this time His Highness being on the chamber-pot and passing choleric and foul matters, caught a cold, and his pulse became weak; however, he felt no chill and no tremor. Seeing this, the Portuguese doctor and Vesalius thought that the lesion was inside, and that the only means of cure was to cut through the bone to the membranes; and such was their opinion so long as a fever was present, and they were opposed to all other means. Excepting for these two, we were all convinced that these symptoms could be ascribed to one or the other of the two following causes: either the bone of the skull was suppurating (and in this case it would be necessary to ruginate) according to these indications, since on Monday the fourth, on Tuesday, and on the other days following the incision, the small [inflamed] spot reappeared; or else the external inflammation had reached the membranes of the brain through the sutures; we were even inclined to favour this latter view. Vesalius had plenty of good reasons to support his opinion, as it is easy to see from the above.

The prince's condition continued to grow worse, and 'at the end of the twentieth day, we were still in doubt with regard to a lesion of the bone, and it was suggested to ruginate'. The result was thus made 'visible to all that there was no lesion in the bone, and none in the corresponding internal part'. 'Thus were dispelled all doubts, so that except for the Portuguese doctor and Vesalius, who never changed their opinion, we were assured that the damage was accidental and solely a result of fever and erysipelas.'[52]

The physicians were eventually rewarded by an improvement in their patient's condition, although Daza Chacon said that there were some who contended that in the case 'success was merely due to chance'. Although Don Carlos continued to improve, it became necessary to incise and drain both of the prince's orbits—a procedure which was carried out at the instigation of Vesalius.

[51] Daza Chacon, op. cit. (15), ii, pp. 190–201: 'True relation of the wound of the head of the Most Serene Prince Don Carlos, our sire, of glorious memory'. The verisimilitude of Daza Chacon's account is attested by the almost verbatim report of another of the attendant physicians, Dr. Olivares, and published in Documentos inéditos para la historia de Espana. Madrid, vol. xv, 1849.

[52] Like Vesalius, the Portuguese doctor, who is never mentioned by name, was apparently an outcast, and it may have been for this reason that he supported the opinion of Vesalius in opposition to the common stand of the Spanish physicians.

Nevertheless, by 5 July Don Carlos had recovered sufficiently to attend a bull-fight in honour of his recovery.

The case had been a tedious one. The rank of the patient, the possible consequence of failure, and even the threatening attitude of the general public, had made it a nerve-racking experience for the physicians. The Spanish physicians appear to have opposed a common front to Vesalius as an alien in their midst. No doubt this was but one of many such instances of jealousy and provincialism, and Vesalius apparently was finding his position at court more and more unpleasant. He had now a considerable personal fortune, while the lure of court life had long since lost its charm for him.

A few months previous to the Don Carlos case he had received Fallopius' gentle criticism of the *Fabrica*, and under its influence a desire seems to have been awakened in him to retire to the academic peace of Padua. This desire was expressed in his reply to Fallopius, completed in the waning of the year, 27 December 1561.

> I sincerely hope that you may long maintain this purpose in that sweet leisure of letters which is yours and in that throng of learned men, whose studies are dear to their hearts, and with whom you can daily compare the concepts of your mind. For I feel that the ornaments of our art originate in that arena from which, as a young man, I was diverted to the mechanical practice of medicine, to numerous wars and to continuous travels ... therefore continue to embellish our common school, whose memory is always most dear to me, with the fruits of your talents and industry.[53]

Whatever may have been the true cause of the departure of Vesalius from the Spanish court and his journey to the Holy Land, nevertheless it seems to have been related to his court service. Paré, mysteriously withholding the actual name of the physician, relates the story of a dissection performed upon a woman suffering from strangulation of the uterus and presumed dead. The signs of life she subsequently exhibited aroused such horror that the physician was forced to seek safety out of the country.[54] This story was repeated by the English physician Edward Jorden, who mentions the name of Vesalius, and suggests that he undertook his pilgrimage as an excuse for leaving Spain.[55] Hubert Languet's account would change the victim of the dissection into a man and make Vesalius liable to the Inquisition, which he avoided only through the protection of Philip II to whom Vesalius made promise of a pilgrimage.[56]

However, other contemporary opinion ignores any such dramatic reason for the departure of Vesalius from Spain and the royal service. There is, nevertheless, the suggestion in several accounts that Vesalius was weary of his court service, and the antagonism of the Galenical school as well as the hostility of the Spanish physicians, and sought some means of discreet withdrawal.[57] Several factors tend to give credence to this view.

[53] Vesalius, *Examen, op. cit.* (30), p. 761.

[54] Paré, *op. cit.* (14), lib. xxiv, c. xlvi, pp. 941–2.

[55] Edward Jorden, *A briefe discourse of a disease called the suffocation of the mother.* London, 1603, ch. iv, fo. 11ʳ.

[56] Melchior Adam, *Vitae Germanorum medicorum.* Heidelberg, 1620; cf. biography of Vesalius, pp. 129 ff.

[57] Pierre Bordey to Granvelle, 4 December 1564, in *Papiers d'état du cardinal de Granvelle,* Paris, 1850, vol. viii, p. 525; de Thou, *op. cit.* (40), vol. iv, p. 632; Giovanni Imperiali, cited in H. Cushing, *Bio-bibliography of Andreas Vesalius.* New York, 1943, p. 205; Charles de Tisnacq, cited in Wauters, *op. cit.* (17), p. 32.

Vesalius was an alien in Spain and apparently regarded in some degree with envy and jealousy by the royal Spanish physicians. There is the suggestion in Daza Chacon's account of the Don Carlos case that Vesalius was obstructed by the Spanish physicians in attendance, and Gachard[58] would go so far as to say that they had even attempted to prevent his coming to Alcalà, and that his efforts were later consciously belittled, while the credit for the prince's recovery was transferred to the miraculous benefit of the long dead Fra Diego, whose body had been exhumed and placed in bed with the unfortunate Don Carlos.[59] That Vesalius was an alien appears to have made it impossible, because of political implications, for him to become the protomedicus, despite that fact that Philip, like his father before him, always turned to Vesalius in time of dire emergency. Nevertheless, the position must have been galling. Furthermore, Charles and Vesalius had been fellow-countrymen, but Philip was more Spaniard than Netherlander. If, as is possible, Vesalius had taken service under Charles as a protection from the consequences of his 'sacrilegious' scientific work and certain sardonic remarks in the *Fabrica* which might have been poorly received by theologians, certainly Philip, far more devout than his father and normally more under the influence of theologians, would have been a far less comforting bulwark against attack, whether national or theological. The statement of Clusius, who reached Madrid on the day when Vesalius departed, that Vesalius had fallen ill and for that reason had been granted royal permission to withdraw from the king's service and undertake a pilgrimage,[60] is in accord with this. Unpleasant conditions of service might well have led to illness, or, at least, a feigned illness would be a convenient subterfuge for withdrawal from an intolerable position.

Finally, it is possible that the appearance of the *Anatomical Observations* of Fallopius reawakened the desire for scientific research which could not be carried on conveniently at court. A pilgrimage to the Holy Land would not only permit Vesalius to withdraw from the royal service, but it would justify an itinerary which would take him to Venice as a port of embarkation. Did he openly seek from the Venetian government his old position at Padua, or did he know that if he returned to Venice it would be offered to him? All we know is that he was offered the position and accepted it with the understanding that he would take up his duties upon his return from his fatal pilgrimage. In this respect Pietro Bizarri's account of the voyage and shipwreck seems most probable in its total lack of the spectacular, and the seemingly authentic source from which it was drawn.[61]

There is one other suggestion for the pilgrimage which is given in a letter written from Cologne by Johann Metel to George Cassander, and which despite a certain weakness of argument, in view of our knowledge of the last years of Vesalius in Spain, nevertheless does lend some slight support to the tradition of the physician's parsimonious nature.

By reason of a certain promise of money by which he would become more wealthy, Vesalius in the previous year set out from Spain for Jerusalem. He did

<hr>

[58] *Don Carlos et Philippe II.* Bruxelles, 1863, pp. 81, 89.
[59] Charles de Mouy, *Don Carlos et Philippe II.* Paris, 1863, p. 64.
[60] de Thou, *op. cit.* (40), vol. iv, p. 632.
[61] Pietro Bizarri, *De bello Cypriaco et Pannonico.* Basileae, 1573, p. 284.

not join up with the merchants but as a companion of the pilgrims, and he provided very meagerly for himself with regard to passage and provisions.   Returning thence, he was met on the journey by a certain George Boucher of Nuremberg, returning from Egypt and the city of Cairo, whom he persuaded to accompany him, so that he left his ship to join [Vesalius] as a companion.   Driven by winds for forty days continuously, and since they were unable to make land, and Vesalius on account of his meanness had provided too meagerly for himself with respect to bread and water, and many were dying and were then thrown into the sea, he having become sick through constitutional weakness and fear, often asked the sailors not to throw him into the sea if he should die.   Finally the little ship reached Zante, and on first disembarking and entering that city he died at its very gate; the one who brought back this information, his companion, erected a monument to him.   Too great love of money, which it may seem to you that his many writings on the understanding of the parts of the human body ought to have quenched, brought this end to so famous a man.[62]

Many have been astonished and would see something almost mysterious in the rejection by Vesalius of his pre-eminent position in the field of anatomy in order to bury himself in the relative obscurity of the Imperial court.   But this is to judge of his motives from the modern point of view.   Vesalius, however, was just as surely conditioned by the common currency of his environment as we are by ours.   Consciously or unconsciously his world was guided by conceptions of a universal order derived from Platonic thinking, and which had their application not only to the universal, but also to the little world of man.   To him, therefore, the ultimate aim of the physician was the perfection of the medical art, attainable only through its practice.   It would be simpler to imagine other more ordinary and mundane motives prompting his change of status, but we would have to ignore the purposeful theme which everywhere unites his writings.   It is true that once his decision was made he found himself entrapped by the court and dependent on royal permission to retire to more fruitful fields, and he recognized his disappointment after scarcely three years of service and saw that he might have obtained his end more fully at Pisa—but too late.   The court period of Vesalius was therefore the complement to his career—his thinking, in a sense, reactionary amidst its progressiveness.

[62] Niceron, *Mémoires*. Paris, vol. v, 1731, p. 140.

JEAN FERNEL'S CONCEPTION OF TUBERCULOSIS

by

ESMOND R. LONG

TUBERCULOSIS has taken a larger toll of life than any other disease. It was a common illness in the cities of ancient Greece and Rome, and has flourished in all succeeding years wherever crowding and poor hygiene favoured dissemination of tuberculous infection.

The first real understanding of its nature is commonly credited to the celebrated seventeenth-century investigators Sylvius de le Boë, Thomas Willis and Richard Morton. There is reason to believe, however, that physicians in the preceding century, not so well known in this particular connexion, contributed significantly to the foundation of knowledge on which the seventeenth-century phthisiologists based their new views. Some of them wrote with assurance on the subject of phthisis, combining observations and conclusions of their own with the firmly entrenched views of the ancients.

It may, therefore, be of more than passing interest to recover the concepts that were prevalent in the first half of the sixteenth century, in the flowering of the Renaissance, when medical scholars were first breaking with the traditions of Hippocrates, Galen and the Arabians. For such a purpose we may turn with confidence and profit to the *Medicina* of Jean Fernel, one of the most distinguished physicians of the period, who has been called by Charles Singer[1] the 'coryphaeus of Medicine' in Paris in that remarkable period when anatomy was in a restless state, about to become a new and precise science, and the beginnings of a discipline of pathological anatomy were already evident.

Fernel was in the formative years of his medical practice in Paris when Vesalius was a resident in that city, when Guenther's published commentaries on the works of Galen were widely used, when Jacobus Sylvius was an influential teacher, and when, as Singer has noted, new texts on Galenic anatomy appeared in the city at the rate of two every month. Fernel, also, was a student of the human frame, but his particular interest was in its physiology, its abnormal functioning, and the treatment of its diseases. Singer has referred to the 'calm, philosophical, eloquent Fernel' as 'the best exponent of physiological views of the century'. His influence on concepts of pathology was perhaps almost as important.

An outline of Fernel's life has been preserved for us by his pupil Guillaume Plancy in a biography presumably written shortly after Fernel's death in 1558, but not published until 1607. According to Plancy, Fernel was born in 1486 (i.e. recalculating Plancy's statement of '1485' on the basis of a more conventional calendar). Actually the date of his birth is uncertain. The interested reader may consult Eloy's *Dictionnaire historique de la medicine ancienne* for the reasons for the uncertainty. The date accepted by many writers is 1497.

---

[1] Charles Singer and C. Rabin, *A Prelude to Modern Science. Being a Discussion of the History, Sources and Circumstances of the Tabulae Anatomicae Sex of Vesalius.* (Publications of the Wellcome Historical Medical Museum, n.s., No. 1.) Cambridge, 1946.

Fernel commenced his studies at the college of Sainte Barbe of the University of Paris, and was first an ardent student of mathematics and philosophy. In 1524 illness forced him to drop his academic activity and leave Paris for a prolonged rest. While he was recuperating new interests developed, and on his return to Paris he devoted himself to the study of medicine. He took his doctorate and was licensed to practise in 1530. For some years thereafter he was more occupied with mathematics and astrology than professional medicine, but finally, about 1535, under the influence of family pressure, he established himself firmly in medical practice.

In the light of these dates which, as noted above, coincided with the great awakening of anatomical science in Paris, it would seem as if Fernel should have been much influenced by new thinking in this subject. He was apparently just too early. Surprisingly little effect of the new developments is evident in his *magnum opus*, the *Medicina*, the first part of which was published in 1542 under the title *De naturali parte medicinae*. The full volume was printed in not quite finished form in 1554. In the dedication of the book to King Henry II, who had an extraordinary regard for Fernel and made him Court Physician, the author noted as the sources of his information Hippocrates, Herophilus, Diocles, Archigenes, Galen, Aretaeus, Aëtius, Paul, Alexander, Actuarius and 'the Arabians'. The list includes no modern. This anatomy, which formed the first part of the *Medicina*, although in no small part based on his own dissections, was essentially the anatomy of Galen.

At this distance it can only be assumed that his views were well set before the new knowledge crystallized. Even Vesalius was a confirmed Galenist when he left Paris in 1536, and the *Fabrica* did not appear until 1543, a year after the first publication of the initial chapters of what was to become the *Medicina*. Additional reasons may be the conservatism of the University, which Singer has stressed in his account of Vesalius' life in Paris, and Fernel's concentration on the classics, which had governed his life since his student days.

Fernel was a serious and outstanding exponent of the Renaissance, but his work reflected its scholarship more than its innovations. Sir Charles Sherrington,[2] who has made a most interesting analysis of Fernel's place in the development of medicine, has called attention to the one-sided effect of Fernel's education and associations. The University of Paris still rested heavily on medieval tradition. No one could have devoted himself more assiduously than Fernel to the great medical texts of antiquity. But he seems to have failed to take advantage of the growing opportunities in Paris for learning new facts through observation and experiment, and expressing new and independent ideas. He was indeed a leader in the revival of learning, but less a modern than Vesalius and others of his Parisian contemporaries in research.

Fernel's service was of a different character. He was first of all a systematist. The *Medicina* in its final form, including the revised and amplified *De naturali parte medicinae*, was a well-organized compendium, divided into three main sections, dealing respectively with physiology,

[2] Sir Charles Sherrington, *The Endeavour of Jean Fernel*. Cambridge, at the University Press, 1946.

pathology and therapeutics. It was the first text in history known to employ the term 'Pathology' in approximately the modern sense. Fernel's biographer Plancy gives Fernel credit for the introduction of the term. The section on Pathology became the most famous part of the *Medicina*. The *Medicina* itself, first published by Andreas Wechel in Paris in 1554, passed through some thirty editions, reprintings and partial translations. The Pathology, as Part II of the *Medicina*, was reissued thirty-six times in little more than a century, and was obtainable as a separate volume of a three-volume edition of the *Medicina* a year after initial publication of the latter. It finally appeared as a wholly independent volume in 1638, and was published in French in 1650. Sherrington has given a comprehensive picture of its content and its influence, and published a bibliographic record of its history.

Fernel's *Pathology* is particularly useful for our present purposes because of its organization into those two branches of pathology now designated as general and special. The first of its seven constituent books is entitled 'On diseases and their causes'. The second is on 'Symptoms and signs', the third on 'The pulse and the urine', the fourth on 'Fevers', and the fifth on 'Diseases and symptoms of special parts'. The last named and the succeeding two are devoted to 'special pathology' in the present sense. The sixth book is on 'Diseases of parts below the diaphragm', and the seventh and last on 'Affections of external parts of the body'.

The subject of phthisis (*tabes* in Fernel's account) appears for the most part in the tenth chapter of the fifth book of the Pathology. The chapter title is 'Symptoms, causes and signs of disease of the lungs'. Fernel divided diseases of the lungs into five main groups: (1) Simple distemper (*intemperies*), (2) obstruction, (3) pneumonia, (4) vomica or abscess and (5) tabes. With the first of these we shall not delay. Among the numerous types of 'obstruction' however—itself a most interesting concept of the ancients in pathology—he included a highly significant account of healed and healing tuberculosis. In discussing asthma and orthopnoea Fernel referred to the 'hardening of a viscous humour into hail-like particles and finally into true stone'. The remarkable fact was that he was drawing on his personal anatomical experience, for he adds: 'In dissections we have occasionally found lungs full of them. Some were very hard and solid, and others of the consistency of old cheese, while others, just beginning to harden, still contained plaster-like pituita. Each was enveloped in its own capsule.'

He referred also to a patient who coughed up small, hard stones which varied from the size of barley grains to that of peas. Similar clinical observations had been made by medical writers many times before, even in ancient times, but never before had they been so clearly correlated with the presence of discrete, encapsulated, calcareo-caseous lesions of the lungs. The description of stages in the process of calcification, including matter with the 'consistency of old cheese' (obviously our 'caseation'), masses of 'plaster-like consistency', and finally nodules that were solid and hard, is not only accurate, but quite as clear and informative as the much better-known descriptions of the next century.

Fernel must have seen a number of cases, for he stated that the abnormality occurred sometimes in people without dyspnoea and occasionally in persons with a kind of orthopnoea with suffocating oppression. We can only speculate as to the identity of the latter type of case; it could have been old fibroid phthisis, although such difficulty in respiration is seldom seen.

It is somewhat tempting to relate Fernel's description of 'crude tubercle engendered from the arteries of the lungs' (*crudum tuberculum pulmonum arteriis adnatum*) (the 'phyma' of the ancients) to phthisis, but such correlation would be far fetched, for the anatomical reference is too vague, and there is little in the symptomatology that Fernel connects with the condition to suggest this disease.

The section on pneumonia also makes reference to phthisis. Fernel noted that in one type of pulmonary inflammation, which 'might be called pneumonia', although it differed symptomatically from the usual disease, the victim was afflicted with cough, difficulty in respiration and lingering fever, finally becoming consumptive without ulceration of the lungs or coughing of blood. This was a conception rather close to that of Rudolf Virchow three hundred years later.

Fernel was perfectly familiar with *vomicae*, or pulmonary cavities, and considered them distinct from phthisis, although he recognized a relationship and stated, quite correctly, that those afflicted with phthisis were disposed to their development. In other words, he considered the cavity a complication, rather than a pathognomonic indication of phthisis, a concept that still holds.

He defined a vomica as a small abscess of the lung, stating that it contained a collection of pus, and noting that it was surrounded by its own membrane. He believed that such a cavity might result in a non-phthisical person from a ruptured vein and subsequent decay of the extruded blood and conversion into pus. This erroneous concept was as old as Galen. He called attention to the fact that such a cavity might be so hidden that the subject of the disability was quite unaware of its existence, 'although all the while harbouring the cause of his death within his chest', a reference that reminds us of the frequent admonitions of experts on tuberculosis to-day on the insidious onset and progress of the disease.

His views on cavities were based on his own observations rather than his reading of the work of the ancients. He referred to the dissection of persons who had died suddenly, in whose bodies no other cause of death was found than a ruptured vomica in the lungs. He believed the pus of the cavity was transmitted to the heart—an old Hippocratic concept—'extinguishing its force', and must have overlooked some other cause of death. He was quite obviously familiar with the cavity, however, as a pathological observation.

Remarkably, two of the victims of this type of demise were distinguished physicians (one would like to know who they were!). They had had no warning in the way of fever, discharge or other symptom. The event reminded him of Hippocrates' reference to hidden suppuration, 'not noticed because of the thickness of pus, and surrounding membrane which prevented the noxious substance from reaching the heart'.[3] Fernel's understanding of the facts before him was overshadowed by preconceived ideas ingrained from long reading and subservience to ancient authority, and one gathers the

[3] *Aphorisms,* vi. 41.

PLATE XXXIV

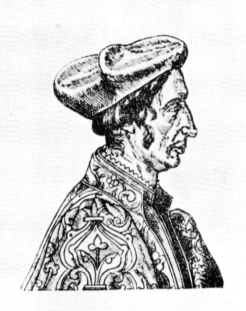

ΙΛΕΡΜΟΣ Ο ΠΛΑΓΚΙΟΣ ΕΣ ΤΟΝ
ΛΑΜΠΡΟΤΑΤΟΝ ΦΕΡΝΕΛΙΟΝ.

Παῖς τε τὰ ζώματ᾽ ἔχλ φύσι, ἠδ᾽ ἐς τοῦσον ὁλιαθι,
Ερϑοι τ᾽ ἰηβϑ, κάλλιον οὔτις ἐρϛ.

FIG. 1. JEAN FERNEL
(In his *Medicina*, Paris, 1554)

PLATE XXXV

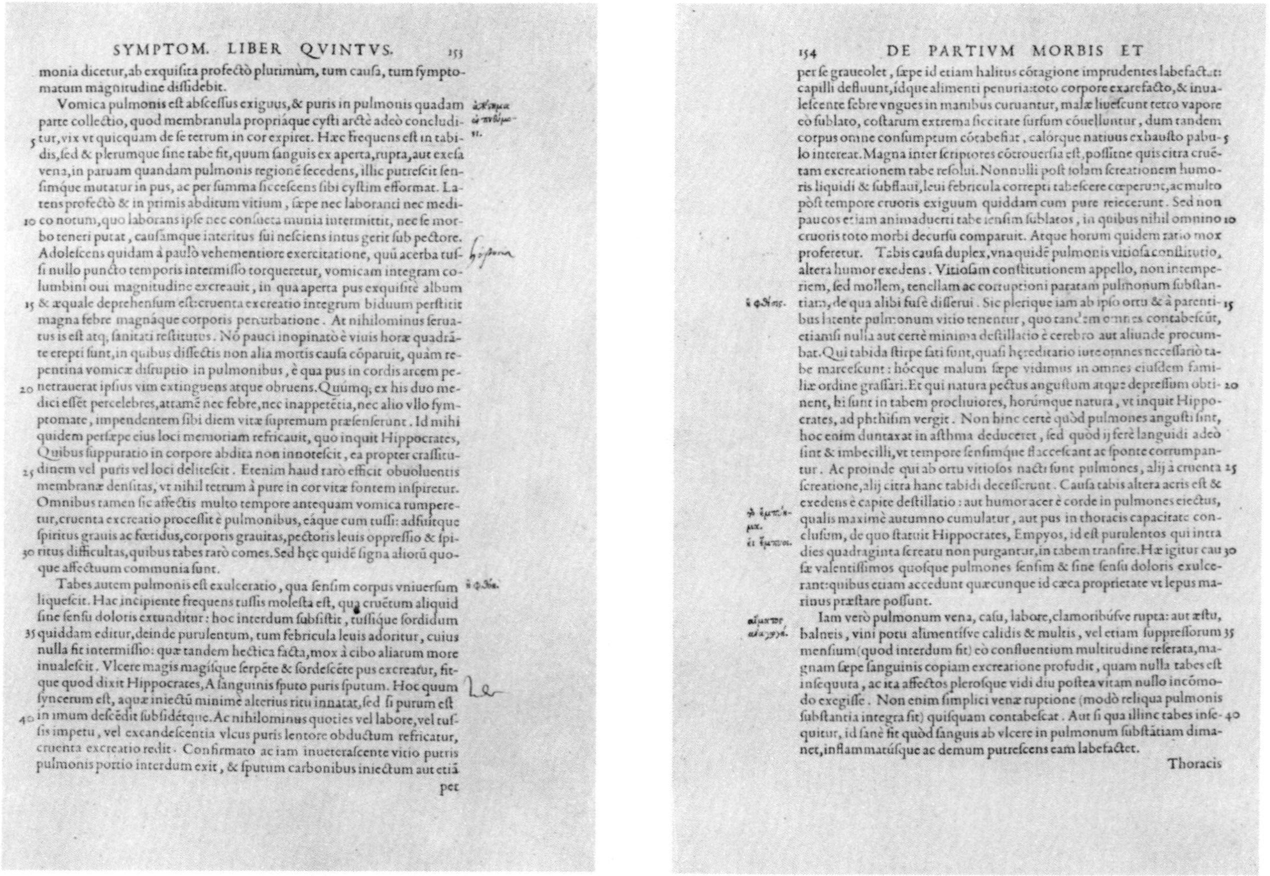

SYMPTOM. LIBER QVINTVS. 153

monia dicetur, ab exquisita profectò plurimùm, tum causa, tum symptomatum magnitudine dissidebit.

Vomica pulmonis est abscessus exiguus, & puris in pulmonis quadam parte collectio, quod membranula propriáque cysti arctè adeò concluditur, vix vt quicquam de se tetrum in cor expiret. Hæc frequens est in tabidis, sed & plerumque sine tabe fit, quum sanguis ex aperta, rupta, aut exesa vena, in paruam quandam pulmonis regionē secedens, illic putrescit sensímque mutatur in pus, ac per summa siccescens sibi cystim efformat. Latens profectò & in primis abditum vitium, sæpe nec laboranti nec medico notum, quo laborans ipse nec consueta munia intermittit, nec se morbo teneri putat, causámque interitus sui nesciens intus gerit sub pectore. Adolescens quidam à paulò vehementiore exercitatione, quū acerba tussi nullo puncto temporis intermisso torqueretur, vomicam integram columbini oui magnitudine excreauit, in qua aperta pus exquisitè album & æquale deprehensum est: cruenta excreatio integrum biduum perstitit magna febre magnáque corporis perturbatione. At nihilominus seruatus is est atq; sanitati restitutus. Nō pauci inopinatò è viuis horæ quadrāte erepti sunt, in quibus dissectis non alia mortis causa cōparuit, quàm repentina vomicæ disruptio in pulmonibus, è qua pus in cordis arcem penetrauerat ipsius vim extinguens atque obruens. Quúmq; ex his duo medici essēt percelebres, attamē nec febre, nec inappetētia, nec alio vllo symptomate, impendentem sibi diem vitæ supremum præsenserunt. Id mihi quidem persæpe eius loci memoriam refricauit, quo inquit Hippocrates, Quibus suppuratio in corpore abdita non innotescit, ea propter crassitudinem vel puris vel loci delitescit. Etenim haud rarò efficit obuoluentis membranæ densitas, vt nihil tetrum à pure in cor vitæ fontem inspiretur. Omnibus tamen sic affectis multo tempore antequam vomica rumperetur, cruenta excreatio processit è pulmonibus, eáque cum tussi: adfuitque spiritus grauis ac fœtidus, corporis grauitas, pectoris leuis oppressio & spiritus difficultas, quibus tabes rarò comes. Sed hęc quidē signa aliorū quoque affectuum communia sunt.

Tabes autem pulmonis est exulceratio, qua sensim corpus vniuersum liquescit. Hac incipiente frequens tussis molesta est, qua cruētum aliquid sine sensu doloris extunditur: hoc interdum subsistit, tussíque sordidum quiddam editur, deinde purulentum, tum febricula leuis adoritur, cuius nulla fit intermissio: quæ tandem hectica facta, mox à cibo aliarum more inualescit. Vlcere magis magísque serpēte & sordescēte pus excreatur, fitque quod dixit Hippocrates, A sanguinis sputo puris sputum. Hoc quum syncerum est, aquæ iniectū minimè alterius ritu innatat, sed si purum est in imum descēdit subsidétque. Ac nihilominus quoties vel labore, vel tussis impetu, vel excandescentia vlcus puris lentore obductum refricatur, cruenta excreatio redit. Confirmato ac iam inueterascente vitio putris pulmonis portio interdum exit, & sputum carbonibus iniectum aut etiā

pet

154 DE PARTIVM MORBIS ET

per se graueolet, sæpe id etiam halitus cōtagione imprudentes labefactat: capilli defluunt, idque alimenti penuria: toto corpore exarefacto, & inualescente febre vngues in manibus curuantur, malæ liuescunt tetro vapore eò sublato, costarum extrema siccitate sursum cōuelluntur, dum tandem corpus omne consumptum cōtabefiat, calórque natiuus exhausto pabulo intereat. Magna inter scriptores cōtrouersia est, possitne quis citra cruētam excreationem tabe resolui. Nonnulli post solam screationem humoris liquidi & subflaui, leui febricula correpti tabescere cœperunt, ac multo pòst tempore cruoris exiguum quiddam cum pure reiecerunt. Sed non paucos etiam animaduerti tabe sensim sublatos, in quibus nihil omnino cruoris toto morbi decursu comparuit. Atque horum quidem ratio mox proferetur. Tabis causa duplex, vna quidē pulmonis vitiosa constitutio, altera humor exedens. Vitiosam constitutionem appello, non intemperiem, sed mollem, tenellam ac corruptioni paratam pulmonum substantiam, de qua alibi fusè disserui. Sic plerique iam ab ipso ortu & à parentibus latente pulmonum vitio tenentur, quo tandem omnes contabescūt, etiamsi nulla aut certè minima destillatio è cerebro aut aliunde procumbat. Qui tabida stirpe sati sunt, quasi hęreditario iure omnes necessariò tabe marcescunt: hócque malum sæpe vidimus in omnes eiusdem familiæ ordine grassari. Et qui natura pectus angustum atque depressum obtinent, hi sunt in tabem procliuiores, horúmque natura, vt inquit Hippocrates, ad phthisim vergit. Non hinc certè quòd pulmones angusti sint, hoc enim duntaxat in asthma deduceret, sed quòd ij ferè languidi adeò sint & imbecilli, vt tempore sensímque flaccescant ac sponte corrumpantur. Ac proinde qui ab ortu vitiosos nacti sunt pulmones, alij à cruenta screatione, alij citra hanc tabidi decesserunt. Causa tabis altera acris est & exedens è capite destillatio: aut humor acer è corde in pulmones eiectus, qualis maximè autumno cumulatur, aut pus in thoracis capacitate conclusum, de quo statuit Hippocrates, Empyos, id est purulentos qui intra dies quadraginta screatu non purgantur, in tabem transire. Hæ igitur causæ valentissimos quosque pulmones sensim & sine sensu doloris exulcerant: quibus etiam accedunt quæcunque id cæca proprietate vt lepus marinus præstare possunt.

Iam verò pulmonum vena, casu, labore, clamoribúsve rupta: aut æstu, balneis, vini potu alimentísve calidis & multis, vel etiam suppressorum mensium (quod interdum fit) eò confluentium multitudine reserata, magnam sæpe sanguinis copiam excreatione profudit, quam nulla tabes est insequuta, ac ita affectos plerosque vidi diu postea vitam nullo incómodo exegisse. Non enim simplici venæ ruptione (modò reliqua pulmonis substantia integra sit) quisquam contabescat. Aut si qua illinc tabes insequitur, id sanè fit quòd sanguis ab vlcere in pulmonum substātiam dimanet, inflammatúsque ac demum putrescens eam labefactet.

Thoracis

FIG. 2. Two pages of Fernel's *Medicina*, Paris, 1554, dealing with his views on phthisis
(From the copy in The Wellcome Historical Medical Library)

impression of confusion at times in reconciling the facts as he saw them in the dead body, or in the clinic, with the statements of Hippocrates.

The final paragraphs of the chapter have to do with his own conception of the disease consumption. 'Phthisis is an ulceration of the lung', he wrote, 'which gradually wastes the whole body.' He summarized the sequence of events in its progression as follows. First there was frequent cough, with painless raising of blood. Later came a type of cough which brought up first a foul and then a purulent material. This was followed by fever, which steadily increased in severity. All this time the ulceration was extending, with continuous production of pus. In this connexion he quoted Hippocrates' dictum, 'from the spitting of blood comes the spitting of pus'.[4] He distinguished several types of sputum, e.g., that which floated on water and that which sank, and described its odour in the natural state and when thrown on live coals, an old test,[5] the foul and odoriferous type characterizing the state when purulent lung itself was coughed up.

Then follows a remarkable statement: 'Often the exhalation corrupts by contagion those who are not careful.' It is not elaborated and we cannot tell whether Fernel is merely repeating, without comment, a vague concept of the ancients or deliberately introducing a view of his own. The idea was not wholly new at the time. Fracastorius had enunciated something like it in his De contagione and had referred to 'contagious phthisis', although not quite in the modern sense.

Fernel proceeded in his description with the familiar Hippocratic picture of hair falling out from lack of nourishment, drying up of the body, increase in fever, curving of the finger nails, lividity of the cheeks, contraction of the ribs, progressive emaciation and finally death—truly a dreadful picture, which in more or less the same form was long current as representing the inevitable course of phthisis, and was dispelled only after a vastly better understanding of the disease was reached.

He went on to say that 'writers' disagreed widely as to whether one could become phthisic without ever having coughed up blood. He took the stand himself that it was possible. In some patients, he pointed out, the disease began with the expectoration of a yellowish liquid humour, followed by fever, and only long afterwards by the raising of blood mixed with pus. Still others, in his own experience, died of phthisis, who had not coughed up blood during the entire illness.

Fernel gave a careful elucidation of his understanding of the etiology of phthisis. To him it was a disease of two causes: (1) a defective constitution of the lungs, and (2) a corrosive humour. He indicated that by defective constitution he meant, not a 'distemper', but rather a soft, delicate lung substance disposed to corruption. He stated unequivocally that some by birth and heredity were tainted with this hidden susceptibility, eventually becoming phthisic even though no distillation of noxious humour took place from the brain or other part of the body. These unfortunates, born phthisic, were inevitably disposed to phthisis by inheritance. He referred to the shape of the chest in this predisposition, citing Hippocrates' view that those

[4] *Aphorisms*, vii. 15.
[5] *ibid.*, v. 11.

who by nature had narrow and depressed chests were inclined to phthisis. Included in the predisposition, with this anatomical defect, was an additional factor in a characteristic listlessness and dullness, which accelerated the withering and deterioration.

The second cause of phthisis was threefold: (1) a corrosive outpouring from the head, (2) a sharp humour from the heart which was expelled into the lungs, particularly in the autumn, and (3) pus enclosed in the cavity of the thorax. Old concepts of Hippocrates will be recognized in all of these factors, including the seasonal enhancement of danger and the supposed relation with empyema.

Fernel referred to the insidiousness with which the process developed, without causing pain even to the most robust lungs. He took sharp exception to the view that rupture of pulmonary veins, resulting from falls, work, shouting, overheating, baths, drinking wine, eating hot foods to excess, or suppression of menses, even though followed by expectoration of great quantities of blood, led to phthisis. He stated that he knew persons who had lived a long time with no discomfort after such an event. No one became phthisic, he said, from simple rupture of a vein as long as the rest of the lung remained intact. If phthisis did result after such an event, it was because of the presence of an ulcer within the lung which became inflamed, began to decay and ended by destroying the lung.

Summary

On the whole Fernel had a limited and inadequate, but not wholly inaccurate, conception of phthisis. He made no reference to the tubercle as the unit of the disease, in spite of the hazy allusions of the ancient Greek authors and Galen to phymata in the lungs and elsewhere in phthisis. The tubercle was not to become established in scientific literature until the time of Sylvius de le Boë. Naturally he could not conceive of a microbial etiology at this very early date in medical science; but there was one extraordinary, although unfortunately isolated and undeveloped, reference to contagion.

On the other hand, he gave a good, although extremely short, clinical description of the course of the disease from its inception to a far-advanced state. Hemoptysis and even as striking a lesion as a cavity were recognized as complications of the disease and not pathognomonic of it.

Much of his conception was based on correlation of observations in the cadaver with the clinical syndrome of cough, fever, hemoptysis, copious, purulent expectoration, hectic flush and emaciation. These he traced to an original ulceration of the lung, and he accepted them as defining the disease.

His theories of the cause were drawn directly from the Hippocratic writers; i.e., the etiological agents were constitutional predisposition and the local effect of acrid humours.

He was well acquainted with the anatomical evidences of healed tuberculosis, as witnessed by his extraordinarily accurate descriptions of caseo-calcareous tubercles, but he quite failed to recognize their origin and relation to phthisis.

In view of Fernel's outstanding position among the physicians of Western Europe, and in view particularly of the extremely wide distribution given to his *Pathology*, there can be little doubt that his concepts were of great influence on the medical profession of his time. It was more than a hundred years before the treatise *De phthisi* of Sylvius de le Boë appeared, and Sylvius was not given to extensive quotation of others in developing his views. There seems little doubt, however, that in the growth leading up to Sylvius' description of phthisis the teaching of Fernel formed an important background. The transition from Fernel to Sylvius was not abrupt. Indeed, much of the text in Sylvius' influential tract is not significantly different from what is set forth in Fernel's *Medicina*.

THE PSYCHIATRY OF PARACELSUS *

by

IAGO GALDSTON

IN his *Paracelsica* Carl Jung says of Paracelsus:

Man kann ihm nicht gerecht werden; man kann ihn immer nur unter- oder überschätzen, und darum ist man mit der eigenen Bemühung, wenigstens einen Teil seines Wesens genügend zu erfassen, stets unzufrieden.[1]

However, despite Jung's perspicacious and somewhat despairing comment, it is very timely to scrutinize the psychiatry of Paracelsus. This not solely because we have entered upon the Atomic Age and thus have realized in an egregious fashion the dream of the alchemist, but also because the atomic bomb has in a rude and compelling manner obliged the scientist to take cognizance of the meaning of life. For in the main, and with but very few exceptions, the scientist has been loath to deal with meanings, and most of all with the meaning of life. With an almost arrogant pride the proverbial scientist announced himself to be agnostic in all such matters. His was the realm of the 'how'. The 'why' he left to the philosophers.

This disassociative process, by which the knowledge of matter was divorced from that of meaning, began at the time of Paracelsus. He was among the last of that small number of learned men who attempted to amalgamate the ancient and modern learnings. As he was unsuccessful in his own time, so with the passage of time he lost meaning for the successive generations of men who clung with increasing desperation to the mensurable data of science, and to whom all that was *unsichtbar* (imperceptible) was mysticism, and hence anathema. On the occasion of the four hundredth anniversary of his death, the Royal Society of Medicine heard this pronouncement on the personality, doctrines, and influence of Paracelsus:

It cannot be said that the abusive rantings of Paracelsus contributed to the general progress of science and medicine that began in the sixteenth century, principally as to the outcome of the diffusion of accurate knowledge by means of printed books. For he was a rude, circuitous obscurantist, not a harbinger of light, knowledge and progress.[2]

A more sympathetic appreciation is that of Charles Singer, who, though he finds Paracelsus violent, dramatic and repellent, is still willing to allow that his 'iconoclasm doubtless did something to deter men from the worship of the old idols.'[3] With genial tolerance Singer takes note of the 'general agreement among the learned and nebulous band of Paracelsists that their

---

* This essay, which was written for this volume, has since been published in the *Bulletin of the History of Medicine*, 1950, xxiv, 205–18, and is reprinted by permission.

[1] 'One cannot do him justice: one can only under- or over-value him, and for that reason one is always dissatisfied with one's own efforts to fathom at least a part of his being.' (C. G. Jung, *Paracelsica. Zwei Vorlesungen über den Arzt und Philosophen Theophrastus.* Zürich and Leipzig, 1942, p. 9.)

[2] H. P. Bayon, 'Paracelsus: Personality, doctrines and his alleged influence in the reform of medicine'. *Proc. Roy. Soc. Med.*, 1941–2, xxxv (Sect. Hist. Med.), 69–76.

[3] C. Singer, *From magic to science.* London, 1928, p. 105.

hero did indeed foreshadow the "new instauration"'.[4] The learned and nebulous band of Paracelsists, however, deems this the lesser of the credits due to their hero. Far more significant is his appreciation of the deficiencies, of the pits and traps that beset the new learning. Paracelsus could not have been either the patron or the disciple of Bacon, though as befits the case, Bacon found something to praise in Paracelsus. Paracelsus was more than suspicious of the persuasion that real knowledge comes through the dismemberment of the whole into its constituent parts. Centuries before the term *holism*[5] was coined to connote to the learned the quality of the whole derived from wholeness, which is greater than that derived from the sum of its parts, and long before *Gestalt* was applied to denote a psychological concept and to label a school of thought, Paracelsus espoused both thoughts in his criticisms of *der todten Anatomie*. 'In der todten Anatomie werdet ihr weder Natur noch Wesen erkennen', wrote Paracelsus. 'In the anatomy of the dead you will discern neither nature nor being. Basically it is of no value [that is, in understanding what goes on inside the living body]. Essence, uniqueness, quality (*Eigenschaft*), being and strength, that which is the highest in anatomy, is dead. This has not been dealt with as yet for it is common practice to disregard the best. But it is the living body that teaches the anatomist [the physician] health and disease, not the dead one: he requires therefore a living anatomy.'[6]

This persuasion, this conviction that only the living scene in all its multiform parts and in its innumerable inter-relations and inter-reactions, can provide some measure of understanding to those who are concerned with well-being and illness, in body and in mind, characterizes and distinguishes the whole of Paracelsus' thinking. This is in essence his challenge to the past and his exhortation to the future. In this light is his preoccupation with the macrocosm and microcosm to be understood. It is this insight that makes his psychiatry so very modern in spirit and viewpoint. 'Er ist nicht veraltet, sondern wächst mit der weiterlaufenden Zeit.'[7] For if modern psychiatry is distinguished in any respect, it is in its integrative character, in its willingness and competence to perceive man in relation to the whole world about him. The spokesmen of modern psychiatry do not employ the terms macrocosm and microcosm, but the essence of what is involved and implied in these terms is reflected in both their criticisms and avowals. Adolf Meyer, speaking on the theme 'The Contributions of Psychiatry to the Understanding

[4] *idem, ibid.*

[5] 'It is quite obvious for any impartial student that Paracelsus was remote from the attitude, methods and outlook of the modern scientist, i.e. the investigator of causality in the modern sense. Van Helmont definitely followed the ideal of the modern scientist, with no little success. Nevertheless, van Helmont realized the paramount importance of entities which are not accessible to causal analysis, especially in Biology, and subscribed, true to Paracelsus' tradition, to "Wholism," "Thinking in Analogies" and Symbolism.' (W. Pagel, *The religious and philosophical aspects of van Helmont's science and medicine.* Supplements to the *Bull. Hist. Med.*, No. 2. Baltimore, 1944, p. 15.)

[6] 'In der todten Anatomie werdet ihr weder Natur noch Wesen erkennen. Nutzt inwendig gar nichts. Essentia, Eigenschaft, Wesen und Kraft, so ist das höchst der Anatomie; ist abgestorben. Die ist bisher noch nicht tractirt worden; denn es ist gemeiner Brauch, das Beste wegzulassen. Aber der lebendige Leib ist es, der Gesundheit und Krankheit anatomatiziren lässt, nicht der todte; er fordert daher eine lebendige Anatomie.' (Paracelsus, *Grosse Chirurgie*, vol. iii, pp. 259–61.)

[7] R. Koch and E. Rosenstock, *Paracelsus. Krankheit und Glaube.* Stuttgart, 1923, p. 5. 'H has not become antiquated, but has grown with passing time.'

of Life Problems', said: 'The human organism can never exist without its setting in the world. All we are and do is of the world and in the world. The great mistake of an overambitious science has been the desire to study man altogether as a mere sum of parts, if possible, of atoms, or now of electrons, and as a machine, detached, by itself, because at least some points in the simpler sciences could be studied to the best advantage with this method of the so-called elementalist. It was a long time before willingness to see the large groups of facts, in their broad relations as well as in their inner structure, finally gave us the concept and vision of integration which now fits man as a live unit and transformer of energy into the world of fact and makes him frankly a consciously integrated psychobiological individual and member of a social group.'[8]

Paracelsus had written 'Der Mensch ist eine kleine Welt, ein Auszug aus der ganzen machina mundi. Im Menschen sind alle Eigenschaften der Welt in eins'.[9]

It is precisely this ample understanding of the little world within the great world, together with all its vast implications, that renders Paracelsus outstanding among psychiatric pioneers. With justice Jung sees in Paracelsus 'einen Bahnbrecher nicht nur der chemischen Medizin, sondern auch der empirischen Psychologie und der psychologischen Heilkunde. . . Er hat . . . in seiner Art die seelischen Phänomene in Betracht gezogen, wie wohl keiner der grossen Aerzte vor oder nach ihm'.[10]

The most common source of psychological conflict, the most common cause of psychopathology, is the emotional dissonance between man and the world he lives in. When the individual and the society in which he lives are not in psychological harmony, the individual is likely to become sick.[11] The psychoanalyst will describe this as a conflict between the *Id* and the *Super-ego*, or as between the primitive drives and the endogenous as well as the exogenous inhibitions. This formulation is fundamental to modern psychiatry and is shared by practically all schools. Paracelsus knew neither the *Id* nor the *Super-ego*, but he did know that those are sick in spirit in whom that which is *mortal* and that which is *immortal*, that which is *intelligent* and that which is *unintelligent*, are not compounded in the appropriate proportions and strengths.[12] He saw man as an amalgam of the divine and the mortal. With superb insight and with comparable vigour Paracelsus expounded his understanding of the human psyche. It is not possible, at least not for me, to translate his words so as to transmit even a

---

[8] A. Meyer, 'The contributions of psychiatry to the understanding of life problems', in *A psychiatric milestone*. New York, 1921, p. 25.

[9] 'Man is a small world (a microcosm) an extract of the whole *machina mundi*. In men are embodied all the qualities of the world.' (Paracelsus, *Astronomia magna*.)

[10] 'A trailblazer not only in medicinal chemistry but also in empirical psychology and psychotherapy. In his own way he took the phenomena of the soul into consideration, as none of the great physicians had done before him or after him.' (C. G. Jung, *op. cit.* (1), pp. 177, 128.)

[11] E. Jones, *Social aspects of psycho-analysis*. Lectures delivered under the Auspices of the Sociological Society. London, 1924, p. 6. 'The pathological states to which psycho-analysts have devoted most attention, the various disorders known as neuroses are themselves not so much diseases in the ordinary sense as forms of individual reaction to social situations, problems and difficulties.'

[12] J. Huser, *Die Bücher und Schriften des . . . Paracelsi*. 10 vols. Basel, 1589–91, vol. ix, pp. 1, 2.

modicum of their vigour and beauty. In the original one hears the overtones of his earnestness, of his fullness, of his eagerness. His words mirror a man of strength and conviction; a man too full of the consciousness of what he needs must say to be halted or gainsaid. 'Fleissig ist ein Aufmerkung zu haben auf die Geist der Menschen, dieweil ihr zween seind, die ihm angeboren anliegen.'[13] Rendered freely, the author counsels a diligent observation of the spirit (*Geist*) of man, 'which is composed of two parts, both of which are native to him. For man should live in the spirit of life and be a man, and should not live according to the spirit of Limbus [the primitive-primeval-chaotic] that will make of him an unintelligent creature. For it is indeed true that man is made in the image of God, and so he has a godly spirit in him. But then he is otherwise (*sonst*) an animal, and as such has an animal spirit; these two are antagonistic, and yet, however, the one must mollify the other. Therefore, man should not be a beast, but a man; to be a man, he must live in the spirit of life, of human life, and suppress (*hinwegtun*) the animal spirit (*viehischen Geist*). Therefore it is necessary to recognize both of the spirits, on the basis of which the true spirit of man is distinguishable from that of the animals'.[14]

In the book *Krankheiten so der Vernunft berauben* Paracelsus describes and distinguishes between different forms of psychopathy, including also the psychoneuroses. 'Viel seind die solch lunatisch Krankheit tragen, deren nicht geacht wird lunatisch zu sein. Denn vielerlei seind Narren, so seind auch vielerlei toub Leut, nicht ein Art, nit auf ein Weg, sondern in viel Weg, in viel Art, in viel Gestalt, und Form.'[15] 'Many are those who are ill who are not thought to be mentally sick (*lunatisch*). For as fools [simpletons, feeble-minded] are of many kinds, so also are there many kinds of crazy people (*toub Leut*) not of one sort, not in one way, but in many ways, of many sorts, in many patterns and forms.'

Paracelsus distinguishes clearly between the feeble-minded and the psychopathic (*die Narren und die Touben*). The former, he says, are born simple in mind, whereas the psychopathic are not born psychopathic. The feeble-minded behave in the wise of an intelligent animal, but the psychopathic in the manner of the irrational (*unsinnige tierische Geist*) animal. To illustrate his meaning, Paracelsus draws upon the analogy of a dog which, while healthy, barks and bites, but does so with the true intelligence of the dog. The feeble-minded may be said to behave in the way of the healthy animal. But the psychopathic behave like a dog deprived of its intelligence—in other words, like a mad dog, for they 'bite everyone and rage' (*wütet in alle Tiere*).

Under the caption of *Wahnsinn* Paracelsus describes mania, of which he recognizes two kinds, that which 'springs up' in the healthy body and that which is engendered by other sickness. The periodicity and self-limiting character of the disorder which he describes, as well as the tendency of its sufferers to recover spontaneously, make it evident that Paracelsus recognized

---

[13] *idem, ibid.*

[14] 'Das seind nun zwei widerwärtige, jedoch aber eins muss dem andern weichen. Nun soll der Mensch kein Tier sein, sondern ein Mensch: Soll er nun ein Mensch sein, so muss er aus dem Geist des Lebens des Menschenleben, und also hinwegtun den viehischen Geist. Nun ist not die zween Geist zu erkennen, auf dass der recht Geist des Menschen unterscheiden werde vor dem tierischen.' (*idem, ibid.*)

[15] *idem, ibid.*

what we to-day call manic-depressive psychosis. Paracelsus furthermore includes under the heading *Wahnsinn* four classes of disorders, which he describes as major psychoses ('die da allzeit bei unsinnigem und unvernünftigem Leben sind'[16]). These he names *Lunatici, Insani, Vesani, Melancholici.* It is not possible, the circumstances being unfavourable, to deal in particular with these four classes of disorders. It is, however, important, since Paracelsus is suspect to the uninformed, to underline the objective and scientific views held by Paracelsus on the origin and causation of the psychiatric disorders which he describes. 'Wir erkennen in den Krankheiten, so der Vernunft berauben, durch Experientirung, dass sie aus der Natur entspringen und kommen.'[17] 'We recognize by experience that the diseases which deprive man of his reason originate and come out of nature [are natural in origin].' In this passage Paracelsus furthermore mocks the priestly clan (*die Götterischen Verweser*) who ascribe such diseases to incorporeal creatures (*uncorporalischen Geschöpfen*) and diabolic spirits. To this belief he will not subscribe, for experience shows that the disorders have their origin in nature.[18]

Nor does Paracelsus prove any less objective and scientific in his approach to psychotherapy. Indeed, he was a psychosomaticist (with apologies for the term)[19] centuries before the concept was re-born and re-christened. Among the general causations of disease he lists as one the *Ens Spirituale*, which can be equated to the psychological factors of disease, somatic as well as psychological. In the section dealing with the effects of the *Ens Spirituale* Paracelsus writes: 'Now, then, you should observe and we point out to you that conscience overcomes the guilty one: similar are the effects of envy and hatred. And we have indicated this to you, so that you should understand how the *Ens Spirituale* so powerfully reigns over the body, that therefore many sicknesses, and all of the kinds of the sicknesses of man can be brought on; therefore you should apply treatment not as in ordinary diseases, but you should treat the spirit [psyche], for it is the spirit that here lies sick.'[20]

Paracelsus dwelt much on the effects of will and imagination on the human body. 'You should know', he wrote, 'that the effect of the will is of major

[16] *idem, ibid.,* pp. 45, 62. 'Those who are permanently afflicted with an insane and unintelligent way of life.'
'Also auch von der *Mania* geredt soll werden, die da ist allein ein Veränderung der Vernunft, und nit der Sinnen: Denn ihnen ist das Sinnen mit Gewalt eingebildet, und aber die Vernunft in ihnen garnichts ist. Und *Mania* kommt in der Gestalt, mit toben und unsinniger Weis, nimmer kein Ruh, viel Unglücks machen, und wird erkennet durch das, dass sie von ihnen selbst wieder nachlassen und aufhören, und zu der Vernunft wieder kommen. Und wiewohl das ist, dass *Mania* viel mal kommt nach dem und sie auch viel hinweg gehet und etlich ist, die nach ihrem Hinweggehn nimmer wieder kommt. Etlich nach dem Mond zufällig ist, etlich nach dem äussern Accidenten sich bewegen. So ist der Manien zwei Geschlecht: Eins, so von gesundem Leibe entspringt, und eins, so von andern Krankheiten erwachset.'

[17] *idem, ibid.,* vol. ix, 'Das siebente Buch in der Arzenei. *De Morbis Amentium*, das ist von den Krankheiten, die den Menschen der Vernunft berauben', pp. 38–92.

[18] *idem, ibid.*

[19] v. 'Biodynamic medicine versus psychosomatic medicine'. *Bull. Menninger Clinic,* 1944, viii, 4.

[20] 'Also wie wir euch anzeigen, sollet ihr merken, dass die Geist den Schuldigen gewältigen: Dergleichen auch die Wirkung verbringen des Neids und Hass. Und haben euch das darumb angezeigt, das ihr verstehen sollet, wie das *Ens Spirituale* so gewaltiglich herrschet über die Leib, dass also viel Krankheiten, und alle Geschlecht der Krankheiten dem Menschen mögen zugefügt werden: Daraufhin nit sollet Arzney brauchen als auf natürlich Krankheiten, sondern ihr sollt den Geist arzneyen, derselbig ist der, der da krank liegt.' (J. Huser, *op. cit.* (12), vol. i, p. 54.)

importance in medicine. For one who does not mean well with himself, and is hateful to himself, it is possible that such a person may be afflicted by the very curse he utters against himself. For cursing derives from the obfuscation (*Verhängung*) of the spirit. And it is also possible that the representations are by curses converted into sicknesses, into fevers, convulsive seizures, apoplexies, and such like so that they are brought about as indicated above.'[21] And with a warning no less timely to-day than when it was written, Paracelsus continues: 'And let this not be a jest to you, you physicians: you know not in the least part the power of the will; for the will is the genetrix of such spirits as the prudent will have no dealings with.'[22]

'Great, too, is the power of belief and of faith, for', wrote Paracelsus, 'belief is of itself capable of making every sort of herb! An invisible nettle, an invisible celandine [balsam], an invisible trioll: and therefore everything that grows in terrestrial nature the power of belief can likewise bring: therefore the power of belief can likewise create every sickness.'[23]

Faith, belief, will, and the passion account in the psychiatry of Paracelsus for many of the ills, and for some of the cures, witnessed in men. Paracelsus is particularly concerned with what we to-day term the primitive drives, and with the anti-social impulsions. He refers to these components of the human personality as *das Viehische im Menschen*—the brute, beast, or animal in man. To the predominance of these he traces the psychological ills in man. Furthermore, he maintains, in a passage of deep and subtle insight, that 'the human intelligence does not become mad, and is not subject to sickness. Hence it is of no profit to search in the human spirit; only in his brute intelligence, therein, reader, peruse. For it is a major achievement to understand the rantings of the lunatic'.[24]

It is only in recent times and largely through the illumination cast upon these matters by Freud and his co-workers that we have come to appreciate the possibility of understanding the 'rantings of the lunatic', and indeed it is 'a major achievement'. So, too, have we learned to understand the 'logicalness' of the paranoid and other psychopathological reasoning processes. The premises and conjunctions are at fault, but the deductions are keenly logical.

It is appropriate at this point to touch upon Paracelsus' use of the magnet in the treatment of somatic ailments, for this bears not only on the influence

[21] 'Aber ihr sollt wissen in euch, dass die Wirkung des Willens ein grosser Punct ist zu der Arzney. Denn einer der ihm selbst nichts Guts gönnet, und ihm selbst hass ist, ist möglich, dass das, so er ihm selbst flucht, ankommt: Denn fluchen kommt aus Verhängung des Geists. Und ist auch also möglich, dass die Bilder verflucht werden in Krankheiten, zu Febern, Epilepsien, Apoplexien, und dergleichen, so sie gemacht sind, wie oben stehet.' (*idem, ibid.*, vol. i, p. 53.)

[22] 'Und lasset euch das kein Scherz sein ihr Aerzte: Ihr wisset die Kraft des Willens nit den mindsten Teil: Denn der Will ist ein Gebärerin solcher Geisten, mit welchen der Vernünftig nichts zu schaffen hat.' (*idem, ibid.*, vol. i, p. 53.)

[23] 'Denn der Glaub vermag in ihm selbst alle Geschlecht der Kräuter zu machen, ein unsichtbare Nessel, ein unsichtbar Schölkraut, ein unsichtbar Trioll: Und also ein jedlich Ding das in der irdischen Natur wachst, das vermag auch die Stärk des Glaubens zu bringen: Also vermag auch der Glaub alle Krankheiten zu machen.' (*idem, ibid.*, vol. i, p. 251.)

[24] 'Denn die menschlich Vernunft wird nicht toub, empfächt auch kein Krankheit. Darum ist in derselbigen Menschen Geist nichts zu suchen, allein in seiner tierischen Vernunft, dieselbig, Leser, durchlies. Denn es ist ein grosses, den touben Wüterich zu verstehn, er ist nicht minder denn ein wütender Hund.' (*idem, ibid.*, vol. ix, pp. 1, 2.)

of the imagination, but is the derivative starting-point of modern psychiatry. The magnet, magnetism, mesmerism, hypnotism, suggestion, psychocatharsis, and psychoanalysis represent a series of stages in the progressive development of modern psychiatric thought and knowledge. The initial impulse to this development came from Paracelsus.

There is no indication that Paracelsus ascribed the influence of the magnet in the treatment of disease to any other quality than the *virtus attractiva macro- et microcosmi*. Imagination, faith, suggestion, did not enter into his account of the powers and operations of the magnet as *specific and separate factors*. Paracelsus was not handicapped by the dichotomy of body and soul that has plagued both philosophy and psychiatry since the advent of the Cartesian science.[25] Paracelsus could not have been guilty of such irrationalities as were uttered by the Commission of the French Academy of Science in its report on Mesmerism: 'L'imagination fait tout: le magnetisme nul.' It was quite sufficient for him to state the rationale of magnetic cures in simple and self-evident terms: 'For in the last analysis it is thus, that we contain within ourselves as many natural powers as heaven and earth possess. Can the magnet draw the iron to itself even though it appears to be a dead thing: so, too, can the dead person draw the living one to himself. Do the climbing vines reach out to the sun, so too well may man in similar manner have access to the sun. Can the planets draw one according to their wishes, so too can the dead body [i.e. the magnet]. These are all invisible works, and yet they are natural.'[26]

Paracelsus was fully cognizant of the existence of both folly and superstition, but he would not grant the existence of both natural and unnatural. Had he been confronted with this paradox, Paracelsus would have responded: 'the natural embraces all else'.[27] With keen insight and as if he were anticipating the criticism of later generations, Paracelsus stated: 'No instructed person ever remained misled, him no one has ever seen superstitious. Where is superstition? Indeed among those that understand nothing. Where is arrogance? But only among those who know nothing. Where is folly? But only among those content in their wisdom and who will seek no further in God's wisdom. And therefore when such an art is expounded and in their thick skulls they cannot fathom it, it must perforce be of the devil and magical.'[28]

Paracelsus recognized the existence of the devil but also that far too much was credited to his works. 'Ere the world comes to an end, many arts now

---

[25] v. I. Galdston, 'Descartes and modern psychiatric thought'. *Isis*, 1944, xxxv, pp. 118–28.

[26] 'Denn endlich ist das also, dass wir in uns haben so viel natürlicher Kräfte, als Himmel und Erden vermögen. Kann der Magnet das Eisen an sich ziehen, und scheint do wie ein tot Ding: So kann auch der tote Mensch den lebendigen an sich ziehen. Gehen die Bettler der Sonnen zu, so mag auch wohl ein Mensch dermassen ein Zugang haben. Können die Planeten einen ziehen nach ihrem Gefallen, so kann auch der tot Cörper dasselb. Das seind alles unsichtbare Werk, und doch natürlich.' (J. Huser, *op. cit.* (12), vol. i, pp. 297-8.)

[27] Goethe's Essay on Nature and its profound effect on Freud.

[28] 'Kein wissender Mann ist nie in Verführung blieben, ihn hat auch niemand aberglaubig gesehen. Wo ist der Aberglauben? Doch bei denen die nichts verstohn: Wo ist die Hoffart? Als allein bei den Unergründten: Wo ist die Torheit? Als allein bei denen, die in ihren Weisheiten bleiben und weiter in Gottes Weisheit nit fahren. Und darum so eine Kunst geoffenbart wird, und sie in ihrem dollen Schädel nit mag unergründet werden, so muss sie teufelisch und zauberisch sein.' (J. Huser, *op. cit.* (12), vol. i, pp. 317, 318.)

ascribed to the work of the devil must become revealed, and it will then be evident, that most of these effects depend upon natural forces.'[29]

It is not possible here to deal amply with the so-called demonology of Paracelsus. Yet it would help to understand *his* devil if we equated him to the *death instinct* of Freud. Between the two there is much in common. Both are destructive forces—the one stands opposed to Eros, the other to God. Jung, who among the contemporary psychiatrists is best equipped to fathom and to interpret the demonology of Paracelsus, astutely observes: 'For us, the so-called moderns, his Homunculi, Trarames, Durdales, Nymphs, Melusine, etc. are certainly close to the crassest of superstitions, but for his time, not at all. These figures were still alive and effective in those times. They were indeed projections; but even of this he had some appreciation, in that, as is evidenced by many passages, he ascribed the origin of the Homunculi and other apparitions to imagination. His primitive perspectives led him to endow the projection with a reality which, in the light of psychological effects, was far more warranted than is our rationalistic presupposition on the absolute unreality of the projected content.'[30]

Paracelsus was not a mystic in the true sense of the word. He mystifies us to-day, but that is largely because our culture has lost the essential skill for dealing with the problems of being in the encompassing manner that was common to his age, and of which he was a master. And here it is pertinent to observe that Paracelsus was not a psychiatrist in the definitive sense of that term. Indeed he probably would have considered such specialization a degradation both of the physician's position and of his obligations. He dealt with mental illness. He studied experience and evolved a classification of the disorders and a rationale of psychopathology. It is proper, therefore, to speak of the psychiatry of Paracelsus. But he nowhere appears to have visualized the speciality of psychiatry. This observation is pertinent to the fact that much of his best psychiatric insight and understanding is revealed in those of his works which do not deal by title or otherwise with psychiatric disorders. It is, for example, most interesting to see how much psychiatric wisdom enters into his writings on 'the female'. 'Darumb so ist die Frau ein ander *Subjectum* denn der Mann. Denn ihr Wurzen dienet zu der Nahrung: Des Mannes stehet still im Mann.'[31] 'Therefore is woman a different subject from man. For her roots serve to nourish; the man's remained fixed in man.' Woman is the 'smallest world' and is quite different from the microcosm-man, 'has a different anatomy, *Theoricam, Causas, Rationes, Curas.* And no matter how much like man in many illnesses, yet

[29] 'Ehe die Welt untergeht, müssen noch viele Künste, die man sonst der Wirkung des Teufels zuschrieb, offenbar werden, und man wird alsdann einsehen, dass die meisten dieser Wirkungen von natürlichen Kräften abhängen.' (Quoted in M. B. Lessing, *Handbuch der Geschichte der Medizin,* Berlin, 1938, p. 366.)

[30] 'Seine Homunculi, Trarames, Durdales, Nymphen, Melusinen usw. sind zwar zunächst krassester Aberglaube für uns sogenannt Moderne, für seine Zeit aber keineswegs. Diese Figuren lebten und wirkten noch in jenen Zeiten. Es waren zwar Projektionen; aber auch davon hatte er eine Ahnung, indem er, wie aus zahlreichen Stellen hervorgeht, um die Entstehung der Homunculi und sonstigem Spuk aus der Imagination wusste. Seine primitive Anschauung schrieb den Projektionen eine Realität zu, welche deren psychologischer Wirkung um vieles gerechter wurde als unsere rationalistische Voraussetzung der absoluten Unwirklichkeit projizierter Inhalte.' (C. G. Jung, *op. cit.* (1), pp. 128–9.)

[31] J. Huser, *op. cit.* (12), vol. i, pp. 194–5.

it is for the physician to distinguish her from the other, that is, from man, for she is a different world.'[32]

Paracelsus evaluates quite fully the role of the procreative function in shaping the physical, the psychological, the nosological, and the psycho-pathological constitution of the female. But there was nothing of the misogynist in Paracelsus; on the contrary, he prized the 'female of the species'. 'Wer kann einer Frauen Feind sein, sie sei gleich wie sie woll?' 'Who can be an enemy of woman, be she as she will. For it is with her fruits that the world is settled, therefore God grants her long life, even though she were a shrew.'[33]

Jung, in his account of the inner personality of Paracelsus, lays much weight upon the fact that Paracelsus was bereft of his mother at the age of nine. This traumatic experience, together with the fact that his father never remarried and remained for many years his son's teacher and companion, undoubtedly did have a profound influence upon Paracelsus' attitude toward womankind.

Perhaps the richest psychiatric yield is to be derived from those of Paracelsus' writings which are concerned with the immortal, the cosmic, the godly, phases of the human being. Here we are confronted not only with the equivalent of the *Super-ego* of modern psychiatry, but we witness also the appreciation which Paracelsus had of the Unconscious, and what in present-day terms is called the phylogenetic components of the psyche.

All of this was not known to Paracelsus, nor yet was it mysterious. It was logically deduced by Paracelsus from his cosmological premises (the relations of macro- to microcosm), and intuitively appreciated. There was a deep impulse operative in Paracelsus to be concerned with such unsettled and undetermined matters, an impulse which the present generation can well appreciate. 'The physician should talk of [treat and be concerned with] the invisible [imperceptible] and know the perceptible.'[34] 'He who knows the imperceptible, is a physician, the imperceptible that which has no name, that which is without substance [insubstantial] and yet has effect.'[35] Paracelsus is deeply concerned with the double nature of man, with his temporality and with his timeless ties with all the universe, with his substantiality and with his immaterial effects upon the universe. He experienced no difficulties in visualizing in what manner this double nature of man could serve to account for health and for illness. In all this he was neither slavish nor fatalistic. The macrocosm rules the microcosm, but the relation is reciprocal. As the Greeks taught that 'character is destiny', so Paracelsus taught 'Der Charakter des Menschen meistert das Gestern' (The character of man masters the stars).

[32] 'Die Frau hat im selbigen ein Gebresten, sie ist die kleineste Welt, und ist ein anders dann der Mann, und hat seine andere Anatomey, *Theoricam, Causas, Rationes, Curas:* Und aber, wiewohl gleich in viel Krankheiten mit dem Mann, das ist aber dem Arzt zu unterscheiden von einander, das ist, vom Mann, denn sie ist ein andere Welt.' (*idem, ibid.,* vol. i, p. 190.)

[33] 'Wer kann einer Frauen Feind sein, sie sei gleich wie sie woll? Denn mit ihren Früchten wird die Welt besetzt, darumb sie Gott lang leben lässt, ob sie gleich gar ein Gall wäre.' (*idem, ibid.,* vol. i, p. 309.)

[34] 'Von dem nun, das unsichtbar ist, soll der Arzt reden, und das sichtbar ist, soll ihm in Wissen stehen. . . .' (*idem, ibid.,* vol. ii, p. 138.)

[35] 'Der ist ein Arzt, der das unsichtbare weiss, das kein Namen hat, das kein Materie hat, und hat doch sein Wirkung.' (*idem, ibid.*)

The whole of Paracelsus' teachings sum up to an effort to perceive and understand man in his physiological and psychological functions, within the framework of nature and the universe, from which he is not set apart, but of which he is rather a component.

Of the Paracelsian treatment of psychic disorders, there is little that needs to be said. His therapy is founded on and conforms to his understanding of the etiology of the disorders. Some have stressed the odd and the bizarre in the Paracelsian therapy, but it can be easily demonstrated that such writers either fail to understand or misconstrue the intent of the treatment they criticize. Blood-letting seems barbaric to us, yet in the instance of mania with much agitation is it any less 'barbaric' to quieten the patient by means of the barbiturates than by blood-letting? Paracelsus advised drilling holes in the patient's skull to let out mania. Is prefrontal leucotomy any less or more rational a procedure? It is, however, not the gross and violent therapeutic procedures advocated by Paracelsus, but his more sedate, basic, common ones that deserve notice. Paracelsus believed in psychotherapy, in the manner practised to-day. He believed in persuasion, exhortation, instruction, fasting, and prayer. He set great value on the therapeutic effects of sleep and advised the use of hypnotics. He believed in the self-healing powers of the soul, *die Heilkraft der Seele*. The violent and hopelessly insane he advised should be incarcerated. In relation to this, it should be borne in mind that Paracelsus firmly believed that every disease was curable, and also that compassion was the physician's crowning gift and virtue. *Barmherzigkeit ist ein Schulmeister der Artzten.*

Coming to the end of this brief sketch of the psychiatry of Paracelsus, I can attest to the validity of Jung's words. *Man ist mit der eigenen Bemühung, wenigstens einen Teil seines Wesens genügend zu erfassen, stets unzufrieden.* How can one be satisfied when the subject is so vast and the man unfathomable, *unerschöpflich*, inexhaustible? Then, too, there is the tantalizing problem of one's interest in Paracelsus, which is never academic, but always freighted with emotions and barbed with psychological implications. My own interest is never in the direction of modernizing Paracelsus. He was, is, and ever will remain, man of the sixteenth century. Nor would I be a follower of that fatuous sport that scans the past for precursors of Freud. To that motley crew of historical scavengers, someone, somehow, should make clear that all the past and all the past holds of men, things and thought, are precursors to every man that follows in the chain of unfolding generations. My interest in Paracelsus has its different roots. It arises out of the appreciation that in his *Anschauung*, in the embrace of his thoughts, there is much that has meaning and inspiration for us to-day. We have come round the bend and completed the circle. Once again we can contemplate heaven and earth, man and the firmaments, within one intelligible framework.

Yet there are those who will not agree. On that score only this need be said. Many among us, confronted with the eternity that is within us (that which Paracelsus termed *unsichtbar*), are frightened, and in their fear, deny what they beheld, and berate those who lifted the curtain.

Finally, I have dealt with the psychiatry of Paracelsus, because it is a psychiatry which, I believe, has taught us and will continue to teach us to understand and to prize the eternal, the unfathomable and *das Unsichtbare* in man.

SIR THOMAS MORE AS STUDENT OF MEDICINE AND PUBLIC HEALTH REFORMER

by

SIR ARTHUR SALUSBURY MacNALTY

SIR EDWIN CHADWICK has been called the Father of English Sanitation; his teaching promoted the study of hygiene, while his 'sanitary idea' has been influential alike in medicine and legislation, and especially in administrative reforms directed to securing wholesome environment and inculcating the gospel of cleanliness.

'There were great men before Agamemnon', and a great forerunner of Edwin Chadwick in public health reform was Thomas More. More is renowned as saint and martyr; he was an eloquent orator, an eminent statesman and legislator, Speaker of the House of Commons, royal ambassador and Lord Chancellor, a master of English prose and a classical scholar. These notable distinctions, these great gifts united in one man, in the very blaze of their glory have obscured Sir Thomas's teaching and work in public health and social medicine.

The study of this somewhat neglected aspect of Sir Thomas More's career is based on Tudor State papers, in passages from his own writings and letters, in the letters and writings of his contemporaries, and in biographies and other books.

Thomas More (1478–1535) was the only surviving son of Sir John More, afterwards a judge of the king's bench, and Agnes, daughter of Sir Thomas Grainger. Sir John is credited with the jest 'that a man seeking a wife is like one putting his hand into a bag of snakes with one eel among them: he may light on the eel, but it is a hundred chances to one that he shall be stung with a snake'. He seems to have been a gentle and upright man and his son, when Chancellor, is said to have invariably visited his father's court to ask his blessing before presiding in his own court.

Thomas went to a City school, that of Saint Anthony's in Threadneedle Street. At the age of thirteen he was placed in the household of John Morton, Archbishop of Canterbury and Lord Chancellor, who prophesied that he would prove 'a marvellous rare man'. Here he took impromptu parts in plays at Christmas and collected material for his life of Richard III from Morton's lips.

The liberal education, beginning at Oxford, which Thomas More received, well equipped him for his future work. For two years (1492–4) he was an undergraduate at Canterbury Hall, Oxford, which was afterwards absorbed in Christ Church. Here he came under the influence of the Humanists, Linacre and Grocyn, who had brought the new learning from Italy. His studies were chiefly Latin, although he may have then been initiated into Greek. Greek was, however, not part of the regular curriculum and was frowned on by the Schoolmen. He also studied French, mathematics and history, and learned to play on the viol and flute. Alarmed at these exotic studies, Sir John More removed his son from the University before he had taken his degree and entered him at New Inn to read law. He became a member of Lincoln's Inn in 1496, was called to the outer bar in 1501 and was appointed reader or lecturer on law at Furnival's Inn.

Thomas had fulfilled his father's hopes by becoming proficient in jurisprudence, but he did not neglect to cultivate the humane studies which had so strongly appealed to him at Oxford and which Bishop Fisher was promoting at Cambridge. His instruction was facilitated by the fact that the Oxford teachers had come to London. William Grocyn was vicar of Saint Lawrence Jewry, Thomas Linacre was tutor to Prince Arthur and a London physician, and Colet was shortly to become Dean of St. Paul's. More wrote to his friend John Holt in 1501:

> You will ask me how I am getting on with my studies. Excellently; nothing could be better. I am giving up Latin and taking to Greek. Grocyn is my teacher.

And he wrote to Colet, his spiritual director, in 1504:

> Meantime I pass my time with Grocyn who is, as you know, in your absence the guide of my life; with Linacre, the guide of my studies; and with our friend Lily, my dearest friend.

More and Lily worked together translating epigrams from the Greek anthology into Latin, though their book was not published until More was forty.

In 1499 More met the Dutch scholar, Erasmus. This was the beginning of a lifelong friendship. He presented Erasmus to Prince Henry, afterwards Henry VIII, then a child of nine years of age. More presented the prince with a poem. This is the first recorded meeting of More with his future royal master.

While enjoying the intellectual companionship of his friends and lecturing on law, More hesitated between Law and Holy Orders. For some four years 'he gave himself to devotion and prayer in the Charterhouse of London'. In the end he decided not to take the vows. This was largely on the advice of Dean Colet, although his father's wishes that he should follow the law no doubt had their weight. But to the end of his life he wore a hair-shirt, scourged himself and practised religious austerities; and he told his daughter, Margaret, in the Tower that had it not been for his wife and children he would long before have closed himself in the cell of a monk. More's religion, as we know from his writings, was the staff and stay of his life.

In 1501, at Grocyn's invitation, he lectured in the Church of Saint Lawrence Jewry on Saint Augustine's *De Civitate Dei*. The lectures were historical and philosophical and possibly criticized the social evils of the time. The chief and best learned men of the City of London came to hear him.

The Influence of Linacre

We know that Thomas More read Aristotle, for he speaks of attending Linacre's course on the *Meteorologica*.[1] This study must not only have trained Thomas in politics, ethics and political economy, but probably interested him in biology and natural history. In Holbein's portrait of

[1] More, *Lucubrationes*, 1563, p. 417 ('Ad Dorpium').

More and his family, the artist has sketched in a small monkey beginning to climb up Lady More's dress. Further evidence of More's love of animals is obtained from Erasmus, who wrote of him:

> One of his great delights is to consider the forms, the habits, and the instincts of different kinds of animals. There is hardly a species of bird that he does not keep in his house, and rare animals, such as monkeys, foxes, ferrets, weasels and the like.[2]

The interest in natural history, as often happens, was associated with an interest in medicine and public health, and it is scarcely an assumption to say that More derived this from his Greek tutor, Thomas Linacre, who was equally renowned as physician and classical scholar. Thomas Linacre (1460 ?-1524), Fellow of All Souls, Oxford, travelled to Italy about 1485-6, in the suite of his old tutor, William de Selling, who was ambassador from Henry VII to the Pope. He went to Florence, where he was cordially received and given full facilities for classical studies by Lorenzo de Medici. A year later, at Rome, the great scholar, Hermolaus Barbarus, introduced Linacre to the study of Aristotle, Dioscorides, Pliny and other medical writers. He graduated as M.D. at Padua with a brilliant disputation, spent some time at Vicenza, and after six years returned to England to be incorporated M.D. at Oxford and to lecture in the University. In 1500 or 1501 Linacre was appointed tutor to Prince Arthur, and soon after the accession of Henry VIII became the royal physician. He received a number of ecclesiastical preferments and after being a deacon was admitted to priest's orders in 1520. He is, of course, famous for the large share he took in elevating the standard of medical education and in the foundation of the Royal College of Physicians in 1518, of which he was the first president. He founded medical lectureships bearing his name at Oxford and Cambridge, for which it is interesting to note that Sir Thomas More, Tunstall, Bishop of London, and two other persons were appointed trustees. He died of the stone and was buried in the old cathedral of Saint Paul. His skill as a physician was high, and he numbered among his patients Cardinal Wolsey, Archbishop Warham and Bishop Fox, besides his own friends, Colet, More, Erasmus, Lily and other scholars.

Linacre wrote several grammatical works and translated Galen into Latin. Erasmus mentions other completed works laid up in Linacre's desk, unpublished. It is not improbable that one or more of these lost works dealt with public health, for both Linacre's pupils, Sir Thomas More and Sir Thomas Elyot, were interested in the preventive aspect of disease and the preservation of health. We can then, I submit, reasonably surmise that More learned much from Linacre, and that this teaching led him to become a pioneer in public health administration.

More's Interest in Medicine

There is an extraordinary and prevalent error that classical studies are antagonistic to the study of science. Thus in public schools there are classical and modern sides, and the intending biologist, chemist, physicist and doctor neglects his general education in order to rush into the laboratory. But

[2] Letter to Ulrich von Hutten, 23 July 1519.

science derives from classical studies.   The Greeks opened the portals of science, and mankind owes them an incalculable debt for this.   Hippocrates was the father of scientific medicine and Aristotle, a great comparative anatomist, urged Alexander the Great to establish a body of learned men with many of the aims of the present Medical Research Council.   It was because the Renaissance embodied the principles of Greek thought and learning that Padua and Montpellier became such famous Universities; and that when the new learning came to England it paved the way for the discoveries of William Harvey and John Hunter, of Jenner, Pasteur and Lister, and so on towards the epoch-making triumphs of medical research and preventive medicine in our own time.   All these wonders can be traced back to the Greeks, but the lesson has been forgotten.   The Oxford humanists were wiser in their own generation.   Richard Fox, Bishop of Winchester, founded Corpus Christi College, Oxford, in 1516 in the interests of the new learning, with provision for a teacher of Greek and a reader in divinity. There was opposition from the Schoolmen, to whom this new foundation was a challenge.   More, with the king's approval, in 1518 wrote a letter to the Fathers and Proctors of the University of Oxford commending the value of Greek studies, and at his request Wolsey sent a royal letter commanding all students in Oxford to study Greek.   That injunction was strictly obeyed for over four hundred years, until the abolition of compulsory Greek in 1920.

In the sixteenth century, the study of Greek not infrequently led on to that of medicine, and Thomas More encouraged this departure in his own household.   The house at Chelsea was always full of scholars and pupils. Nicholas Kratzer, Henry VIII's astronomer, was a frequent visitor, and so were Erasmus and other scholars from overseas.   More believed in the higher education of women and his daughters were liberally educated. Erasmus wrote to Ulrich von Hutten in the letter to which previous reference has been made:

> I should rather call his house a school, or universitie of Christian religion, for there is none therein but readeth or studieth the liberall sciences; their speciall care is pietie and vertue, there is no quarelling or intemperate words heard, none seen idle, which household that worthy gentleman doth not govern by proude and loftie words, but with all kind and courteous benevolence: everybody performeth his dutie; yet is there always alacratie; neither is sober mirth anie thing wanting.

There are at least three instances of members of More's learned household studying medicine.   The first is Margaret Gigs, the foster-sister of More's daughter Margaret, who was to him 'as dear as though she were a daughter'. As a child she committed small faults in order to have the pleasure of a gentle reproof from More.   She was a Greek scholar, fond of mathematics, and studied medicine.   More relates in the *Second Booke of Comfort against Tribulacion*, that when he lay in a tertian fever, symptoms arose which baffled his two physicians, but Margaret Gigs, then a young girl, identified the condition in Galen's *De differentiis febrium*.   More made Margaret Gigs his almoner for his out-door charities, and she married John Clement, whom she had known from a child, and helped him in his medical work and classical studies.   She was cast in an heroic mould.   In 1535 ten Carthusian monks who refused to acknowledge Henry VIII as head of the Church were barbarously imprisoned in Newgate. They were kept standing bolt upright, tied with iron collars fast by the necks to the posts of the prison, and great fetters fast rived on their legs with great iron bolts; so straitly tied that they could neither lie nor sit nor otherwise ease themselves, and they were left without food to die. For many days Margaret Clement fed them, having bribed the gaoler to allow her to enter the prison with food, disguised as a milkmaid. At length the terrified gaoler refused to admit her any more and all but one of these unfortunate men died. On her death-bed, in exile at Mechlin in 1570, Margaret told her husband that these monks stood about her bed and bade her come away with them.

I must refer next to one illustrious Tudor physician, perhaps the most lovable of them all. John Clement, M.D. Oxon, was brought up in the household of Sir Thomas More. More took Clement with him on his embassy to Bruges, and said of him: 'He is so proficient in Latin and Greek that I have great hopes of his becoming an ornament to his country and to literature.' That aspiration was fulfilled. In 1519 Clement settled in Corpus Christi College, Oxford, having been appointed Wolsey's rhetoric reader in the University and later professor of Greek. More wrote to Erasmus:

> My Clement lectures at Oxford to an audience larger than has ever gathered to any other lecturer. It is astonishing how universal is the approbation and love he gains. Even those to whom classical literature was almost anathema attend his lectures and gradually modify their opposition. Linacre, who, as you know never praises any one very much, admires him greatly, so that if I did not love Clement so much, I should be almost tempted to envy the praise he wins.

In 1521 Clement went abroad to study medicine and classical literature at Lyons, Padua and Siena. Clement's wife and former pupil, Margaret Gigs, was deeply read both in Greek and medicine, and helped him in his work. He became F.R.C.P. in 1528, and in the following year was one of the physicians sent by Henry VIII to Wolsey when he lay ill at Esher after his fall from power. In 1544 Clement was elected President of the College of Physicians. Constant, like More, in his attachment to the old faith, Clement retired to Louvain when Edward VI ascended the throne. He returned to England in Mary's reign, but the accession of Elizabeth drove him once more abroad. He died at Mechlin in 1572. His writings relate to classical studies,[3] and he does not seem to have given the world the benefit of his medical knowledge.

More's third medical protégé was Richard Hyrde. He was tutor to More's children, and when Margaret Roper translated Erasmus' *Treatise on the Pater Noster*, Hyrde contributed an introduction in English which justified the right of women to a scholarly education. Hyrde's study of Greek authors attracted him to medicine. As physician he accompanied Bishop Gardiner on his embassy to the Pope in 1528 and died of a chill.

Now it is clear that this study of medical authors and constant intercourse with the best physicians of the day were essential features in the development of Thomas More as an enlightened public health reformer. Edwin Chadwick,

---

[3] Clement wrote a criticism of Gallus. He was the author of *Carmina et Epigrammata, lib. I.;* of *Translations of the Epistles of St. Gregory Nazienzen;* of the *Homilies of Nicephorus Calixtus;* and of the *Epistles of Pope Celestin to Cyrillus, Bishop of Alexandria.*

great as he was, necessarily based his legislative reform on the reports of Southwood Smith, Arnott, Kay and other medical pioneers, and in the process acquired much medical knowledge. Later still, Sir Robert Morant was a walking encyclopaedia of medical knowledge collected from many sources.

Like these great civil servants, Thomas More was no mean amateur in medicine. When his daughter, Margaret, fell so ill of the sweating sickness, probably in 1528, that 'by no invention or devices she could be kept from sleep, so that both physicians and all other there despaired of her recovery and gave her over', More, on his knees in prayer, thought of a remedy which, when he told the physicians, they marvelled that they had not themselves remembered. The remedy was administered—unfortunately we are not told its nature—and the patient was restored to perfect health.[4]

More's writings contain many illustrations and comparisons drawn from his medical knowledge. This is strikingly exemplified in his unfinished treatise, *De Quatuor Novissimis*, 'The Four Last Things', written in 1522 when he had just been knighted and was Under-Treasurer. It is a meditation on death, and he described the book as 'a short medicine, containing only four herbs, common and well known, that is to wit, death, doom, pain and joy'.

> For what would a man give for a sure medicine that it should all his life keep him from sickness, namely, if he might by the avoiding of sickness be sure to continue his life one hundred years.

In Sir Thomas's last book, *A Dialoge of Comfort against Tribulacion*, written in 1534 when he was imprisoned in the Tower of London, there are again many instances culled from the author's medical lore. Extracts from these two books will sufficiently indicate the medical cast of Sir Thomas's mind.

Of apothecaries and medicines. An allusion to the polypharmacy of the time:

> The physician sendeth his bill to the apothecary and therein writeth sometime a costly receipt of many strange herbs and roots, fetched out of far countries, long lien drugs, all the strength worn out, and some none such to be gotten. [*D. Q. N.*]

More compared pagan philosophers with apothecaries:

> Some good drugs have they yet in their shops for which they may be suffered to dwell among our poticaries, if their medicines be not made of their own brains, but after the bills made by the great physician God, prescribing the medicines himself, and correcting the faults of their erroneous receipts. For without this way taken with them, they shall not fail to do, as many bold blind poticaries do: which either for lucre, or of a foolish pride, give sick folk medicines of their own devising, and therewith kill up in corners many such simple folk, as they find so foolish to put their lives in such lewd and unlearned blind bayardes[5] hands. [*Dialoge of Comfort.*]

Speaking of the spiritual medicine for sin he writes:

> This short medicine is of a marvellous force, able to keep us all our life from sin. The physician cannot give no one medicine to every man to keep him from sickness,

---

[4] Roper (see bibliography).
[5] Bayarde—one recklessly blind to the light of knowledge.

but to divers men divers, by reason of the diversity of divers complexions. This medicine serveth every man. The physician doth but guess and conjecture that his receipt shall do good; but this medicine is undoubtedly sure.

Treacle as a prophylactic.   More speaks of the prevalent belief that treacle was a prophylactic against infectious disease:

For folk fare commonly as he doth that goeth forth fasting among sick folk for sloth rather than he will take a little treacle before.

And again,

Now if a man be so dainty-stomached, that going where contagion is, he would grudge to take a little treacle, yet were he very nicely wanton if he might not at the leastwise take a little vinegar and rose-water in his handkerchief. [*D. Q. N.*]

Idiosyncrasies in diet:

Like as a sick man feeleth no sweetness in sugar, and some women with child have such fond lust that they had liefer eat terre [earth] than treacle, and rather pitch than marmalade, and some whole people love tallow better than butter, and Iceland loveth no butter till it be long barrelled.   [*D. Q. N.*]

Mind and body.   More often speaks of the influence of mind over matter, for instance:

The spiritual pleasure is of truth so sweet that the sweetness thereof many times darketh and minisheth the feeling of bodily pain . . . and credible is it that the inward pleasure and comfort, which many of the old holy martyrs had in the hope of heaven, darked and in manner overwhelmed the bodily pains of their torments. [*D. Q. N.*]

Nor let no man think strange, that I would advise a man to take counsel of a physician for the body in such a spiritual passion.   For sith the soul and the body be so joined together, that they both make between them one person, the distemperance of either other, engendereth some time the distemperance of both twain.   [*Dialoge of Comfort.*]

The pains of death.   He describes the pains of death:

lying in thy bed, thy head shooting, thy back aching, thy veins beating, thy throat rattling, thy flesh trembling, thy mouth gaping, thy nose sharping, thy legs cooling, thy fingers fumbling, thy breath shorting, all thy strength fainting, thy life vanishing, and thy death drawing on!   [*D. Q. N.*]

It is a vivid and accurate picture, and Shakespeare, when he put into the mouth of Mistress Quickly that account of Falstaff's death-bed, may have borrowed from it.

A medical allegory.   More, in *De Quatuor Novissimis*, defines a medicine as such a thing as, either applied outwardly to thy body or received inward shall preserve thee against that sore or sickness that else would put thee or some part of thee in peril.

and for the purpose of his allegory he regards our life as an incurable sickness with meat and drink as a medicine:

by which is resisted the peril and undoubted death that else should in so few days follow by the inward sickness of our own nature continually consuming us within.

He refers later to leprosy, the falling sickness, colic and the stone, and the itch of a sore leg.

Treatment of the primary infective focus.   Thomas More knew that in treating disease it was necessary to treat the primary infective focus, the *fons et origo mali.*   He wrote:

> It is in physic a special thing necessary to know where and in what place of the body lieth the beginning and as it were the fountain of the sore from which the matter is always ministered unto the place where it appeareth (for, the fountain once stopped, the sore shall soon heal of itself, the matter failing that fed it, which continually resorting from the fountain to the place, men may well daily purge and cleanse the sore, but they shall hardly heal it).   [*D. Q. N.*]

A medical dissertation on gluttony.   The chapter on gluttony, in which he includes alcoholic excess, is a medical excursus on the subject.   I give two extracts in illustration.

> If God would never punish gluttony, yet bringeth it punishment enough with itself; it disfigureth the face, discoloureth the skin, and disfashioneth the body, it maketh the skin tawny, the body fat and fobby, the face drowsy, the nose dropping, the mouth spitting, the eyes bleared, the teeth rotten, the head hanging, and the feet tottering, and finally no part left in right course and frame.   And beside the daily dulness and grief that the unwieldy body feeleth by the stuffing of the paunch so full, it bringeth in by leisure the dropsy, the colic, the stone, the strangary, the gout, the cramp, the palsy, the pox, the pestilence and the apoplexy— diseases and sickness of such kind that either shortly destroy us, or else, that worse is, keep us in such pain and torment that the longer we live the more wretched we be.

> Thus fare we, saith Plutarch, that through intemperate living drive ourselves into sickness and botch us up with physic, where we might with sober diet and temperance have less need of physic and keep ourselves in health.   [*D. Q. N.*]

In his keen observation, in his reflection and deductions and in his dislike of over-drugging, More had all the endowments of a wise physician.   From the quotations I have given, it is apparent that he would have been a great one if he had chosen medicine as his profession.   Evidently, he was intensely interested in medical studies and in the art of healing.

Commissioner of Sewers

On 3 September 1510 the young lawyer, Thomas More, was appointed one of the Under-Sheriffs of the City of London.   His appointment was made on account of his legal knowledge, for the Under-Sheriff was the legal permanent official who advised the Sheriff in those numerous cases which came under his jurisdiction.   In addition, this office gave him opportunity to advise the City Fathers on measures of sanitary reform, in which he was so much interested, and this interest was further shown by his appointment in 1514 as one of the Commissioners of Sewers along Thames Bank between East Greenwich and Lambeth.   Though much of the work was riparian in character and directed towards preventing encroachments of the sea, flooding of low grounds and maintenance of river banks, regulations were also made against trade effluents, deposits of rubbish in rivers, and pollution of rivers, streams and wells.   The larger towns were provided with a regular water system with public stand-pipes, and water sometimes was laid on to the houses. London for a long time had been well supplied with water, but under the Tudors seven or eight more conduits were set up from which fresh water was hawked about the streets in barrels. The improvement of London's water supply was much in More's mind when he described the river of Anyder on which Amaurota, the chief city of Utopia, was situated. Anyder, like the Thames, is a tidal river:

> When the sea floweth in, for the length of thirtie miles it filleth all the Anyder with salte water, and driveth back the freshe water of the ryver. . . . They have also another river which indede is not verie great. But it runneth gently and pleasauntly. For it riseth even oute of the same hill that the citie standeth upon, and runneth down a slope into the middes of the citie into Anyder. And because it riseth a little withoute the citie, the Amaurotians have inclosed the heade springe of it, with stronge fences and bulwarkes, and so have joyned it to the citie. This is done to the intente that the water should not be stopped nor turned away, or poysoned, if their enemies should chaunce to come upon them. From thence the water is derived and conveied downe in cannels of bricke divers ways into the lower partes of the citie. Where that cannot be done, by reason that the place wyll not suffer it, there they gather the raine water in great cisternes, wiche doeth them as good service.

These are the words of an enlightened public health administrator, and throughout his career More, despite the claims of high office, continued with his work for the improvement of England's water supplies. In 1526 he was again appointed Commissioner of Sewers by the coast of Thames, from East Greenwich to Gravesend,[6] and, as Lord Chancellor, he probably initiated the important Act of Parliament (23 Hen. VIII, c. 5) which appointed Commissioners of Sewers in all parts of the Kingdom. The water of England was notoriously unsafe. Henry VII in a letter to Ferdinand and Isabella said it was undrinkable, and therefore the young princess, Katherine of Aragon, betrothed to Prince Arthur, should be accustomed to drink wine. 'Water is not wholesome, sole by it selfe, for an Englysshe man', wrote Andrew Boorde. Thomas More endeavoured to improve the purity as well as the number of water supplies.

Utopia

On 3 May 1515 the Court of Aldermen permitted More to occupy his office of Under-Sheriff by deputy, whilst he went 'on the kinges ambasset into Flaunders'. His embassy was to the Archduke Charles, afterwards Charles V, and its purpose was to settle a dispute between London merchants and foreign merchants resident in London. He visited Bruges, Brussels and Antwerp. In the latter city he became the friend of Peter Giles, to whom he dedicated Utopia. While abroad More wrote the second part of this work and added the introduction or first part on his return to England. The book was published in December 1516 by Tierry Martin of Louvain. Utopia is 'No-Where', the imaginary Commonwealth of the Renaissance idealists. It contains many allusions to the state of England at the time, the harm done to agricultural labourers by the enclosure of arable land as pastures for sheep, the unreasonable savagery of the penal code, and advocates

6 *Letters and Papers* (Henry VIII), iv, No. 2758.

many desirable social reforms. But it is also a remarkable treatise on public health administration, so far-seeing indeed that its teaching has been insufficiently appreciated by even the most recent of More's biographers. Inspired by his knowledge of the principles of Greek medicine and influenced by the need for sanitary reform, which he had observed in the City of London, More applied his learning and experience to a description of public health provision in Utopia, for its citizens esteemed health as 'the greatest of all pleasures'.

He envisaged a well-built city with gardens and open spaces, a public water supply, drainage and cleansed streets, with public abattoirs outside. Public hospitals were provided for the treatment of rich and poor and isolation hospitals for cases of infectious disease. Other amenities included communal meals, the safeguarding of maternity with municipal nurses for infant welfare, nursery schools (or crèches) for children under five, free universal education for all children with continuation, adolescent and adult schools; religious instruction, industrial welfare, enlightened marriage laws and eugenic mating and obedience to the laws of health, including fresh air and sunlight and active occupation without undue fatigue. It is a comprehensive programme of social medicine which, written in the sixteenth century, expresses many of the aspirations of to-day.

A marvellous book written by a marvellous man. John Burns, a collector of More's writings, told me that he dated his interest in social reform and his political career from the accidental purchase of a copy of *Utopia* at a second-hand bookstall. And under John Burns, when President of the Local Government Board, began the social health services. Thus the written words of More exert their humane influence in modern times.

Interest in Care for the Sick and Infirm

Before turning to further aspects of More's work in public health administration, I would like to show that his interest in medicine and the prevention of disease was joined with a kind and charitable heart, which was touched by all forms of human suffering. This is revealed in the words of Thomas Stapleton, whose Life of More appeared in 1588.

More was used, whenever in his house or in the village he lived in there was a woman in labour, to begin praying, and so continue until news was brought him that the delivery had come happily to pass.

The charity of More was without bounds, as is proved by the frequent and abundant alms he poured without distinction among all unfortunate persons. He used himself to go through the back lanes and inquire into the state of poor families; and he would relieve their distress, not by scattering a few small coins, as is the general custom, but when he ascertained a real need, by two, three or four gold pieces.

When his official position and duties prevented this personal attention, he would send some of his family to dispense his alms, especially to the sick and the aged. [This office, as already mentioned, was frequently performed by Margaret Gigs.] He very often invited to his table his poorer neighbours, receiving them . . . familiarly and joyously; he rarely invited the rich and scarcely ever the nobility. Not a week passed without his taking some poor sufferer into his house and having him tended. In his parish of Chelsea he hired a house, to which he gathered many infirm, poor and old people, and maintained them at his own expense. When More was away, his eldest daughter, Margaret . . . had the care of this house.

He even received into his household and supported a poor widow named Paula, who had spent all her money on a lawsuit.

The relief of the destitute and care of the sick were largely in the hands of the religious houses, and it was not until after the Dissolution of the Monasteries that the poor became a State problem, necessitating Poor Law legislation. More, in his wisdom and humanity, would have devised a sound system of poor law relief. The Poor Law legislation of Henry VIII and Edward VI put the onus of relief on the charity of local districts, and the problems of unemployment and destitution were not handled effectively until the celebrated Poor Law Act of Elizabeth in 1601.

In More's *Dialoge of Comfort against Tribulacion* he speaks of the duty of providing not only for children, but for servants and other dependants in sickness or in old age, as he himself had already done as far as he was able.

Meseemeth also that if they fall sick in our service, so that they cannot do the service that we retain them for, yet may we not in any wise turn them out of doors and cast them up comfortless, while they be not able to labour and help themself. For this were a thing against all humanity.

More as a Health Administrator

There was much epidemic disease in Tudor times. Outbreaks of typhus fever appeared in Europe and began to be frequent in the towns and overcrowded gaols of this country. Typhoid, dysentery and malaria were endemic. Sir Thomas himself suffered from a tertian fever. Creighton notes an epidemic of influenza in 1510. The deadliest epidemics were plague and the 'sweating sickness'.

Plague had remained endemic in England since 1349, the terrible year of the Black Death, which destroyed two million people, half the existing population. At the beginning of the sixteenth century there was a general recrudescence of plague. After nearly depopulating China, it spread over Germany, Holland, Italy, Spain and Britain in the first decade of the century. In 1500 the plague was so severe that Henry VII retired to Calais. From 1511 to 1521 there is not a single year without some reference to the prevalence of plague in the letters of Erasmus and elsewhere.

The sweating sickness was one of those mysterious maladies, like influenza and encephalitis lethargica in our own time, which suddenly appear, wreak havoc and destruction for a time, and then as suddenly disappear. The disease was first noted in August 1485, and was also brought to England in the army of Henry VII, which landed at Milford Haven.[7] It spread to London, where it caused great mortality. In 1502 it seems to have been prevalent in the West Country, and Prince Arthur probably succumbed to it at Ludlow, when Katherine of Aragon was attacked but recovered. In 1507 a milder outbreak occurred. There were severe epidemics in 1517, 1528 and 1551. The last epidemic was described by Dr. Caius. The disease has been identified by

[7] See Thomas Forrestier, M.D., Brit. Mus., Addit. M.S. 27582 ; also C. Creighton, *History of epidemics in Britain*, Cambridge, vol. i, 1891, p. 237.

Dr. Creighton, the epidemiologist, and Dr. Michael Foster with 'miliary fever' (*schweissfriesel, suette miliaire*, or 'the Picardy Sweat'), a malady repeatedly observed in France, Italy and South Germany, but not in the United Kingdom. It was characterized by intense sweating and an eruption of vesicles, lasted longer than sweating sickness, occurred in limited epidemics and was usually not fatal. The first epidemic was seen in 1717 and it continued to 1906 and even later. Dr. Michael Foster and Sir Henry Tidy saw cases of the disease in France during the war of 1914–18.[8]

In the summer of 1517, London was visited by a virulent outbreak of the disease, which spread by the following year all over the country and especially in the crowded towns. Colet succumbed to the infection, Wolsey had more than one attack and Andreas Ammonius, Henry VIII's Latin secretary, died of it. More wrote to Erasmus on 19 August:

> We are in the greatest sorrow and danger. Multitudes are dying all round us; almost everyone in Oxford, Cambridge and London has been ill lately, and we have lost many of our best and most honoured friends; among them—I grieve at the grief I shall cause you in relating it—our dear Andrew Ammonius, in whose death both letters and all good men suffer a great loss. He thought himself well fortified against the contagion by moderation in diet. He attributed it to this that, whereas he met hardly anyone whose whole family had not been attacked, the evil had touched none of his household. He was boasting of this to me and many others not many hours before his death, for in this sweating sickness no one dies except on the first day of attack. I myself and my wife and children are as yet untouched and the rest of my household have recovered. I assure you there is less danger on the battlefield than in the city. Now, as I hear, the plague has begun to rage in Calais just when we are being forced to land there on our embassy, as if it was not enough to have lived in the midst of contagion, but we must follow it also. But what would you have? We must bear our lot. I have prepared myself for any event. Farewell in haste.

More noted the danger of relapse in sweating sickness. 'Considering there is, as physicians say, and as we also find, double the peril in the relapse that was in the first sickness.'[9]

Plague was also prevalent, and the disease terrified King Henry, who fled from London to Windsor and thence to Abingdon. In April 1518 both plague and sweating sickness were rife in Oxford. The king appointed More, who had returned from the embassy to Calais, to supervise the health measures to be taken in this emergency. On the 28 April Master More certified from Oxford to the king at Woodstock that three children were dead of the sickness, but none others; he had accordingly charged the mayor and commissary in the king's name 'that the inhabitants of those houses that be and shall be infected, shall keep in, put out wispes [of hay] and bear white rods, according as your Grace devised for Londoners'. They were also forbidden to keep animals in their houses, and officers were required to keep the streets of the town cleansed and to burn refuse.

---

[8] M. G. Foster, 'Sweating sickness in modern times', in *Contributions to medical and biological research, dedicated to Sir William Osler.* New York, 1919, vol. i, p. 52; also H. Tidy, *Brit. Med. Journ.,* 1945, ii, 63, 196.

[9] *The pitiful life of King Edward the Fifth.* Camelot edition, p. 230.

Here we see notification and segregation used for the prevention of epidemic disease and Thomas More controlled it by these means. The King's Council approved these measures, and in June 1518 Pace wrote from the Court at Woodstock to Wolsey that 'all are free from sickness here, but many die of it within four or five miles, as Mr. Controller is informed'.

On the 18 July More wrote:

> We have daily advertisements here, other of some sweating or the great sickness from places very near unto us; and as for surfeits and drunkenness we have enough at home.

In the severe outbreak of 1528 More's daughter, Margaret, as already related, nearly succumbed to the sweating sickness. Anne Boleyn was attacked by it, and her royal lover hastily left her for several weeks.

More's excellent sanitary regulations, no doubt, helped to prevent more wide-spread infection and to diminish the virulence of these pestilences. The first plague order was issued in the thirty-fifth year of Henry VIII in 1543 and, as Creighton remarked, contains the germs of all subsequent preventive practice. More had then been dead for eight years, but the order codified his previous regulations and instructions. Instead of wisps of hay the sign of the cross is to be set on every house which should be afflicted with the plague, and there continue for forty days. Segregation, disinfection—chiefly by burning straw pallets, etc., and scouring and the bearing of white rods by plague contacts—are enforced, and this additional humane regulation breathes the spirit of Thomas More:

> That no housekeeper should put any person diseased out of his house unless they provided housing for them in some other house.

The more one delves into State papers of the time of Henry VIII, the more one reads Sir Thomas More's books, treatises and letters, and studies the account of his work in the letters of Erasmus and other contemporaries, the more one marvels at his wisdom and his outlook upon hygiene and public health.

Hospital Reform

This admiration for More is further enhanced when we examine his views on hospitals. He was a protagonist of hospital reform. In *Utopia* he sets forth a hospital scheme in these words:

> For in the circuite of the citie, a little without the walls, they have iiii hospitalles, so bigge, so wyde, so ample and so large, that they may seme iiii little townes, which were devised of that bignes partely to thintent the sycke, be they never so many in numbre, should not lye to thronge or strayte, and therefore uneasely and incommodiously: and partely that they which were taken and holden with contagious diseases such as be wonte by infection to crepe from one to another, myght be layde apart farre from the company of the residue. These hospitalles be so wel appointed, and with al thinges necessary to health so furnished, and more over so diligent attendaunce through the continual presence of cunning phisitians is geven, that though no man be sent thether against his will, yet notwithstandinge there is no sicke persone in all the citie, that had not rather lye there then at home in his owne house.

Sir Thomas More, when he wrote on theological or religious subjects, was often prolix, but in this account of the best form of hospital, its amenities and advantages, he is wonderfully concise. Yet all the points are there, situation, provision for all sick persons, proper furnishing and equipment, medical specialists in regular attendance, everything indeed that we are now endeavouring to obtain for the sick in the middle of the twentieth century. Oh, great Sir Thomas More!

Throughout the greater part of More's life the sick were nursed in the hospitals maintained by the religious houses. We know from a Chadwick Lecture, delivered in 1933 by Mr. Percy Flemming, that these hospitals were built with reasonable regard to hygiene and sanitation. In London the five priories of Austin Canons, Holy Trinity or Christ Church just within Aldgate, Saint Bartholomew's in West Smithfield, Saint Mary Overies, Saint Mary Spital and Saint Mary's Elsing Spital, had maintained hospitals for the sick and infirm. They were Saint Mary Spital, Saint Mary's Elsing Spital, Saint Bartholomew's and Saint Thomas's in Southwark. Saint Mary of Bethlehem (Bethlem, Bedlam) for insane patients was outside Bishopsgate on the site now occupied by Liverpool Street Station.

In 1529 Sir Thomas More succeeded Wolsey as Lord Chancellor. It was an anxious time, for Henry was pressing on with his plans for divorcing Queen Katherine and marrying Anne Boleyn, and More made no secret of his disapproval. He accepted office on the understanding that the king would grant him liberty of conscience and not employ him in the divorce proceedings. This promise Henry eventually broke. More's appointment was a popular one. The Imperial Ambassador, Eustace Chapuys, wrote to the Emperor Charles V:

> The Chancellor's Seal has remained in the hands of the Duke of Norfolk till this morning, when it was transferred to Sir Thomas More. Everyone is delighted at this promotion, because he is an upright and learned man, and a good servant of the Queen.

There was not only the affair of the divorce to trouble the new chancellor, but it was clear, as the French ambassador wrote, that after the fall of Wolsey, the king and nobles meant to attack and plunder the Church. This was foreshadowed before More became chancellor, in a scurrilous pamphlet called the *Supplication of the Beggars* by one Simon Fish, a lawyer of Gray's Inn and a friend of Tyndale. It was sent to Anne Boleyn, who gave it to the king. It advocated and recommended the wholesale confiscation of Church property and endowments, and included the abolition of the hospitals maintained by the monks for the benefit of the sick poor. Fish had the effrontery to pretend that this would be for the benefit of the poor. Henry apparently referred the pamphlet to More, who in 1529 published a counterblast to it, entitled a *Supplication of Souls in Purgatory*. This pamphlet is written supposedly by holy souls in protest against Fish's denial of purgatory, and pleads for continued prayers on their behalf. More demonstrates the folly of abolishing the hospitals in the following words:

> Then cometh he at the last unto the device of some remedy for the poor beggars. Wherein he would in no wise have none hospitals made, because he saith that therein the profit goeth to the priests. What remedy then for the poor beggars?

He deviseth and desireth nothing to be given them, nor none other alms or help requireth for them, but only that the king's highness would first take from the whole clergy all their whole living, and then set them abroad in the world to get wives, and to get their living with the labour of their hands and in the sweat of their faces . . . . and finally to tie them to the carts to be whipped about every market town till they fall to labour. . . .

He showeth himself that he nothing else intendeth but openly to destroy the clergy first, and after that covertly, as many as have aught above the state of beggars. What remedy findeth the proctor for them? He will allow them no hospital. . . . They must not be given money, nay not a groat; for the priests would get hold of that.   What other thing then?   Nothing in the world will serve but this . . . that everything should be taken from the clergy. . . . Is not this a goodly mischief for a remedy? Is not this a royal feast to leave the beggers meatless and then send more beggars to feast with them.

More alludes to the benefits conferred by the hospitals in diminishing the amount of sickness among the destitute. He admits and laments he has no statistics to quote, but neither, he observes, has Fish.

If we should tell you what number there was of poor sick folk in days passed long before your time: ye were at liberty not to believe us. Howbeitt he cannot yet on the other side for his part neither, bring you forth a bederoll of their names; wherefore we must for both our parts be fain to remit you to your own time and yet not from your childhood (whereof many things men forget when they come to far greater age) but unto the dates of your good remembrance.

Here we can remark on More's appreciation of the value of case records and of vital statistics, which were lacking in the case under consideration.

He considers that the number of the sick through hospitals are less than in times past, though he will not quarrel with those who have a contrary impression, 'for sorry sights stick in the memory'. But he cites the French pox:

And then of the French pockes thirty year ago went there about sick five against one that beggeth with them now. . . . As for other sickness the incidence is not greater than in times past.

Fish did not think the monastic alms were sufficient to prevent the necessitous from being famished, and becoming sick and dying from hunger.

We verily and truly think he shall seek far and find very few, if he find any at all, for albeitt the poor householders have these dear years made right hand shift for corn; yet our lord be thanked men have not been so far from piety as to suffer poor impotent persons die at their doors for hunger.

In his cupidity and want of humanity for his necessitous subjects, Henry ignored More's wise counsel.   By 1539 the total number of suppressed religious establishments was 655 monasteries, 90 colleges, 2,374 chantries and free chapels and 110 hospitals.

The Corporation of London foresaw the evil that would result and, in 1538, Sir Richard Gresham, the Lord Mayor, asked that the three remaining hospitals, Saint Mary Spital, Saint Bartholomew's and Saint Thomas's and, also, the Abbey of Tower Hill, might be placed with their revenues at the disposal of the mayor and aldermen so that 'all impotent persons not able to labour might be relieved'. Nothing was done until 1544, when Henry refounded Saint Bartholomew's Hospital, though he afterwards resumed possession of it. Henry's physicians said the only way of getting the king to listen to reason was to have him fall ill. This was exemplified on his death-bed in 1547, when he made the comprehensive agreement with the citizens, which led to his posthumous, if unmerited distinction as first founder of the 'Royal Hospitals'. At last the citizens obtained their hospitals.

The blow struck at the treatment of the sick in the provinces by the suppression of the hospitals was more deadly. A few of the old hospitals were refounded, but twenty-three of the principal English counties had no hospital until the eighteenth century. It is a deplorable story, for Henry VIII wilfully sinned against the light when he paid no attention to More's plea for retention of the hospitals.

The Martyrdom

Sir Thomas More was Lord Chancellor of England for only two years and seven months. As Miss Routh observes: 'Neither time nor occasion was his to carry out great reforms; from the first he realized how precarious was his position; how warily he must balance himself to maintain it.'

He cleared off the arrears of work left by Wolsey, which may have included certain measures of sanitary reform, and he preserved Christ Church for Oxford. Disagreeing with Henry's policy of disestablishing the papacy in England and making himself supreme head of the Church, More resigned his office on 16 May 1532, and retired to Chelsea to engage in religious controversy. This further annoyed Henry, as did also More's refusal to attend his marriage with Anne Boleyn. In 1534 Sir Thomas More was committed to the Tower for refusing to take any oath that should impugn the Pope's authority or assume the justice of the divorce. Cranmer advised he should be allowed to take a modified oath of fealty, but Cromwell and Anne Boleyn made the king adamant. More aged during his fifteen months' imprisonment; he wrote in the Tower his *Dialoge of Comfort against Tribulacion* which, as we have seen, contains many medical similes, and treatises on Christ's passion.

On 1 July 1535 he was indicted for high treason at Westminster Hall, found guilty on the perjured evidence of Rich, the Solicitor-General, and executed on Tower Hill on 6 July.

In the shadow of death, More did not lose his sense of humour. 'I pray thee see me safely up', he said to the lieutenant at the scaffold, 'and for my coming down let me shift for myself.' He put aside his beard from the block saying that 'it had never committed treason'.

More's execution shocked Christendom. Charles V declared then or previously that he would have preferred to lose his best city than have lost such a worthy counsellor. Sir Thomas was beatified on 9 December 1886 by Pope Leo XIII.

More's Personal Appearance

We have two accounts of More's appearance. The first, written by Erasmus in 1519, reads:

To begin, then, with what is least known to you, in stature he is not tall, though not remarkably short. His limbs are formed with such perfect symmetry as to leave nothing to be desired. His complexion is white, his face fair rather than pale, and though by no means ruddy, a faint flush of pink appears beneath the whiteness of his skin. His hair is dark brown or brownish black. The eyes are greyish blue, with some spots, a kind which betokens singular talent, and among the English is considered attractive. . . . His countenance is in harmony with his character, being always expressive of an amiable joyousness, and even an incipient laughter and, to speak candidly, it is better framed for gladness than for gravity and dignity, though without any approach to folly or buffoonery. The right shoulder is a little higher than the left, especially when he walks. This is not a defect of birth, but the result of habit, such as we often contract. In the rest of his person there is nothing to offend. His hands are the least refined part of his body.[10]

The second account I take from Lord Campbell. It describes More's appearance on his last days:

On the morning of the trial, More was led on foot in a coarse, woollen gown through the most frequented streets from the Tower to Westminster Hall. The colour of his hair, which had become gray since he last appeared in public; his face, which, though still cheerful, was pale and emaciated; his bent posture and his feeble steps, which he was obliged to support with his staff, showed the rigour of his confinement and excited the sympathy of the people, instead of impressing them, as was intended, with dread of the royal authority.[11]

As the curtain falls on that tragic closing scene on Tower Hill, when we consider the splendour of Sir Thomas More's talents, the greatness of his acquirements and the innocence of his life, with Lord Campbell, 'we must still regard his murder as the blackest crime ever perpetrated in England under the form of law'.

Comparison Between More and Chadwick

There are certain remarkable points of comparison in the careers of Sir Thomas More and Sir Edwin Chadwick as public health reformers. They both derived their interest in social reform from philosophers, More from Linacre and Chadwick from Jeremy Bentham. Both men had a broad outlook on the problems of health and disease. 'Chadwick', says Sir Benjamin Ward Richardson, 'treated all professions with equal freedom, when any subjects connected with his own pursuits were under discussion; so that they who listened often wondered, when they were not intimate with him, what his own profession might be.'

Sir Thomas More, as we have seen from *Utopia*, devised a most complete system of health and social reform, which was greatly in advance of his time and in some respects in advance of our own time. His fame as public health reformer, therefore, rests more on planning and prophecy than on achievement. He was, however, a great administrator, and reference has been made to his practical measures as Commissioner of Sewers in regard to water supplies and to his distinction in initiating the control of epidemic disease and plague. Had England then been ruled by an enlightened monarch, interested in the welfare of his subjects, public health reform would have been inaugurated on

[10] Letter to Ulrich von Hutten, *op. cit.* (2).
[11] *Lives of the Lord Chancellors*, 1856, chap. xxx, 'Life of Sir Thomas More'.

wise lines in the sixteenth century, for Sir Thomas had the root of the matter in him. Henry VIII was well educated, something of a scholar, and knew he had a loyal servant and talented minister in Sir Thomas. Tyranny, greed and opportunism made the king shut his ears to wise counsel. Henry's disregard of More's advice to retain the hospitals is a glaring instance of his callous indifference to suffering. Previously, in order to build a royal manor and to make a park for hunting, he had seized a leper hospital and evicted the inmates. Such was the origin of Saint James's Palace and Park.

Chadwick was more fortunate than More in that he succeeded in bringing about enduring measures of sanitary and social reform. His zeal in this matter outran his discretion, and for the latter years of his long life he had to stand aside and to see others reap the rewards of his labours. In retirement he wrote assiduously, as did More; pamphlets, presidential and other addresses, reviews and critiques came from his pen at frequent intervals. But unlike More he had an unattractive prose style and was no orator.

Edwin Chadwick learned much medicine and public health from Dr. Southwood Smith and Dr. Arnott. He was, however, too optimistic in anticipating that environmental hygiene would soon bring about a golden age in which doctors, 'those necessary evils', were not very likely to last and would neither be able to live—nor die! Sir Thomas More had a higher opinion of the work and value of doctors in preventive medicine.

Both these public health reformers were advocates of liberty and the right of free speech. It was Sir Thomas, when Speaker of the House of Commons, who petitioned the king in 1523 for freedom of speech by members of parliament and secured a large measure of success for this request. Chadwick was regarded as an autocrat, but he said he advocated centralization for the protection of liberty. He held that 'Liberty is a right with a corresponding obligation to respect it. Liberty consists of the power of doing anything which does not hurt another'. Edwin Chadwick in many ways rekindled the torch of public health reform which had fallen from the lifeless hands of Thomas More and lay smouldering for some three centuries.

Sir Thomas More's activity in the prevention of disease and public health, which we have considered, was only one aspect of a full and busy life devoted to God and the King. Witness his last words: 'I die the King's servant, but God's first.'

This interest was sanctified by his religion and his love of humanity. I cannot end better than by quoting the words of Dr. Maynard Smith concerning Sir Thomas More:

> He was a man of infinite charm, a loving father and a chivalrous friend. He was an enthusiast for learning and an enthusiast for justice. He was a friend to the poor and a champion for the oppressed. He loved this world and all that was in it, but he gladly died for something of more value, for what he believed to be the cause of God and truth.[12]

[12] H. Maynard Smith, *Pre-Reformation England*. London, 1938, p. 484.

BIBLIOGRAPHY OF SIR THOMAS MORE

The life of Sir Thomas More, by William Roper, edited by E. V. Hitchcock. London, 1935.

The life and death of Sir Thomas More, by Nicholas Harpsfield, edited by E. V. Hitchcock, with historical notes by R. W. Chambers, 1932. (First edition.)

The Rastell Fragments, printed as an Appendix to Harpsfield's *Life,* 1932.

The Paris News Letter, describing More's death, printed as an Appendix to Harpsfield's *Life,* 1932.

Vita Thomae Mori, in the *Tres Thomae* of Thomas Stapleton, 1588. The Cologne edition of 1612 is the most accessible. English translation by Mgr. Philip Hallett, 1928.

The life of Sir Thomas More, by his great-grandson (Cresacre More). Ed. of 1726.

The life of Blessed Thomas More, by T. E. Bridgett. London, 1891.

Thomas More, by R. W. Chambers. London, 1935.

Sir Thomas More and his friends, by E. M. G. Routh. London, 1934.

Utopia in Latin and English, with notes by J. H. Lupton. Oxford, 1895.

The workes of Sir Thomas More, wrytten in the Englysh tonge. London, 1557.

The English works of Sir Thomas More, edited by W. E. Campbell, with introductions and notes by A. W. Reed, R. W. Chambers, and W. A. G. Doyle-Davidson. London, vol. i, 1931, etc. (*In progress.*)

Thomae Mori Lucubrationes. Basel, 1563.

The Four Last Things by the Blessed Martyr Sir Thomas More, Kt. Edited by D. O'Connor. London, 1935.

Opus epistolarum Des. Erasmi Roterodemi, recognitum per P.S. et H. N. Allen. Oxford, 1906, etc. (*In progress.*)

The epistles of Erasmus, arranged by F. M. Nichols. London, 1901–17. A translation with commentary of the letters to Dec. 1518.

Calendar of letters and papers, foreign and domestic of the reign of Henry VIII. Vols. i–iv, ed. by J. S. Brewer, vols. v–xxi, ed. by J. Gairdner. London, 1862–1910.

State papers, published under the authority of His Majesty's Commission. Vol. i, King Henry VIII. London, 1830.

A calendar of the correspondence of Sir Thomas More, by Elizabeth F. Rogers, *English Historical Review,* 1922, xxxvii, 546–64.

E. Wenkebach, *John Clement, ein englischer Humanist und Arzt des sechzehnten Jahrhunderts.* In *Studien z. Gesch. d. Med.,* Leipzig, 1925, pt. xiv.

John Clement, in W. Munk, *The Roll of the Royal College of Physicians.* Second edition. London, 1878, vol. i, p. 25.

The social life and theories of Sir Thomas More, by Richard O'Sullivan, K.C. Reprinted from *The Dublin Review.*

BOOK IV

THE NEW PHILOSOPHY

ON MISUNDERSTANDING THE PHILOSOPHY OF FRANCIS BACON

by

BENJAMIN FARRINGTON

THE tercentenary of Francis Bacon's death fell twenty-four years ago. The occasion did not pass without a number of tributes. I shall recall two.

Professor Broad wrote a witty and high-spirited essay characteristic of much of the Cambridge philosophy of the period, but came to the depressing conclusion expressed in his closing sentence: 'So far as I can see, the actual course which science has taken, even if it has been in accord with Bacon's principles and has led to the results which he desired and anticipated, has been influenced little if at all by his writings.'[1] This seems an odd application of a doctrine that did not need to be made odder, the parallelism between mind and matter. Bacon wrote to influence the development of science. Science followed the course that he desired. But the events are not connected. It is perhaps necessary to start off on the wrong foot to arrive at so lame a conclusion. The purpose of this paper is to suggest a closer connexion between the thought of Bacon and the course of history than Professor Broad admits.

Professor Broad, in his tribute, confined himself to Bacon the logician. He considered only 'his claims to be the Father of Inductive Philosophy'. A similar limitation was imposed on himself by the second panegyrist, the late Professor A. E. Taylor. Taylor was much more serious than Broad and, it must be admitted, much more dull. He did not come to the paradoxical conclusion that Bacon's writings have counted for nothing. On the contrary he set him on a pedestal. Unhappily it is an inappropriate pedestal in an inappropriate part of the gallery. A problem had been set the year before by Dr. Adolfo Levi, to determine the relation of the thought of Francis Bacon to Cartesianism.[2] Taylor attacked this problem, and, relying more on Whitehead than on history to assist his analysis, came to the conclusion that the proper niche for Bacon is between Plato and Leibniz.

> In truth [says Taylor], it is in . . . the recognition of the discovery of 'forms' as the true problem of science and the identification of the 'forms', so far as the physical sciences are concerned, with space-time patterns, that his real significance for living thought must be found. . . . Foremost on the list of the forerunners of a philosophy of nature at once organic and mathematical, should stand the names of the two great mathematical metaphysicians of the ancient and modern world, Plato and Leibniz. Between them, as a connecting link, for all his personal want of mathematical equipment, might well stand Bacon, who found in Plato an anticipator of himself, as he was in turn recognized with generous appreciation by Leibniz.[3]

[1] C. D. Broad, *The philosophy of Francis Bacon.* Cambridge, 1926.

[2] A. Levi, *Il pensiero di F. Bacone considerato in relazione con le filosofie della natura del Renascimento e col razionalismo cartesiano.* Turin, 1925.

[3] A. E. Taylor, 'Francis Bacon' (Annual Hertz Lecture on a Master Mind). *Proc. Brit. Acad.,* 1926, xii, 273 ff.

Taylor was perhaps more distinguished for ingenious learning than for judgement. Notoriously Bacon did not find in Plato an anticipator of himself. Nor can the effort to cover up Bacon's ignorance of mathematics by describing it as a *personal* want of mathematical equipment carry us very far. Would Taylor have us suppose that in some *impersonal* way Bacon knew what he did not know? These are desperate expedients of one determined to find for Bacon a place among the metaphysicians and logicians, which is not where he belongs.

The urge to make of Francis Bacon something other than he was did not begin with Taylor. It was in the 1830's that there appeared the essay in which Macaulay exalted Bacon as the apostle of utility, comfort and material well-being.[4] This view, though not adequate, is well-founded and tells an essential truth. But it shocked contemporary opinion, and Baconian scholarship has ever since been trying to live it down. Even the great edition of Spedding, Ellis and Heath, a superb monument of scholarship, is not free from this preoccupation.[5] Heath, who edited the legal remains, need not concern us here. But Ellis, who had undertaken the philosophical writings, had occupied himself mainly with mathematical studies and was never quite at home with Bacon. Though his labours as editor were soon terminated by ill health, his bias had been imparted to the whole edition. It was finally upon Spedding that the whole editorial responsibility, except for the legal remains, devolved. Spedding's devotion to Bacon had begun in the 1840's with a repudiation of Macaulay's estimate of Bacon's character, and the editing of Bacon remained his main employment for over thirty years. There can be no question but that he did his job extraordinarily well. Spedding's editorship is the main event in the history of Baconian scholarship. But Spedding, too, had his weak side. He deliberately limited his studies, both historical and philosophical, to the Baconian period. He had a playful habit of exaggerating his ignorance of all other periods, which should not deceive us. But this professed indifference to wider historical studies indicates a certain failure to appreciate the significance of Bacon. Bacon, who felt himself to be the precursor of a revolution not so much in human thought as in human life, is not to be understood except against a background of three thousand years, which is perhaps the reason why the historian Macaulay understood certain truths about him which eluded the philosophers.

Spedding, however, eventually came to a much clearer understanding of Bacon's purpose than Ellis ever had. Ellis thought that the chief originality of Bacon's work lay in his contribution to logic, although he completely exploded the error Taylor sought to revive, that Bacon's main concern was the doctrine of 'forms'.[6] Spedding saw that it lay in a certain programme of Bacon's for a vast organization of research. Ellis thought that the *Novum Organum* was Bacon's most important work. Spedding thought that the *Parasceve* or *Preparation for a Natural and Experimental History* was not

---

[4] Macaulay, Essay on Bacon.
[5] *The Works of Francis Bacon*. Ed. by J. Spedding, R. L. Ellis and D. D. Heath. New edition. London, 1870-2.
[6] *ibid.*, vol. i, pp. 21-67.

only regarded by Bacon as the more important work but was in fact so. There is no doubt in my mind that Spedding was right. His Preface to the *Parasceve*[7] is the single most useful contribution to the interpretation of Bacon's thought. It gives us something that is not to be found in the later valuable editions of the *Novum Organum* by Brewer[8] and Fowler.[9] The fault with these books is that they are too bookish. Perhaps they are right in treating the *Novum Organum* as Bacon's most important contribution to thought. They do not sufficiently regard the fact that Bacon intended, as he said, a contribution not to contemplation but to action, not to thought but to life.

That Francis Bacon felt himself to stand in a symbolic relation to his age appears in a hundred passages of his writings, not least in those in which he seeks to disarm suspicion of pride. His sense of having a message of overwhelming importance to deliver to mankind is first revealed in the lost tract written in his twenties, *Temporis Partus Maximus*.[10] The feeling that on him devolved the role of prophet, if not indeed of midwife, for the successful accomplishment of this birth remained with him while life lasted, providing the inspiration in particular for his intense activity in his last five years. There is at times a burning zeal in him that reminds one of Lucretius, a solemnity of utterance that recalls the Roman poet. Among the lineaments of his character is discernable 'an aspect as if he pitied men'. He seems one that has a priceless boon to confer, but cannot win acceptance for it. With admirable persistence he seeks to gain his end, but even *his* wit, *his* learning, *his* eloquence are insufficient. In the end he is beaten, for what he wants done is something that no man can do alone. He rarely finishes a book, for his ambitions are not in the domain of authorship. His writings are a means to an end which needs the help of others, and collaborators are not immediately forthcoming. But what his own generation has failed to produce posterity may provide. Accordingly he either himself writes in Latin or has translated into Latin such portions of his writings as he thinks it most urgent to preserve, for he doubts whether English has a world future but is sure that Latin has. What was it he wanted done?

Ellis and all those who think like him answer that the main ambition of Bacon was to found a new science of logic in order to redeem the human mind from error. In this, of course, they are not wholly wrong. Bacon did attempt to found anew the rules of induction. Furthermore, as they rightly point out, he thought he had made a contribution to logic of supreme importance; and when it is objected that there is nothing very novel in the rules of Baconian induction, they urge that it is not fair to judge the *Novum Organum* as it stands, since it is but a fragment. In the second book Bacon tells us what the completed work was intended to contain. 'I propose to treat', he writes, 'of Prerogative Instances, of the Supports of Induction, of the Rectification of Induction, of Varying the Investigation according to the nature of the subject, of Prerogative Natures, of the Limits of Investigation or a Synopsis of all Natures in the Universe, of the Application to Practice or of Things in their relation to Man, of Preparations for Investigation, and

[7] *ibid.*, pp. 369–90.
[8] J. S. Brewer, *Francisci de Verulamio Novum organum*. London, 1856.
[9] Bacon's *Novum organum*. Ed. by T. Fowler. 2nd edition. Oxford, 1889.
[10] Bacon's *Works, op. cit.* (5), vol. i, pp. 104–5.

finally of the Ascending and Descending Scale of Axioms.'[11] Here are nine main divisions of the projected work, only the first of which was adequately treated. But, if Ellis is right, it was to the completion of this scheme that Bacon should have devoted all his energies. Did he do so? Nothing of the sort. The *Novum Organum* was published in 1620 when Bacon was fifty-nine. He was then at the height of his intellectual vigour and beginning the most active period of his literary career, but he deliberately left the logic incomplete and took up a different portion of his plan, namely the *Parasceve* or *Preparation for a Natural and Experimental History with a view to the founding of Philosophy*. This deliberate choice definitely disproves, as Spedding says, the conclusion of Ellis that Bacon's main concern was with his rules of induction.

The importance attached by Bacon to his *Natural and Experimental History* is more clearly understood in the light of his career as a whole. He was admitted to Trinity College, Cambridge, when twelve and there soon developed his distaste for the disputatious philosophy of Aristotle. At the age of fifteen he accompanied the English ambassador to Paris and spent there two or three years. Not long after his return, while still in his early twenties, he produced the lost *Temporis Partus Maximus*. There is proof that this contained in some form the programme of what was later to be called by Bacon *The Great Instauration*. The next twenty years and more of his life are filled with professional and public affairs. He becomes a Member of Parliament, a Bencher of Gray's Inn and the friend of Essex, and, after various changes of fortune, rises to be Lord Chancellor. But the early ambition is only covered over, not dead. In 1605 appeared *The Advancement of Learning*. About two years later, when Bacon was forty-seven years of age, it appears that he had finally settled the plan of *The Great Instauration*. From 1607 he begins to refer to it by this name.

The *Great Instauration*, according to the account Bacon gave of it in the writing called *Distributio Operis*,[12] was to be in six parts. First was to come a description and classification of the existing sciences with analysis of their insufficiency and hints for filling the gaps. The already published *Advancement of Learning* was to be taken as supplying this part. Second was to come the *Novum Organum* or *Directions for the Interpretation of Nature*. The third part, the *Parasceve*, was designed to be a sort of preliminary catalogue of the Universe, an encyclopaedia of Nature and the Arts. The purpose of this vast assemblage of information was to supply material to which the rules of induction could be applied, Bacon's main criticism of the logic of Aristotle and the Schools being that it concerned itself with such a paucity of facts. Fourth was to come *The Ladder of the Intellect*, which was to consist of demonstrations in certain limited and specially significant fields of the correct application of the logic. The fifth part was to offer certain *Anticipations of Philosophy*, that is to say tentative forecasts of the new knowledge and power that would belong to man when the Great Instauration was complete. The sixth part was no mere book but a new form or stage of human society, which Bacon must be left to describe in his own words.

<hr>

[11] *ibid.*, p. 268.   [12] *ibid.*, pp. 134–45.

The sixth part of my work, for which the rest are but the preparation, will introduce and reveal the philosophy which is the product of that legitimate, chaste and severe method which I have taught and prepared. But to perfect this last part and bring it to issue is a thing both above my strength and beyond my expectation. What I have been able to do is to give it, as I hope, a not contemptible start. The destiny of the human race will supply the issue, and that issue will perhaps be such as men in the present state of their fortunes and of their understandings cannot easily grasp or measure. For what is at issue is not merely a contemplative happiness but the very reality of man's well-being and all man's power of action. Man is the helper and interpreter of Nature. He can only act and understand in so far as by working upon her or observing her he has come to perceive her order. Beyond this he has neither knowledge nor power. There is no strength that can loosen or break the causal chain. Nature cannot be conquered but by obeying her. Accordingly these twin goals, human science and human power, come in the end to one. To be ignorant of causes is to be frustrate in action.[13]

These are proud words. The conclusion of Bacon's work is not to be distinguished from the destiny of mankind. It is not to be a chapter in a book but a chapter in history. Such a claim would amount to insanity were it not for the fact that Bacon claimed no other greatness for himself than to be the voice of his age. He did not claim to be the maker of a new world but the herald of its coming. Nothing is more remarkable about Bacon than the extent to which his mind was penetrated by history, and this characteristic had been present from the first literary expression of his genius in his twenties in *Temporis Partus Maximus*. It is not too much to say that he saw such an intimate connexion between true thought and the active life of men, that he despised all thinking that had no effect on the material condition of mankind. True thinking for Bacon ended not in contemplation but action. It was part of history, not only of the history of thought. It is this Baconian connexion between thought and life that Broad and Taylor ignore or deny.

In the writing called *Sic Cogitavit* Bacon says that his purpose is to restore 'that comerce of the mind with things, which is the most important of all earthly concerns'.[14] In the *Parasceve* he puts the same thought in other words. He tries to rouse men, as it were, from a deep sleep, so that they may at last understand what it means 'to consult nature about nature'. These ideas are for him so charged with historical meaning that he does not shrink from saying that 'the brute beasts by their natural instincts have made many inventions while all the arguments and rational deductions of men have produced little or nothing'.[15] He amplifies this thought in the *Parasceve*: 'The universe is not to be narrowed down to the limits of the understanding, which has been men's practice up till now, but the understanding must be stretched and enlarged to take in the image of the universe as it is discovered.'[16] Bacon is convinced that the universe is infinitely richer and more complex than the human mind, and that the mind must not impose itself on matter but instruct itself from matter. He will not have as the basis of deduction axioms which are spun out of the mind, but only such axioms as are won by his kind of induction, that is 'by attention to sense evidence, by closing

[13] *ibid.*, p. 144.   [14] *ibid.*, p. 121.
[15] *ibid.*, p. 183.   [16] *ibid.*, p. 397.

with nature, by hanging over her operations and almost taking a hand in them'
('inductionem . . ., quae sensum tuetur et naturam premit et operibus
imminet ac fere immiscetur').[17] From this kind of induction are eventually to
be wrung axioms which 'are not notional, but which Nature would recognize
as being really her first principles, and which cleave to the very marrow of
things'.[18] Finally, conceiving this to be the historical relation between man's
mind and matter, he does not hesitate elsewhere to conclude that 'the material
and mental progress of mankind are one and the same thing'.[19] In this sense
we must understand both his youthful characterization of his philosophy as the
birth of time, and his mature identification of the sixth and last stage of his
philosophy with the destiny of the human race. For Bacon man is not
essentially a rational animal. His definition is *homo, Naturae minister et
interpres*,[20] and this for Bacon is a truth in time. Through serving and
interpreting Nature man becomes more truly man.

In a paper published in 1914 Sir Thomas Clifford Allbutt[21] threw out the
suggestion that Bacon's first impulse to his peculiar philosophy of nature
was derived from the famous French potter Palissy. It was not many years
after his return from Paris that Bacon produced the lost tract containing
a preliminary sketch of what was later to become *The Great Instauration*.
From 1575 to 1584, which covers the time during which Bacon was in Paris,
Bernard Palissy lectured to a large and distinguished audience on agriculture,
chemistry, mineralogy and geology, and did so with a collection of natural
objects about him. In 1580 he published his *Discours Admirables* in the
Preface to which we read:

> . . . Comment est il possible qu'un homme puisse sçavoir quelque chose et parler
> des effects naturels, sans avoir veu les livres Latins des philosophes? Un tel propos
> peut avoir lieu en mon endroit, puis que par practique je prouve en plusieurs
> endroits la théorique de plusieurs philosophes fausse, mesmes des plus renommmez
> et plus anciens, comme chascun pourra voir et entendre en moins de deux heures,
> moyennant qu'il vueille prendre la peine de venir voir mon cabinet, auquel l'on verra
> des choses merveilleuses qui sont mises pour tesmoignage et preuve de mes escrits,
> attachez par ordre et par estages, avec certains escriteaux au dessouz, afin qu'un
> chacun se puisse instruire soy mesme: te pouvant asseurer (lecteur) qu'en bien peu
> d'heures, voire dans la première journée, tu apprendras plus de philosophie naturelle
> sur les faits des choses contenues en ce livre, que tu ne sçaurois apprendre en
> cinquante ans, en lisant les théoriques et opinions des philosophes anciens.[22]

This is the very heart of Bacon's message. This is the commerce of the
mind with things. Sir Clifford Allbutt was surely right in detecting in
Palissy and his scientific museum at least a striking congruity with the spirit
of the future author of *The Great Instauration*. To the precocious lad in
his teens who had already learned to despise 'Aristotle', the appeal from
books to nature herself would have come as a revelation. There is, of course,
no actual proof that Bacon ever listened to Palissy and examined his *cabinet*.

---

[17] *ibid.*, p. 136.   [18] *ibid.*, p. 137.
[19] *ibid.*, vol. iii, p. 612.   [20] *ibid.*, vol. i, p. 157.
[21] Sir T. Clifford Allbutt, 'Palissy, Bacon and the revival of natural science'. *Proc. Brit.
Acad.*, 1913–14, vi, 233 ff.
[22] B. Palissy, *Discours admirables*. Paris, 1580. See the 'Advertissement aux lecteurs', quoted
from *Les oeuvres de Palissy*. Paris, 1880, p. 166, ll.16–31.

But the probability is very great and is strengthened by the veiled allusion in the *Novum Organum*:

> There is another great and powerful cause why the sciences have made but little progress. It is not possible to run a course aright when the goal itself has been wrongly set. The true and lawful goal of the sciences is none other than this, that human life be endowed with new inventions and powers. But of this the great majority have no feeling, but are merely hireling and professorial. Only occasionally it happens that some artisan of unusual wit and covetous of honour applies himself to a new invention, which he mostly does at the expense of his fortune.[23]

This fits well the story of the potter who, in his quest for the secret of the white enamel to glaze his pots, had broken up his furniture to feed his kilns.

Palissy taught that every art, if thoroughly studied, has a fulness of science in it. 'Would you like me to tell you in what book of the Philosophers I read these beautiful secrets? It was in a pot half full of water . . .' Such statements occur everywhere in his writings. He is never done emphasizing his debt to things and not to books. 'I am neither Greek nor Jew, neither poet nor rhetorician, only a simple, humble-minded ill-educated craftsman; . . . but I had rather utter truth in my peasant's speech than lies in the language of the rhetorician.'[24] That Bacon almost certainly knew Palissy justifies Allbutt in connecting his doctrine of the commerce of the mind with things with the practice of the French potter and gardener. But it is wrong to look for an exclusive connexion. The thing was in the air, as has long been apparent to more advised historians of the development of ideas.[25] Still more wrong, and not to be passed over without vehement protest, is Allbutt's contention that Bacon spoiled what he borrowed while suppressing the name of the humble man to whom he was indebted. This is to see things altogether out of focus. It is probably true that Palissy had a surer grasp of scientific method than Bacon, and it is certain that he achieved a vastly greater number of positive results. The mistake is to compare them, for their achievements lie in different fields. For Palissy the doctrine of the commerce of the mind with things meant a simple rejection of book-learning, and the setting of himself up as a humble handicraftsman against the pretensions of the philosophers. For Bacon it constituted a different challenge arising from his wider opportunities. He had the knowledge of the classical tongues from which Palissy was shut out. That is to say, he had the key to history. He could do what Palissy could not, he could set the new ideal of the commerce of the mind with things against the long history of the domination of syllogism.

Students of the *Novum Organum* will remember the amazing historical perspectives opened up in the passage which begins: 'The sciences which we possess come for the most part from the Greeks.'[26] Here powerful and original judgements crowd thick and fast upon one another, but they are historical judgements and do far more to constitute the principles of the history of science than to establish a correct theory of experiment. Bacon is

[23] Bacon, *op. cit.* (5), vol. i, p. 188.

[24] Palissy, *op. cit.* (22), p. 187; and the 'Dédicaces' to the *Recepte véritable*. Rochelle, 1563 (quoted from the same ed., p. 13).

[25] e.g. Taine, *History of English Literature*, vol. ii, 3, 1.

[26] Bacon, *op. cit.* (5), vol. i, p. 181.

on Palissy's side, but he is so as a student of the whole course of human
history. The older Greeks are preferred to the later by reason of their
closer contact with nature. The whole of classical antiquity is contrasted
unfavourably with modern times by reason of the shortness of the historical
record and the narrower confines of the known world. A new criterion of the
truth of philosophy is set up, that science like religion is to be judged by its
fruits. The philosophical scepticism of the ancient schools is castigated,
not because it hinders belief, but because it hamstrings action. The duration
of the memory of the human race, as supported by written records, is set at
twenty-five centuries, but it is remarked that not all of these were fruitful.
'Time, like space, hath its deserts and wastes, and only three revolutions
and periods of learning can properly be reckoned, one among the Greeks,
the second among the Romans, and the last among us, that is to say, the
nations of Western Europe, and to each of these periods scarce two centuries
can be assigned.' Climates of opinion unfavourable to the development of
natural philosophy are recognized and defined. Pagan antiquity is blamed
for absorption in morals and politics, Christianity for absorption in theology,
and both ages for a contempt of manual labour which has excluded from the
purview of the philosopher the sciences concealed in the crafts. With this
last attitude Bacon connects the exaggerated reliance placed in logic and
mathematics, although, as he says, logic can only give consistency and not
new knowledge, while mathematics ought to be called in to give definiteness
to knowledge, not to generate it and give it birth.

Such were the historical judgements which resulted from Bacon's studies
and meditations. These, of course, were outside the scope of a Palissy.
Bacon did as much as any one man who ever lived to deepen the historical
consciousness of mankind. Historians of science have still something to
learn from him. It was because he was able to set the new spirit, which
was manifested not only in Palissy but in others at this time, against the
background of the human achievement to date, that Bacon spoke not with the
shrill personal assertiveness of a Palissy but in the austere, lofty, animating
tones of history itself, styling the new doctrines not the product of wit but the
product of time. Sir Clifford Allbutt fell below the level of his subject when
he saw beneath such phrases nothing but the Lord Chancellor of England
adding another to his meannesses by stealing the credit of the French
working-man.

If by reason of his learning Bacon passed an historical judgement on the
new attitude to nature, by reason of his prominent position in public affairs
he was led to consider the political and social implications of putting the new
knowledge into practice. Bacon lived in the midst of an industrial revolution,
in a period when the idea of the application of science to industry was
beginning to strike the minds of men with overwhelming force. 'There
have been two industrial revolutions in England, not one', writes John U. Nef.
'The first occurred during the hundred years that followed the dissolution
of the monasteries, in 1536 and 1539. . . . By the reign of Charles I, from
1625–1642, England was on the point of becoming, if she had not already
become, the leading nation of Europe in mining and heavy manufacturing.'[27]

[27] J. U. Nef, *Industry and commerce in France and England, 1540–1640.* Memoirs of the
Amer. Phil. Soc., 1940, vol. xv.

This revolution was felt also on the Continent. Biringuccio's *Pirotechnia* (1540), which for originality compares with Palissy's writings, was plundered by Georg Agricola, translated out of its native Italian into learned Latin, and incorporated in the *De re metallica* (1556), a book which sets the whole mining industry on a sound scientific basis and discusses its relation to human well-being with knowledge and vision. Bacon was acquainted with this book and shares its spirit. Science for Bacon, as for Agricola, is applied science; it means industry and the investment of capital. Bacon sees the old philosophy of the schools as a shackle on the limbs of the young giant industry. When he inveighs against philosophical scepticism he complains that by these false doctrines 'men are easily dissuaded from venturing their fortunes and exertions on mere speculative opinions which must for ever defy solution'.[28]

The eighty-eighth aphorism further unfolds the implications of this statement. It postulates a connexion between the progress of human knowledge and human industry, and claims that knowledge lags because industry is lacking in enterprise. The lack of enterprise is laid at the door of traditional philosophy.

> The philosophy now in vogue [he writes], if carefully examined will be found to advance certain points of view which are deliberately designed to cripple enterprise. Such are the opinions that the heat of the sun is a different kind of thing from the heat of fire, or that men can only juxtapose things but cannot like nature make them act upon one another. The effect and intention of these arguments is to convince men that nothing really great, nothing by which nature can be commanded and subdued, is to be expected from human art or human labour. Such opinions, if they be justly appraised, will be found to tend to nothing less than a wicked effort to curtail human power over nature and to produce a deliberate and artificial despair. This despair in its turn confounds the promptings of hope, cuts the springs and sinews of industry, and makes men unwilling to put anything to the hazard of trial.

Here we see in all its concrete actuality what Bacon meant when he said that his philosophy was designed to produce not new arguments but new arts. Such a passage is inexplicable in an academic treatise on inductive logic. The eager polemic tone of the passage is at once explained when we read the description of the period in Nef: 'All over Europe the ecclesiastical foundations, with their religious objectives, were less inclined than laymen to use their funds for the development of heavy industry.'[29] Nef sees clearly that in attacking Scholasticism Bacon was clearing the decks for the application of science to industry. He does not so clearly understand Bacon's attitude to the throne. 'It was chiefly English merchants', he writes, 'with interests in trade, mining, or manufacture, who perceived a connexion between freedom from government interference and the material improvement sought for by the "new philosophy". Francis Bacon, the greatest popularizer of that philosophy, missed the connexion. He was a king's man in politics and took an active part in promoting royal monopolies.' He was a king's man, it is true. But in the vision he had of the future of science he needed the help of kings. A *regium opus* he called his great plan.

---

[28] Bacon, *op. cit.* (5), vol. i, p. 184.
[29] Nef, *op. cit.* (27), p. 141.

With the background that has now been supplied it is easy to understand why Bacon left his logic incomplete and turned to a different portion of his plan. It was in 1620 that the *Novum Organum* appeared, and at the end of the first book he reveals that he has changed his opinion of the relative importance of parts of his project.

It is time for us to prescribe rules for the interpretation of nature. But to this body of rules we attribute neither necessity as if nothing could be done without it, nor perfection, although we think our precepts are most useful and correct. For we are of opinion that if men had at their disposal a proper *Natural and Experimental History* and would apply themselves to it they might by the proper exertion of their minds fall into our way of interpretation without the aid of any body of rules. For interpretation is the true and natural act of the mind when all obstacles are removed.[30]

This natural and experimental history to which he now began to attach primary importance he conceived of as a great co-operative work. Observers all over the world were to gather material in accordance with a pre-arranged plan, and this material was subsequently to be sifted and interpreted by experts. Of this plan he writes in the *Parasceve*:

I must repeat here what I have so often said that though all the wits of all the ages should meet in one, though the whole human race should make philosophy their sole business, though the whole earth were nothing but colleges and academies and schools of learned men, yet, without such a Natural History as I am going to describe, no progress in philosophy and the sciences worthy of humanity could be made. But if such a history were once provided and well-ordered, with the addition of such light-giving experiments as the course of the interpretation would itself suggest, the investigation of Nature and of all sciences would be the work of only a few years. Either this must be done or the business must be abandoned. For in this way and in this way only can the foundation be laid of a true and active philosophy.[31]

Two years later, in the *Auctoris Monitum* prefixed to the *History of the Winds*, which is one of the most witty, passionate and eloquent of all Bacon's writings, he tells us how he sees in his mind's eye, scattered throughout Europe, men fit for collaboration in the great plan for the regeneration of mankind by the application of science to nature, and he reflects that 'even if the logic were finished and given to them it would not help them much to complete the Natural and Experimental History, whereas the history, even without the logic, would greatly promote the restoration of the sciences'.[32]

The History on which Bacon now rested all his hopes was to be not merely natural but experimental. The word 'experimental' is misleading and serves to keep our historians of science still off the plain path to the understanding of Bacon. It suggests the laboratory, but what Bacon had in mind was the workshop. The modern equivalent of the word would be 'industrial'. Bacon thought this the most novel and the most important part of his plan.

[30] Bacon, *op. cit.* (5), vol. i, p. 223.
[31] *ibid.*, p. 394.
[32] *ibid.*, vol. ii, pp. 15–16.

It is only now, now, I say, for the first time and never before that such a work has been put in hand. Neither Aristotle nor Theophrastus nor Dioscorides nor Pliny, much less any of the moderns, set before themselves the aim of which we speak.[33]

The ancients wrote much natural history, but neglected the enquiry into the mechanical arts. Yet it is the mechanical arts that give the better insight into the secret places of nature. Nature with her profusion and spontaneity dissipates the powers of understanding and by her variety confounds them. In mechanical operations the attention is concentrated, and the modes and processes of nature, not only her effects, are seen.[34]

Prejudice has stood in the way of research into nature through the avenue of the mechanical arts, but we must lay aside such pride. Among the arts we must prefer those which exhibit natural bodies and the materials of things, and which change and adapt them. Such arts are agriculture, cooking, chemistry, dyeing, glass-making, enamelling, sugar-refining, powder-making, the manufacture of fire-works, paper and so on.[35]

The history we are compiling, then, is not only of nature as she exists free and unconfined, when she flows along spontaneously accomplishing her tasks. Such is the history of the heavens, of meteorology, of earth and sea, of minerals, of plants, of animals. But much more we seek the history of nature constrained and vexed, that is to say of nature thrust from her original state, mastered and modified by the art and agency of man.[36]

The scope of the Natural and Experimental History Bacon had in mind is indicated in his catalogue of particular enquiries to be comprehended in it, which is digested under one hundred and thirty separate heads. About half of these fall under the description of natural science as it had been written by the Greeks and their followers. The other half belong to experimental or industrial history. Bacon's conception was that the phenomena of nature and industry should be rapidly catalogued under the heads he ventured to suggest, in order to expel from men's minds the grotesque misconceptions that prevailed.

We are attempting to set up in the mind a real model of the world such as it is found to be, not such as it is dictated by any man's reason. This cannot be done without dissecting and anatomising the world most diligently. We declare it to be necessary to destroy utterly the foolish little models, the apish imitations, which have been formed in various systems of philosophy by the fancies of men.[37]

For the construction of this model Bacon wanted the help of a multitude of workers. The desideratum being an encyclopaedia of nature and the arts, he saw no reason why the average man should be unable to supply him with some of the necessary facts. He wanted records of hail, snow and frost all over the world. He wanted data about tides. He wanted to know about metals and mining, about the growth of the human child, about pottery, printing and gardening. He saw no reason why the merchant and sailor, the miner and the engineer, the smith, the potter, the printer and the gardener, not to speak of any intelligent father of a family, should be unable to supply him with some relevant information. All, under suitable direction, could help in gathering the facts. The facts, when collected, were

---

[33] *ibid.*, vol. i, p. 395.   [34] *ibid.*, vol. iii, p. 686.   [35] *ibid.*, vol. i, p. 399.
[36] *ibid.*, p. 141.   [37] *ibid.*, p. 218.

to be sorted and interpreted by men of wider knowledge and more philosophical outlook. For the conduct of the enquiry the material to be investigated was to be divided up according to the different arts and crafts. But since the object of the whole endeavour was not the mercenary promotion of already existing arts, but the constitution of a true philosophy of nature which would then be fruitful of new and unimagined arts, the material when collected was to be arranged on a new principle, according to the light it threw on the physical structure of different bodies. *Inquisitio per artes, dispositio per corpora.* Bacon, of course, had not realized all the complexity and difficulty of his breath-taking programme. But that it was the destined path of progress is proved by the experience both of the French Encyclopaedists and of the British founders of the Royal Society, who were his true followers.

It is hardly worth arguing against those who reproach Bacon with being 'merely practical', with being 'basely utilitarian', with 'subordinating truth to practice'. We may satisfy ourselves with translating one of his more eloquent passages.

> Wherefore, if there be any humility towards the Creator, if there be any reverence and praise of his works; if there be any charity towards men and zeal to lessen human wants and human suffering; if there be any love of truth in natural things, any hatred of darkness, and desire to purify the understanding; men are to be entreated again and again that they should dismiss or at least for a moment set aside those inconstant and preposterous philosophies which prefer theses to hypotheses, which have led experience captive and triumphed over the works of God; that they should humbly and with a certain reverence draw near to the book of creation; that they should there make a stay, that on it they should meditate, and that then washed and clean they should in chastity and integrity turn them from opinions.[38]

The path forward in Baconian studies and criticism would seem not to lie in quarrelling with his criterion of truth, *quod in operando utilissimum, id in sciendo verissimum*, but in following the development in the thought of later writers of his pregnant insight into the connexion between human destiny and human control over nature by the application of science.

[38] *ibid.*, vol. ii, pp. 14–15.

THE ATTITUDE OF FRANCIS BACON AND DESCARTES TOWARDS MAGIC AND OCCULT SCIENCE

by

LYNN THORNDIKE

THE purpose of this paper is to indicate briefly the attitude towards magic and occult science of two men who have commonly been regarded as initiating, the one modern experimental science, and the other modern philosophy, Francis Bacon and René Descartes. What was the position of the man who demanded 'an absolute regeneration of science', and of the man who would first apply the sponge to the previous painting and raze to the ground the previous edifice—what was their position with regard to the traditional mass of magical and occult lore which had been so indissolubly intermingled with the science and thought of the past?

Bacon declaimed against 'learned but idle and indolent men' who had 'received some mere reports of experience, traditions, as it were, of dreams'. Just as the naturalist, Aldrovandus, in the sixteenth century, aimed to exclude *nugae* from his portly folios, so Bacon tried to exclude fables, marvels, curiosities and traditions from his experiments. Did he succeed?

Traces of the astrological point of view are still manifest in Bacon's pages. To the Moon he assigned such influences as the eduction of heat and induction of putrefaction, moistening, exciting the spirits in bodies—of which action lunatics were the great example. He believed that the new moon and the full moon affected winds and weather; that conjunctions of the planets were preceded and followed by windy weather, unless the Sun was a participant in the conjunction, in which case the weather was fair; and he listed other weather signs from the constellations. Incidentally we may remark that he also still believed in storm-producing wells, that is, if one cast a stone into them. He criticized the art of astrology at some length, but believed that it should be expurgated rather than utterly rejected.

Bacon's biology was still interlarded with tales of inventions made by brute animals or instances of marvellous sagacity on their part. He further marvelled that venomous animals should like the shade of 'odorate and wholesome herbs'. It did not seem to occur to him that they stationed themselves there to catch and kill insects, although in another passage he asserts that the chameleon does not subsist entirely on air, but also devours flies which it catches with its long tongue. The prevalence of putrefaction was manifest long after a recent outbreak of the plague in the generation of toads with tails two or three inches long. For Bacon still believed in 'living creatures that come of Putrefaction'.

Like Telesio in the previous century, Bacon resorted to 'spirits' to explain any natural, or supposedly natural, phenomena for which he could not otherwise account. These spirits, it is true, were not demons but neither were they tangible bodies, although they existed in all tangible bodies. They were neither vacuum, air, heat nor fire. They were very fine and subtle, rarefied to the point of being invisible, and yet not immaterial. They differed from one another as much as tangible bodies did; would easily dissipate, evaporate, infuse or boil away; and were almost never at rest. Nitre, though cold, cleans clothes because it has a subtle spirit. Quicksilver is the coldest of metals because it is the fullest of spirit. 'The leaf of burrage hath an excellent spirit to repress the fuliginous vapour of dusky melancholy, and so to cure madness.' In animate bodies vital spirits are added to those of inanimate bodies. The force of explosives convinced Bacon that a small amount of spirits in the brain and sinews would readily move the entire body. The effects of motion on the body were also accounted for by these spirits, and the reason that to an intoxicated person the whole room seems to be going round is that the spirits are revolving in his brain. Infectious diseases are more in the spirits than in the humours, and putrefaction is produced by the effort of the spirits to get out of the body. 'Surely the cause that blows and bruises induce swellings is that the spirits, resorting to succour the part that laboreth, draw also the humours with them.' The spirits are susceptible to heat, which refines them and, for example, make the cock bird a better singer than the hen. Cats and owls could not see at night, unless there were still a little light, 'proportionable' to their 'visible spirits'. Human beings see better with one eye closed, because then the visual spirits unite more. Worms, flies and eels continue to move after they have been cut to pieces, because their vital spirits are diffused almost all over their bodies, while human beings perspire more in the upper parts of their bodies, because these are fuller of spirit. Tears are caused by a contraction of the spirits of the brain, 'and this contraction . . . causeth also wringing of the hands, for wringing is a gesture of expression of moisture'—a very pat instance of the logic of magic and of magical association of ideas. The splendour of gems shows that they contain fine spirits, and Bacon even concedes that 'they may work by consent upon the spirits of men to comfort and exhilirate them'. He denies, however, their particular properties, yet a few pages later explains the notion that wearing a blood-stone checks nose-bleed by astriction and cooling of the spirits. He then raises the question whether the jewel found in the toad's head is not of like virtue, 'for the toad loveth shade and coolness'—another example of magical logic and association of ideas. The fact that children and some birds learn to speak so easily, and in darkness as well as in light, made Bacon wonder if there was not some transmission of spirits from the teacher to the learner predisposing the latter to imitate the former. Thus the supposed action of the spirits borders on the occult, on fascination and the evil eye, on natural magic. As an attempt to explain nature they may represent something of an improvement on the occult virtues and specific forms of the scholastic period, but it is a slight one. They are still semi-occult themselves.

Bacon held that the confessions of witches were not to be rashly believed and that imagination played a large part in them, but he repeats the old theory of natural divination without unfavourable comment. He rejected the explanation why certain plants grew best near certain others, and not near yet others, that they were sympathetic or antipathetic, for the more sensible reason that plants requiring different nourishment from the soil grow best near each other. But he believed that bears grew fat while hibernating, although they ate nothing then, and that earth taken from the Nile valley grew heavier when the river rose. Also that the skin of a wolf cured colic by some sympathy, perhaps because the wolf was 'of great edacity and digestion,' and so parts of the animal would comfort the bowels. Also that warts were cured by rubbing them with a bacon rind and hanging it up in the sun. Yet he censured the appeal to occult virtue as slothful. But he experienced the same difficulty as Pliny had in his *Natural History* of excluding the magical lore of the past, and gave the same excuse for letting some of it pass, 'lest our incredulity may prejudice any profitable operations in this kind, especially since many of the ancients have set them down'. So, while he had said that methods of doctoring herbs to make them medicinal or to alter their colour or aroma were mere fancies, he finally set some of them down. He also repeated such time-worn legends as those of the maiden fed on poison and the bezoar stone.

Bacon's medicine somewhat savours of magic or at least of charlatanry. He was, however, more interested in the prolongation of life and health than in the cure of disease. He was somewhat sceptical as to the efficacy for this purpose of the flesh of harts and serpents, or that Artesius had prolonged his life artificially for one thousand and twenty-five years (as recorded by Roger Bacon). But his 'Grains of Youth' were compounded of four of nitre, three of ambergris, two of orris powder, one quarter poppy seed, one half saffron, with water of orange blossoms and a little tragacanth. His 'Methusalem Water' was the result of repeated washing, steeping, drying and powdering of shells, tops of rosemary, pearls, ginger, white poppy seed, saffron, nitre, ambergris, cucumbers sliced in milk and stewed in wine, vinegar, spirits of wine, etc. A simpler prescription was wine in which gold had been quenched. Again, Bacon tells of a great man whose custom it was to have 'a clean clod of earth' brought to him every morning before he got up and to sit in bed holding his head over it for some time. Bacon further recommended 'divers creatures bred of putrefaction, though they be somewhat loathsome to take, . . . as earthworms, timber-sows and snails . . . . And since we cannot take down the lives of living creatures, which, some of the Paracelsians say, if they could be taken down, would make us immortal,' the next best thing is 'to take bodies putrefied such as may be safely taken'.

Gilson has said that the Cartesian philosophy was in large part a clear explanation of facts which do not exist. Descartes still denied the existence of a vacuum. He still tried to answer such questions as why children and old people weep easily. He still posited the existence of animal spirits in the brain. He still repeated, without acknowledgement, Costa ben Luca's tenth century physiological explanation of thought as centring in the movement of the pineal gland. He still endeavoured to explain why the sea was not increased by the rivers flowing into it, by supposing the return of its water to the tops of mountains through underground passages, although Jacques Besson in the previous century had maintained that evaporation and rainfall sufficed to supply all springs and streams. Descartes still discussed bitumen and *minium*, earthquakes and volcanoes and comets, and the other natural phenomena which had been staple topics of scientific treatises for centuries. He suggested a possible explanation for the reputedly inextinguishable lamps which burned hundreds of years without the addition of new fuel. In general he was concerned with the same problems, topics and notions as had occupied

science and philosophy for ages past.   But when he came to specialize, it was in
fields such as geometry and dioptrics, which offered much less opportunity for
the infiltration of magical and occult detail than the natural history and
experiments of Francis Bacon.   In *The Search after Truth* Descartes explained
that it would not be possible for him to treat in detail the various experimental
sciences; that would require examination of all the herbs and stones from the
Indies, sight of the phoenix, and acquaintance with all the marvellous secrets
of nature.

If, however, we ask whether the Cartesian attitude of doubt and mechanistic
interpretation of nature was directed against astrology, the doctrine of occult
virtue, and the like, and whether it was responsible for the abandonment of such
views or of superstition generally, the answer will have to be rather in the negative.
Descartes, it is true, felt that he was above being deceived 'by the promises of
an alchemist, the predictions of an astrologer, the impostures of a magician,
the artifices or the empty boastings of any of those who make a profession of
knowing that of which they are ignorant'.   Yet he was credulous as to the
wounds of a corpse bleeding at the approach of the murderer and as to instant
warnings, in dreams or waking, of the afflictions, danger or death of distant
friends and kindred.   In *The Search after Truth* Epistemon is especially
curious concerning 'the secrets of the human arts, apparitions, illusions, and,
in a word, all the wonderful effects attributed to magic.   For I believe it to be
useful to know all that, not in order to make use of the knowledge, but in order
that one should not allow one's judgement to be beguiled into admiration of an
unknown thing'.[1]   And Eudoxus promises, 'after having struck wonder into
you by the sight of machines the most powerful and automata the most rare,
visions the most specious, and tricks the most subtle that artifice can invent, I
shall reveal to you secrets which are so simple that you will henceforward
wonder at nothing in the works of our hands'.[2]   Both the phenomena here
alluded to and the explanation promised were commonplaces of natural magic.
Again, in his *Principles* Descartes affirms that there are no qualities so occult, no
effects of sympathy or of antipathy so marvellous or strange, nothing in nature so
rare, but that his principles will explain it, provided it proceeds from a purely
material cause. His chief suggested explanation is that long, restless, string-like,
little particles of the first element, existing in the intervals or interstices of
terrestrial bodies, may be the cause, not only of the attractions exerted
by the magnet and amber, but of an infinity of other marvellous effects.
'For those that form in each body have something particular in their figure
that makes them different from all those that form in other bodies,'[3] and they
may pass to very distant places before they strike matter which is disposed to
receive their action.   Since Descartes was so confident of his ability to think up
a rational and mechanical explanation for all such seemingly occult phenomena,
he would seem likely to encourage rather than to discourage the belief in
them.   Furthermore, his tendency to advertise the results of his method as
marvellous as well as easy savours more of magic than of science.

[1] *The Philosophical Works of Descartes rendered into English by Elizabeth S. Haldane and
G. R. T. Ross.* Cambridge, 1911, vol. i, p. 310.
[2] *ibid.*, p. 311.
[3] Descartes, *op. cit.* (1), *Principles of Philosophy*, vol. iv, p. 187.

ASTRONOMY IN THE SIXTEENTH AND SEVENTEENTH CENTURIES

by

HERBERT DINGLE

A PERIOD of scientific activity presents itself to the historian under two aspects. It is primarily the scene of a succession of discoveries, ideas, theories, originating in various places and various minds, which call for chronicling; on the other hand, it is also visible as a stage in a process, a fragment of a continuously developing system of thought, with respect to which the individual discoveries, ideas and theories are seen as sign-posts, serving mainly to mark out the track of development.

The scientist who assumes the role of historian tends by instinct to regard his subject under the former aspect. It is safer; it affords scope for his familiar technique for distinguishing fact from error; and it is objective, yielding results whose certainty or probability depends as little as possible on the personal characteristics of the investigator. To attain scientific precision the object must be viewed *sub specie temporis*; to see it *sub specie aeternitatis* is to invite endless, and only too often profitless, controversy.

Nevertheless, in this essay the astronomy of the sixteenth and seventeenth centuries is regarded chiefly from this more hazardous point of view, and this for several reasons. In the first place, except to the enthusiast in astronomy it is much more interesting. It is doubtless important to know whether Galileo or Scheiner or Fabricius or Harriot was the original discoverer of sun-spots, and the whole essay might easily be occupied by an evaluation of their claims, but it is unlikely that many readers would feel their pulses throbbing faster as the drama approached its climax. Secondly, when the period under discussion is as remote as that with which we are now concerned, there is some justification for turning its remoteness to advantage. The passage of time makes more and more difficult the discovery of what occurred and what it meant to those who experienced it, but it makes more and more clear the significance of the period in the evolutionary process. The subjectivity of the interpretation, never perhaps wholly removable, is tempered by the tangible evidence of subsequent events. Thirdly, the occasion merits something more original than a summary of well-established facts easily accessible elsewhere, and since I have no qualification for the spade-work of the historian, interpretation only is left to me as a legitimate task. Finally, and perhaps most important of all, astronomy in the sixteenth and seventeenth centuries had a more vital influence on the direction of intellectual development in the widest sense than any science has had since the beginning of history, with the possible exception of the advance of general science at the present time, which must be left to future generations properly to assess. To record the events of this crucial period without regard to their larger implications would be equivalent to writing the life of Luther without considering the Roman Church, or to estimating the career of Napoleon as a brief interruption of the history of the French monarchy.

The effect of the astronomy of these two centuries was indeed profound. We can see it best by comparing typical examples of men's views of the universe taken from the beginning and end of the period respectively. Fig. 1. is a diagram which appeared in Apian's *Cosmographia* in 1539 and represented,

LIBRI COSMO.   Fo.V.

Schema huius præmiffæ diuifionis Sphærarum.

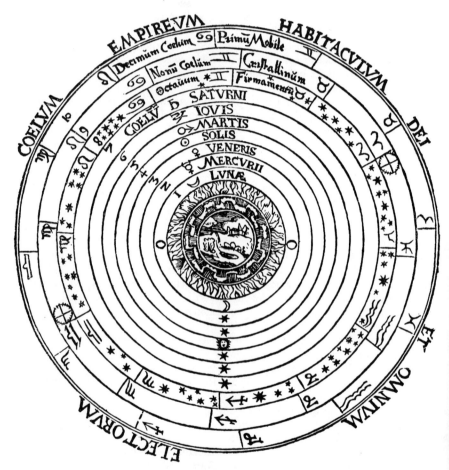

Fig. 1. Diagram of the Universe (From Apian's *Cosmographia*, 1539).

practically without variation, the unquestioned belief of the whole of Europe at that time. At the centre is the Earth, and surrounding it are the other 'corruptible' elements, water, air and fire. All this was stationary, and round it moved the rest of the universe, comprising the spheres of the Sun, Moon, planets and fixed stars. Each sphere had a simple circular movement, but the heavenly bodies, which were in themselves insignificant, each shared the movements of several spheres and so pursued a complex path, which served as a clue to the astronomer intent on discovering the motions of the invisible but much more fundamentally important spheres. The world-view of this time is well represented in the Elizabethan poets, whose thought it informed and whose expression it shaped, although in their day it had already been marked for oblivion. Marlowe, perhaps, most conspicuously, and Shakespeare most familiarly, preserve it for us. Puck's fairy wandered 'everywhere, swifter than the Moon's sphere', not swifter than the moon, which was simply borne along by the rolling sphere. 'O Sun', cries Cleopatra, 'burn the great sphere thou mov'st in!' Everyone knows the famous passage in *The Merchant of Venice* in which the Pythagorean notion of the music of the spheres, unheard by mortal ears just as the spheres themselves were unseen by mortal eyes, is associated with even the smallest of visible orbs. The universe, consisting of the things which were unseen, unheard and eternal, was bodied forth by the things which were seen and heard and would dissolve leaving not a wrack behind.

Nevertheless, the real world, though hidden, was not inaccessible ; it was both finite and intelligible, within the grasp of man's reason. The whole was circumscribed in time and space, and man, fixed for a short term of years at the centre of the vast machine, could master the working of the whole and aspire to reach the abode of the blessed beyond the outermost stellar sphere. Nor was he merely a spectator. His career and destiny were, to some extent at least, determined by the influence of the spheres, and astrology in the Middle Ages was a respectable university discipline. The universe was vast, but it was not unconcerned with human affairs.

I can find no warrant, however, for the frequently expressed view that in the medieval scheme the Earth was the glory and end of Creation, and that the tragedy of the Copernican revolution lay in its abasement.[1] The truth seems rather to be that the Earth played at least as small a part in the Aristotelian as in the Copernican organization. It was thought at rest not because of the dignity belonging to quiescence, but because observation seemed to show that it was at rest. Such a state, moreover, was not dignified; uniform circular motion was the mark of perfection, and this was possessed neither by the Earth itself nor by bodies moving on the Earth. The central position of the Earth also was demanded not by necessity but by observation, and, in fact, the scheme required that the Earth was not at the centre of most of the spheres, but only of the outermost. It was celestial matter, again, which was ingenerable and incorruptible. It was impious to believe in sun-spots, but everyone confessed to earth-spots. To a much greater extent than is commonly believed, the world-view of the Middle Ages was a common-sense view, based on observation and formed by the interpretation of observations in the light of a few Aristotelian and scriptural *a priori* principles.

To sum up, then, we see the universe at the end of the fifteenth century as a finite system, enigmatic but ultimately intelligible, unseen but symbolized by

---

[1] For example, as expressed in J. W. Draper, *History of the conflict between religion and science*. New York, 1874.

visible forms, immeasurably vast but extending its influence into the details of earthly things. It was a unified system, whose study was indivisible into categories of thought such as astronomy, cosmology, theology. Astronomy was cosmology—there was no study of separate bodies for their own sakes— and cosmology was inseparable from theology, for the abode of the blessed was as much a part of the system as were the crystalline spheres. Man, the lowly inhabitant of the central depth, could rise to the supreme height; his greatness lay not in his actuality but in his potentiality. He was bounded in a nutshell, but he could become king of space.

I would like to be able to give a corresponding diagram of the universe at the end of the seventeenth century, to show the change that had come about, but in truth the essence of the change is contained in the fact that this cannot be done. The universe had ceased to be picturable; there had indeed ceased to be a universe in the traditional sense, for in place of an intelligible system there was nothing but an infinite void, populated by none could say how many wandering, unordered, unsupported bodies, without effect on human concerns, and beyond knowledge and understanding. Gone were the spheres, gone the boundary of the universe, the abode of the blessed. Cosmology no longer responded to the impulses of the spirit; it showed a dumb, purposeless chaos, cold, barren and inscrutable, in which the aspiring soul not only could find no answer to its prayers but became aware of an overpowering menace, the crushing oppressiveness of infinite indifference. The successor to Apian's cosmography is the cry of Pascal: 'Le silence éternel de ces espaces infinis m'effraie!'

The profundity of the division thus created between the intellectual and the spiritual, emotional, religious—call it what you will—approach to the world of experience can scarcely be exaggerated. I think we have not even yet to any appreciable extent begun to heal it. Throughout the nineteenth century we hear a recurring cry of despair at the unresponsiveness of nature to the irrepressible yearnings of the human spirit, and it was a twentieth-century poet who felt a stranger and afraid in a world he never made. This incompatibility between the view of the universe which satisfies intellectual curiosity, and that which meets the demands of instinctive spiritual restlessness, remains our greatest problem, and I would hazard the opinion that some modern philosophies, such as Nietzscheanism on one hand and Dialectical Materialism on the other, the success of whose appeal to many intelligent minds can scarcely be accounted for on rational grounds alone, owe their popularity mainly to the fact that they do make some semblance of restoring the ancient unity of outlook to a people subconsciously unable to choose between alternative and irreconcilable world-attitudes. Be that as it may, however, our immediate concern is with the intellectual approach alone, and here it must be said that even by the end of the seventeenth century some recovery had been made from the initial bewilderment. An infinite universe had been found not necessarily inapprehensible by the inquiring mind, even if deaf to the appealing spirit. What was banishment to one was already felt as emancipation by the other, and a start was made on the road which we are still treading. That will appear in due course. We must now turn to the events of the period itself.

When Copernicus[2] in 1543 launched his geostatic system upon the world, he had no consciousness that he was ending an epoch in thought. His problem was the old one of deducing the movements of the spheres from the appearance of the stars and planets, and he accepted implicitly the *a priori* principles by which the inferences were to be controlled, and made them, in fact, the justification for his scheme. His universe was finite, it contained the traditional spheres, and it exhibited only the uniform circular movements proper to celestial matter. Its novelty was that it reduced the spheres of the Sun and fixed stars to rest and gave their apparent movements to the Earth.

The scheme appealed to many of those able to understand it by virtue of its simplicity, but it was ridiculed by the masses because of its absurdity. Was it not obvious that the Earth was stationary, and was not the movement of the Sun and the stars plain for all to see? For fifty years after the death of Copernicus the new idea made slow progress, but it met with little opposition for any but purely observational reasons. There were, it is true, objections on scriptural grounds,[3] but there were also answers to those objections on the same grounds, and in the end nothing of any significance emerged from such discussions. The determining factors in the controversy took shape independently, in the passion for exact observation of Tycho Brahe and the equally intense passion for systematization of Kepler. These men produced the evidence that was to make the triumph of the Copernican system inevitable, and at the same time shatter the preconceptions which had inspired its construction.

For, despite the revolution in thought justly associated with his name, Copernicus was not by nature an adventurous thinker. It was the mathematician, not the pioneer, in him that revealed itself in the change of view-point which he introduced, and, simplicity having been achieved, he appears to have had no impulse to work out the implications of his new idea. Kepler remarked that he did not know his own riches and tried to interpret Ptolemy rather than nature.[4] A more daring mind would have seen at once that the proposed change would demand the most radical reform of world-view. For example, the Copernican scheme required that the stars must be at an enormous distance from the Earth, otherwise they would suffer an apparent annual displacement owing to the Earth's revolution round the Sun. But since, at that time, it was universally believed that the stars appeared not as points but as discs having finite diameters, great distance implied great dimensions, immeasurably beyond anything thought possible. This consideration, which does not seem to have occurred to Copernicus, weighed so heavily with Tycho Brahe that, in spite of the enormous advantages of the Copernican system, which he fully realized, he could not accept it but proposed instead a compromise between it and the system of Ptolemy, which left the Earth stationary.[5]

[2] N. Copernicus, *De revolutionibus orbium coelestium*. Norimbergae, 1543.

[3] For example, Luther's argument that it was the Sun and not the Earth that Joshua bade stand still (see Luther's *Table Talks*). See also C. Singer, *A short history of science*. Oxford, 1941, p. 182; and J. L. E. Dreyer, *History of the planetary systems*. Cambridge, 1906, pp. 352–3.

[4] J. Kepler, *De motibus Stellae Martis*, 1609, chap. xiv, in *Opera omnia*. 8 vols. Francofurti a.M., 1858–71, vol. iii, p. 234.

[5] Tycho Brahe, *Astronomiae instauratae progymnasmata*. Uranienborg, 1587, vol. ii, chap. viii.

Again, and still more important, although Copernicus had never questioned the existence of the crystalline spheres, he had destroyed all reason for assuming it. So long as the stars were believed to revolve round the Earth it was incredible that thousands of separate bodies at various distances from the axis should move independently in precisely the same period. There was no rational alternative to the hypothesis that the motion was that of a sphere, on the surface of which the stars were fixed, and by analogy spheres would naturally be postulated for the planets also. But when the stars were reduced to rest, the function of the spheres collapsed. There were no similar motions to correlate, but only a single movement of the Earth. The whole substance of the medieval universe became a phantom of the imagination, and in its place was left nothing—a void with no boundary.

The realization of what had happened spread gradually as the sixteenth century wore on, and it was assisted by more than one kind of circumstance. Daring, speculative philosophers, like Bruno, realized quite clearly that Copernicus had, in effect, annihilated the spheres, and that the universe expanded to infinity, could contain nothing which could claim the distinction of being stationary, and hence nothing which could be said absolutely to move.[6] The relativity of motion had been discovered, though it was not fully to be comprehended for another three hundred and fifty years. Limitless space meant limitless multitudes of worlds and limitless possibilities of life. The effect of the new vistas was overwhelming on minds accustomed to near and clear horizons, and the inheritors of the spirit of precise calculation turned away from systematizing the universe to cultivate their own gardens.

It thus came about that in astronomy proper the result of the new freedom was paradoxically to restrict the scope of activity. The time-honoured problem—the invention of complexes of spheres—was taken away, and in its place was left little but the task of compiling more accurate tables of the positions of the heavenly bodies. It happened, however, that here also the spheres were to receive a death-blow. It was the very precision of the measurements which Tycho Brahe made of the comet of 1577 that convinced him of its great distance and of its motion through the material of the spheres if they existed.[7] Two momentous conclusions followed: the spheres were imaginary, and the perfect, immutable translunar matter could suffer change. Astronomy, forced back into its lair, dealt the medieval cosmology as fatal a blow as any struck by liberated and rampant philosophy.

Apart from these wider and unexpected issues, however, the domestic tasks of astronomy had an importance of their own. On them depended, among other things, the establishment of a practicable calendar, and the Gregorian reform, introduced in 1582, was the product of great labour, curtailed but by no means reduced to anything like simplicity by the Copernican change of view-point. The value of the results was limited less by the methods of analysis of the observations than by the inaccuracy of the observations themselves, and what above all things was needed, both for the evident and for the yet unrealized work that lay ahead, was the precise and

---

[6] G. Bruno, *Cena de le ceneri, Della causa principio ed uno, De l'infinito universo e mondi.* Venice, 1587.

[7] *op. cit.* (5).

trustworthy determination of celestial positions. The need called forth the man, and in the period from 1568, when Tycho Brahe conceived the plan of his first giant quadrant, to 1601 when, on his death-bed, he entrusted the results of his work to his pupil Kepler, the vitally important advances in astronomy lay in dogged and patient measurement, not in transcendental thinking.

Astronomical observation in this pre-telescopic age was mainly a matter of the construction of bigger and better instruments. Actual observing skill, in the modern sense of the term—the instinct for correct interpretation of things imperfectly seen and for selection of the essential needle from the superfluous bundle of hay—was in small demand. The star or planet, a point of light, was seen through two widely separated 'pin-holes' or 'sights', and once it had been seen, the accuracy of the observation depended on the perfection with which the instrument was graduated and mounted. Tycho possessed that combination of vision, patience, enthusiasm and ability to persuade a patron to provide the necessary money which his task required, and in his work the word 'accuracy' acquired a new meaning.

Of course, judged by modern standards, even Tycho's measurements appear crude, though it is doubtful whether, without the telescope, they could even now be greatly improved upon; but astronomy provides many examples of the deduction of precise results from rough data, and of these none is more striking than the one before us. Until the present generation, and perhaps even now, Newton's law of gravitation stood at the high-water mark of exactness in science, and it is not often realized that it was extracted from data which the modern observer would reject out of hand. Tycho's observations with 'sights' and Galileo's with water-clocks were the raw material out of which was shaped the greatest scientific generalization in history. The fact is not without significance.

Tycho was far from being unskilled in the reduction of his observations, and he performed one service for at least the convenience of astronomers in finally destroying belief in an illusory movement of the stars known as *trepidation*.[8] It is Kepler, however, to whom we owe the greatest fruits of Tycho's labours. This extraordinary man stands outside any systematic account of the development of Renaissance thought. Fundamentally he was a new Pythagoras, dominated by a passion for finding harmony in nature and capable of incredible toil on the slightest hint of a possible mathematical relation. Equally strong cases could be made out for writing him down as an inspired genius or as a hopeless lunatic, were it not that he never relaxed his hold on the one final arbiter of all his imaginings—the observations of Tycho. Of the instinct for distinguishing the fertile from the barren soil of thought, so characteristic of Copernicus, he had nothing. On the other hand, from the tyranny of *a priori* metaphysical principles, which dominated Copernicus, he was almost entirely free. He was in consequence faced by an infinite, undifferentiated field in which to labour, with no guiding voice to tell him where he should or should not plough. He had only infinite industry, immense mathematical skill, and a standard by which to test the products of his work. It is not surprising that he produced many tares; the miracle is that he could show such a superabundance of wheat.

[8] Tycho Brahe, *Astronomiae instaurata mechanica.* Wandesburgi, 1598.

Kepler's three laws give the essential regularities of the solar system. Adopting the Copernican scheme, he was able to state the shape of a planetary orbit, the law of variation of speed in the orbit, and the connexion between the period of revolution of a planet and its mean distance from the Sun.[9] These laws completed the reformation which Copernicus had begun, in a way which Copernicus could never have foreseen and would scarcely have approved. The dogma of uniform circular celestial motions was discredited: the orbits of the planets were not circles but ellipses, with the Sun at a focus, and the velocities were not uniform but varied continuously with the distance of the planet from the Sun. These two laws were at the same time the death-knell of medieval metaphysics and the herald, as yet not recognized, of modern physics. The third law, however, was wholly constructive; it established a system where there was none before. Until this law was discovered there was no reason for grouping the spheres of the planets into a separate community from the spheres of the fixed stars; the diurnal motion of the latter, in fact, was transmitted to the planetary spheres also. There was, it is true, a wide-spread medieval fancy of a cosmic dance, which implies some sort of communal movement—Copernicus himself speaks of his system as explaining 'the ballet of the planets'—but this conception was quite independent of astronomical descriptions of the motions: it was metaphysical in character and appears to have comprehended the whole universe, stellar and planetary spheres alike. It was left to Kepler to discover a true solar system, with orbits mathematically related to one another, standing out as a compact unit against the inaccessible stars.

The most momentous effect of Kepler's work was to bring the long history of traditional astronomy to an abrupt and inescapable end. The spheres had gone, the stars had been relegated to regions infinitely beyond reach, and now the mechanism of the planetary system, the only remaining object of possible research, was finally interpreted. The ephemerides might be improved, and the passage of time might enable the scale of the system to be more accurately determined, but, except for these minutiae, nothing conceivable remained to be done. Astronomy was at its period, and there was nothing left remarkable above the visiting Moon.

It is doubtful, however, if anyone realized this at the time, except possibly Kepler himself, in whose ecstatic jubilation we may indeed glimpse an awareness that the last secret had been read. 'The book is written', he exclaimed, 'to be read either now or by posterity, I care not which. It may well wait a century for a reader, as God has waited six thousand years for an observer.'[10] But Kepler's was a solitary note, and for this there is more than one reason. In the first place, the speed of progress during the sixteenth century, measured against the background of the history of the preceding fourteen hundred years and the magnitude of the conceptions involved, had been breath-taking. Unbridled speculation on one hand, and dogged conservatism on the other, were common enough, but, apart from Galileo, we find no one with the mental power and poise requisite for a sober assessment of the

[9] The first two laws were published in *De motibus Stellae Martis* (*op. cit.* (4)) (1609), the third in *Harmonices mundi*. Lincii, 1619.

[10] *Harmonices mundi, op. cit.* (9).

position, and Galileo, as we shall see, was otherwise preoccupied. Again, the necessary basis of Kepler's laws—the Copernican view of the universe— was still for the most part an object of ridicule; here also enlightenment awaited Galileo's labours and persecution. And finally, even before the candles had been lit round the sanctified corpse of the old astronomy, the new had been born, and the Nunc Dimittis was lost in the Magnificat.

Goethe—no mean authority—has declared that there is no pleasure equal to that of being on with the new love before one is quite off with the old. If that is so, the astronomers of the early seventeenth century are to be envied. In two separate and independent directions, new and endless paths of inquiry revealed themselves, and it is to Galileo that we owe our recognition of both. The first originated with the invention of the telescope, the second with the invention of modern science. It has often been regretted that two contemporary astronomers of such outstanding genius as Kepler and Galileo should have been so indifferent to one another's achievements, but in truth it could scarcely have been otherwise. When one has for the first and last time discovered the eternal laws laid down by God at the Creation, and has for the first time and for ever opened the ears of the human mind to the divine harmonies, is he likely to be impressed by a new toy or by the childish timing of balls running down grooves? And when another has found the keys of new and unimagined realms of discovery, and sees day by day unfolding before him fresh wonders and ever-increasing possibilities of knowledge hitherto undreamed of, is he likely to be impressed by the final rounding off of a played-out theme? That Kepler and Galileo were contemporaries was the merest accident. In temper, outlook and achievement they were centuries apart.

The remainder of our period belongs to Galileo and his successors, but no history of this time, however brief, can omit a reference to Kepler's one successor, Jeremiah Horrocks. This extraordinary youth—he died in 1641 in his twenty-second year—entirely self-taught in astronomy, working in obscurity and in what little time his duties as a clergyman allowed him, discovered, among other things, certain discordances in the 'perfect' harmony of Kepler's ellipses, unravelled the orbit of the Moon, and, on the basis of his own improved tables, predicted and observed the transit of Venus of 1639, of the occurrence of which no other save his friend Crabtree, to whom he had revealed his calculation, was aware.[11] We can only speculate on what he might have achieved had he lived. Grant conjectures that the history of physical science in the seventeenth century would have read very differently from what it does now, and seeing what he was able to do in the dry tree, we can indeed set no limits to his powers in the green. He is among the inheritors of unfulfilled renown.

We may conveniently consider the early history of the new science under the separate headings of telescopic and mathematical astronomy, for the two held little discourse with one another. They broke through the barrier terminating the older astronomy by two distinct types of assault. The telescope showed that, within the solar system at least, positions and motions were not the only possible objects of study. When their mysteries had been

---

[11] Jeremiah Horrocks, *Venus in sole pariter visa.* Dantzig, 1662. (Written in 1640.)

solved there remained the nature of the heavenly bodies themselves to be determined—those stones rejected by the builders of the spheres, and now become the head of the corner; their surfaces could be scrutinized and their changes observed: new objects could be discerned, and that apparently without limit as the degree of perfection of the instrument advanced. Astronomy detached itself from cosmology and began to exist in its own right. But with the stars, the effect of the telescope was simply to emphasize the hopelessness of the problem. The false discs were destroyed and mere points of light remained. Bruno's daring speculation of an infinite plurality of worlds was all but confirmed. There was little doubt that the very magnitude of the stellar universe placed it beyond hope of intellectual comprehension; the finite mind could not grasp the infinite expanse of star-filled space.

It was here that the second discovery came to the rescue, the discovery of modern science, of 'scientific method', of 'inductive generalization'—the name is comparatively of little moment. This, though started by Galileo, came to full realization only with Newton. What it did in effect was to provide a means by which the finite mind *could* grasp the infinite creation. The device was to turn from cataloguing the path of each body and to seek instead *principles of behaviour* which were exhibited by all, no matter how numerous they might be. If such principles existed, they could be deduced from experiments performed on a few bodies, tested by application to others, and then applied 'by induction' to the whole, finite or infinite. This was the new task to which Galileo set himself in his experiments with falling bodies. It is the process we now carry on under the name of 'science'.

Let us begin with the telescope. This was invented by Galileo, though not before he had heard of its previous accidental construction by an obscure Dutchman. He immediately saw its possibilities in astronomy, and proceeded to realize them. He was rewarded beyond all possible expectation. In a short space of time the Earth-like surface of the Moon, the composition of the Milky Way and the inexpressible richness of the stellar universe, the satellites of Jupiter, sun-spots and the Sun's rotation, the phases of Venus, the apparent triplicity of Saturn—all these things were added to knowledge and hailed as a foretaste of greater revelations yet to come.[12] Throughout the century they did come, though naturally the pace slackened rapidly after the initial outburst. A few illustrative examples must suffice.

I shall not dwell on the development of the telescope itself, although, of course, that was an essential factor in the progress of this branch of astronomy, or on the growth of observatories to exploit the new instrument, of which our own at Greenwich, established in 1675, has a special interest for us. Our concern now is with ends, not means, and of these the most obvious was pursued by Hevelius who, by his chart of the Moon's surface, founded the systematic study of lunar topography.[13] A more dramatic story, however, is that of the gradual elucidation of the structure of Saturn's rings, which reflects the steady improvement in technique, and at the same time introduces us to some of the great names in seventeenth-century astronomy. To Galileo, Saturn had at first appeared as a triple body; his telescope was unable to

[12] Galileo Galilei, *Sidereus nuncius*. Venetiis, 1610.
[13] Cf. R. Grant, *History of physical astronomy*. London, 1852, p. 229.

show the true character of the appendages. On a later occasion, when, as it happened, the Earth was in the plane of the rings, he looked again and saw merely a simple disc like that of Jupiter.[14] This strange anomaly greatly perplexed him, but he never reached an explanation. It was reserved for Huygens in 1656, with a better telescope and a longer series of observations, to show the true form of this unique planet. But Huygens saw only one ring.[15] Not until 1675 was it discovered, this time by Cassini, that the ring was double, a narrow dark division separating a bright inner from a duller outer portion.[16] To carry the story further, to the discovery of a third ring and the fragmentary nature of all, would take us beyond our scope, but the development is worth mentioning in order to show the entirely new character that astronomy had assumed as a result of this one invention.

Another consequence of telescopic observation, whose importance cannot be over-estimated, was Roemer's deduction in 1676 of the finite velocity of light.[17] Of all his discoveries with the telescope, that of Jupiter's satellites gave the greatest pleasure to Galileo, but even his prophetic soul could scarcely have divined that they would bring the knowledge which was not only to provide Bradley with the first observational confirmation of the motion of the Earth,[18] but also, much later, to deceive us with the expectation that the motion of the Earth could ever be observed.[19] The paradox, as everyone knows, has been resolved by Einstein: we merely note here that Galileo's so ingenuous 'Medicean stars' have, in the end, brought far greater perplexity than his apparently inexplicable Saturn. This example illustrates also the advantage to the historian of a remote view-point. I have said that the importance of this deduction of Roemer's cannot be over-estimated, and I do not think anyone would now question this. Yet Grant, in writing his history of astronomy in 1852, already nearly two hundred years after the event, does not deem it worth a place among the eight references to Roemer in the index. In the text the discovery is dismissed in two lines.[20]

We turn to the second of Galileo's legacies, the inductive process of modern science, and this leads us straight to Newton. The subject, of course, transcends astronomy in the narrow sense (if astronomy *has* a narrow sense), but its origins were astronomical and astronomy provided the first great example of its application. We see its nature best by contrasting the outlook of Copernicus with that of Newton—the *De revolutionibus* with the *Principia*. Let us look at one or two salient features of the contrast.

To begin with, both modes of approach to the problem took observation as their starting point, but they dealt with observations in very different ways. To the medieval mind the observed positions of the heavenly bodies were data to be fitted into a preconceived type of pattern. The orbits were necessarily

[14] Galileo, letter to Velser, December 1612. English translation in D. Brewster, *Martyrs of science*. London, 1841, pp. 51–2.

[15] C. Huygens, *Systema Saturnium*. Hagae-Comitis, 1659.

[16] J. D. Cassini, *Journ. des Sçavants (1677)*, Paris, 1718, 32–4; *Mém. de l'Acad. des Sci. (1666–99)*, Paris, 1730, x, 582–4.

[17] O. Roemer, *Journ. des Sçavants (1676)*, Paris, 1717, 133–4; *Mém. de l'Acad. des Sci. (1666–99)*, Paris, 1730, x, 575–7.

[18] James Bradley, *Phil. Trans. Roy. Soc.*, 1727–8, xxxv, 637.

[19] See, for example, A. A. Michelson and E. W. Morley, *Phil. Mag.*, 1887, 5s., xxiv, 449.

[20] Grant, *op. cit.* (13), p. 461.

circular, the velocities necessarily uniform, and the motions had to be accommodated to those of spheres satisfying certain conditions. These conditions were imposed *a priori*, their sanction, apart from their having been laid down by Aristotle, being their appeal to a sense of fitness. The heavens must be perfect, and circularity, sphericity and uniformity were attributes of perfection.

The Galilean-Newtonian method likewise sought to interpret observations in terms of general principles, but its essential characteristic was that the principles were not pre-established but were left to be suggested by the observations themselves. Nothing was excluded as illegitimate, nothing imposed as necessary. The derivation of the principles—an act of imagination, of induction—was the end and not the beginning of philosophical inquiry, and all attempts to limit or control the suggestions of phenomena themselves, whether by idly imagined entities or by supposed primary necessities, were regarded as inventions of 'hypotheses' and flatly rejected.

The rejection was emphatic with both Galileo and Newton, but its form varied according to the characters of the men. To Galileo, *a priori* principles and occult influences appeared as mere names mistakenly regarded as things, and he tried to discredit them by exposure and satire.

> We [says Simplicius, the Aristotelian, in the *Dialogues*], confining our selves to the terms of Art reduce the cause of these and other the like natural effects to *Sympathy*, which is a certain agreement and mutual appetite which ariseth between things that are semblable to one another in qualities; as likewise on the contrary that hatred and enmity for which other things shun and abhor one another we call *Antipathy*.
>
> And thus [replies Sagredus] with these two words men come to render reasons of a great number of accidents and effects which we see not without admiration to be produced in nature. But this kind of philosophating seems to me to have great sympathy with a certain way of Painting that a Friend of mine used, who writ upon the *Tele* or Canvasse in chalk, here I will have the Fountain with *Diana* and her Nimphs, there certain Hariers, in this corner I will have a Hunts-man with the Head of a Stag, the rest shall be Lanes, Woods, and Hills; and left the remainder for the Painter to set forth with Colours; and thus he perswaded himself that he had painted the Story of *Acteon*, when as he had contributed thereto nothing of his own more than the names.[21]

Newton, in an age which had known Puritanism, was sterner, chastizing where Galileo had ridiculed:

> Whatever is not deduced from the phenomena, is to be called an hypothesis; and hypotheses, whether metaphysical or physical, whether of occult qualities or mechanical, have no place in experimental philosophy . . . . Give me leave to insinuate, Sir, that I cannot think it effectual for determining truth, to examine the several ways by which phenomena may be explained, unless where there can be a perfect enumeration of all those ways . . . . The *Aristotelians* gave the Name of occult Qualities, not to manifest Qualities, but to such Qualities only as they supposed to lie hid in Bodies, and to be the unknown Causes of manifest Effects: Such as would be the Causes of Gravity, and of magnetick and electrick Attractions, and of Fermentations, if we should suppose that these Forces or Actions arose from Qualities unknowne to us, and uncapable of being discovered and made manifest. Such occult Qualities put a stop to the Improvement of natural Philosophy, and therefore of late Years have been rejected. To tell us that every Species of Things

[21] Galileo, *Dialogues concerning the Two Great Systems of the World* (Salusbury's translation 1661), Dialogue iii.

is endow'd with an occult specific Quality by which it acts and produces manifest Effects, is to tell us nothing: But to derive two or three general Principles of Motion from Phaenomena, and afterwards to tell us how the Properties and Actions of all corporeal Things follow from those manifest Principles, would be a very great step in Philosophy, though the Causes of those Principles were not yet discovered.[22]

Another important characteristic of the new science was that it shifted the emphasis from passive observation to active creation. The older astronomer could do nothing but discover; at the very highest, as in Kepler, he thought God's thoughts after him. The new astronomy, for all its humility in the face of facts, laid on its devotees the task of inventing a scheme of the universe, and so called for an act of creative imagination. It was all very well to let phenomena suggest their own principles, but phenomena were dumb. Their way of directing science was to show themselves and then require the astronomer to propose a scheme, to which they would merely rap out the answer, yes or no. Even that exaggerates their contribution. They might signal 'No', but 'Yes' could only be inferred from their immobility. Newton's great scheme of universal gravitation, for instance, was his own creation. He knew no more of the facts than many another, but he alone could create the principles with which to confront nature. And he could never get the final approval of nature. The most that he could expect was that all his importunity would never provoke her to dissent. That is the inescapable penalty of induction. You may surmount the barrier of the infinite by generalizing from the particular to the universal, but you can never know that you have generalized rightly. Newton's supreme achievement passed the tests of nearly a quarter of a millenium, and then, by the tiniest shake of the head, nature interposed her veto, and the whole fabric was shattered.

We are learning now not to reject induction on that account, but rather to revise our expectations. Not only do we find it better to travel hopefully than to arrive, but we are beginning to understand that what is gathered on the journey remains a permanent possession. Newton's gravitational force has followed the celestial spheres into the limbo of curiosities, but, unlike the spheres, it has left a permanent legacy of knowledge which has been transfigured but not destroyed. We hail its successor no longer with any illusion of finality, but with a well-founded hope of further progress.

That, however, is a modern attitude. On the intellectual side the seventeenth century closed in a blaze of glory. In less than a hundred years the new science had brought forth the greatest co-ordination of knowledge in history, and while, by its very perfection, it might seem to close the door to further generalization as irrevocably as Kepler had closed the door to further geometrical description, the possibilities of application to concrete problems were unlimited, and there were fields of inquiry other than astronomy in which the same methods might be expected to yield the same success. Achievement in the new endeavour was no longer an end but a beginning.

The final appraisal of the work of these two centuries is still a task for the future. To the men of the time it was an utter impossibility, and even to us, after the passage of two hundred and fifty years of unparalleled progress, there is much that remains uncomprehended. We no longer share the

---

[22] I. Newton, *Opticks*. 4th edition. London, 1730, p. 377.

extravagant enthusiasm which saw only that God had let Newton be and all was light. Our eyes have adapted themselves to the light, and we see dark corners and a marked deficiency of certain colours. There is more than a suspicion of space absorption, and our eyes are not altogether free from aberrations. On the other hand, we are to some extent released from the illusions of those to whom the light was light invisible, who saw only that science had given a star and taken a Sun away. We recognize the inductive process of science as the source of all subsequent natural knowledge, and the more it teaches us, the better we are able to understand its nature. It is not our task here to examine it in its fuller maturity. We have seen it started on its career, and we may wish it God-speed.

FIRE AND THE FLAMMA VITALIS:
BOYLE, HOOKE AND MAYOW

by

DOUGLAS McKIE

Introduction

FROM early times it was known that air was necessary for the maintenance both of fire and of life. The ancient Egyptians used the blow-pipe and the bellows to increase the heat of their furnaces by a more copious supply of air.[1] Cicero spoke of *cibus animalis* as the nourishment that the lungs draw from the air.[2] In a simple way this knowledge was applied in classical antiquity, and Vitruvius described how men digging wells let down a lighted lamp into the shaft to test the air before going down; if the flame continued to burn, they might safely descend.[3] In this way arose the phrases *flamma vitalis, flammula vitæ*, the vital flame, the flame of life, the fire of life, and so on, the literary imagery in which these simple facts were expressed.

In the period during which modern science arose, the chemical facts relating to combustion and respiration were gained only slowly, and what is very common knowledge in our own time took over a century to establish. In this essay we shall discuss the chemical researches of two of the outstanding seventeenth-century investigators of these problems, Boyle and Hooke, make

---

[1] See J. R. Partington, *Origins and development of applied chemistry*. London, 1935, pp. 8, 15, 21–2, and other references in subject-index under 'blow-pipe' and 'bellows'.

[2] Cicero, *De natura deorum*, ii. 55: 'In pulmonibus autem inest raritas quaedam et adsimilis spongiis mollitudo ad hauriendum spiritum aptissima, qui tum se contrahunt adspirantes, tum in respiratu dilatantur, ut frequenter ducatur cibus animalis quo maxime aluntur animantes.'

[3] Vitruvius, *De architectura*, viii. 6: 'Hoc autem quibus rationibus caveatur, sic erit faciendum. Lucerna accensa demittatur; quae si permanserit ardens, sine periculo descendetur.'

brief reference to the work of Mayow, and attempt to disentangle a history that has become confused in the interval of almost three hundred years that now separates us from their work.

Boyle's Experiments on Combustion (1660)

The Hon. Robert Boyle (1627–91) carried out many experiments on combustion and respiration in the receiver of his 'Pneumatical Engine', as he called the air-pump invented and constructed for him in 1658–9 by Robert Hooke (1635–1703). With these experiments both problems entered upon their modern history by the experimental establishment of the relevant chemical facts. Lighted candles and wax tapers put into the receiver went out when it was evacuated of its air; if it was not emptied of its air, they burned much longer before going out.[4] 'Kindled Wood-coals' and 'a piece of Match, such as Souldiers use' behaved similarly, but the 'coals' could be rekindled if quickly taken out of the receiver and swung about in the air, and the 'Match' was re-ignited if air was admitted.[5] Boyle noted, of course, that in the open air these combustibles burned for a longer time than in the unevacuated closed receiver. It was thought that fire died away in enclosed spaces because it was extinguished by its own fumes. The experiments did not bear this out, because the fire died out on removal of air which gave room for the fumes. To make this proof complete, Boyle included in the receiver a bladder partly filled with air and tied closely at the neck; the fire went out and the fumes seemed to fill the receiver, but the air in the bladder expanded, and hence the fumes could not have prevented the residual air in the receiver from expanding.[6] After a number of unsuccessful attempts, the gunpowder in a pistol was fired even in an evacuated receiver, though Boyle did not feel assured that some small amount of air had not remained in the receiver[7]; but combustibles in the evacuated receiver could not be ignited by a burning-glass from outside, although he thought that this might have been due to the thickness of the glass of the receiver.[8] At the conclusion of this work, he forbore for the moment to make any conclusions.[9]

Boyle's Experiments on Respiration (1660)

In this same work Boyle reported similar experiments on respiration. A lark, a sparrow and a mouse were successively placed in the receiver with results similar to those obtained in the experiments on combustion. Life was extinguished by removal of the air, although this evacuation removed also the 'fuliginous Steams' discharged from the lungs and alleged by some to act in like manner to the fumes produced in combustion.[10] Moreover, a mouse was found to live through a whole night when left in the unevacuated receiver, so that animals died from want of air, not from the 'steams' they produced when enclosed in the receiver.[11] Boyle felt that he was unable to draw any conclusions; his experiments, he thought, were too few, and respiration

---

[4] Robert Boyle, *New Experiments Physico-Mechanicall, touching the Spring of the Air, and its Effects (made for the most part, in a New Pneumatical Engine)*, etc. Oxford, 1660, pp. 74–8.

[5] *ibid.*, pp. 78–83. [6] *ibid.*, pp. 84–8.

[7] *ibid.*, pp. 88–102 (pp. 90–9 omitted in pagination).

[8] *ibid.*, pp. 102–5. [9] *ibid.*, p. 104.

[10] *ibid.*, pp. 328–34. [11] *ibid.*, p. 334.

PLATE XXXVI

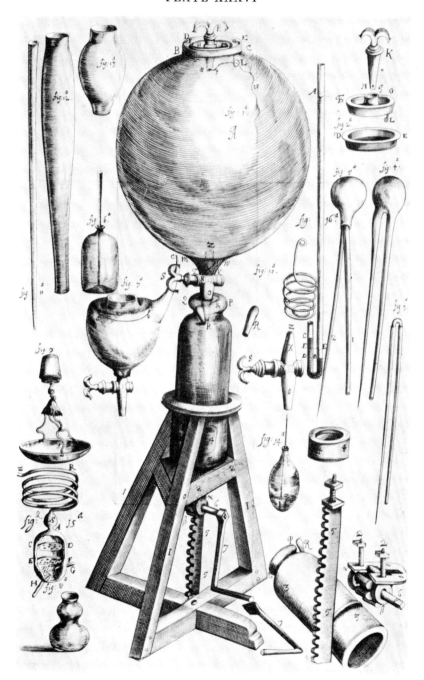

FIG. 1. Boyle's air-pump, designed and constructed by Hooke
(R. Boyle, *New Experiments Physico-Mechanicall*, Oxford, 1660)
(From the British Museum copy)

appeared to be rather more than less mysterious than it did before.[12] He seemed persuaded, however, that in respiration the air did more than merely remove what was thrown out of the blood in its passage through the lungs.[13] Current explanations and opinions were not very amenable to experimental study; but he recalled an opinion of Paracelsus that the lungs consumed part of the air and rejected the rest, as the stomach concocted meat, making part of it useful to the body and rejecting the other; and from this opinion it appeared that air contained 'a little vital Quintessence', a small part of useful matter in a much greater quantity of unserviceable material.[14] This needed, said Boyle, not assertion, but proof. He made some further experiments with a new-born puppy, an eel, a snail and various insects,[15] and postponed speculation, contenting himself with the opinion that the air played some part in respiration which had not yet been explained.[16] He had, however, noted a resemblance between fire and life, since he had found in his experiments that the flame of a lamp persisted no more than did the life of an animal in his receiver on evacuation of the air; and he was inclined to accept the opinion expressed by some that air was needed 'to ventilate, and cherish the vitall flame, which they do suppose to be continually burning in the heart'.[17]

Hooke's Theory of Combustion (1661–1664)

In a tract[18] published shortly after Boyle's *New Experiments*, etc. had appeared in 1660, Robert Hooke, who had invented and constructed the air-pump for those experiments and who had been Boyle's paid assistant during the time in which they were carried out, asserted that in the wicks of lighted candles and lamps the oil or spirits or melted tallow 'is dispersed and carried away by the Flame (which what it is, and how it consumes bodies, I shall on some other occasion by many luciferous Experiments manifestly prove)'. Hooke's interest in the problem of combustion may have been aroused by his association with Boyle. He was a bolder thinker than Boyle, but this mere hint is all that he allowed himself to express in 1661. Until the publication of his *Micrographia* in 1665, we have to seek for his ideas in the minutes of the meetings of the Royal Society as published in Birch's *History of the Royal Society*. These minutes record several discussions and some experiments, before the publication of the *Micrographia*, on such matters as the extinguishing of a lighted candle under a cupping-glass and the maintenance of flame in a vessel under water, but these date before Hooke's appointment as curator of experiments on 12 November 1662. At the meeting of 3 December 1662, at which Hooke was present, a paper was presented by Power[19] on the subject of 'damps' in coal-mines which reveals the opinions then held about the substances we now know as 'gases'. There were, said Power, 'three sorts of damps; or rather, three degrees of the same damp'. The 'common damp' put out a candle, but did not suffocate

---

[12] *ibid.*, p. 335.
[13] *ibid.*, p. 359.
[14] *ibid.*, p. 362.
[15] *ibid.*, pp. 368–73, 377–81.
[16] *ibid.*, p. 383.
[17] *ibid.*, pp. 365–7.
[18] Robert Hooke, *An Attempt for the Explication of the Phænomena, Observable in an Experiment Published by the Honourable Robert Boyle, Esq.*, etc. London, 1661, p. 45.
[19] T. Birch, *The History of the Royal Society of London*, etc. 4 vols. London, 1756–7, vol. i, pp. 133–6.

the miners; the 'suffocating damp' was, as its name implied, fatal to the miners, and dogs or lighted candles were used to test for its presence; and the 'fiery damp' was most dangerous and explosive. Here 'damps' were considered as merely qualitatively different, but essentially the same; and for long afterwards this idea persisted, the substances we now know as 'gases' and recognize as different chemical entities being similarly regarded as qualitatively different varieties of air, as air slightly altered and with different properties. Shortly after this, Hooke turned to experiment before the Society; and he found by using a bladder that the same sample of air would serve for human respiration, without a supply of fresh air, for only five inspirations, and that with difficulty (21 January 1662/3).[20] On this date Hooke made a suggestion for an important experiment, the result of which was later on to cause much difficulty for many years, namely, the enclosing 'of an animal and a candle together in a vessel, to see whether they would die at the same time or not'.[21] A week later, on 28 January 1662/3, the experiment was made with a burning lamp and a chick: 'and the lamp went out within two minutes, the chick remaining alive, and lively enough.'[22] Thus the first significant experiment bearing at once on the related problems of combustion and respiration had produced a result that suggested difference rather than similarity in these processes. On 4 February 1662/3, further experiments were made on the continued respiration of the same air and some figures were obtained, not of any great interest.[23]

On 25 February 1662/3, Hooke, having been instructed at the meeting held a week previously to bring in a 'scheme of experiments' concerning air, brought in a 'scheme of inquiries' about the air numbering about a hundred.[24] The Society instructed him to set about the making of suitable experiments on the first 'head' of his scheme of inquiries, namely, the constitution and substance of the air. We cannot say what effect this heavy demand had upon Hooke, but he does not appear to have shown any readiness to put it into operation, although it must be remembered that at this time he was working at his microscopical observations, and that it was only on the completion of these and of the printing of the *Micrographia* towards the end of 1664 that he resumed his activities on the problems of combustion and respiration. Meanwhile, during the years 1663 and 1664, the Society witnessed experiments on the effect on fishes of the removal of air from the water in which they had been placed, and on the breathing of a mouse in condensed air and of various birds in common, rarefied and condensed air: after an initial failure with compressed air, the bird being taken out dead, it appeared that a bird lived longer in compressed than in common air.[25] Hooke had taken part in these experiments, but not very actively until late in 1664, when, on 2 November, he suggested the famous experiment of displaying the thorax of a dog, inserting a tube in the wind-pipe and blowing air into the lungs.[26] A week later, on 9 November 1664, he reported the result of the experiment; the dog's heart had continued to beat, life persisting for over an hour, so long as

[20] *ibid.*, vol. i, p. 179.   [21] *ibid.*, vol. i, p. 180.   [22] *ibid.*

[23] *ibid.*, vol. i, p. 192.   [24] *ibid.*, vol. i, pp. 202 ff.

[25] *ibid.*, vol. i, pp. 214, 216, 218, 244, 309, 389, 392, 395, 401, 404, 408, 418, 423, 427, 428.

[26] *ibid.*, vol. i, p. 482.

the lungs were distended by supplies of fresh air,[27] whereby it was evident that life depended on the continuous supply of that air, and not on any mere mechanical motion of the respiratory organs.

Combustion in Hooke's 'Micrographia' (1665)

However, when the *Micrographia* was printed, it was clear that Hooke had been formulating his theory of combustion which was set out in Observation XVI, entitled '*Of* Charcoal, *or burnt* Vegetables'.[28] Proceeding from the observation that wood heated in a closed vessel was converted into charcoal, but not consumed unless air was admitted, Hooke argued that the air acted as a menstruum or solvent of 'sulphureous', i.e. combustible, bodies, provided the bodies were heated sufficiently. This dissolution produced great heat, commonly called 'fire', and therefore fire was not an element; sometimes the action was so violent as to put the particles of the burning body into that rapid motion that produced the 'action or pulse of light' in the air. But the most striking point in Hooke's theory was '*that the dissolution* of sulphureous bodies is made by a substance inherent, and mixt with the Air, that is like, if not the very same, with that which is fixt in *Salt-peter*, which by multitudes of Experiments that may be made with *Saltpeter*, will, I think, most evidently be demonstrated'.[29] Moreover, 'the dissolving parts of the Air are but few, that is, it seems of the nature of those *Saline menstruums*, or spirits, that have very much flegme mixt with the spirits, and therefore a small parcel of it is quickly glutted, and will dissolve no more; and therefore unless some fresh part of this *menstruum* be apply'd to the body to be dissolv'd, the action ceases, and the body leaves to be dissolv'd and to shine, which is the Indication of it, though plac'd or kept in the greatest heat; whereas *Salt-peter* is a *menstruum*, when melted and red-hot, that abounds more with those Dissolvent particles, and therefore as a small quantity of it will dissolve a great sulphureous body, so will the dissolution be very quick and violent'.[30] 'Therefore . . . , it is observable', he went on, 'that, as in other solutions, if a copious and quick supply of fresh *menstruum*, though but weak, be poured on, or applied to the dissoluble body, it quickly consumes it: So this *menstruum* of the Air, if by Bellows, or any other such contrivance, it be copiously apply'd to the shining body, is found to dissolve it as soon, and as violently as the more strong *menstruum* of melted *Nitre*.'[31] The 'shining transient body which we call *Flame*' was, added Hooke, a mixture of air and the 'volatil sulphureous parts of dissoluble or combustible bodies'.[32] This hypothesis he had 'endeavoured to raise from an Infinite of Observations and Experiments, the process of which would be much too long to be here inserted, and will perhaps another time afford matter copious enough for a much longer Discourse, the Air being a Subject which (though all the world has hitherto liv'd and breath'd in, and been conversant about) has yet been so little truly examin'd or explain'd, that a diligent enquirer will be able to find

---

[27] *ibid.*, vol. i, pp. 485–6.

[28] Robert Hooke, *Micrographia: or Some Physiological Descriptions of Minute Bodies made by Magnifying Glasses with Observations and Inquiries thereupon.* London, 1665, pp. 100–106. The book was printed in 1664, but not published until 1665.

[29] *ibid.*, p. 103.   [30] *ibid.*, p. 104.   [31] *ibid.*, pp. 104–5.   [32] *ibid.*, p. 105.

but very little information from what has been (till of late) written of it. . . .'[33] Elsewhere, he said, he would show the use of the air in respiration, but here he had only time to give a hint of his hypothesis.[34]

Hooke's theory marks a great advance; it is the first step towards the modern theory of combustion. It supposes the air to consist of parts that differ in their chemical behaviour. One of these parts is active in combustion, and later Hooke was to say that the same part was active in respiration; and the active part was like, if not identical with, something that was contained in saltpetre. Hooke was clearly probing his way, in great difficulty and out of due time, towards that constituent of air that was active in combustion and respiration and also present in saltpetre, the substance we now know as oxygen. Despite this clear trend towards a discovery that was still over a century ahead, we must note that, when Hooke considered the action of air on particles of iron dropped through a flame, he concluded that the air acted on a part of the iron, on 'a very *combustible sulphureous* Body' contained in it, so that iron was not elementary, but compounded of differing parts.[35] We may recall, in concluding this account, that the experiment on the living dog had shown that life persisted so long as the lungs were distended by supplies of fresh air.[36]

Hooke's Theory at the Royal Society (1665–1670)

After the printing of his *Micrographia*, Hooke began to expound his theory at the meetings of the Royal Society. Many experiments were made, and the same experiment was often shown at successive meetings, but we shall note here only the historically significant experiments. The discussions that took place afford strong evidence of the degree to which Hooke had outrun his contemporaries in his study of this problem. On 4 January 1664/5,[37] Hooke made the experiment with a live coal in a glass vessel; the fire died away, but revived when the coal was brought out into the air; and the experiment was intended to show 'that air is the universal dissolvent of all sulphureous bodies, and that this dissolution is fire', and that this is done 'by a nitrous substance inherent and mixt with the air'. To the objection that it was the agitation of the air driving the igneous particles into the combustible body that made it burn and consume, Hooke replied that a burning body was extinguished when not supplied with fresh air, and that a red-hot combustible would not be consumed until air was admitted to it. Boyle, who, it must be remembered, had, as we have seen, made a number of decisive experiments on the necessity of air for the maintenance of flame and fire, proposed the trying of an experiment in which a burning coal was to be put inside a receiver connected with a pair of strong bellows, 'with the clack stopt, and the nose made fast with cement' to the receiver, the bellows to be worked to see if the resulting 'wind' would make the coal burn.

At the next meeting, on 11 January 1664/5,[38] Hooke showed that red-hot sulphur in a sealed tube did not burn until air was admitted; and charcoal heated red-hot in a sealed tube did not burn. Moreover, charcoal covered with sand and 'kept in a very great heat for about two hours' in a crucible was

[33] *ibid.*   [34] *ibid.*   [35] *ibid.*, p. 45.
[36] *loc. cit.* (27).   [37] Birch, *op. cit.* (19), vol. ii, p. 2.   [38] *ibid.*, vol. ii, p. 4.

after cooling found to be 'scarce sensibly diminished'. Objection was made that the air in the vessel was 'superonerated' with the 'steam', that is, the smoke, of the wood, and that this was the reason why the charcoal did not burn; but Hooke replied that this called for an experiment in which the air was evacuated from the vessel, thus making the smoke fall down, whence it would appear that it was lack of air which prevented combustion. Such an experiment had already been carried out by Boyle.[39]

At the meeting of 18 January 1664/5,[40] an experiment on the lines suggested by Boyle on 4 January was made, the bellows and the coal being enclosed in a box. After ten or twelve minutes the coals went out, despite the working of the bellows, 'nor could they be revived by any blowing of the included air upon them', but as soon as fresh air was admitted and the bellows plied, burning began again. Discussion followed. The President, Lord Brouncker, considered that the experiments had answered the objection about the agitation of the air, and thought that an experiment might be made to show 'that it was not the filling of the pores of the air with exhalations, and the rendering it thereby unable to receive more of them, that made it go out'. Sir Robert Moray apparently still considered that the extinction of the fire might be caused by the compression of the air and suggested an experiment to decide this. Hooke countered with the argument that, since it had been found that highly rarefied air extinguished burning bodies, condensed air would keep them burning longer. Boyle suggested three experiments: (1) to try to kindle combustible matter or to convert it into smoke by a burning-glass from outside in the air in which the coals would no longer burn, and, among other combustibles, to try finely-powdered coals of the same kind as those extinguished; (2) when sunbeams could not be used, to let fall a red-hot iron on the extinguished coals from which the smoke was to be raised; and (3) to distil finely-powdered charcoal and examine the products to see if it was correct that such coals would afford ' no more steams'. We may perhaps sense an acidulous note in Hooke's expression of a desire 'that some experiments might be suggested, that were not solvable by the hypothesis of fire proposed by him'. Moray then made a further suggestion that Boyle, 'who had long since considered this subject of fire, and flame, and heat, might give the society his thoughts thereof', but Boyle was busy with other matters which he felt would not give him time to review what he had previously written. We quote this discussion as typical of the reception that Hooke's ideas met with; experiments were repeated and further discussions ensued, but it is clear that Hooke's theory was not well received. Little purpose would be served by further quotations and we shall limit ourselves to brief reference to the many other experiments that were made. A lamp burned five times as long in compressed as in common air;[41] a red-hot iron could not re-kindle coals extinguished in a closed glass receiver until air was re-admitted;[42] charcoal and nitre enclosed in a glass were found to burn,[43] and sulphur dropped on red-hot nitre in a receiver exhausted of air inflamed;[44] Hooke argued on 27 June 1667,[45] that air was fit for respiration because there

[39] loc. cit. (6).

[40] Birch, op. cit. (19), vol. ii, pp. 7–8.

[41] ibid., vol. ii, p. 10.

[42] ibid., vol. ii, p. 12.

[43] ibid., vol. ii, p. 15.

[44] ibid., vol. ii, p. 19.

[45] ibid., vol. ii, p. 184.

was in it 'a kind of nitrous quality', which being spent made the air unfit for respiration; a bird lived much longer in compressed than in common air;[46] and on various dates in February and March 1670/1, Hooke himself was enclosed in an apparatus and found that he was not affected on the withdrawal of a part of the air, recorded on an included gauge, by anything except some pain in the ears.[47] In the five years following its publication in the *Micrographia*, Hooke's theory does not appear to have gained any adherents among the Fellows of the Royal Society.

A New Experiment by Boyle on Respiration (1670)

In 1670 Boyle reported two new series of experiments on respiration. In the first of these,[48] he showed that suffocation by drowning killed various animals a little sooner than evacuation of the air in which they were enclosed in a receiver, but he noted that the destructive action in drowning was applied at once, whereas the removal of the air from the receiver was gradual; however, he was able to improve his technique so that a mouse was killed in the receiver by removal of the air in less than half a minute. The second series[49] included an experiment with an important result; a mouse was included in a glass vessel together with a mercury gauge, the vessel was sealed and the respiration of the mouse continued for over two hours with no apparent change in the pressure of the air, so that 'Air, become unfit for Respiration, may retain its wonted pressure'. The experiment was described by Boyle as follows:

'We took a Mouse of an ordinary size, and having (not without some difficulty) conveyed him into an Ovall Glass, fitted with a somewhat long and considerably broad neck, which we had provided, that it might be wide enough to admit a Mouse in spight of his struggling. We conveyed in after him a Mercurial Gage, in which we had diligently observed and marked the Station of the Mercury, and which was so fastned to a Wire reaching to the bottom of the Ovall Glass, that the Gage, remaining in the neck, was not in danger to be broken by the motions of the Mouse in the Oval part: The upper part of the long neck of the Glass was, notwithstanding the wideness of it, hermetically sealed by the help of a Lamp and a pair of Bellows, that we might be sure, that the imprisoned Animal, should breathe no other Air, then that which filled the Receiver at the time when it was nipped up. This done, the Mouse was watched from time to time, and though by reason of the largeness of the Vessel in comparison of so small an Animal, he seemed to me rather drooping then very near death at the end of the second hour; yet coming to look upon him about half an hour after, he was judged by the Spectators quite dead, notwithstanding our shaking of the Vessel to rouze him up. This made me cast my eyes upon the Gage, wherein I could not perceive any sensible change of the Mercuries Station.'[50]

The mouse, however, recovered on the admission of fresh air, and the humane Boyle set him at liberty, although not before he had tried another experiment with him. But the result of the experiment quoted cannot have

[46] *ibid.*, vol. ii, p. 304.
[47] *ibid.*, vol. ii, p. 470.
[48] Robert Boyle, *Phil. Trans. Roy. Soc.*, 1670, v, 2011–31.
[49] *ibid.*, pp. 2035–56.
[50] *ibid.*, pp. 2046–7.

provided much support for Hooke's theory, since there appeared to be no decrease in the pressure of the air; if a reduction in pressure had been observed, that theory might have gained a striking confirmation; the experiment was made, however, in a receiver, and not over water, and hence there was no change in pressure, since the carbon dioxide, produced in respiration, contains, as we now know, its own volume of oxygen.

Boyle on 'Flame and Air' (1672)

Shortly after the publication of the two memoirs referred to in the preceding section, Boyle made further experiments described in some tracts prepared in 1671 but not published until 1672. These are concerned to some extent with the 'vital flame' that some of Boyle's contemporaries supposed to reside in the heart of animals and to the preservation of which, as of other flames, air was necessary. Boyle reveals himself in these tracts as not so certain as some of his contemporaries that air was so necessary to the production and conservation of all kinds of flame as his previous experiments had led them to conclude.[51] The experiments now reported on combustibles placed in a receiver, which was then exhausted of its air, scarcely call for much comment. Sulphur would not ignite in vacuo either by contact with red-hot iron or by heating the containing vessel on coals;[52] burning sulphur was extinguished in vacuo, but rekindled with 'divers little flashes', though not with a constant flame, on readmission of a small amount of air;[53] gunpowder in vacuo was not fired by a burning-glass;[54] gunpowder let fall on a hot iron in vacuo did not take fire, but Boyle noticed a slight explosion when air was admitted;[55] on one occasion some gunpowder, carefully heated in an evacuated vessel on the ashes above a charcoal fire, did not fire, but seemed to be partly kindled and gave a considerable flame, Boyle observing that it was 'the sulphureous ingredient' that had been 'in part kindled';[56] gunpowder in a pistol fired in a vacuum did not explode, but a small residue of powder in the pan of the pistol took fire when the experiment was tried again after readmission of the air;[57] and aurum fulminans was fired in vacuo by a burning-glass and also by a hot iron (at night, the flash was visible).[58] Since it was easier to preserve flame in a body already kindled than to produce it in the first place, Boyle tried some experiments to see whether bodies actually burning might not be kept so without the concurrence of air. Kindled sulphur,[59] the 'fumes' (hydrogen) from 'saline Spirit' and steel filings,[60] and spirit of wine 'impregnated with a metal'[61] all went out when the receiver was evacuated, but it is significant of Boyle's attitude that he seems to have felt himself that in some cases the flame survived the exhaustion for some time, although he credits some of the observers with this opinion.[62] Gunpowder packed in a goose-quill or 'a piece of a Tobacco-pipe' burnt under water.[63]

---

[51] Robert Boyle, *Tracts written by the Honourable Robert Boyle, containing New Experiments, touching the Relation betwixt Flame and Air*, etc. Oxford, 1672, pp. 16–17. (Printed in London, published in Oxford.)

[52] *ibid.*, pp. 21–4.   [53] *ibid.*, pp. 29–30.   [54] *ibid.*, pp. 33–4.
[55] *ibid.*, pp. 35–8.   [56] *ibid.*, pp. 39–40.   [57] *ibid.*, pp. 42–4.
[58] *ibid.*, pp. 46–9.   [59] *ibid.*, pp. 54–8.   [60] *ibid.*, pp. 63–6.
[61] *ibid.*, pp. 67–8.   [62] *ibid.*, p. 58.   [63] *ibid.*, pp. 71–9.

Boyle's Experiment on the Burning of Gunpowder under Water (1671)[64]

The result of this last experiment, confirmed in various vessels, could not fail to bring Hooke's theory very prominently into Boyle's thoughts. We shall refer to his comments below. First, it is interesting to quote, if only for its appeal to the chemist, Boyle's own description of this striking experiment on what he called 'wildfire': 'The way of making the Experiment is this: We took of Gunpowder three ounces, of well burnt Charcoal one drachm, of good Sulphur or flower of Brimstone a little less than half a drachm, of choice Salt-petre near a drachm and a half: Which Ingredients being well reduc'd to powder, and diligently mingled without any liquor; *either* a large Goose-Quil, whose feathery part was cut off, *or* a piece of a Tobacco-pipe of two or three inches long, and well stop'd at one end, had its cavity well fill'd with this mixture, (instead of which, beaten Gunpowder alone might serve, if it did not operate too violently, or waste too soon:) For the kindling whereof, the open orifice of the Quil or Pipe was carefully stopt with a convenient quantity of the same mixture, made up with as little Chymical Oyle or Water, as would bring it to a fit consistence. This Wild-fire was kindled in the Air, and the Quill or Pipe, together with a weight, to which 'twas tied to keep it from ascending, was slowly let down to a convenient depth under water, where it would continue to burn, as appeared by the great smoak it emitted, and other signs, as it did in the air; because the shape of the Quil or Pipe kept the dry mixture from being accessible to the water (that would have disorder'd and spoil'd it) at any other part than the upper Orifice; and there the stream of kindled matter issued out with such violence, as did incessantly beat off the neighbouring water, and kept it from entering into the cavity that contain'd the mixture, which therefore would continue burning till 'twas consumed.'[65]

Boyle had already noticed a possible criticism and dealt with it: 'And that there might be no suspicion, that whilst the mixture continued under water, it did only as it were vehemently ferment, or suffer a violent agitation of its parts without having them kindled, till in their ascending they were actually fired by the contact of the air, incumbent on the surface of the water; To obviate this suspicion (I say) we were careful to try the Experiment, not only in other Vessels, but in a large Glass, the transparency of whose Sides, as well as that of the contained water, would permit us to see for a while the burning of our composition, which was sometimes with a weight detain'd, and sometimes with a *Forceps* held, till 'twas consumed, a good way under the surface of the Water.'[66]

It was a new and important result.

Boyle on Hooke's Theory (1672)

Boyle's comments on the striking experiment that he had so successfully made show that he had Hooke's theory in mind. He wrote: ''Tis probable, that most men will conclude from this Experiment, that Air is not so absolutely necessary to the duration of Flame, as some other of our Tryals seem to argue; and that there ought to be a difference made between ordinary

---

[64] The *Tracts*, etc., 1672, *op. cit.* (51), were ready for publication in 1671, and it seems reasonable to date the experiment as 1671 rather than 1672.

[65] *Tracts*, etc., 1672, *op. cit.* (51), pp. 74-5.

[66] *ibid.*, pp. 73-4.

Flames, and those that burn with an extraordinary vehemency. But my design being, as I long since intimated, rather to relate Tryals than debate Hypotheses, I shall only add, that it may be pretended on the behalf of the opinion that this experiment seems to disprove, that, not to mention the Air that may lurk in the Pores of the Water, or that which may be intercepted between the little grains of Powder whereof the mixture consists, the Saltpetre it self may be suppos'd to be of such a texture, that in its very formation the corpuscles, that compose it, may intercept store of little aereal particles between the very minute solid ones which those Corpuscles are made up of. And this inexistence of the Air in Nitre may be probably argued from the great windiness of the flame that is produced upon the deflagration of Nitre. According to this surmise, though our mixture burns under water, yet it does not burn without air, being supplied with enough to serve the turn by the numerous eruptions of the aereal particles of the dissipated Nitre it self.'[67]

Boyle's opinion was therefore that nitre might well contain particles of air enclosed among its component corpuscles,[68] and therein he differed from Hooke who regarded air and nitre as containing a common constituent. Moreover, Boyle had, as he pointed out here, formerly tried 'to remove this suspicion' by preparing nitre in a vacuum: 'On this occasion I remember, that in another Paper I relate, that for divers purposes, and among them to remove this suspicion, I successfully tried to reproduce Nitre *in Vacuo Boyliano*, that there might not be any Air, or at least any quantity worth heeding, intercepted between the convening particles, that by their coalitions made up the nitrous Corpuscles, which in favour of the necessity of Air to Flame may be pretended to be but so many little empty bubbles close stop'd, whose moister parts may by the fire that kindles the nitre be exceedingly rarified, and in that estate emulate air, and violently burst their little prisons, and throw about the fragments of them with force, and in numbers enough to make their aggregate appear such a flame, as is wont to be made by unctuous and truly combustible Bodies; and yet this rarifi'd substance, that thus shatters the nitrous particles, may really be no true and lasting air, but only vehemently agitated vapours, which presently, upon the cessation of the heat, return to liquor; as we see, that the vapours of an Æolipile, that issue out after the aereal Particles have been expell'd, *though* they make a great noise and a temporary wind near the hole they stream out at, and would perhaps, if that hole were close stopt, break the Æolipile; *yet* are not true and permanent Air, but at a small distance off the Instrument return into water.'[69] Boyle added that he could suggest 'other suspicions and conjectures about the inclusion of Air between the particles of Salt-petre', but forbore the mention of them 'in a Writing design'd to be chiefly Historical'.[70]

Boyle's Further Experiments on Flame in the 'Tracts' (1672)

Other experiments in the *Tracts* of 1672 showed that it was difficult to kindle one body with the flame of another *in vacuo*;[71] as to how Boyle was able

[67] *ibid.*, pp. 76–7.

[68] Boyle had previously obtained bubbles of air both from water and from mercury (*New Experiments Physico-Mechanicall*, etc., 1660, *op. cit.* (4), pp. 147–62).

[69] *Tracts*, etc., 1672, *op. cit.* (51), pp. 77–9.

[70] *ibid.*, p. 79.   [71] *ibid.*, pp. 89–93.

to kindle the first body *in vacuo*, it seems that he had a 'well-disposed parcel of Sulphur' that, he said, could be ignited *in vacuo*;[72] as he had been working so much with nitre, possibly some contamination may have occurred. It appeared therefore that flame could not be communicated without the help of air. A train of gunpowder could be kindled here and there *in vacuo* by a burning-glass, but the flame would not pass along the train.[73] Gunpowder enclosed in two separate glass vessels, one partly and the other carefully evacuated of air, exploded in both cases on being heated, although in another experiment, in a small evacuated vessel carefully heated, it did not go off or burn,[74] and the explosion of the powder in both the evacuated and the unevacuated vessels seemed to contradict what might be inferred from the previous experiments.

Boyle's Experiments on Respiration in the 'Tracts' (1672)

Turning to study what he called 'the relation betwixt air and the *flamma vitalis*' of animals, Boyle dealt more exhaustively with the phenomenon that we have already noticed as a difficulty in the solution of the related problems of combustion and respiration,[75] namely, that animals placed in closed vessels together with kindled combustibles easily outlived the flames, even when the flames were put out by gradual evacuation of the air from the vessels. He described the first experiment as follows: '. . . we took the small Glass-lamp . . . , and having lighted it, we plac'd both it and a small Bird (which was a Green-finch) upon the Brass-plate, and in a trice fastned it to the lower orifice of the Receiver, and then watched the event; which was, that within two minutes (as near as we could estimate by a good minute-watch) the flame, after having several times, almost quite disappear'd, was utterly extinguished; but the Bird, though for a while he seem'd to close his eyes as though he were sick, appear'd lively enough at the end of the third minute; at which time, being unwilling to wait any longer by reason of some avocations, I caused him to be taken out.

'After he had for a pretty while, by being kept in the free-Air, recovered and refreshed himself, the former tryal was repeated again, and at the end of the second minute the flame of the Lamp went out; but the Bird seem'd not to be endanger'd by being kept there a while longer.

'After this, we put in together with the same Bird two lighted Lamps at once, (*viz.* the former and another like it) whose flames, according to expectation, lasted not one whole minute before they went out together. But the Bird appear'd not to have been harmed, after having been kept five or six times as long before we took off the Receiver.'[76]

Other experiments followed, similar results being obtained with a mouse enclosed with a lamp burning spirit of wine, and again with a wax-candle; then Boyle used a bird with a candle and then with a taper without evacuating the receiver, followed by a bird with a candle and then a taper, and then a bird with kindled charcoal; and in all cases life survived the extinction of

[72] *ibid.*, p. 88.　　　　　　　　　　[73] *ibid.*, pp. 94–7.
[74] *ibid.*, pp. 101–4.
[75] See references 21 and 22.
[76] *Tracts*, etc., 1672, *op. cit.* (51), pp. 110–12.

fire.[77] He described the experiment with the bird and the lighted candle as follows:

'We took a Green-finch and a piece of Candle of twelve to the pound, and included them in a great capp'd Receiver, capable of containing about two Gallons or sixteen pound of water, which was very carefully cemented on to the Pump, that no Air might get in or out. In this Glass we suffer'd the Candle to burn till the flame expired, (which it did, in more than one Tryal, within two minutes or somewhat less;) at which time the Bird seemed to be in no danger of sudden death; and, though kept a while longer in that clogg'd and smoaky Air, appeared to be well enough when the Receiver was removed. Afterwards, we put the same Bird into the Receiver with a piece of a small wax Taper, whose flame though it lasted longer than the other, yet the Bird outlived it; and 'twas judged he would have done so, though the Flame had been much more durable. After this, we included the same Bird with the first-mention'd Candle in the Receiver, which we had caused to be often blown into with a pair of Bellows, to drive out the smoak and infected Air; and then beginning to pump out the Air, we found, that the Flame began more quickly to decay, and the Bird to be much more discomposed than in the former Experiments; but still the *Animal* outlived the Flame, though not without Convulsive motions.'[78]

The other experiments gave similar results and Boyle summed up as follows:

'Whether this survival of Animals, not only to a flame that emits store of fuliginous steams, as in this tryal; but to that which is made of so pure a fuel as Spirit of Wine, that affords not such steams (as in the former experiment;) *Whether*, I say, this survival proceed from this, That the Common flame and the Vital flame are maintained by distinct substances or parts of the Air; *or* that common Flame making a great waste of the Aereal substance, they both need to keep them alive, cannot so easily as the other find matter to prey upon, and so expires, whilst there yet remains enough to keep alive the more temperate Vital flame; *or* that both these causes, and perhaps some other, concurr to the *Phænomenon*, I leave to be consider'd.'[79]

In other words, the experiments had thoroughly established what had previously been observed eight years earlier in a single experiment suggested by Hooke on 21 January 1662/3, and made on 28 February of that year, well before the publication of Hooke's theory,[80] namely, that animals could respire air in which flame had died out; and this at once led to the possibility of there being two different substances in the air, one maintaining the common flame of fire and the other cherishing the vital flame of life, though it might be that the common flame used up more extensively an aereal constituent which nourished both the common flame and the vital flame, whence the common flame expired first. The evidence could not be readily explained on Hooke's theory except by this latter explanation; and, in any case, Boyle was hesitant about deciding between two explanations on the evidence before

---

[77] *ibid.*, pp. 112–17.   [78] *ibid.*, pp. 114–16.   [79] *ibid.*, pp. 117–18.

[80] See references 21 and 22. A similar experiment made on 8 February 1664/5, in which a bird was enclosed with burning coals, showed that the bird began to die about the same time as the coals went out (Birch, *op. cit.* (19), vol. ii, p. 12): thus, what Boyle established here was really new, since it was previously uncertain.

him, which could scarcely be regarded as definitely pointing one way or the other.

Hooke's Work on Combustion (1672–1674)

We turn now to consider Hooke's work during the years from 1672 to 1674 as recorded in Birch's *History*. We have just seen what opinions Boyle had formed on the problems of combustion and respiration and how these differed from those advanced by Hooke. At the meeting of the Royal Society held on 26 June 1672, Hooke said that he considered the principal use of respiration was to convey into the blood something from the air essential to life, and to remove from the blood something noisome that was discharged back into the air.[81] On 13 November 1672, Hooke suggested that an attempt be made to find out whether air was consumed or increased by burning, and Boyle, probably mindful of their differing opinions on the problem, proposed an inquiry as to whether or no air was 'intercepted and compressed' in the making of saltpetre.[82]

The experiment to find out whether air increased or decreased in burning was tried before the Society at the next meeting, on 20 November 1672,[83] and it failed; it was decided to try it again on the following Saturday at Hooke's lodgings in Gresham College, before some of the Fellows who used to meet there, the result to be reported to the Society at the next meeting, but no report is recorded by Birch. At the next meeting, held on 27 November,[84] it was tried again, but 'the success not proving satisfactory', Hooke was ordered to repeat it at the next meeting. At the next meeting, on 4 December 1672, when the experiment was called for, Hooke reported that he had made the experiment and had found neither increase nor decrease of the air, but when the experiment was done before the Society, it miscarried and a repetition at the next meeting was ordered.[85] It miscarried again on 19 February 1672/3,[86] and Hooke 'was desired to fit it better for the next meeting'. The apparatus failed again on 5 March 1672/3, and Hooke 'was ordered to fit it with care'.[87] On 19 March 1672/3, Hooke read a discourse in which he reported that he had made the experiment and had found that the air was diminished by one-twentieth; and he was desired to continue and to report further results from time to time, and also to bespeak some of the Fellows to assist in the experiments.[88] And there the matter seems to have rested. It is to be remarked that this important experiment was not carried out successfully before the Society and that we have no details of the apparatus, of the design of the experiment or of the materials used. We now know the significance of the fact it tended to establish; that may not have seemed so significant at that time, except perhaps to Hooke, and we have to remember that in 1670 Boyle had found no decrease of air in respiration.[89]

Boyle's Theory of Combustion and Respiration (1674)

In 1674 Boyle set out in some further *Tracts* his views on the air and his theory of the part played by it in combustion and respiration. The air, he said,

---

[81] Birch, *op. cit.* (19), vol. iii, p. 55. [82] *ibid.*, vol. iii, p. 61. [83] *ibid.*
[84] *ibid.*, vol. iii, p. 63. [85] *ibid.*, vol. iii, p. 68. [86] *ibid.*, vol. iii, p. 76.
[87] *ibid.*, vol. iii, p. 77. [88] *ibid.*, vol. iii, p. 78. [89] See reference 50.

was commonly recognized as having the qualities of heat, cold, dryness and moisture, but it had also been found to possess other qualities, such as gravity and elasticity, and the power of refraction of light and so on; and it might, he suspected, have other different and more latent qualities and powers due to the parts of which it consisted. For atmospherical air 'is not, as many imagine, a Simple and Elementary Body, but a confus'd Aggregate of Effluviums from such differing Bodies, that, though they all agree in constituting, by their minuteness and various motions, one great mass of Fluid matter, yet perhaps there is scarce a more heterogeneous Body in the world':[90] it was a 'great receptacle or rendevouz of Celestial and Terrestrial Effluviums'.[91]

Proceeding, Boyle expounded his theory of combustion and respiration as follows:

'The Difficulty we find of keeping Flame and Fire alive, though but for a little time, without Air, makes me some times prone to suspect, that there may be dispers'd through the rest of the Atmosphere some odd substance, either of a Solar, or Astral, or some other exotic, nature, on whose account the Air is so necessary to the subsistence of Flame; which Necessity I have found to be greater, and less dependent upon the *manifest* Attributes of the Air, than Naturalists seem to have observed. For I have found by tryals purposely made, that a small flame of a Lamp, though fed perhaps with a subtil thin Oyl, would in a large capacious glass-Receiver expire, for want of Air, in a far less time than one would believe. And it will not much lessen the difficulty to alledge, that either the gross fuliginous Smoak did in a close Vessel stifle the flame, or that the pressure of the Air is requisite to impel up the aliment into the wieck: For, to obviate these objections, I have in a larger Receiver imploy'd a very small wieck with such rectified Spirit of Wine, as would in the free Air burn totally away; and yet, when a very small Lamp, furnished (as I was saying) with a very slender wieck, was made to burn, and, fill'd with this liquor, was put lighted into a large Receiver, that little flame, though it emitted no visible smoak at all, would usually expire within about one minute of an hour, and, not seldom, in a less time; and this, though the wieck was not so much as sing'd by the flame: Nor indeed is a wieck necessary for the experiment, since highly rectified Spirit of Wine will in the free Air flame away well without it. And indeed it seems to deserve our wonder, what that should be in the Air, which inabling it to keep flame alive, does yet, by being consum'd or deprav'd, so suddenly render the Air unfit to make flame subsist. And it seems by the sudden wasting or spoiling of this fine Subject, whatever it be, that the bulk of it is but very small in proportion to the Air it impregnates with its virtue. For after the extinction of the flame, the Air in the Receiver was not visibly alter'd, and, for ought I could perceive by the ways of judging I had then at hand, the Air retain'd either All, or at least far the greatest part of its *Elasticity*, which I take to be its most genuine and distinguishing property.

'And this *undestroy'd springyness* of the Air seems to make the necessity of fresh Air to the Life of *hot* Animals, (few of which, as far as I can guess after

[90] Robert Boyle, *Tracts: containing I. Suspicions about some Hidden Qualities of the Air*, etc. London, 1674, p. 2.   [91] *ibid.*, pp. 4–5.

many tryals, would be able to live two minutes of an hour, if they were totally and all at once deprived of Air,) suggest a great suspicion of some *vital substance*, if I may so call it, diffus'd through the Air, whether it be *a volatile Nitre*, or (rather) some *yet anonymous* substance, Sydereal or Subterraneal, but not improbably of kin to that, which I lately noted to be so necessary to the maintenance of other flames.'[92]

The 'yet anonymous substance' was present in the air in very small proportions, since the air retained 'at least far the greatest part of its Elasticity', both after combustion and after respiration; and, it is to be noted, it is not regarded as an ingredient of nitre, because Boyle had already concluded that air itself might be intercepted between the corpuscles composing nitre.[93] And it is in this latter respect that Boyle's theory differed from Hooke's. The problem seems to have attracted little further serious attention at the meetings of the Royal Society, so far as Birch's *History* goes, Hooke's theory not being discussed there again until 1679, when, on various dates, his experiments were repeated without, it would seem, any significant purpose except to show that air was necessary for the maintenance of fire. Birch's *History* goes no further than the year 1687.

Mayow's 'Tractatus Quinque' (1674)

The work of John Mayow (1641–79)[94] has been studied critically by Patterson,[95] who has shown that Mayow's data on combustion and respiration were extensively borrowed from Boyle and Hooke and that his speculations were very confused and contradictory. However, in his *Tractatus quinque* of 1674, Mayow made use of the experiment in which a lighted candle was placed in air contained in a vessel, a cupping-glass, inverted over water and a decrease in the volume of the air observed, which Mayow regarded as a result of the combustion,[96] not as had been more usually said of this ancient experiment, which has a history reaching back at least to Philo of Byzantium,[97] that it demonstrated Nature's *horror vacui*. It is curious that we have no record of any observations of this old experiment made by the Fellows of the Royal Society at their meetings, with the exception of vague entries in Birch's *History* for three dates in 1661: on 5 June,[98] the first of these, 'A discourse was held concerning the extinguishing of a lighted candle in a vessel like a funnel or blind head';[99] on 13 June, 'It was ordered, that the experiment of

---

[92] *ibid.*, pp. 24–7.

[93] See references 67 and 69.

[94] Mayow was born in Cornwall in 1641, not, as is usually stated, in London with various dates. See D. McKie, *Phil. Mag.*, 1942, xxxiii, 51–60.

[95] T. S. Patterson, 'John Mayow in contemporary setting.' *Isis*, 1931, xv, 47–96, 504–46.

[96] John Mayow, *Tractatus quinque medico-physici*. Oxford, 1674, pp. 98–9; English translation, *Medico-physical works*. Edinburgh, 1907 (Alembic Club Reprint No. 17), pp. 68–9.

[97] Some very interesting references to the medieval history of this experiment will be found in Duhem's 'Roger Bacon et l'horreur du vide' in *Roger Bacon—Essays*, edited by A. G. Little. Oxford, 1914, pp. 241–84. The experiment was described by many authors, including J. B. van Helmont (1577–1644) in his *Ortus medicinæ* (Amsterdam, 1648), where also an account is given of the experiment so often used by Hooke to illustrate his theory, the charring or incombustibility of coals heated in a closed vessel.

[98] Birch, *op. cit.* (19), vol. i, p. 26.

[99] A 'blind-head' was a vessel, used by chemists, about the same size and shape as a 'cupping-glass' (see R. Boyle, *A Continuation of New Experiments Physico-Mechanical. . . . The I Part*, etc. Oxford, 1669, p. 122).

PLATE XXXVII

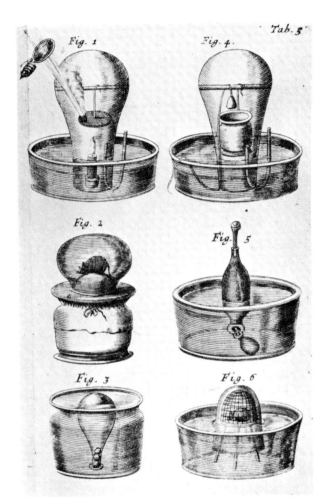

FIG. 2. Mayow, *Tractatus quinque*, 1674. Tab. V
(From a copy in the Wellcome Historical Medical Library)

the cupping-glass and lighted candle be made at the next meeting';[100] and on 26 June, 'The experiment of the cupping-glass and light was made, and succeeded according to expectation'.[101] No other details are given either of the experiment or the 'expectation'. It seems strange that this experiment was not mentioned, so far as we are aware, when the problem of air and combustion was considered from time to time. Of course, Hooke was not active in the Society[102] at the time of the references to the experiment given above; and it is possible that when it was then discussed, discussion may have been directed to the problem of the air and its pressure which was a leading topic in 1661. As for Boyle, he does not seem to have referred to the experiment in his studies on combustion, but he had experimented with a cupping-glass and had ascribed its action to the pressure of atmospheric air.[103]

In other places in the *Tractatus quinque*, Mayow claims a decrease of about one-thirtieth in the volume of air contained in the same cupping-glass when camphor was burnt in it by means of a burning-glass.[104] By suitably arranging a mouse on a support inside the glass, he claimed to have found a decrease of one-fourteenth of the air.[105] Mayow's explanation was that air contained 'nitro-aerial particles', which were consumed in combustion and respiration. In the other work that we have been considering up to this point, no decrease of the air in respiration had been established and, in fact, the absence of any reduction of pressure by respiration had been experimentally demonstrated by Boyle,[106] who had included a pressure gauge in a closed receiver containing a mouse, but who had not experimented over water, while Hooke had reported an unverified decrease of one-twentieth of the air in burning, without any experimental details or description of apparatus.[107] But Mayow's experiments were made in a vessel inverted over water, while Boyle's were made in the receiver of his air-pump or other closed receivers, but not over water, and hence Boyle's apparatus and method, as we have already pointed out,[108] concealed a decrease in the volume of the air where Mayow's revealed it. Mayow also observed[109] a decrease in the volume of the air, again in the same apparatus, by producing in it, by the action of spirit of nitre on iron, the gas we now know as nitric oxide, which in the hands of Priestley a century later was to play a part in the discovery that air was composed of more than one 'air' or gas. The decrease observed by Mayow amounted to one-fourth, a very good result. All these decreases in air were observable as a result of the method of experimenting over water. Mayow showed the decrease in the volume of air in respiration by another ingenious method, by placing a mouse in a bell-jar on a moistened bladder stretched over the open end of a cylindrical vessel; the decrease in the volume of the air in the bell-jar

[100] Birch, *op. cit.* (19), vol. i, p. 29.

[101] *ibid.*, vol. i, p. 31.

[102] Hooke was proposed as curator of experiments on 5 November 1662, and appointed on 12 November (Birch, *op. cit.* (19), vol. i, pp. 123–4): he was elected Fellow on 20 May 1663 (*ibid.*, p. 240) and on 3 June of the same year he was 'elected a fellow of the society by the council, and exempted from all charges' (*ibid.*, p. 250).

[103] Robert Boyle, *A Continuation of New Experiments*, etc. 1669, pp. 118–24.

[104] *Tractatus, op. cit.* (96), pp. 100–101: *Medico-physical works*, pp. 70–1.

[105] *Tractatus, op. cit.* (96), pp. 104–5: *Medico-physical works*, pp. 72–3.

[106] See reference 50.   [107] See reference 88.   [108] See reference 50.

[109] *Tractatus, op. cit.* (96), pp. 136–8: *Medico-physical works*, pp. 94–5.

containing the mouse was evident from the bulging of the stretched bladder into the jar.[110]

Boyle's Later Experiments on Respiration (1677)

In an experiment made on 17 June 1677, Boyle studied the respiration of a mouse in compressed air (two atmospheres) and of another mouse in common air: the mouse in compressed air lived much longer than the one in common air, but Boyle stated that in the case of the mouse in common air he had observed a decrease of one-thirtieth in the pressure of the air,[111] which is possibly a malobservation since the experiment does not appear to have been done over water. Previously, as we have seen,[112] Boyle had found that there was no reduction of pressure in air by respiration. The result was confirmed in another experiment made on 21 July 1677, the amount of air consumed being somewhat less; but, on leaving the apparatus to stand, much air was produced and so Boyle stated 'that *living* Animals do consume air, but *dead* ones produce new'.[113]

Hooke's Theory (1677–1682)

In the years from 1677 to 1682, Hooke made some interesting references to his theory on three occasions. In his book *Lampas*, he applied the theory to explain the consumption of oil in the wicks of lamps; the air 'dissolved' the heated particles of the oil and the dissolution produced light. He stated that 'many Authors' had made use of his theory and asserted it, 'nor have I yet met with one considerable objection against it'.[114]

In his 'Lectures of Light', read in May 1681, he stated: '. . . 'tis the fresh Air that is the Life of the Fire, and without a Constant supply of that it will go out and Die. Somewhat like this is observable in the Life of Animals, who live no longer than they have a constant supply of fresh Air to breath, and, as it were, blow the Fire of Life; for so soon as that supply is wanting, the Fire goes out, and the Animal dies, and all the other vital Functions cease; as any one may presently see, if he puts a small Animal as a Bird, or the like, into a small Glass and covers it close; for in a short time the Air becomes satiated, and is no longer fit for Respiration; but though the Animal breath it as before, and Pant and move his Lungs as before; yet if the Air be not fresh, the Fire of Life will extinguish. Some Learned Philosophers and Physitians have been of the Opinion, that the use of Breathing was for nothing else, but that by the Motion of the Lungs the Blood might be kept circulating which past through them, or that the Steams of the Blood might be carried off, which it could not do when it was full of Steams; but by many Trials I have proved that neither of those are at all the Cause of the Death of the Creature, but only the want of fresh Air.'[115]

[110] *Tractatus, op. cit.* (96), pp. 103–4: *Medico-physical works*, p. 72.

[111] Robert Boyle, *A Continuation of New Experiments Physico-Mechanical . . . The Second Part*, etc. London, 1682, pp. 74–5: the experiments are dated. The first edition of this work appeared in Latin as *Experimentorum Novorum Physico-Mechanicorum Continuatio Secunda*, etc. London, 1680.

[112] See reference 50.   [113] *op. cit.* (111), pp. 80–1.

[114] Robert Hooke, *Lampas : or Descriptions of some Mechanical Improvements of Lamps*, etc. London, 1677, p. 1.

[115] *Posthumous works*, etc., edited by Richard Waller. London, 1705, p. 111.

Again, in his 'Discourse of the Nature of Comets', read before the Royal Society in 1682, he asserted 'that the Air it self is no farther the *Menstruum* that dissolves Bodies by Fire and Flame, than as it has such a kind of Body raised from the Earth, as has a Power of so dissolving and working on Unctuous, Sulphureous or Combustible Bodies: And this is the Aerial or Volatile Nitrous Spirit, which, provided it be supplied to the Body to be so dissolved, as by Fire, will work the same effect, even without Air. This is obvious in Compositions made with Salt of Nitre and other combustible Substances, as in Gunpowder, and the like, which will actually burn without the help of Air, as may be tried with it under Water; nay in an exhausted Receiver, as I have often tried, wherein the Effects are much the same, as if the same Accensions had been made in the open and free Air; though where this Nitrous part is wanting, no Combustion, Dissolution or actual Fire will be produced, be the Heat never so great'.[116]

Conclusion

The active history of Hooke's theory seems to end with these pronouncements of its author in 1682. Boyle's experiments of 1677, published in Latin in 1680 and in English in 1682,[117] seem also to mark an end of his work. The difference between their theories has been made clear above. It seems to us that, for Boyle, there was some uncertainty about whether gunpowder could be fired in a vacuum. He had explained its burning under water as possibly due to particles of air enclosed within the corpuscular fabric of the nitre itself,[118] an explanation that he could have applied equally well to its inflammation *in vacuo*. But reviewing his experiments on the latter, we sense some doubt in his mind as to whether gunpowder could really be fired *in vacuo*, that is, without the concurrence of air. In 1660, he was not sure of the result that he obtained when he tried to fire gunpowder in a pistol in the evacuated receiver; most of the attempts failed, and only once did the experiment succeed, on which occasion he mentions that some small amount of air might have remained in the receiver, since pumping could never entirely extract it all;[119] and in 1672 he mentions this experiment again and the possibility of there being some small residue of air in the receiver, in spite of the great rarefaction.[120] Moreover, in 1660, he noted in 'blank' tests with the unprimed pistol in the evacuated receiver that the cock in striking the steel 'struck out of it as many and as conspicuous parts of Fire, as, for ought we could perceive, it would have done in the open Air'[121]: and yet all the attempts but one to fire the gunpowder in the pistol *in vacuo* failed.

Again, in 1672,[122] Boyle made reference to an experiment with combustible matter made in 1660,[123] when he stated that gunpowder could not be fired *in vacuo* by a burning-glass. He thought that it might be argued 'that Brimstone, which is one of the ingredients of Gunpowder, appears by several tryals to be sometimes capable of accension [i.e. of being set on fire] in our *Vacuum*, and therefore probably may kindle the rest'.[124] This seems to be based on the property of the 'well disposed parcel of Sulphur' that he had referred

---

[116] *ibid.*, p. 169.
[117] See references 111 and 113.
[118] See reference 67.
[119] See reference 7.
[120] *op. cit.* (51), pp. 40–2.
[121] *op. cit.* (4), p. 89.
[122] *op. cit.* (51), pp. 33–4.
[123] *op. cit.* (4), pp. 102–5.
[124] *op. cit.* (51), p. 32.

to;[125] but still the gunpowder did not burn in the absence of air, and he adds that 'the newly recited experiment was not the single one, we made about that time, that discover'd a great indisposition even in Gunpowder to be fir'd in our Vacuum'.[126]

Further, in 1672, gunpowder was not fired *in vacuo* by a red-hot iron, although the sulphur in it appeared to burn;[127] although gunpowder, he noted, had a great disposition to take fire, it would not do so without air, and, in repeating this experiment, he let in the air and after a time 'the powder suddenly went off with a great flash'.[128] Some gunpowder in an evacuated vessel carefully heated on ashes or coals did not take fire, although here also the sulphur in it 'was in part kindled'.[129] In 1672, the experiment with the pistol failed again, but succeeded when air was re-admitted:[130] he found that once again gunpowder heated in an evacuated vessel did not take fire, but he obtained some contradictory evidence when, having put gunpowder into two vessels, one evacuated and the other partly filled with air, he found that explosions occurred in both vessels on heating.[131]

These experiments on the firing of gunpowder *in vacuo* can have given no assurance of the fact to so careful and skilled an experimenter as Boyle; and he seems to have doubted whether gunpowder could be fired without the concurrence of air. This may possibly explain why he did not adopt Hooke's theory. It must be admitted, however, that at a meeting of the Royal Society on 15 February 1664/5, Boyle is reported as having affirmed that gunpowder burned very well in a receiver from which the air had been extracted;[132] there seems little of this confidence in Boyle's own writings, and the record of this statement made by him in 1664/5 makes no reference, it may be noted, to any explanation that he may have suggested; and we have drawn attention above to the way in which he thought the burning of gunpowder under water might be explained.

Hooke, however, had no doubts on this point, as the quotations that we have given make amply clear. But his theory was born out of due time, and had to wait for the invention of a method of collecting the gaseous products from burning bodies, and for the isolation and recognition a century later of the constituent common to air and to nitre. Meanwhile, the idea that air contained something that was active in combustion and respiration found acceptance, and indeed became enshrined in the immortal *Principia*, in which Newton stated that its source might be found in those strange wanderers the comets, whose apparently erratic journeys across the heavens he had brought under the sway of his laws of motion and gravitation:

'Porrò suspicor spiritum illum, qui aeris nostri pars minima est sed subtilissima & optima, & ad rerum omnium vitam requiritur, ex Cometis præcipue venire.'[133]

[125] See reference 72.   [126] *op. cit.* (51), p. 34.   [127] *ibid.*, pp. 35–6.
[128] *ibid.*, pp. 37–8.   [129] *ibid.*, pp. 39–40.   [130] *ibid.*, pp. 42–4.
[131] *ibid.*, pp. 102–3.   [132] Birch, *op. cit.* (19), vol. ii, p. 15.   [133] *Principia*, 1687, p. 506.

THE REACTION TO ARISTOTLE IN SEVENTEENTH-CENTURY BIOLOGICAL THOUGHT

CAMPANELLA, VAN HELMONT, GLANVILL, CHARLETON, HARVEY, GLISSON, DESCARTES

by

WALTER PAGEL

Introduction

SEVENTEENTH-century scientific thought is often represented as the fruit of antagonism to Aristotelian and scholastic philosophy. In the light of the material submitted in the present paper such view calls for qualification—at all events in the sphere of seventeenth-century biology. For the biological philosophies of Harvey and Glisson are based on Aristotelianism, to which even their scientific work seems palpably indebted.

Nevertheless, opposition to Aristotle and the Schoolmen, their methods and conclusions, formed a strong incentive to independent research, and indeed to a biological view of the world such as was conceived by van Helmont. It was, however, often the letter rather than the spirit of Aristotelian doctrines, their system as transmitted by the Schoolmen rather than the original, against which the attacks of early biologists appear to be directed.

Three such anti-Aristotelian currents will be presented, partly in autobiographical accounts, and will be compared with the Aristotelian biological philosophies.

I

Then I became frightened because not truth, but rather falsehood instead of truth, seemed to me to dwell in the Peripatus, and I examined all Greek, Latin and Arabic commentators of Aristotle and began to start at their doctrines even more, and felt the urge to find out whether what they said was to be read in Nature, which, as I knew from the Sages, was the live book that God has written. As the doctors could not satisfy my doubts, I decided to study myself all the works of Plato, Pliny, Galen, the Stoics, the followers of Democritus, and in particular those of Telesio, and to compare them with the primordial book of Nature, in order to recognize from the original, written by God's own hand, where they had copied right and where wrong. . . . Neither in my public discussions at Cosenza, nor in private talks with my brethren, did I find much ease by their responses; but Telesio delighted me, for the freedom in his philosophy, and because he made the nature of things, not the dicta of men, his master.

Anxious about the truth of a matter, study its whole history. . . . He who wants to study Physiology must first learn the natural history of minerals, plants and animals, elements and composite things from Pliny, Agricola, Gesner, Aldrovandi, Imperatus, Dioscorides, Theophrastus and the like; it is because of their ignorance of the history of the things which constitute a branch of learning that the Schoolmen hang on to battles of words and are led astray from things to words. . . .

But take care not to become entangled in any sect of philosophers or jurists believing that they are immune from error, for everybody is capable of falsehood, either from ignorance or from malice or from fear: God alone is true. What is a testimony from God, you can thus recognize: by finding out whether it is inherent in the nature of things (the first divine document) or in the Holy Books. . . . Read all men's books and do not prematurely reject what defies your understanding. Many things believed to be false have come true, for example that there are inhabitants beyond the equator, or that there is another hemisphere to the earth. . . . Hence one must give credence to those who testify rather than to those who vent opinions, rather to Columbus than to Lactantius and Procopius . . . for many things appear to be impossible which nevertheless verily exist. Hence you, Naudaeus, rightly contend in your *Apology*[1] that many illustrious men were by no means necromancers, but that it is a story put out by the ignorant who, failing to grasp the reason behind things, say that what nature does, happens by supernatural action. It is the stupid who talk many lies and call the wise men diabolic or angelic; yet they could not arrive at this opinion unless nature and politics revealed with certainty that angelic and diabolic men do exist. Nor can the illusions which inspired such writers as Apuleius, Lucian and Agrippa do away with the fact that magicians really existed in the world. Nor will the poetic fables about Pegasus and Bellerophon discredit what Suetonius submits about Simon Magus. Nor is true prophecy negatived because gypsies and astronomers are mendacious; just as it cannot be denied that some gold is pure because there is some mixed and very much false—chymical-gold. . . . Finally if a proposition strikes you as impossible, such as that the sun stands still in the centre and the earth rotates, do not at once believe and declare that it is impossible, but reserve your judgment until you have collected the arguments from all sides and established the truth.

It is thus that Thomaso Campanella (1568–1639)[2] airs his diffidence about Aristotelianism, and indeed about all doctrines that are not borne out by the 'Book of Nature'. He thus associates with opposition to Aristotle an urge for empiricism. Nature, the universal source of the empiric, derives its authority from its divine creator; it is the 'Codex mundi originalis et autographus'. Hence empiricism should be the attitude of the God-fearing, who will attain truth by the investigation of real objects rather than by wordy arguments. The pious modesty of the empiric will require a full 'history', i.e. observation and description of his subject, for it is 'history' which prevents dogmatism, i.e. the overrating of human reasoning. This is liable to err, while God alone is true. In other words, scepticism engenders empiricism. Certain facts do exist in spite of all human lies, illusions and errors. They are within the grasp of the sober observer, the 'witness', and of those who weigh their evidence impartially.

This is undoubtedly the spiritual atmosphere which enabled science to develop. Its elements are here set out in an autobiographical account of the manner in which scepticism was aroused in the mind of a young philosopher, by the perusal of the works of Aristotle and his commentators. Opposition to the wordy arguments and altercations of the peripatetic Schoolmen, associated with a yearning for empirical truth, is a strong current typical of the spiritual motives by which the forerunners and initiators of modern science were actuated.

---

[1] Gabriel Naudé (1600–53), to whom these lines were dedicated, graduated in physic at Padua, was made librarian to Cardinal Bagni and to Barberini, and subsequently called by Richelieu and Mazarin, over whose library he presided. He wrote: *Apologie pour les grands hommes soupçonnés de Magie* (English: *The History of Magick by way of Apologie, for all those eminent Persons who have unjustly been reputed Magicians*. Trans. by Davis. London, 1657).

[2] Thoma Campanella, *De libris propriis et recta ratione studendi. Syntagma ad Gabrielem Naudaeum Parisin*. In *Grotii et aliorum dissertationes de studiis instituendis*. Amsterodami (Elzevir), 1645, pp. 368–413.

The same emerges from another autobiographical account which, though more colourful in detail, reveals the same combination of empiricism, scepticism and piety on one hand, with antagonism to overbearing human reason and to Aristotelianism on the other. It is the life and academic record of Jean Baptiste van Helmont, as given by himself in the introductory treatises to his 'Rise of Medicine'.[3]

II

At the age of seventeen I had finished my course in philosophy, and it was then that I noticed that nobody was admitted to the examination who was not masked in his gown and hood, as if the robes warrant scholarship. The professors made a laughing stock of the academic youth that was to be introduced to the arts and learning, and I could not help wondering at a sort of delirium in the behaviour of professors, nay of everybody as much as the simplicity of the credulous youth. I retired into a deliberation in order to judge myself how much I was of a philosopher and had attained truth and science. I found myself inflated with letters and, as it were, naked as after partaking of the illicit apple—except for a proficiency in artificial wrangling. Then it dawned upon me that I knew nothing and that what I knew was worthless. I did astronomy, logic and algebra for pleasure, as the other subjects nauseated me, and also the Elements of Euclid, which became particularly congenial to me as they contained the truth. . . . But I learned only vain eccentricities and a new revolution of the celestial bodies,[4] and what seemed hardly worth the time and labours I had spent. . . . Having completed my course, I refused the title of Master of Arts since I knew nothing substantial, nothing true; unwilling to have myself made an arch-fool by the professors declaring me a Master of the Seven Arts, I who was not even a disciple yet. Seeking truth and science, though not their outward appearance, I withdrew from the university. I was promised a wealthy canonry on condition that I would only devote myself to theology; but St. Bernard warned me against living on the sins of the people. I prayed, however, to the Lord that he might make me worthy to receive my vocation as would please him best. This was the year in which the Jesuits began to teach philosophy at Louvain, against the will of the king, the notables and the university. When this was prohibited by Clement VIII, they attracted the more wealthy, in addition to the crowds of students who had gathered to study for their degrees in the commendable subject of geography. One of their professors, Martinus del Rio, first a judge in charge of a Spanish military detachment,[5] then retiring from the Senate of Brabant and joining the Jesuits, expounded his Disquisitions on Magic. I attended both courses with great zeal. But what I reaped in the end was empty straw and poor senseless prattle. In the meantime, in order to let no hour pass in vain, I became engrossed in Seneca, who pleased me immensely, and so even more did Epictetus. I thus seemed to have found the marrow of truth in moral philosophy. . . . I prayed to the Prince of Life for the stamina to contemplate the naked truth and love it per se—a desire that was intensified by Thomas à Kempis and later by Tauler. Then I ardently hoped to

[3] J. B. van Helmont, 'Studia authoris' in Ortus medicinae. Amsterodami (Elzevir), 1648, pp. 16 ff.

[4] The Copernican theory.

[5] A detailed account of the controversial points in Del Rio's biography is found in Nève de Mévergnies, Jean-Baptiste van Helmont. Philosophe par le Feu. Paris, 1935, p. 115, footnote 8. The author rejects the reading: 'Judge of Turma in Spain.' This probably derives from the spelling of 'Turma' with a capital T in the first and following editions of the Ortus medicinae, and from the English translation by Chandler (London, 1662, p. 12), rather than from the interpretations of Rommelaere and Redgrove, as Nève de Mévergnies seems to believe.

attain Christian perfection by following Stoicism. Some time later, being fatigued by these exercises, I fell into a dream in which I saw myself as an empty bubble extending from earth to heaven. Above me hovered a tomb; below, however, in the place of earth was an abyss of darkness. Immensely frightened I lost consciousness of everything, including myself. When I recovered, I realized at once, that we live, move and exist in Christ Jesus.... I became certain that, except by special grace, nothing but sin awaits us in any activity. Then I recognized that my Stoicism kept me an empty and inflated bubble, between the abyss below and the necessity of imminent death. It struck me that my studies were making me arrogant, though affecting to be moderate. Confident of the freedom of my will, I would readily forego divine grace, as if we are the arbiters of our destiny. Away with such monstrous blasphemy, I said. I renounced Stoic philosophy as hateful and beneath the dignity of a Christian, and tired and disgusted with too much reading, I amused myself by browsing in Mathiolus and Dioscorides—in the belief that nothing is so necessary to mankind as God's grace, admiring how in the plants it provides their appropriate needs and ripens their fruit. I soon noticed that botany has in no way progressed since the days of Dioscorides; that even to-day his pictures, nomenclature and descriptions of plants are after all these years the recognized basis of every discussion, but that no advance had been added, about their virtues, properties and use, except for the fictions of the later authors as to the grades of elemental qualities to which the whole composition of the plant was ascribed. But I knew that about two hundred plants, though identical in quality and grade, are quite different in virtues, and that a number of others, different in quality and grades, act synergically. So not the herbs (the seals of divine love), but the herbalists fell into disrepute with me. I enquired whether there was a text-book of the axioms and rules of medicine, for I believed that this could be taught like any art or science and was not merely a gift of grace.... I was told that all particulars of the effects of plants, from the cedar to the hyssop, were to be found in Galen or Avicenna. But as I was not credulous nor found the desired certainty in the books, I well nigh suspected that it lay in the truth that He who created medicine remained its continuous distributor. Anxious and uncertain about which profession I should choose, I studied the customs and laws of nations, and the decisions of sovereigns. I saw that law is made up of human traditions, uncertain, unstable and devoid of truth. As there was no stability in human things and no core of certainty, I saw that my life would be useless were I to base it on human decisions.... On the other side I was impressed by the misery of human life and the will of God, whereby everybody must sustain himself as long as he can. With a singular avidity I turned to the most gentle study of nature, and as the soul is enslaved by its inclinations I lapsed unconsciously into natural science. I read the institutions of Fuchs and Fernel which led me through the whole of medicine by way of a survey, and found myself amused. Is this the way medicine is taught—without theory, and a teacher who has received the gift of healing from a master? Is it not in this way that the whole of natural history is obstructed by the qualities and elements ? I, therefore, read Galen's works twice, once Hippocrates, whose aphorisms I knew almost by heart, the whole of Avicenna and about a total of six hundred Greek, Arabic and modern authors, seriously and attentively, and compared and abstracted them. Then, I re-read the collection of my notes and recognized my poverty, and the labours and years I had consumed angered me.[3]

Van Helmont sees the root of the evil in the 'heathen' doctrines of Aristotle, whom he has found 'utterly ignorant of the principles of nature and poor in his knowledge of physics, who has ridiculously described time, locality,

PLATE XXXVIII

3⁵¹

THOMÆ CAMPANELLÆ
D E
LIBRIS PROPRIIS
& rectā ratione studendi.
SYNTAGMA,
AD GABRIEL. NAVDÆVM
Parisin.

PROOEMIVM.

NON immeritò te Philosophorum
Mercurium vocai posse cense-
mus, perspicacissime *Naudæ,* cum
videamus te sapientum dogmata,
vitas , mores, rationem dicendi,
atque docendi studiose perscruta-
ri, examinare , promulgare , & in mundi senis
personare, & quid boni, quid mali latet in scien-
tiis, ac sophistarum in lucem pandere, ut uni-
cuique quod suum est non deceptæ amplius tri-
buant scholæ, & procul à calumniis , procul ab
adulatione fiant; Quapropter ego cujus commen-
tarios ferme omnes perlegisti, aſque tuis appro-
basti scriptis editis, abs te stimulatus, adjuratis-
que, ut omnium librorum meorum numerum
ac rationem tibi patefacerem usque ad schedas;
puras enim ex his, & modum dicendi, & arcana
rerum introspiciendi, & æmulationem peruti-
lem sic eruere; petitionibus tuis generosis de-
esse nolui, quamvis non tantum , talemque me
intelligam , unde exemplar nisi ærumnarum se-
rearum homine accipiant. Dixit Æneas Asca-
nio filio apud Virgilium :

Disa

FIG. 2.   The first page of Campanella's Autobiography,
in the 1645 edition of Grotius' *Dissertationes*

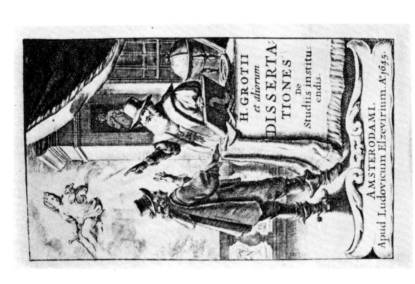

H. GROTII
et diuorum
DISSERTA-
TIONES
De
Studiis instituend-
endis.

AMSTERODAMI,
Apud Ludovicum Elzevirium. A.1645.

FIG. 1.   Title-page of Grotius et al., *Dissertationes de studiis
instituendis,* Amsterdam, 1645

vacuum, infinity, chance and similar abstractions absolutely alien to the realm of nature, as if they were physical objects'.[6]

Van Helmont thus summarizes his view of Aristotelian cosmology in his treatise 'On Time' in which he develops an original, 'biological', time conception. It is of special interest that most of van Helmont's contemporaries, however hostile to Aristotle, either followed the latter's concept of time or criticized it, but did not arrive at a new solution of the problem. In Aristotle's philosophy time played but an ancillary role—it was subservient to motion; it measured motion. In antiquity Plutarch and above all Plotinus had objected to this degradation of time. Before van Helmont's age, Cardan[7] had admitted the Aristotelian position that time is the measure of motion. He had denied, however, the concreteness of time altogether. Although time 'belongs' to nothing, everything is *in* time, and time is inherent in everything. For, time generates and destroys everything, it is the author of life and death. Yet, although time accompanies us incessantly, we never recognize it. Although æons of time lie before us, the loss of a single moment in the past is of infinite significance, as nothing can be undone. Time never is, but ever proceeds into infinity. We, therefore, comprehend not time, but what happens in it, what has happened and what remains. Time itself is not accessible to sensual perception, but a product of imagination whereby it is recognized. Van Helmont's contemporary Campanella[8] said that the Aristotelian definition of time as the measure of motion does not define time, but the use to which we put it. The motion of the Sun measures time, rather than time measures it. Aristotle was ignorant of the essence of time which happens to be used by us as a measure. Patrizzi, a decided adversary of Aristotelianism, subordinates time to 'world', and submits to its definition as measure of motion.[9] In Giordano Bruno's cosmology there is no place for the Aristotelian view of time. With the infinity and plurality of worlds which Bruno postulates, no finite time, no division of time into past, present and future, no limitation of time to a finite world can be compatible.[10] Where the Aristotelian Cosmos ends, new worlds begin. There is space again, and although infinitely bigger, it is similar to that which contains our own world. There are matter and form and indeed physical objects, for 'locus' demands 'locata'. Where there are located objects, however, there is 'duration'. It is the duration of objects in space which constitutes time. Therefore, no real and general norm of all times can exist.[11] Time is not bound up with motion.

[6] *De tempore*, 1 ff.: *Ortus medicinae, op. cit.* (3), p. 630. See for translation and commentary the present author in 'J. B. van Helmont, *De tempore* and biological time'. *Osiris*, 1949, viii, 346–417, notably p. 382.

[7] Hieronymus Cardanus, *De subtilitate libri xxi nunc demum recogniti et perfecti.* Lugduni, 1554, p. 523.

[8] Campanella, *Realis philosophiae epilogisticae partes quattuor.* Francofurti, 1623, pp. 16–17.

[9] Franciscus Patritius, *Nova de universis philosophia libris l comprehensa.* Venetiis, 1593. v. 'Hermetis Trismegisti mens, ad Hermetem', lib. x, fo. 20v°, col. 1.

[10] Giordano Bruno, *De immenso et immensurabilibus*, lib. i, cap. 12. Latin edition by F. Fiorentino. Naples, 1884, vol. i, I, p. 244; *De triplici minimo et mensura lib. v.* Francofurti, 1591, p. 22. See also D. W. Singer, 'The Cosmology of Giordano Bruno'. *Isis*, 1941, xxxiii, 187.

[11] Bruno, *De immenso, op. cit.* (10), lib. vii, cap. 7, p. 256. Aristotle who failed to find 'time' in this world, doubted its existence outside it. For he has linked it up with the 'Primum Mobile', i.e. the eighth sphere. For it was supposed to be the measure of all motions owing to its continuity, regularity and simplicity. In the same way Aristotle failed to find 'space' in this world and doubted its existence outside it.

It exists when everything is at rest. Hence motion measures time rather than time measures motion, and not time itself, but its recognition is linked up with motion.[12] 'Duration' is infinite, 'a beginning without end and an end without beginning. The whole of duration is, therefore, an infinite instant that is at the same time beginning and end'.[13] Van Helmont made all this negative criticism of the Aristotelian conception his own, added many new arguments and proffered a new theory of time. According to him time is devoid of succession and does not admit of division. It is independent of motion and change, and cannot therefore serve as measurement for anything. Being inseparable from eternity, it has a universal character, but also inheres in the individual objects with which 'it is more intimate than they are with themselves'. It is the entity which endows beings with a specific life-rhythm and determines their length of life. This is specific for each individual and depends upon the length and intensity of their functions, i.e. the *specific* duration of motions.

Van Helmont, thus linking time with the individual being, seems to approach Bruno's concept of time as the duration of objects in space. In Bruno's cosmology, however, time is subjected to 'worlds' and to 'space'. As these are infinite, time must be likewise. As space postulates things in space, there must be time in order to define their duration. Van Helmont's view is different. It is religious and at the same time biological. It visualizes time as the rhythm of individual life. This is a derivative of the eternal life of God. It is therefore divine and bound up with eternity. Time is the mediator, effecting the link between the individual and the divine in that it distributes schedules of life to beings. Hence time is responsible for specificity, i.e. the essential differences of one being from the other.

Generally speaking, van Helmont's main objection against Aristotelianism and the Schoolmen is their broad employment of mathematical symbolism, and the formal logic of 'entia rationis', where really existing objects and phenomena of Nature are under consideration. Taking all phenomena, observed and reported, in a naïve way as subjects of investigation, van Helmont often displayed a credulity which offered a welcome target to his sometimes more critical, though much less ingenious and meritorious adversaries. Yet, his trends of thought were legitimate from the scientific point of view, in that he aimed at a natural explanation of apparently supernatural phenomena. There was no obscurantism in van Helmont's treatment of the subject, and, dealing with such superstitions as the 'magnetic cure of wounds', he developed theories which were the forerunners of modern immunological thinking.[14]

The majority of his enemies, however, were in no way concerned with a scientific handling of the matter. They did not even put the 'quaestio facti' or deny the possibility of the phenomena in question. They introduced the action of the devil and thus condemned those whom they called his disciples: i.e. Paracelsus and van Helmont.

---

[12] Bruno, *Acrotismus s. Rationes articulorum physicorum adversus Peripateticos Parisiis propositorum.* Viteb. 1588, *v. loc. cit.* (10), Napoli, 1879, pp. 53 ff.; p. 146, Artic. xxxix.

[13] Bruno, *De immenso, op. cit.* (10), p. 21.

[14] Van Helmont, *De magnetica vulnerum curatione, op. cit.* (3), p. 602. W. Pagel in *J. B. van Helmont.* Berlin, 1930, p. 100.

This combination of antagonism towards the Aristotelian Schoolmen with the quest for empirical research has in van Helmont's case a strong mystical and religious-pragmatical accent. The formally-logical altercations and arguments employed by the Schoolmen he exposed as but the fruit of lower functions of the human mind, which will never lead it to the essence of objects and phenomena, i.e. to reality and truth. This is divine, and therefore not accessible to complacent human reasoning, but is disclosed to the humble who can read the 'Book of Nature' and is open to the grace of illumination. This attitude yielded some palpable results for the foundation and progress of science, and of biology in particular. It was van Helmont who went out to search for the divine spark in beings and discovered a chemical entity—Gas. He devised one of the early thermometers, used the balance in quantitative experiments, taught the indestructibility of matter, determined the specific gravity of urine, and based on this a diagnostic test; he established acid as a digestive factor in the stomach and alkali in the duodenum; he based pathology on the local changes in the organs and exogenous pathogenic agents as their causes.[15]

There is every reason to believe that Giordano Bruno in his opposition to the Schoolmen was actuated by similar motives—i.e. his antagonism to exaggerated rationalism and a dogmatic non-mystical religion.[16]

III

The seventeenth century saw the revival of Atomism and Epicureanism, which bore its most significant fruit for Science in Robert Boyle's new conception of matter. It was bound to arise out of antagonism to Aristotle's anti-atomistic doctrines of the elements, and indeed to his whole philosophy. There is hardly a better witness voicing these contemporary currents and fashions of thought than Boyle's admirer, the sceptic divine and essayist, Joseph Glanvill (1636–80). He says: 'And indeed by some all men are accounted Scepticks, who dare dissent from the *Aristotelian* Doctrines, and will not slavishly subscribe all the Tenents of the *Dictator* in *Philosophy*, which they esteem the only true and certain Foundations of Knowledge . . . for the great *Gassendus* is charged with so much Scepticism on this account, that he writ an Exercitation against Aristotle', and it was said, '*those that slight* Aristotle's *Grounds must of necessity, being always in quest of Principles, ever fall short of Science*'. To reject the ancient philosophers as sources of true knowledge, and 'to seek Truth in the great Book of Nature' will brand such great men as Bacon, Descartes and the scientists of the Royal Society as 'Scepticks'. 'This is Scepticism with some; and if it be so indeed, 'tis such Scepticism, as is the only way to sure and grounded knowledge, to which confidence in uncertain opinions is the most fatal Enemy'.[17]

[15] W. Pagel, *Nature*, 1944, cliii, 675; *idem, Brit. Med. Journ.* 1945, i, 59; *idem, Osiris*, 1949, viii, 347.

[16] On the view of the Copernican Theory as a 're-emergence of ancient Pythagorean and mystical truth' as cherished by Bruno and his sympathizers in England, see F. A. Yates, 'Giordano Bruno's conflict with Oxford'. *Journ. Warburg Instit.*, 1939, ii, 227; and 'The religious policy of Giordano Bruno'. *ibid.*, 1940, iii, 181.

[17] 'Of scepticism and certainty.' Essay ii in Joseph Glanvill, *Essays on several important subjects in philosophy and religion.* London, 1676, p. 44.

'Knowledge is capable of far greater Heights and Improvements', says Glanvill, 'than it hath yet attain'd; and there is nothing that hath stinted its Growth, and hindered its Improvements more, than an over-fond, superstitious opinion of Aristotle, and the Ancients, by which it is presumed that their Books are the Ne Ultra's of learning, and little or nothing can be added to their discoveries: So that hereby a stop hath been put upon Inquiry, and men have contented themselves with studying their Writings, and disputing about their Opinions, while they have not taken much notice of the great Book of Nature, or used any likely Endeavours for further acquaintance with it.' But a real advance in Science can be achieved by 'enlarging the History of Things. . . . The History of Nature is to be augmented, either by an investigation of the Springs of Natural motions, or fuller Accounts of the grosser and more palpable Phenomena'; and it is precisely this which Glanvill sees pursued in his own age in 'Chymistry, Anatomy and the Mathematicks' with the aid of 'multitudes of excellent instruments, which are great Advantages to these later Ages', such as the microscope, telescope, thermometer, barometer and the air-pump—which were 'either not at all known, or but imperfectly, by Aristotle and the Ancients . . . some of which were first invented, all of them exceedingly improved by the Royal Society'.[18] Aristotle appears as the '*Tyrant of Stagyra*',[19] or with Thomas Aquinas as one of the 'great Troublers of the World who have vex'd it by the Wars . . . of the Brain', who have 'so dear and so precious a memory', while the first discoverer of such 'excellent mystery' as the compass and so many experimenters who have really advanced knowledge remain unknown.[20] Glanvill draws up a catalogue of the results accruing from contemporary research, notably by members of the Royal Society, in order to mark the progress achieved.[21] This is followed by a special account of Boyle's work.[22] The essay concludes with a further deprecation of Aristotle, who, according to the remark of Francis Bacon, 'did not use and imploy Experiments for the erecting of his Theories; but having arbitrarily pitch'd his Theories, his manner was to force Experience to suffragate and yield countenance to his precarious propositions'.[23] In subsequent essays on 'Pious Science', Glanvill defends Science against the suspicion of Atheism and endeavours to show the 'usefulness of real Philosophy to Religion' and the 'Agreement of Reason and Religion'—a discussion maintained at the level of shallow Deism. In spite of all enlightenment and progressive words, Glanvill, defending the reality of witchcraft against what he calls 'Modern Sadducism',[24] displays little less credulity and obscurantism than do van Helmont and most of his scientific contemporaries.

What strikes the most impressive note in these essays is the consciousness of the author and his contemporaries of the entirely new and unheard of aims of his time, and the actual advance already made towards their new scientific ideals. Earlier, Paracelsus and van Helmont had proclaimed a

---

[18] Glanvill, 'Modern improvements of useful knowledge'. Essay iii in *op. cit.* (17), p. 2.
[19] *ibid.*, p. 10.   [20] *ibid.*, p. 33.   [21] *ibid.*, pp. 3–34.
[22] *ibid.*, pp. 38–45.   [23] *ibid.*, p. 49.
[24] *idem*, 'Against modern sadducism in the matter of witches and apparitions'. Essay vi in *op. cit.* (17).

PLATE XXXIX

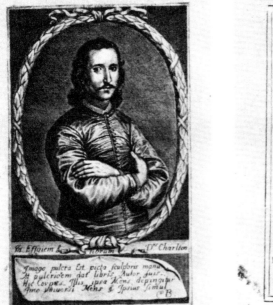

FIG. 3. Title-page and portrait of Walter Charleton in his *Immortality of the Human Soul*, 1657

FIG. 4. The passage in Charleton's *Immortality of the Human Soul*, 1657, in which he discusses the shift of interest from religious to scientific subjects

relentless defection from the ancient ways, but emphasized the novelty of their individual endeavours rather than that of their period. Even more than in Glanvill such consciousness of the age and its peculiar aims is recognizable in Walter Charleton (1619–1707).[25] He had started as an admirer of van Helmont, some of whose treatises he had translated. He then developed atomistic and Epicurean leanings, but took pains to forestall the suspicion of atheism—chiefly in his two dialogues on 'The Immortality of the Human Soul, demonstrated by the Light of Nature'.[26] This, not unlike Glanvill's essay, contains a catalogue of recent scientific work, as carried out under the auspices of the Royal College of Physicians, notably by Harvey and Glisson, as well as of work in physics and mathematics by Oxford scholars.[27] And it is in this work that we find even a discussion of the historical causes of the new tendencies of the age and their special cultivation in England. How could, asks the host of the interlocutors, all this be achieved 'in a land yet wet and reaking with blood . . . in a Nation so lately opprest by the Tyranny of Mars, and scarce yet free from the distractions of a horrid Civil War'? Athanasius (Charleton) answers: 'Every Age hath its peculiar Genius, which inclines men's minds to some one study or other, and gives it a dominion over their affections proportionate to its secret influence.' Moreover, he says, it was just 'our late Warrs and Schisms' that have powerfully influenced this development, in that they have 'almost wholly discouraged men from the study of Theologie; and brought the Civil Law into contempt. The major part of young Schollers in our Universities addict themselves to Physick; and how much that conduceth to real and valid knowledge, and what singular advantages it hath above other studies, in making men true Philosophers, I need not intimate to you'.[28] And, as the second interlocutor remarks, 'why may we not refer these Innovations in Philosophy, Physick and the Mathematicks . . . rather to the English Humour of affecting new Opinions, than to any real defects or errors in the Doctrine of the Ancients?', Charleton (pointing to the Copernican system) retorts: 'Neither have we introduced any Alterations in Natural Philosophy, Physick and other parts of Human learning, but what carry their utility with them, and are justifiable by right reason, by autoptical or sensible demonstration, and by multiplied experience. So that every intelligent man may easily perceive, that it hath been the Reformation, that drew on the Change; not the desire of Change which pretendeth the Reformation . . . . The Reformers . . . followed that Counsel of the Scripture which injoynes us, to make a stand upon the Ancient way, and then look about us, and discover, what is the straight and right way, and so to walk in it.'[29]

[25] For a short biography and bibliography of Charleton see Sir H. Rolleston, 'Walter Charleton, D.M., F.R.C.P., F.R.S.', *Bull. Hist. Med.*, 1940. viii, 403.

[26] W. Charleton, *The immortality of the human soul*. London, 1657.

[27] *ibid.*, pp. 34–48.

[28] *ibid.*, p. 49.

[29] *ibid.*, pp. 50–2. This is the very topic to which modern studies in sociological history have been devoted, notably Robert K. Merton's 'Science, technology and society in seventeenth century England'. *Osiris*, 1938, iv (2), 360–632. Merton has given a quantitative estimate of the shift of emphasis and interest from theological to scientific studies which took place between 1600 and 1700 and which Charleton witnessed. The D.N.B. data on which Merton based his research indicate an almost continuous and unbroken decline of interest in the ministry as an

It is well known how anti-Aristotelianism reached its philosophical climax in the work of Francis Bacon. In his writings, Aristotle's name stands for all that he finds fault with in a philosophy that had been used as a basis of science from antiquity up to his own time. To Bacon, Aristotle personifies all *idola theatri*, i.e. all prejudices that are due to blind obedience to authority. Against Aristotelian syllogism Bacon establishes induction, for syllogism makes words, but cannot invent; it serves the *munus professorium*, not the *'regnum hominis'*. True induction must take the place of pseudo-induction, i.e. the crude 'Aristotelian' empiricism which remains a descriptive collection of material, but falls short of discovering the laws and causes in nature. Regulated induction, which leads from step to step in a continuous chain from simple observations to general axioms, should replace the method of invention so far in common use, to wit the jumping from the simple to the highest and from the particular to the Universal.[30]

IV

From the foregoing account, antagonism to Aristotelian philosophy appears as the common denominator of all the varied motives, currents and trends of thought which made for the foundation and advancement of modern science in the seventeenth century. Yet, William Harvey, who, by the discovery and scientific demonstration of the circulation of the blood, founded modern physiology and biology, felt himself deeply indebted to Aristotle. He says: 'The authority of Aristotle has always such weight with me that I never think of differing from him inconsiderately'.[31] It is the sovereignty of the heart, its independence of the brain in sense and motion, its supremacy in being 'the first part which exists, [its containing] blood, life, sensation, motion, before either the brain or the liver were in being'[32]—in other words the main

occupation, and as a contemporary source is cited John Eachard's *The grounds and occasions of the contempt of the clergy*. London, 1670. Among the reasons for the shift the religious factor claims pride of place, notably the prevalence of protestant and puritan ethics with the emphasis laid on 'meritory works', blessed reason, profitable education, the study of God as the 'great author of Nature' in his works, in other words religious pragmatism. 'Religion is one expression of cultural values, and in the seventeenth century a clearly dominating expression' (Merton, *loc. cit.*, p. 414). 'But perhaps the two most important elements in the culture which account for the acceptance of progressivism are changes in the social organisation and the application of canons of utilitarianism. This was a period of rapidly increasing vertical mobility; the bourgeois class was coming into power. Wealth was becoming ever more effective as a means of obtaining prestige . . . the cultural soil of XVIIth Century England was peculiarly fertile for the growth and spread of science.' (*ibid.*, pp. 596–7.)

[30] See Kuno Fischer, *Franz Baco von Verulam. Die Realphilosophie und ihr Zeitalter.* Leipzig, 1856, p. 140; T. Fowler, *Bacon's Novum Organum.* Oxford, 1878, pp. 72 ff. ('The reaction against the authority of Aristotle'—Valla, Rud. Agricola, Agrippa, Vives, Paracelsus, Nizolius, Ramus, Telesius, Patricius, Bruno, Campanella, Severinus, Cabeus, etc., etc.)

[31] 'Tantopere . . . apud me semper valuit Aristotelis autoritas, ut non temere ab illa recedendum puto.' Harvey, 'On generation', xi. *Works.* Eng. trans. by R. Willis. London, Sydenham Soc., 1847, p. 207 (Latin text from *Bibl. Anat.* ed. Manget and Le Clerk, Geneva, 1685, vol. i, p. 614.)

[32] 'Nec minus Aristoteli de principatu cordis assentiendum; a cerebro motum, et sensum non accipere, nec a jecore sanguinem? sed principium venarum et sanguinis esse et hujusmodi . . . quod cor nempe primum subsistens sit, et habeat in se sanguinem, vitam, sensum, motum, antequam aut cerebrum aut jecur facta erant, vel plane distincta apparuerant, vel saltem ullam functionem edere potuerant. Adde, suis propriis organis ad motum fabricatis, cor tanquam animal quoddam internum, diutius consistit: quasi, hoc primo facto, ab ipso postea fieri, nutriri, conservari, perfici, totum animal tanquam hujus opus et domicilium, natura voluisset.' *Exercit. anat. de motu cordis et sanguinis*, cap. xvii. *Bibl. Anat.* ed. Manget and Le Clerk, Geneva, 1685, vol. ii, p. 62. *Works, op. cit.* (31), p. 83. See also 'Second disquis. to John Riolan jr.', *Works, ibid.*, p. 137.

tenets of Aristotle's physiology—which Harvey feels he has proved. The stroke of genius by which Harvey welded the multitude of his observations and arguments into the concept of blood circulation, he himself describes as follows:

> I began to think whether there might not be a motion, as it were, in a circle. Now this I afterwards found to be true; ... Which motion we may be allowed to call circular, in the same way as Aristotle says that the air and the rain emulate the circular motion of the superior bodies; for the moist earth, warmed by the sun, evaporates; the vapours drawn upwards are condensed, and descending in the form of rain, moisten the earth again; and by this arrangement are generations of living things produced; and in like manner too are tempests and meteors engendered by the circular motion, and by the approach and recession of the sun.
>
> And so, in all likelihood, does it come to pass in the body, through the motion of the blood; the various parts are nourished, cherished, quickened by the warmer, more perfect, vaporous, spirituous, and, as I may say, alimentive blood; which, on the contrary, in contact with these parts becomes cooled, coagulated, and, so to speak, effete; whence it returns to its sovereign the heart, as if to its source, or to the inmost home of the body, there to recover its state of excellence or perfection. Here it resumes its due fluidity and receives an infusion of natural heat—powerful, fervid, a kind of treasury of life, and is impregnated with spirits, and it might be said with balsam; and thence it is again dispersed; and all this depends on the motion and action of the heart. ...
>
> The heart, consequently, is the beginning of life; the sun of the microcosm, even as the sun in his turn might well be designated the heart of the world; for it is the heart ... which ... is indeed the foundation of life, the source of all action.[33]

Here, the circulation of the blood is visualized as the microcosmic copy of a general cosmological pattern and principle. It no longer remains a discovery of scientific detail, but obtains a position in a view of the world which is based on two main tenets of Aristotle: the excellence of the circular motion and the parallelism of the macrocosm and microcosm, that is, the universe and the living organism. We need not, therefore, be surprised that the first approval of Harvey's discovery came from the mystic Robert Fludd (1574–1637), who called Harvey his 'friend, colleague and compatriot well versed not only in anatomy but also the deepest mysteries of philosophy', and his theory a demonstration that the spirit of life retains an impression both of the planetary system and of the zodiac.[34] In other words, he regarded the genuine Aristotelian idea of the 'fountain of life' in the living body imitating the circular movement of the 'common parent and producer' in the bigger world of the universe, the Sun, as an essential requisite of Harvey's work. It should be borne in mind that at this time Harvey was widely disbelieved and attacked by the exponents of 'scientific' and professional medicine, as then understood.

In his first book, that on the circulation of the blood (1628), Harvey had already shown an inclination to regard the blood as the original part formed, and therefore the source of life:[35] this view is not advanced as being at variance

[33] 'Motion of the heart', viii. Eng. trans., *op. cit.* (31), pp. 46–7. Also: 'On generation', l. *ibid.*, *Works*, p. 367.

[34] The present writer was the first to draw attention to Fludd with reference to Harvey's discovery: W. Pagel, 'Religious motives in the medical biology of the XVIIth century'. *Bull. Hist. Med.*, 1935, iii, 277.

[35] 'Motion of the heart', iv, *Works*, *op. cit.* (31), pp. 29, 30.

with that of Aristotle, and we have mentioned how he extols the heart in the true Aristotelian tradition. But in his later work—that on Generation (1651)— he expressed a disagreement with Aristotle, and definitely placed the heart second in dignity to the blood. Referring to the authority of the Pentateuch, he says the blood is the residence of life 'because in it life and the soul first show themselves and at last become extinct'.[36] He says also: 'I maintain, against Aristotle, that the blood is the prime part that is engendered, and the heart the mere organ destined for its circulation.'[37]

It should be emphasized that it was not a materialistic tendency by which Harvey was actuated in according the blood a position of primary importance, in the sense that it 'constitutes the vital principle itself'. This is the wording of Willis's translation. A more accurate version would probably be: 'in it the vital principle inheres'.[38] That such a materialistic twist was really intended by Harvey is hardly possible, as it is at variance with his many other utterances as quoted below. If it were so, it would be antagonistic to Aristotle's conception of the 'vital principle', the *anima* which may be defined as follows: Owing to its material composition and organization a natural object contains life and function—*potentially*. It may attain *reality* by the action of the *anima*, evidently a functional impulse which 'perfects' the body by enabling it to step out into reality. The *anima* indicates for instance a plan inherent in the form and function of a vital organ such as the eye. It is not, however, a material body such as the heart, let alone something dependent on it such as the blood.[39]

It is more than doubtful whether Harvey really meant to identify 'soul' with 'blood'. He admittedly says it is not as improbable as it seems that 'blood is the soul itself in the body'.[40] But this sentence is an isolated instance. Moreover, it is not meant in a material, but in a functional sense. For, Harvey continues, it is only when the circulation, its causes and vital importance and the other 'secret functions' (*arcana*) of the blood are considered that blood appears to be the very 'soul' of the body. In most places he speaks of life residing, revealing itself and the soul in the blood where there are 'the lares and penates of life enshrined', and 'the vital principle itself has its seat'.[41] Rather than the embodiment of the soul, the blood appears to be, according to Harvey, its vector. This, however, is not meant in the sense of Scaliger and Fernel, who believed that the vital principle (soul), i.e. 'heat' and 'spirits', are *added* to the blood which, by itself, cannot display any activity superior to that of its elementary constituents. It is, in the present author's opinion, because of its materialistic implications that Harvey deprecates such view. In the same way he militates against the elemental

---

[36] 'On generation', li. *Works*, *op. cit.* (31), p. 376.

[37] *ibid.*, p. 374.

[38] *ibid.*, p. 376. The Latin text runs as follows: 'Nec sanguis solum pars primigenia et principalis dicendus est, quod in eo, et ab eo motus, pulsusque principium oriatur; sed etiam quia in eo primum calor animalis innascitur, spiritus vitalis ingeneratur et anima ipsa consistit. Ubicunque enim primo immediatum et principale vegetativae facultatis instrumentum reperitur: ibi quoque animam primo inesse indeque originem sumere, verisimile est, quoniam illa a spiritu, et calido innato separari nequit.' *Bibl. Anat.*, *op. cit.* (31), vol. i, p. 664.

[39] Aristotle, *De anima*, ii. 1; 412^a (trans. J. A. Smith, Oxford, 1931) and *ibid.* i. 2; 405^b (rejection of the theory that the soul is blood).

[40] 'On generation', lii, trans. by Willis, *op. cit.* (31), p. 309.

[41] *ibid.*, p. 376.

faculties being held responsible for the excellence of the blood. Just as there exists in the semen, says Harvey, something which makes it generative and exceeds the powers of the elements in building an animal, there dwells in the blood some power which acts beyond the power of the elements, its chief function being nutrition and preservation of the parts of the body. It is a nature and indeed a 'soul' inherent *in* the blood, neither a fire, nor something that takes its origin from fire or from an astral element.[42]   Harvey is sceptical towards the role of the elements, and indeed to their existence in the sense of the ancient and contemporary doctrines, thereby closely following the vitalistic argument as advanced by van Helmont,[43] and later taken up, on the strength of further empirical (chemical) findings by Boyle. 'The so-called elements are not prior to those things that are engendered, but rather are subsequent thereto; they are remainders rather than principles. Neither Aristotle himself nor anyone else has ever demonstrated the separate existence of the elements in the nature of things, or that they were the principles of bodies which consist of parts similar to one another.'[44]

If, then, blood and 'soul' are identical, the latter, however, being neither the product of the elemental constitution of the blood nor of something 'ethereal' ('heat', 'spirit' or 'astral body') added to it, 'soul' can mean nothing but the natural function inherent in blood which acts as the material substratum necessary for the appropriate effects to be obtained in physical life. Only as far as the blood displays a certain function ('virtues and powers'), i.e. not blood substance by itself, but blood flowing in its proper channels, can it be called 'spirituous' or 'celestial'.[45]

As Joseph Needham has pointed out, Harvey's leanings were vitalistic and 'he argues against both those who wished to deduce generation from properties of bodies (like Digby) and the Atomists (like Highmore).'[46]   In other words, his views were anti-materialistic in the true Aristotelian tradition. Harvey says:

> It is a common mistake with those who pursue philosophical studies in these times, to seek for the cause of diversity of parts in diversity of the matter whence they arise. Thus medical men assert that the several parts of the body are both engendered and nourished by diverse matters, either the blood or the seminal fluid. . . . Nor do they err less who, with Democritus, compose all things of atoms; or with Empedocles, of elements. As if *generation* were nothing more than a separation, or aggregation, or disposition of things. It is not indeed to be denied, that when one thing is to be produced from another, all these are necessary, but generation itself is different from them all. I find Aristotle to be of this opinion; and it is my intention, by-and-by, to teach that out of the same albumen (which all allow to be uniform, not composed of diverse parts,) all the parts of the chick, bones, nails, feathers, flesh, &c. are produced and nourished. Moreover, they who philosophize in this way, assign a material cause [for generation], and deduce the causes of natural things either from the elements concurring spontaneously or accidentally, or from atoms variously arranged; they do not attain to that which is

[42] *ibid.*, pp. 505–7.
[43] See W. Pagel, 'The religious and philosophical aspects of van Helmont's science and medicine'. *Bull. Hist. Med.*, 1944, Suppl. ii, pp. 3 ff.
[44] 'On generation', lxxii. *Works, op. cit.* (31), p. 517. (Willis's trans. here slightly emended.)
[45] *ibid.*, lxxi, pp. 507, 510.
[46] Joseph Needham, *History of embryology*. Cambridge, 1934, p. 120.

first in the operations of nature and in the generation and nutrition of animals; viz. they do not recognize that efficient cause and divinity of nature which works at all times with consummate art, and providence, and wisdom, and ever for a certain purpose, and to some good end; they derogate from the honour of the Divine Architect, who has not contrived the shell for the defence of the egg with less of skill and of foresight than he has composed all the other parts of the egg of the same matter, and produced it under the influence of the same formative faculty.[47]

Harvey thus establishes the immateriality of the vital principle in the sense of Aristotle, against the crude materialistic and pseudo-idealistic ('animistic') theories of his time.

A further point which may be mentioned in this connexion is Harvey's denial of the entry of air into the blood, the 'concoction' of the latter in the lungs, and the diversity of arterial and venous blood in quality. As Curtis has shown,[48] the transit of the blood through the lungs was no essential requisite for the discovery of the circulation. But apart from that it is tempting to suggest that Harvey's ulterior motive for his denial of the above points was the tendency to remove all reasons for a materialistic derivation of the vital function of the blood from air entering it.

To divest the 'vital principle' from all such materialistic notions is clearly the aim of Aristotle's treatise *On the soul*—in spite of the 'life giving' qualities which the philosopher attributed to the 'psychical' or 'generative' heat of the sun and animals elsewhere in his writings.[49] Harvey's adherence to the Aristotelian interpretation of the 'soul' as something functional, which he located in the blood, seems thus to be the result of his philosophical convictions rather than the fruit of despair to which 'the lifelong thinker upon the meaning of the circulation' (Curtis)[50] was driven by his ignorance of the oxygenation of the blood. We agree, however, with Curtis that Harvey saw both circulation and 'the prodigious history of generation' in the same light, and, as the present author would add, as the fundamental microcosmic cycles which determined the position of the smaller world of the organism in the macrocosmos of the celestial bodies.

It was this philosophical view which, to Harvey, consummated the ultimate meaning of these biological processes. Boyle tells us that Harvey was led to his discovery by the reflection 'that so provident a cause as nature had not so plac'd many valves without design',[51] that is, without a consideration of final causes in the true Aristotelian sense—for it was Aristotle who had said that 'Nature, like Mind, always does whatever it does for the sake of something, which something is its end'.[52] But, to Harvey, adherence to Aristotelian philosophy did not mean the subjection of empiricism to reasoning, for he refers to Aristotle's advice: 'Faith is to be given to reason if the matters demonstrated agree with those that are perceived by the senses; when things

---

[47] 'On generation', xi. *Works, op. cit.* (31), pp. 206–7.

[48] J. G. Curtis, *Harvey's views on the use of the circulation of the blood.* New York, 1915, pp. 38–53. See also W. Pagel, *Isis,* 1951, xlii, 22.

[49] *De generatione animalium,* 736^b–737^a (ed. by A. L. Peck, Loeb Library, p. 170) and 762^a. 18–24 (Loeb, p. 356).

[50] Curtis, *op. cit.* (48), p. 152.

[51] W. Pagel in *op. cit.* (34), p. 309.

[52] *De anima,* ii. 4; 415^b.

PLATE XL

T R A C T A T U S
De
Natura Substantiæ

ENERGETICA,

Seu de

VITA NATURÆ,

Ejúsque

Tribus primis Facultatibus,

I. PERCEPTIVA,
II. APPETITIVA, & naturalibus, &c.
III. MOTIVA,

Authore FRANCISCO GLISSONIO, Medicinæ Doctore, & Regio in florentissima Cantabrigiæ Academia Professore, celeberrimíque Col. Med. Lond. Socio, nec non illustrissimæ Societatis Regalis Collegâ.

L O N D I N I,

Typis E. Flesher. Prostat venalis apud H. Brome sub signo bombarda in Cœmeterio Paulino, & N. Hooke ad insignia Regia in vico Little Britain. M DC LXXII.

FIG. 6. Title-page of Glisson's *Tractatus de natura substantiæ energetica*, 1672

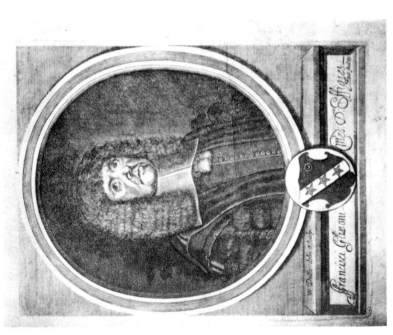

FIG. 5. Portrait of Francis Glisson in his *Tractatus de natura substantiæ energetica*, 1672

PLATE XLI

CAP. VII.

De Irritabilitate Fibrarum.

1. Motiva fibrarum facultas, nisi Irritabilis foret, vel perpetuò quiesceret, vel perpetuò idem ageret. Actionum igitur earum varietates & differentiæ, earundem Irritabilitatem clarè demonstrant. Hæc autem supponit perceptionem & appetitum, ut de novo fibra excitetur. Datâ verò Perceptione, appetitus & motus lege naturæ consequuntur: ita ut declaratio foliis Perceptionis fibrarum ad earum Irritabilitatem manifestandum sufficiat. Interim, cùm frequenter sensus, necnon appetitus sensitivus, cum perceptione naturali in hac Irritatione fibrarum complicentur, operæ pretium fuerit, ecquid Perceptio naturalis sola, ecquid cum sensu conjunctâ, ecquid denique ab appetitu sensitivo impulsâ, ad motum Fibrarum contribuat, & quid, investigare. Hoc quò facilius fiat, Perceptionem ad Fibrarum motum spectantem, in tres species, tentandi gratiâ, distinguere & easdem sigillatim describere, atque adeò examinare, visum est. Perceptionem itaque Irritationis ad fibras relatam (sive reipsâ ita sit, sive fecta) esse triplicem supponimus, naturalem, sensitivam, & ab appetitu animali regulatam. Prima, naturalis, ea est quâ fibra alterationem sibi illatam, sive gratam, sive ingratam, percipiens, ad eam appetendam, vel fugiendam, & conformiter ad fe movendam, excitatur. Secunda, sensitiva, est ea quâ fibra sensu alterationem in externo organo factam advertens, & aliquid appetendum, seque conformiter movendam, impellitur. Tertia, ab appetitu animali regulata, ea est quâ cerebrum fibras musculorum ad ea quæ appetit exequenda, ab intûs commovet. De his ordine pauca.

2. De naturali Perceptione fibras irritante, an sit, aliqui fortasse dubitabunt; sed alibi realitatem naturalis Perceptionis in genere afferuimus, nempe libro De Vita naturæ, quam qui agnoscent, multò faciliùs eandem fibris, spiritibus insitis & influentibus, hisque vitalibus, imbutis, indulgeant. Utcunque,

V 2

[Marginal notes: Irritabilitas supponit perceptionem. Modus de naturali perceptione requirenda. An naturalis Perceptionis infita.]

TRACTATUS

DE

VENTRICULO

ET

INTESTINIS.

Cui præmittitur alius,

DE

PARTIBUS CONTINENTIBUS

in genere; & in specie,

DE IIS

ABDOMINIS.

Authore *FRANCISCO GLISSONIO*, Medicinæ Doctore, & Regio in florentissima *Cantabrigiæ* Academia Professore, celeberrimique Coll. Med. Lond. Socio, necnon illustrissimæ Societatis Regalis Collegâ.

LONDINI,

Typis *E. F.* Prostat venalis apud *Henricum Brome* sub signo Bombardæ in Cœmeterio *Paulino*. MDCLXXVII.

Fig. 7. Title-page of Glisson's *Tractatus de ventriculo et intestinis*, 1677

Fig. 8. The passage in Glisson's *Tractatus de ventriculo* discussing the application of the philosophical theory of perceptibility in matter to the anatomy and physiology of fibres

have been thoroughly scrutinized, then are the senses to be trusted rather than the reason.'[53] Moreover, he says against those who had attacked him for having refuted the authority of Galen: 'The facts cognizable by the senses wait upon no opinions, and . . . the works of nature bow to no antiquity; for indeed there is nothing either more ancient or of higher authority than nature.'[54]

V

The biological insight which Harvey derives from his actual work as well as from Aristotelian philosophy thus culminates in the demonstration of the immanence of life and function in organized matter, neither of which can exist independently of each other. 'Soul' or 'life' is the 'actuality', i.e. the actual function of an organ: the organ needs the actuality in order to be alive, but in the same way the soul cannot exist, act or manifest itself without material organization. This conception of immanence stands in decided contrast to all dualistic doctrines, which visualize the soul as a separate 'immortal' entity which enters an independent material substratum from outside and leaves it when death occurs. In this view the body remains a lifeless aggregate of particles, which is kept together and preserved from decay by the action of the soul *on* it. The view of immanence, however, will not recognize such inert matter at all, but sees even the lowest objects in nature, such as dust or stone, endowed with some sort of dynamical impulse.

This is precisely the view of another Aristotelian biologist, Francis Glisson (1596–1677), and, most probably, through him that of Leibniz (1646–1716).[55] Glisson, who uses neo-scholastic methods of demonstration even in his anatomical works, first of all objects to the atomic concept of matter. The difference in the arrangement of particles in the gaseous, fluid and solid state of a substance does not affect its 'species', its virtues, as recognizable for example in the odour of rose water, which remains the same in the volatile as in the fluid substance.[56] The yolk and albumen of eggs, blood, milk and humours of widely different classes of animals are very similar to each other in colour, shape and consistence, i.e. in the arrangement of particles and texture, yet fundamentally different *specie naturae*, i.e. in function and potentialities. The chemical differences of substances and elements are real and essential, and not only due to variations in the arrangement of particles of a homogeneous and uniform inert matter. If this were true it

---

[53] *De generatione animalium*, iii. 10; 760ᵇ (Loeb, *op. cit.* (49), p. 344). Harvey, 'Second disquis. to Riolan'. *Works, op. cit.* (31), p. 131 and introd. to 'On generation', *Works*, p. 158.

[54] 'Naturae opera facta manifesta sensui, nullas opiniones, nullamque antiquitatem morari: natura enim nihil antiquius, majorisque auctoritatis.' 'Second disquis. to Riolan', *Bibl. Anat., op. cit.* (31), vol. ii, p. 73; *Works, op. cit.* (31), p. 123.

[55] On Glisson as a precursor to Leibniz see H. Marion, *Franciscus Glissonius quid de natura substantiae s. vita naturae senserit et utrum Leibnitio de natura substantiae cogitanti quidquam contulerit*. Thèse, Paris, 1880. The present writer hopes to resume this question at a later date. The work in which Glisson sets out his cosmology and philosophy is the *Tractatus de natura substantiae energetica s. de vita naturae ejusque tribus primis facultatibus, i. perceptiva, ii. appetitiva, iii. motiva, naturalibus*. Londini, 1672. The subject of this treatise is taken up again in his *Tractatus de ventriculo et intestinis*. Londini, 1677, with special reference to irritability and 'sensitive appetence', their anatomical and physiological significance and their location in the fibres of the abdominal organs (see pp. 147 and 157 ff. of this treatise). In fact Glisson had started writing it in 1662, but wanted it to be preceded by the philosophical treatise of 1672.

[56] *Tractat. de natura substant., op. cit.* (55), pp. 181 ff.

should be much easier to convert them into each other, for example, salt and 'spiritus pinguis' (distillates from plants) should be mutually convertible just as easily as ice becomes water or a vapour is converted into a liquid.[57] Chemical processes alter the density, rarity, tenacity, friability, asperity, levity, hardness and softness of a substance—in other words the texture of its particles, its 'schematismus', but not its specific properties.[58] It is, therefore, idle to try to produce the specific odour of plants or to 'isolate' specific substances by the 'philosophy through fire', i.e. by chemical operations. For fire and analysing destroy specific virtues rather than generate them. It is not a confluence of separately existing elements that generates a composite object, for the 'semina' of plants and animals are obviously 'mixed' in the same ratio as the body substance of the adult individuals.[59] The requisite necessary for generation is therefore a predetermined elementary mixture rather than a fortuitous confluence of single elements in seed and soil. It is thus that matter does not serve merely as a passive inert dough. It actively and vitally collaborates with the 'generans' in that it undergoes certain 'predispositions'. These remove all that is inimical in it to the 'idea' of the 'generans', and enable matter to restrict the 'generans' to one particular and specific form, i.e. that of the individual to be generated. In the true Aristotelian sense, form makes out of the potential matter of a horse the actual here and now existing horse; it is the actuality, the realization of a certain potentiality of matter. But it is the latter that predetermines and limits its form to that of a horse and nothing else.[60]

The 'vitality' and significance of matter are not restricted to organic beings in Glisson's philosophy. Dynamical impulses, a 'primordial' and 'primeval' life appertain to matter in general. It is inalienably bound up with such 'life' and not subject to death.

This 'vita insita' is not a kind of sensation. Campanella had visualized a 'sensus rerum' in all objects of nature. Glisson objected that any sensual faculty is bound up with the function of a 'specific' organ, with an 'organica facultas'. Hence a stone or dead body cannot be endowed with it. There is, however, a simple (not sensual) 'natural perception', and 'energetic nature' in 'substance'.[61] This is 'simple', in that it does not permit of a distinction in

---

[57] ibid., p. 179.

[58] ibid., p. 181: 'Mutatio schematismi non variat speciem.'

[59] ibid., pp. 176 ff., 'An elementa praefuerint in misto'; p. 179, 'An elementa sint materiae schematismi'.

[60] ibid., p. 136: 'Previous dispositions in matter'; 'Immanence of form in matter'; 'Forma non esset natura, nisi ab intus manaret'. p. 140: 'Forma non educitur, donec materia sponte suscipit et quasi eligit seu in se elicit naturam ei generantis similem. Existimo enim solam materiam intrinsice attingere versionem formae extrinsecus oblatae in naturam suam atque operationem hanc esse actionem vitalem rei se perficientis. Materia, cum nolit annihilari, in extremis angustiis dictamini generantis ultro obsequitur, novamque legem essendi et operandi, novam indolem s. naturam additionalem sibi asciscit: atque adeo eductio formae in ultimo ejus actu non est pura passio, sed immanens quaedam actio s. actus vitalis.' p. 144: 'An generatio activa sit modus materiae.' Generation is 'eduction', i.e. the process by which matter generates 'form'. p. 145: 'Unicum inter materiam et formam modum pono eumque in materia' (in opposition to the scholastic doctrines as expounded by Suarez). p. 146 ff., 'De causa formae materiali'. 'Est ergo generatio causalitas materiae exercita et spectat ad partes materiae, non ad partes formae.' p. 161: Matter gives form its 'Esse', but form determines and limits the action of matter. Out of the potential matter of a horse, form makes the actual matter of the horse which exists here and now.

[61] ibid., p. 208.

it between a 'fundamental' substratum devoid of functional impulse and the 'energetic substance' by means of which matter acts. Such a distinction between a 'magma' which gives matter its empirical existence and its activity, its 'life', its function, is merely the result of human reasoning and analysis. Our intellect is limited, it is weak. It cannot adequately and distinctly grasp objects as they are in themselves and in all their aspects at once ('Res integras adaequate et distincte simul comprehendere'[62]). It therefore resorts to differentiation that is not based on diversities immanent in the objects themselves, but sets up 'entia rationis', i.e. 'inadequate concepts' which may serve as working hypotheses.

Glisson thus conceives of matter as bound up with primeval *'perception'*. It harbours incorruptible 'life' and constitutes 'Nature', in that it contains the principle which directs all function. It is in this sense that Hippocrates called 'Nature' the healer of disease. It is the 'principium operationis' of Aristotle and his scholastic followers, notably Suarez.

No further research has been undertaken, however, into the way Nature acquits herself of these duties. Motion has been assumed to be the way in which this is achieved, but motion that comes from inside the object and does not act on it; motion which is the 'life' of matter has so far only been recognized in organic beings. In Glisson's opinion motion is inherent in matter at large. Matter, as far as it is 'energetic substance' and releases motion from inside itself, 'lives'. Yet life is not simply motion, for it is more intimately connected with its substance than is an 'accident' such as motion. But life is the 'principle' of motion, it determines the kind and type of motions that take place. This is seen for example in plants which are devoid of motions vital to animals, such as the pulse and the circulation of the blood and animal heat.[63]

'Nature', embracing substance and matter at large, organic as well as inorganic beings, 'has therefore a claim to an even more eminent title, namely that of the Vital Principle of Function or of Life-Inherent-in-Substance'.[64] This life has no more than one aspect, and in it there can be no question of distinction between things physical and spiritual; it is therefore 'simple', and because it is simple, it is perpetual; for decay is the separation of component parts, and only composite things are liable to corruption. This indissoluble unity of 'substance' and 'life' Glisson denotes as *biousia*. Its elementary functions, common to *all* objects in nature, are : Perception, appetence and motion. 'Substance' first engenders a perception of what has to be done ('opus aggrediendum'); the object perceived is then desired and the desired end consummated. Organic life develops by virtue of a 'duplication' or 'triplication' of these functions. 'Simple', 'natural' perception requires no specific organs, nor is it limited in distribution and scope by organization. 'Animal perception', however, needs membranes, humours, nerves and brain whereby simple perception is enabled to become sensation, i.e. duplicated (perceived) perception ('perceptio perceptionis'). Such duplication cannot take place, for example, in lesions of the nervous system

---

[62] *ibid.*, pp. 186 ff., and *Introductio* and *Dedicatio*, pp. 1 ff.
[63] *ibid.*, p. 191.   [64] *ibid.*, p. 191.

when simple perception is recorded by the eye, or another sense organ, but not dealt with by the brain.[65]

The simplest form of organic life, i.e. of 'duplication' of the primitive life of matter, is seen in plants which are endowed with a 'vis plastica'. Such organic life requires the co-operation of the vital functions that take place in the organs and tissues ('vita insita') with the action of the vital humours ('vita influens'). Not merely contact, but the intimate union of these two 'lives' is necessary to bring about 'duplicated', i.e. organic life. For without the 'vita influens' the functions of the organs and tissues remain dormant, as it were 'fixed' or 'crystallized' inside the rigid anatomical structures. They are not unlike colours which require light in order to act and to be seen. It is this union with the subsequent 'excitation' of life inherent in the tissues ('spiritus insiti') which elicits all the functions essential to organic life, such as preservation from decay, invigoration, tonus, activity and maintenance of the right chemical composition. A still higher perfection of life, its 'triplication', obtains in animals in which the 'vita insita' unites with two 'vitae influentes', covering vegetative functions as well as sensation and voluntary motion. A 'rational soul' which is independent of matter is briefly discussed but without significance in Glisson's work.

As organic life represents the duplication or triplication of the incorruptible 'primeval' life of matter, death amounts to dissolution of the duplication of life in plants and of its triplication in animals. In the latter the 'triuna sensitiva' perishes when it is suppressed in the brain or heart. 'We, therefore, deny', Glisson continues, 'an emigration of anything in the nature of a soul belonging to the material substance when living beings die, and maintain that the death of the sensitive soul is but a dissolution of the threefold confederation of life ... and that the simple primeval life of nature can neither perish nor change'.[66]

This definition of death repeats implicitly Glisson's philosophy of life. It shows precisely the stand he takes against Dualism. Descartes, who proclaimed it, had not denied that the ordinary and especially the involuntary functions are the result of the organization of the bodily machine, and therefore not attributable to the action of the soul. Ignorance of anatomy and mechanics, of the extremely fine organization of living beings which enables them to carry out all their varied movements, he says, have led people to resort to the soul as the universal cause of these functions; as has also the observation that the same parts which we see in the living are also present in the dead, where nothing seems to be amiss but the soul. The soul, however, being a substance different from the body, emerges in cogitation, will, imagination, perception and sensation alone, and any function that can be ascribed to it is 'cogitationum species'. Other functions such as the motion of the heart and arteries, digestion of food, etc., which have nothing to do with 'cogitation', are but physical motions. Moreover, the soul requires sound organs in order to display its functions, as is seen, for example, in the impairment of volition which follows nervous lesions, and in convulsions; while, on the other hand, a body with all its organs tuned up to a movement needs no soul to bring it about. It is not the soul that causes spontaneous

[65] ibid., p. 211.   [66] ibid., p. 235.

functions and movements, although, when the soul deserts the body at the time of death, functions cannot take place any longer. Hence we may conclude that the departure of the soul from the body is due to the same cause as the cessation of the functions of the latter. The body remains a machine comparable with a clock, in which nobody will see a soul at work indicating the hours.[67]

The dualistic doctrine thus recognizes some functions as immanent in organization, but not *all* functions. It is his endeavour to demonstrate the identity of all functions in principle which separates Glisson by a wide gulf from Descartes. The latter concentrates on a soul which leaves the body at death and is responsible for certain functions. To Glisson, 'soul' is but one aspect, one grade of the living, i.e. of the 'energetic substance'. There is no difference in kind between these aspects and grades, from the lowest stage of matter endowed with the most 'dim perceptions' to the higher forms of consciousness in the living animal. In Glisson's philosophy, matter appears as much 'spiritualized' as 'soul' is 'materialized', so that the contrast between them is only artificial. As the present author has tried to show, van Helmont, before Glisson, had embarked on these lines which were to lend the basis to the 'dynamic' system of Leibniz. His world consists of Monads, i.e. the smallest centres of energy that are different in quality and range, from those endowed with dim perception—such as primary matter with no more than the passive power of resistance—to the highest monads which direct self-conscious and thinking beings. But *all* monads are alive, as they all follow intrinsic schedules of function and aim. Life thus appears as the common denominator of all objects in nature, and solves the perennial problem of the relationship between body and soul. Biological units with physical and psychical aspects rather than 'bodies' and 'souls' constitute the world. It is obvious that this philosophy favours the vitalistic point of view. We have seen how Glisson was led to it by his insight into the immanence of functions in organized matter. The same emerged from Harvey's observations and reflections. In both Harvey and Glisson a strong influence of Aristotle, the father of Vitalism, is recognizable.

Van Helmont searches for the hall-marks of 'specificity' in Nature; he endeavours to uncover and isolate the created 'semina', the monads that are hidden in natural objects, and direct them to the specific functions and destinations whereby they 'live'. His religious mind cannot see them as the result of fortuitous changes in the quantity and local arrangement of smallest particles which are identical in quality. Matter, *qua* created, must have something divine immanent in it, to wit its specific disposition. This he believes to be represented in the Gas into which an object can be converted. Gas, therefore, means spiritualized matter of a certain individual entity or species, the material vector of specificity. It demonstrates the virtual unity of matter and dynamic impulse, the 'life' of all organized matter. This is, in fact, Glisson's concept of the 'energetic nature of substance'. It is the vitalistic point of view. In his results, van Helmont thus closely approaches the Aristotelian lead. It appears that his opposition was directed not against

[67] Descartes, *Tractatus de homine et de formatione foetus.* (Ed. Lud. de la Forge. Amsterodami (Elzivir), 1677, pp. 191–4.

the vitalistic and biological implications of Aristotelianism, but against the broad employment of syllogisms and mathematical patterns; he fought against materialistic notions, such as that of a certain heat from the Sun (the 'fifth element') acting as generating power in the semen, and against the ancient theories of the elements, humours and temperaments. Van Helmont is interested in the *empirical* isolation and demonstration of the 'vital principle' by means of chemical methods, rather than the *ontological* clarification of its 'position' in the philosophy of Nature. In this respect, Glisson approaches much more to Aristotle and the Schoolmen; nor was Glisson actuated by religious motives—unlike van Helmont who was inspired by Saint Augustine, an inspiration which may well have been transmitted to him by his neighbour at Ypres, Jansen, whom he mentioned, and whose religio-political ideals he shared. Yet, in the vitalistic results of his work, van Helmont stands in one line with Glisson and Harvey, the Aristotelian biologists and thinkers.

This cannot be said of such men as Charleton and Glanvill, who combine a genuine anti-Aristotelian attitude with an adherence to the doctrines of Descartes.[68] The latter, declaring the body to be a pure machine, decidedly separated from the soul, was bound to initiate the mechanistic point of view in the seventeenth century. Consequently Charleton advocates—against Aristotle—the separate existence of the vegetative soul, which enters the body from outside and animates it like a soldier whose arms spring to life when he uses them. Moreover, he voices such mechanistic views as that of the soul agitating heart and blood, and thereby preventing the putrefaction which would follow the sedimentation of the humours.[69] Glanvill is even more definite in his dualism.

> The natures of Soul and Body [says Glanvill] are at the most extreme distance . . . nor is there any appearance of likeness between them: For what hath Rarefaction, Condensation, Division, and the other properties and modes of Matter, to do with Apprehension, Judgment and Discourse, which are the proper acts of Spiritual Being? We cannot then perceive any congruity by which they are united: nor can there be any middle sort of Nature that partakes of each . . . so that what the cement should be that unites Heaven and Earth, Light and Darkness, viz. Natures of so diverse a make, and such disagreeing Attributes, is beyond the reach of any of our Faculties. . . . And we can give no better account how the Soul moves the Body. . . . We know as little, how the Soul so regularly directs the Animal Spirits and Instruments of Motion which are in the Body. . . . That they are conducted by some knowing Guide is evident from the steadiness and regularity of their motion. . . . That the soul hath Life and sense; but that the Body in strictness of speaking, hath neither the one nor other.[70]

---

[68] In Glanvill's case adherence to Descartes' philosophy was slightly tempered by his sceptical rejection of any dogmatism, Aristotelian or Cartesian. But he certainly subscribed to the dualistic separation of Body and Soul, which to him not only meant the 'nous' but also the 'anima vegetativa'. In Charleton there is no trace of scepticism. On the contrary, he freely borrows in an eclectic and not very critical way from various sources. His choice as a motto to 'The immortality of the soul', of Aristotle's phrase 'It remains, then, that Reason alone enters in, as an additional factor, from outside' (*De generatione animalium*, 736^b, *op. cit.* (49), p. 170) leads him to attribute his own (Cartesian) Dualism to the Father of Vitalism ('Immortality, *op. cit.* (26), p. 172). The same conclusion was drawn by Glanvill (Essay ii, *op. cit.* (17), p. 56).'

[69] *op. cit.* (17), p. 174.

[70] Glanvill, Essay ii in *op. cit.* (17), p. 56.

This is indeed the position 'upon which all the Philosophy of Des Cartes stands'.

Guided through seventeenth-century thought by the contemporary attitude towards Aristotle, we arrived at a distinction between two main biological currents. One of these is the vitalistic trend, as represented by Harvey and Glisson, the Aristotelian scholars, and by van Helmont, whose opposition to Aristotelianism was not directed against its vitalistic purport. We endeavoured to show how this vitalistic biology culminated in the vitalistic philosophy of Leibniz, and how Glisson can be visualized as the link between van Helmont and the Philosophy of Monadology. Their insight into the immanence of 'life' in matter forms the common ground of these biological philosophies. Dualism, on the other hand, which separates 'life' and 'soul' from matter and body by a wide gap, leads to the mechanistic point of view as established by Descartes and followed by English Deists. Tempting as it is, it would be beyond the scope of this paper to follow these trends through biological philosophy in the eighteenth and early nineteenth centuries where they are still recognizable, and to examine their influence on 'progress' in science. That they can indeed claim such significance for seventeenth-century science is shown by the examples of Harvey, of van Helmont, of Glisson. The prime importance of the heart, from which the blood, the vector of life, goes out and to which it returns, 'Gas' as the vector of specificity, and the intrinsic life of fibres and sphincters, their 'irritability'—all these fundamental discoveries are but scientific correlates of the philosophical insight into the immanence of 'vital' impulses in matter, into the 'energetic nature of substance'. We wish to add, however, that in dealing with such philosophical theories, we are not primarily actuated by the desire to demonstrate their usefulness, or otherwise, for what is visualized as lines of scientific progress from a modern point of view. We feel that the history of the science of biology as such cannot dispense with these aspects, for, as Bacon has warned us:[71] 'Historians should not be like critics who spend their time praising or blaming, but the facts themselves should be represented plainly and descriptively, with not more than sparse insertion of opinions. The material should be drawn not from the works and opinion of others, but all the main sources which are extant from a certain period should be consulted; not, however, merely read, but digested and understood in the peculiarity of their propositions, style and methods whereby the literary genius of that age as if by a magic formula should be raised from the dead.'

The author wishes to acknowledge his indebtedness to Mr. Bernard Pagel, of the Observatory, Cambridge, to Mr. F. N. L. Poynter, of the Wellcome Historical Medical Library, and to Dr. Ch. H. Talbot, of the Warburg Institute, University of London, for valuable suggestions and bibliographical help.

---

[71] 'De augmentis scientiarum', ii. 4; Bacon, *Opera*. Francofurti, 1665, pp. 49–50.

THE ELUSIVE HUMAN ALLANTOIS IN OLDER LITERATURE

by

A. W. MEYER

AS Hyrtl emphasized in 1880, the story of the allantois, like that of many other things, is lost in prehistory.[1] Moreover, its history in the vertebrates exceeds my powers and the time and space at my disposal. I shall hence confine this delineation to man and largely exclude discussions of the confusion of the allantois and yolk-sac with the chorion, and of the allantois with the extra-amnionic space and its contents, on the part of great men such as Albinus, Colombus and Harvey, and of lesser ones such as Velpeau, Seiler and others.

The avian and ungulate allantoids must have obtruded themselves upon the attention of the earliest observers, but the existence of the human long eluded and perplexed them. Although it was sought ardently, its nature and presence were not established until about two generations ago. Indeed, the final controversy regarding it occurred late in the nineteenth century and involved some of the most prominent European zoologists and anatomists, apparently, however, without resolving all doubts, for Schäfer in 1890 merely stated that 'there is reason to believe that it is found in the human embryo at a very early period—indeed the earliest human embryos that have hitherto been described already possess an allantois'.[2]

Since some of the predecessors of Vesalius believed in the presence of an allantois in man, it is not surprising that he too described it. He wrote in 1543:

> The next covering of the fœtus from the likeness to sausages (stuffed things) is very aptly called allantois by both those—Galen and later ones who had truly investigated (learned) it. For while dissecting, this outermost covering was gently rubbed away from the uterus, and blood, black as if burned, black and greenish, flowed forth from that (uterus), and no other covering of the fœtus having been broken, the fœtus is delivered from the uterus, it shows the form of some sausage, not indeed an oblong one, which is formed from the thin, the small intestine, but a short one, made from the thicker larger intestine sewed together above and below, not indeed so much obstructed by a noose, for the second covering corresponds to the intestine: the fœtus, moreover, and everything which this covering embraces, upholds the idea of their having been stuffed into an intestine. For the second covering is a real membrane and is interwoven with certain true arteries, almost in the same manner in which the adhering white or tunic of the eye is endowed with them.[3]

The odd illustration of the allantois from the second edition (1555) is reproduced here as Fig. 1.

Although Rueff in 1554 also designated an outer, fœtal membrane as allantois, stating, according to Needham, that one of his illustrations, (*b*), 'shows

[1] Joseph Hyrtl, *Onomatologia anatomica*. Vienna, 1880.

[2] E. A. Schäfer in *Quain's Elements of anatomy*. Tenth edition, ed. E. A. Schäfer and G. D. Thane. Vol. i, pt. i (Embryology), London, 1890, p. 44.

[3] Vesalius, *De humani corporis fabrica*. Basileae, 1543, p. 542.

the same mass in the uterus and wrapped round with the three coats, amnion chorion, and allantois', Needham suitably added that it was 'a lamentable but interesting misrepresentation of the facts'.[4]

Colombus wrote in 1559 of the amnion as a third membrane, but mistook the placenta for chorion and the membranous chorion for allantois.[5]

Arantius is said to have believed that the urachus is a continuation of the allantois and always persisted but not as an evident canal.[6] In spite of this, however, and of his knowledge of the occurrence of human, urinary, umbilical fistulae, he (like Fallopius[7]) seems to have denied its occurrence in man. His pupil Fabricius, who likewise was aware of the occurrence of congenital, umbilical, urinary fistulae, and who thought that the urachus in man 'is split up into numerous very minute filaments, which transmit urine to the chorion by a process of filtration, as it were',[8] also denied the existence of the human allantois in the fifth chapter of the second book of his *De formato foetu*[9] of 1604. In this chapter on the need for an allantois Fabricius wrote:

> Therefore—as nature does nothing uselessly—it is well worth our while to inquire *why* nature did not permit the urine to be contained (retained) in the chorion of *all* animals, while it, nature, did so permit in man, dog, cat and some others, but permitted it not in the sheep, ox, goat and other animals of their kind; and to inquire also why in these later-named animals nature caused a third membrane to be added to the others, the so-called allantois, destined for the collection of the urine. It is to be answered thereto that nature willed that for the umbilical vessels sometimes a third coating be provided, because for these animals such was mostly indicated or necessary in the fœtus. The vessels in this third coating, in the chorion, are sometimes scattered in the whole extent of the chorion which is bound up with a fleshy substance, which extends beneath the other parts of the chorion— otherwise it is bare of all other vessels, like in man and others. Therefore it becomes obvious that in those animals which have the umbilical vessels dispersed all over the chorion, there be prepared a third membrane, for, if nature should have thrown the urine into the chorion, the vessels through contact with the urine would become drenched (saturated) and therefore distended also easily cooled down—or, what would be of still greater importance—might become endangered because of the distention caused by the amount, for even the arteries would absorb some of the urine, all of which cannot happen to a chorion that is devoid of all such vessels.[10]

Aldrovandus,[11] who reproduced some of the fanciful figures of Rueff, apparently without due credit, and pictured the allantois as illustrated in Fig. 2, wrote:

> Truly from excess moisture of this, two other tunics result which are well guarded; one of these called allantoides is exceedingly sinuous—into it flows urine and sweat of the fœtus where they are held to the time of birth; when the

[4] Joseph Needham, *Chemical embryology*. Cambridge, 1931, p. 120; *idem, A history of embryology*. Cambridge, 1934, p. 92.

[5] Realdus Columbus, *De re anatomica*. Venetiis, 1559.

[6] J. C Arantius, *De humano foetu*. Venetiis, 1595. [Also the edition published at Lugd. Bat., 1664.]

[7] Gabrielus Fallopius, *Observationes anatomicae*. Venetiis, 1562.

[8] Trans. by Howard B. Adelmann in *The embryological treatises of Hieronymus Fabricius of Aquapendente*. Ithaca, N.Y., 1942, p. 269.

[9] H. Fabricius, *De formato foetu*. Venetiis, 1600.

[10] *ibid.*, p. 130. Trans. by Louis Rigert, 1933. [Unpublished.]

[11] Ulysses Aldrovandus, *Monstrorum historia*. Bononiae, 1642. Tab. vi, p. 44.

infant separates off the urine not through ureters but through certain umbilical courses. The third tunic, exceedingly soft and called the amnea, surrounds the whole foetus, so that it may be repelled by (? first) teeth. The present figure shows the differences of these tunics with a mixture of the birth (*geniturae*) of each.

Riolan, whom Hyrtl credited with the doubtful honour of having introduced many incorrect terms into anatomy, rejected the idea of Arantius that the urachus is merely a ligament, but likewise declared against its presence in man.[12] Spigelius, on the other hand, held to its presence but failed to represent or describe it, although his interest lay largely in late rather than in early foetal anatomy. Although the conclusions of Spigelius were not based on first hand observation of young human conceptusses, his discussion is quite representative of the attitude of many of the older investigators. In the fifth chapter of his *De formato foetu*, on the allantois, he wrote:

The Allantois, a membrane placed below the Chorion, derives its name from the Greek 'Allanta', because of its resemblance to the figure of an 'Alanta' (Greek), by which word the ancients designated a certain form of sausage, which Apitius called Lucanic sausage and thus also did he call this intestinal part. The first question which will arise will be: whether this membrane occurs also in the Human Foetus. Against Galen there are several old and very learned and, in matters of dissections Anatomical, very experienced men, who flatly deny this, and who have indeed found it in the foetus of the sheep, the ox, and the goat; wherefore they are of the opinion that the old Anatomists described as the Human Foetus the foetus of one of these animals. And, with some merit, one could conjecture that the Ancients really had described the Goat, or the Sheep or other Animals of this kind, when we consider that Theophilus in his book of the Constitution of the Human Body taught in Chapter XIX each single part that belongs to the Foetus, as well as the three membranes (teguments), and orders for that purpose that a pregnant goat be in all form of Art (with all ingenuity) dissected. So, Aëtius (Tetrvib. iv, ser. iv) asks the reader: If anybody would with all application (ingenuity) inspect all that belongs to a Foetus, he could dissect for that purpose either a goat, a cow or a deer. And, while the opinion of these men is a new one, it is certainly one worthy of a thoroughgoing research, especially as we will find in corroboration of it the authority of the famous Rufus of Ephesus. Herein the older Galen, and others cited with much praise at different times by him, in his first book, *Of the nomenclature of the several parts*, writing in his last Chapter of the Human Foetus, and principally of the membranes of the Chorion and the Amnion, remembers as much, and declares on his own authority that in his autopsies he had found a fluid or semi-fluid flowing into the Chorion, while of the Allantois he makes no mention whatever. Hereafter, almost all the others, who thus far and herein have become renowned, have assigned the Allantois to the Human Foetus, either following herein the authority of the Ancients or of the Moderns. To put myself up as an Arbiter in the dissensions of such renowned men of science is so much more displeasing to me, as I have not, like them, become gray and venerable in Anatomic dissections. Nevertheless, guided by these reasons I am of the belief that the Allantois can be found in the Human Foetus. For, in the very first place, there is just as much need of this membrane in the Human Foetus as in the Foetus of the other Quadrupeds. It certainly did not behoove Nature so much to segregate the Urine from other fluids of sweat, and to collect all of it in its proper (own) places, that is between the Chorion and the Amnion, but it behooved Nature very much better to have it all contained in its proper

[12] Jean Riolan, *Anatomica humani foetus historia*. Paris, 1618.

PLATE XLII

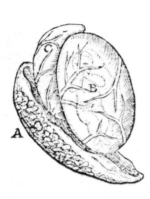

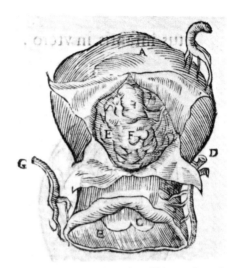

FIG. 1. A conceptus, after Vesalius, 1555, in which C is said to represent the allantois, human by implication

FIG. 2. The allantois after Aldrovandus, 1642

E is said to be the 'Tunica and allantoide' which is said to be 'well hidden and exceedingly sinuous'. Urine and sweat of the foetus are said to flow into it to the time of birth. F. Parenchyma foetus.

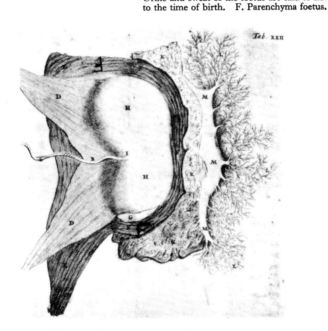

FIG. 3. The allantois after de Graaf, 1677

Tab. xxii, as seen in an abortus of three months.

'G. Allantoidis portio amnio nudata.
H.H. Allantoidis sive membranae urinariae pars inflata quatennus sub amnio collocatur.
D.D. Membranae amnii duae partes expansae.
F.F. Amnii et chorii partes complicatae.' ('F', 'F' retouched.)

membrane, like in a proper receptacle, in the space between the Chorion and the Amnion, which is sufficiently large . . . . One other reason for our contention is one which my celebrated countryman, Vesalius, in his Commentaries on Anatomy has represented to us heretofore, saying: that in the Human Fœtus there be an intestine which looks like the tubes out of which sausages were made, this intestine being situated between the Chorion and the Amnion, by which arrangement the Urine of the Fœtus would be conserved (held back) in the womb (uterus). In regard now to the solution of other opinions to the contrary and especially in regard to the opinion which claims that in dissections no Allantois ever could be found, it must be said here that it certainly can be found if they would dissect the placenta earlier in the pregnant woman and in the same way as Vesalius had done, as otherwise certainly, because of extreme thinness this membrane would immediately be broken loose even by the most careful handling. And, although the authority of Rufus of Ephesus is of a very high degree with me, it nevertheless is not so great that I would rather give him the preference over Galen, even if Galen really never dissected a pregnant womb, as in those times it was so strictly forbidden to dissect human bodies; however, he followed the opinion of many eminent Anatomists, who had dissected Humans, following the example of Herophilus, who himself from the anatomy of apes and other quadrupeds, concluded that the good faith of others were worthy enough to be retained in his own commentaries, very often being herein lead by the very best opinions and demonstrations, so that what he himself could not find in dissections of humans, he still believed, and therefore presupposed the good faith of the researchers and in such a degree, that he himself came to believe that the Allantois really could be found in a Human Fœtus. The Ancients quite frequently had been describing the Fœtus of sheep or of goats, not because they never dissected a pregnant woman, as even for doing that there would have been very few opportunities, so that earlier Anatomists, before they started dissecting an Human Fœtus, trained themselves beforehand in the dissections of Sheep Fœtuses; and they gave to the several membranes such names as they saw fit to give; and so it has happened that the Allantois membrane got its name from the Sausage, because of the resemblance to the intestines used in making sausages, or to the intestines out of which sausages were manufactured. Now, if we inflate the Allantois of a sheep, it very plainly assumes the form of a Lucanic sausage. Now, the Allantois of the Human Fœtus is reported to us (by the Ancients) to be a rather oblong bladder like a sausage, and therefore it is designated as the oblong intestine, so much so that for this reason Vesalius was of the erroneous belief that the name of Allantois should not be given to this bladder, but to the Chorion with the fleshy and inverted Placenta, as it was on all sides enveloped therein. The Allantois is an extremely thin or fine membrane, white and soft, in the sheep, provided with extremely thin veins and arteries or arterioles for its nourishment; situated in the middle between the Chorion and the Amnion, and wholly therein contained where the Placenta, too, is fully covered, connected beside that also with the Meatus, which is called the Urachus, by which the bladder also receives the Urine; and its function is to keep apart and to conserve the Urine of the Fœtus from any sweat (Sudor).[13]

William Harvey, who declared he had never seen an urachus in man also felt that one should be present. In the chapter on 'The Membranes and Fluids of the Womb', which is appended to his *De Generatione*, Harvey referred to Fabricius as describing a third membrane 'called Allantoides

---

[13] A. Spigelius, *De formato foetu*. Patavii, 1626, ii, cap. v. [Also *Opera omnia*, Amsterdam. 1645.]

that is intestinal, because it looks like an intestinal sausage, and does therefore not envelop the fœtus, but lies below the part of the thorax and the abdomen and stretches out to both horns of the uterus'. Harvey continues:

He maintains that this membrane could be found only in the fœtus of sheep and cattle, and he says also that it is connected with the urachus and that through the latter it receives urine from the bladder. Therefore, says he further, 'in horned animals, who have this allantoid tunic, the urachus is so large and straight, that it resembles a small intestine; it sensibly becomes thinner toward the fundus of the bladder, so that it makes the impression that its origins were rather toward the intestines than toward the bladder. But in man, and other animals that have a double row of teeth, and which are devoid of an allantoide, the mentioned largeness of the urachus does so diminish, that when it alone comes forth from the fundus of the bladder as a single tube, it soon splits off in extremely thin fibres, which then together with the vessels go farther than the umbilicus, and transmit the urine into the chorion, so as almost to escape sight'. For this reason he accuses Arantius of a double error: once, because he denies that the urachus could be found in man, and, because he asserts that the fœtus gave off urine through the pudenda.

But in this regard, I will frankly confess that I share in Arantius' error, if such it be. As a matter of fact, I am sure that through the compression of the bladder in a greater fœtus (be it of man or animals) urine flows out through the pudenda. But an urachus I have never seen, nor did I observe that urine because of the compression of the bladder was transmitted into the secundines. But I saw in sheep and deer, between the umbilical arteries, something like a continuation of the bladder, containing urine, but not such as an urachus is described.

But I would hardly so temerariously deny the existence of the Allantoides: these inside membranes, so far yet, are very thin and transparent (as we have seen between the two albumens) so that they may escape our sight. Really in the hen's egg, between the colliquamentum and the albumen (that is between the amnion and the chorion) there is some whitish excrement, nay, sometimes even true fæces from the rectum are found there, as we have said above and as Coiter, too, observed.

Furthermore, regarding that tunic of the colliquamentum in which the chick is swimming, although it be pellucid, thin and so subtle that even in the opinion of Fabricius it could not be thought any thinner, it would be possible—as by the same witness all these membranes, although being very thin, are nevertheless double—that nature was forced to deposit between its double membranes some urine or something else. I will gladly agree with Fabricius that such an allantois exists; but a sausage, stretched out to both horns, I cannot find in the secundines of cloven-hoofed animals, nor anything else beyond the conceptus itself. I find, as I already have said, only some prolongation between the umbilical arteries which contains some excrementitious fluid, which prolongation is bigger in some, smaller in others.

For this reason, in my opinion, the tunic which Fabricius calls the allantoides, is in fact the chorion. But the ancients named it allantoides because of the figure of a double sausage which it has. The external membrane, which like an overcoat, in the middle constricted, reaches out to both (horns) extremities and constricts the womb lying in between (or the connexion of both horns), is the chorion; to sheep, deer, dames (fallow deer) and other cloven-hoofed animals it is proper, and can easily be extracted whole when apprehended by the hand in the middle of its tract; and for this reason we call that the concept of these animals, or their egg. In the manner of the egg, it contains a double fluid, the foetus and anything that belongs to it and has the same attributes as Aristotle gives to the egg; namely, that in the beginning, an animal consists of the same substance the remainder of which later becomes its food.

But I think that the tunic which Fabricius called the Allantois is rather the chorion, or else the reduplication of the two tunics has come about praeternaturally. Therefore, it is found only in a few animals, and not always even in these. At the beginning (of generation) it is not found at all; later on it appears bigger in some animals; in others less conspicuous, and in not a few it can be discerned only as a prolongation of the bladder. Nay, even Fabricius did not think that it envelops the fœtus, but thought that it were needed to contain urine. And I would believe for sure that he mentioned the allantois rather in order to remain true to the doctrine of the ancients, than that he could have believed that it really could be found and that it really served any purpose. As a matter of fact it is believed by the ancients and likewise by the whole Medical Fraternity, that the chorion contains urine, and he himself says, that two fluids were around the fœtus; the one, the sweat in the amnion, the other fluid, the urine, in the chorion.

It appears obvious, therefore, that the ancients understood under these two names the one and the same thing, namely in cloven-hoofed animals, in which alone it can be found, they called it allantois because of its form; in others, though, they called it chorion from its very office, the retention of urine. And therefore, they do not pretend that in man or any other animals (than the aforementioned) this tunic could be found. Also, what good would a second tunic for the retention of urine serve, when this service is already rendered by the chorion, as follows from their own sentence?

There can really not be adduced any likely reason why in the sheep, the goat and other cloven-footed animals this tunic can be found, but not in the dog, the cat, the mouse and others. For, as a matter of fact, if this tunic were present for the retention of urine, it would be necessary also in the fœtus of the sheep or bovines as there is a greater quantity of urine than in those with double rows of teeth, or else it would be necessary that there should be three different fluids, or else that two tunics should be destined for receptacles of urine. For, I am sure that the chorion, even from its formation, is full of water. But it is not meet to drive this contention still farther; I would rather narrate what my observations have shown me.

It is one thing to explain the already perfected form of the concept or of the embryo, as Fabricius has done, and it is another thing to describe its generation and first schematism; as too it is one thing to describe an apple or ripe seeds of plants, and again, another thing to make clear its production from the first germs. We, for this reason, shall bring to light how the concept becomes perfected step by step, so that from doing so, it becomes clearer what can be stated of the membranes and other parts that belong to the fœtus.[14]

A reference to Fig. 3 after de Graaf reveals that he too believed that the amnion and allantois formed a fused layer.[15] His illustration reminds one of the figures of Bidloo and of others, except that de Graaf put the letters designating the allantois on the inside of the amnion. However, I do not feel that he, or others before or after him who represented things as they thought they

---

[14] William Harvey, *Exercitationes de generatione animalium.* London, 1651, pp. 277 ff. Trans. by Louis Rigert, 1933. See also *The works of William Harvey*, trans. by Robert Willis. London, 1847, pp. 551-4.

[15] The illustration is a portion of Tab. xxii in Regner de Graaf, *De mulierum organis generationi inservientibus tractatus novus.* Lugd. Bat., 1672. (The introduction to this work is dated 30 May 1671.)

were, are especially blameworthy. A little reflection will remind everyone that that is exactly what we are doing to-day, and what our successors undoubtedly will do, whenever the facts are not sufficiently known.

Figs. 4a and 4b are reproduced from 'The Anatomy of Humane Bodies By Will.[m] Cowper, Surgeon'.[16] Cowper's description of 'The Fifty-eighth Table' (Fig. 4a) says that it 'Shews the External Convext Surface of the *Placenta Uterina* free'd from the *Uterus*'. The letters EE are said to designate

The Urinary Membrane call'd *Alantoides*, lying immediately under the *Chorion*, and cleaving to it by Vessels and Fibers; it Environing the whole *Foetus*, according to *Bidloo*. The Existence of this Membrane is much Doubted of in Humane Bodies. I must confess I never met with a Subject in which I could Discover it. The Midwives take Notice of a *By-Water*, as they call it, near the Time of the *Partus*; which I am apt to think is the Contents of this Membrane breaking forth, which often happens some Weeks before the Birth, and no ill Consequence follows.

In his comments on Table 59 (Fig. 4b here) Cowper further said that CC represents

Part of the Urinary Membrane not free'd from the *Chorion*: In Cows and other Quadrupedes, it is Long and Unequal; whence it's call'd *Allantoides* or *Farciminalis*: it is plac'd between the *Amnios* and *Chorion*, and receives the Urine from the Bladder by the *Urachus* thro' the Umbilical Rope. The *Urachus* of Humane Bodies is scarce Pervious. I must acknowledge in the Subjects I have Examin'd, I could never make the Wind pass from the Bladder of Urine into the *Urachus* in the Umbilical Rope; but I have constantly found the *Urachus* evidently Hollow from the Bottom of the Bladder to the Navel in a *Foetus*, and very little further.

Nothing could illustrate the search for the human allantois better than the case of 'Rich [*sic*] Hale, M.D.', 1701.[17] Hale began the report of his erroneous and puzzling discovery of it, by saying that the ancients knew it only in brutes and that it was 'sufficiently described' in them by the 'excellent Anatomist', Dr. Needham,[18] who 'also first discovered part' of it in man, but that 'neither he, nor any other, has taken the right method of finding it entire'.[19] Hale added:

Dr. *Needham* says, that after the *Amnios* is cleared, and left fixed to the *Umbilical Rope*, you may divide by the fingers, or knife, the remaining part of the *Involucra* into two Membranes. The *exterior* he truly calls the *Chorion*, the *interior* he takes to be the *Allantois*.

[However, Hale maintained that] . . . by these ways of separation, you will presently tear the *Allantois*, and be able to discern only some small pieces of it. Besides, the *Allantois* is at first sight, so like the *Amnios*, that many who suppose the *Amnios* double, and that its Coats are easily separable, have taken these pieces of the *Allantois*, for broken parts of one of the Coats of the *Amnios*. Whereas having first found the *Hole* whence the Urine came forth (if the *Allantois* is not too much torn) you may blow up the *Allantois* with a Pipe to its full dimensions, and then

[16] William Cowper, *The anatomy of humane bodies, with figures drawn after the life by some of the best masters in Europe.* London, 1698. (The title quoted in the text is from the engraved title-page.)

[17] Rich[ard] Hale, 'The human allantois fully discovered, and the reasons assigned why it has not hitherto been found out, even by those who believed its existence'. *Phil. Trans. Roy. Soc.*, 1701, xxii, 835–50.

[18] Walter Needham, *Disquisitio anatomica de formato foetu.* London, 1667.

[19] *ibid.*, p. 836.

PLATE XLIII

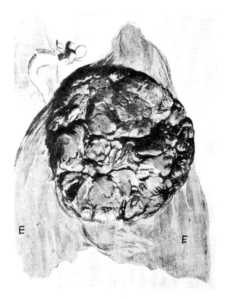

FIG. 4*a*

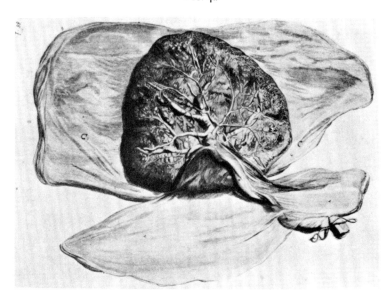

FIG. 4*b*

FIG. 4*a* and *b*.   The allantois after Cowper-Bidloo, 1698

4*a* (Tab. 58) EE is said to represent the 'Urinary Membrane call'd *Alantoides*, lying immediately under the *Chorion*, and cleaving to it by Vessels and Fibers; it Environing the whole *Fœtus*'.

4*b* (Tab. 59) CC is said to designate 'Part of the Urinary Membrane not free'd from the *Chorion*'.

see its true Shape, the *Fundus*, the *Crevix* [*sic*], the insertion there of the *Urachus*, its relation to the other Membranes, *&c.* Be the *Allantois* never so much torn, yet this way you may easily separate many Inches of it, from the *Chorion*, and *Amnios*. Which easie separation demonstrates a distinction of Membranes, since no double Membrane can be divided by the breath alone.[20]

Hale considered de Graaf's figure, reproduced here as Fig. 3, 'to be fictitious', and charged de Graaf with adding the allantois of a colt 'to the *Secundines* of a *Humane Fœtus*', just as Vesalius had added 'the *Secundines* of a *Whelp*' to such a fœtus. In concluding, Hale declared:

Lastly, 'Tis most evident that *De Graaf* knew nothing of the true Shape of this Membrane, and that he had never seen one entire, because he consents to *Needham*'s description of it as true, which yet is false in several particulars. For 1st, the *Urinary* Membrane does not cover the whole *Fœtus* (as he affirms) but only that part of it, which respects the *Chorion*, and does not lie on the *Placenta*; for the *Allantois* can be extended at farthest but to the edges of the *Placenta*, where the *Amnios* and *Chorion* are so closely joined by *Fibres*, that no Membrane can come between them. Wherefore 2dly, the the [*sic*] *Allantois* is not every where fastned to the *Chorion*. And consequently 3dly, the *Allantois* can't be of the same Shape that the other Membranes are of, nor be like the *Allantois* of a *Colt*, which contains the *Fœtus* in the *Amnios*; all which nevertheless *Needham* asserts. In short, Dr *Needham* had seen only pieces of the *Urinary* Membrane, but never an entire one, and so could only guess at the Shape, *&c.* of it, from what he had observed in *Mares*, and *Glanduliferous* Animals. He might have made a better guess at the figure, site, *&c.* of a *Humane Allantois* from that of a *Whelp*, which does not every where encompass the *Fœtus*, as he observes.[21]

Hale held that three membranes can easily be discovered in women who die late in labour, and declared that Tyson found that number in such a case, some years before, when 'he saw *two Bladders*, containing Liquors of different colours', after dividing the chorion. 'This observation fully satisfied that great Anatomist, to as [*sic*] the existence of an *Allantois*; and its figure, texture, site, *&c.* might also have been discovered by him, had not the less curious Spectators been impatient to pass on to other parts of the Dissection.'[22]

Hale claimed that the urachus is always pervious to urine whether it has a lumen or not, and that urinous fluid is always found in its substance. He further held that if the abdominal muscles contract before birth, urine could more easily pass through the substance of the urachus and into the allantois than out through the open urethra! Hale, apparently a preformationist, held further that

Since all the parts are perfectly formed before *Impergnation* [*sic*] not very long after Impregnation they may begin to perform their Offices. No doubt they begin as soon as there is occasion for any separation, and a separation of Urine is necessary, when the *Fœtus* is first nourished by the *Umbilical Arteries*.[23]

Hale also claimed that the amnion is twice as thick as the allantois, that one allantois may suffice for twins, that the urachus extends throughout the cord and 'seemed as big as a common Knitting Needle', it was 'of a darker substance

---

[20] *ibid.*
[22] *ibid.*, p. 839.
[21] *ibid.*, p. 838.
[23] *ibid.*, p. 842.

than the *Placenta*', and 'appear'd in every respect like that part of the *Navel-string*, which is allowed by all Anatomists to be the *Urachus*'.[24] Hale further declared: 'These two are the only entire *Urinary* Membranes that I have prepared. Yet in the many *Secundines* that have come to my hands, I have ever found three distinct Membranes easily separable.'[25] He says he owes it to the assistance of Mr. Cowper 'that the figures belonging to these papers appear correct', and added that Cowper used the occurrence of 'By Waters' as an argument for the existence of an allantois.

Hale represented an allantois from an early abortion, as shown here in Fig. 5 reproduced after Hale, and closed his article with the following observation:

> Perhaps some less curious Persons may think such *discoveries* as these of no use. But these may consider that hence we can better explain some *Phœnomena*, as voiding *Urine* by the *Navel*, and the *Breaking of Waters* from Women half gone with Child, and tell the consequences of such accidents; as also better account for those *Waters*, and *Bladders* Midwives meet with, and direct them in their doubtful Operations, &c. 'Tis something likewise to have cleared Points thus long controverted by the greatest Anatomists, &c.[26]

Since Haller had written an article upon a pervious urachus and a human allantois in 1739,[27] one is surprised to find him saying in his *First Lines of Physiology*, which was issued in 1747, 1751, 1767, 1771, 1779, and 1780, that man has no allantois. But in the English edition of 1786 (translated from an earlier Latin edition) the following passage appears:

> It may then be demanded, whether there is any allantois? since it is certain that there passes out from the top of the bladder a duct called the *urachus*, which is a tender canal, first broad, covered by the longitudinal fibres of the bladder as with a capsule; and afterwards, when those fibres have departed from each other, it is continued thin, but hollow, for a considerable way over the umbilical cord, yet so that it vanishes in the cord itself. Whether this, although it be not yet evident in the human species, is not confirmed by the analogy of brute animals, which have both an urachus and an allantois? But as for any proper receptacle continuous with the hollow urachus, it either has not yet been observed with sufficient certainty, or else the experiment has not been often enough repeated, to render the opinion general in the human species; and those eminent anatomists who have observed a fourth kind of vessel to be continued along the umbilical rope into its proper vesicle, will not allow that vessel to be called the urachus, and very lately have referred it to the omphalo-mesenteric genus[187];[28] and in the human fœtus, the urine is separated in a very small quantity: but it perhaps may be no

---

[24] *ibid.*, p. 849.

[25] *ibid.*, p. 850.

[26] *ibid.*

[27] Albrecht von Haller, *De uracho pervio et allantoide humana*. Gottingae, 1739.

[28] Footnote (187) in the original reads as follows:

'[187] Since I first made a drawing in my anatomical descriptions of the embryo, after Albinus and Boehmer, concerning the bladder resembling the allantois, which Hunter and Sandifort have confirmed by an elegant figure, I have twice had an opportunity of seeing the same with a similar filament. I filled another fœtus with wax; and that filament which might impose upon us for the urachus was likewise filled: the artery certainly ran from the vessels of the omentum to the cord, and was distributed in very small branches through the cellular texture of the rope and upon the bladder.'

It is of special interest that it was Wrisberg who annotated the fifth edition of Haller's *First Lines*, as quoted in Hunter's *Animal Oeconomy*, and wrote the above comment.

PLATE XLIV

FIG. 5.   The human allantois after Hale.

'Fig. 1 represents the *Secundines* of *Twins*, to shew the *Allantois*, and its Relation to the other Membranes, &c. after the parts were prepared and dryed.

A A A   A Part of the *Chorion* expanded.
B B B   a *Line*, expressing the edges of the *Placenta*.
C C C   the *Amnios*, which is united to
D   the *Allantois*, at
E E E   the Line of *Union*.
F   the *Cervix* of the *Allantois*.
G   a *Hole* at the *Fundus* of the *Allantois*, whence the *Urine* came forth, and where the *Allantois* was blown up.
H   Part of that half of the *Allantois*, which lies under the *Line of Union*, and immediately covered the *Foetus's*, unless it is supposed that the *Amnios* is continued under the *Allantois*.'

'Fig. 2.   V that part of the *Allantois* which is below the *Line of Union*, near its neck F.'

'Fig. 3.   Shews an entire *Allantois* of a very small *Abortion*. N.B.   This *Allantois* was easily separated from the other Membranes between which it lay; and the *Amnios* remained an entire *Bladder* or Membrane under the *Allantois*.
Now some to whom I have communicated these *Figures* object, that what is called the *Line of Union* can be on(e) real thing.' [sic].

[Note.   In Figs. 1–5 certain letters which would not have reproduced clearly have been retouched or repeated.]

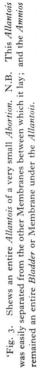

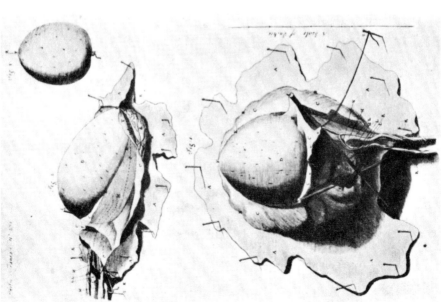

improbable conjecture, that some portion of the urine is conveyed to a certain extent into the funiculus umbilicalis, and there is transfused into the spungy cellular fabric that surrounds it; and therefore, that, of all animals, man has the longest umbilical cord, because he alone has no allantois. But then this can take up but a small space, terminating in the funis, and hardly ever seems to reach as far as the placenta. Sometimes, even in an adult person, this open duct has brought the urine to the navel.[29]

According to Teacher,[30] William Hunter denied the existence of an allantois in man[31] and made the lack of suitable magnification the excuse for not having done more about the matter. In the *Gravid Uterus*, Hunter, in his description of Fig. vii, Pl. xxxiv, referred to 'the cavity or space between the amnion and chorion', without however calling it the allantois.

In a manuscript copy of a description of the human gravid uterus by William Hunter which is in the Cushing Collection at Yale, there is a fuller statement upon the subject. Under the heading 'Of the Allantois and Urachus', Hunter, according to the writer, apparently said:

It was very natural for such Anatomists, as were conversant with the secondines of quadrupeds only, to suppose that there was an human allantois, or reservoir of urine for the foetus, among the secundines with a urachus or conduit leading to it from the bladder: & they would more readily adopt this opinion, when they observed in the human body & especially in children a ligamentous substance passing from the bladder to the navel, which is commonly enough called the remains of the urachus. But that men who have had opportunities of enquiring into the fact should in spite of the evidence of their senses be ready to believe that man must have because the quadruped hath an allantois appears to me founded too much upon loose reasoning. In reality, the argument, drawn from the brute creation, appears to have more force towards disproving than towards establishing the human allantois. It might be stated thus: quadrupeds great and small have an allantois: in all of them the membrane itself is distinctly seen; the urachus is easily seen; any fluid thrown into the bladder, passes without difficulty along the navel string into the allantois; the two collections of [a cancelled word here] fluid viz the liquor amnii & urine are seen & distinguished at first sight. From these facts we might presume a priori that there were similar appearances in the human subject & these as much more striking [cancelled word] in a human foetus than they are in a kitten, as that is larger than this. But in fact none of these appearances are seen in the human subject & therefore we must conclude from analogy that the similar parts do not exist.

Among all the dissections which I have made of the gravid uterus & of conceptions which have been thrown off in an intire state (except in very young conceptions, when the vesicula umbilicalis is turgid) I have never seen anything like two distinct bags of water; nor any membrane between the Chorion and Amnion; nor any passage leading from the bladder along the navel string to the rest of the secundines. The observations give me a conviction that there is no human allantois. What there is in the very early part of pregnancy, in the navel string, besides the blood vessels above described, is not now the question. Neither have I ever seen in the human subject anything like ompalo-mesenteric vessels,

---

[29] Haller, *First lines of physiology*. Trans. from the Latin, with notes by Professor Wrisberg. 2 vols. 5th edition. Edinburgh, 1786, vol. ii, pp. 217–8.

[30] John H. Teacher, *The anatomical and pathological preparations of Dr. Wm. Hunter*. Glasgow, 1900, p. lix.

[31] William Hunter, *Anatomia uteri humani gravidi tabulis illustrata*. Birmingham, 1774.

or any membrane analogous to that in a dog or cat through which these Vessels are distributed.

The coat or covering of the navel string which has a smooth or polished surface, is composed of the united membranes chorion & amnion & is almost inseparably united with the parts which it encloses. The ligament which goes from the bladder of the fœtus to its navel between the umbilical arteries, commonly call'd the urachus or its remains grows more slender as it passes along: In the navel string it is hardly perceptible, except near the fœtus; it is like a fine thread a little more white & opake than the rest. When you have found it near the fœtus, by taking a little pains you may trace it sensibly almost the whole length of the string. Mr. Cruickshank first observed this to me.[32]

John Hunter apparently agreed with his famous brother for, under 'Observations on the Placenta of the Monkey', he stated as a conclusion: 'There is no urachus, and of course no allantois, not even the small ligament that appears to be a drawing in of the bladder at its attachment to the navel, the bladder here being rounded.'[33]   These words of John's recall Cowper's statement: 'I must acknowledge in the Subjects I have Examin'd, I could never make the Wind pass from the Bladder of Urine into the *Urachus* in the Umbilical Rope; but I have constantly found the *Urachus* evidently Hollow from the Bottom of the Bladder to the Navel in a *Fœtus*, and very little further.'[34]

Since Meckel and von Baer represented vesicular allantoids in early human conceptusses, the question of its existence in man was revived and finally evoked a very spirited controversy in the 80's of the nineteenth century. As the further discussion of the subject will show, its final resolution had to await the invention of new technical methods.[35]

---

[32] [William Hunter], 'A description of the human gravid uterus and its contents'.   [n.d.] (An anonymous MS., apparently a student's notes, now in the Cushing Collection at Yale University.)   See *Harvey Cushing Coll. of Books and MSS.*, New York, 1943, MS. 38.   The quotation above is from fo. 78 ff.

[33] John Hunter, 'Observations on the placenta of the monkey', in *Observations on certain parts of the animal oeconomy*. London, 1786, p. 138.

[34] *op. cit.* (16), sig. Gg^v (text to Tab. 59).

[35] This essay is from the Department of Anatomy of Stanford University.   It forms the first part of a history of the human allantois.   The second part, dealing with the later history, will be published in a further communication.

THE ACADEMY OF THE INVESTIGATORS

by

MAX H. FISCH

Prelude

THE quarrel of ancients and moderns in Italy[1] occupied the sixteenth and seventeenth centuries and the first half of the eighteenth. At the beginning of the seventeenth century the ancients were still in almost complete possession of the universities. In medicine, for instance, the texts were selected writings of Hippocrates, Galen and Avicenna, and the lectures were commentaries on those texts. In spite of the work of Vesalius and other pioneers of the sixteenth century, anatomical dissection remained for the most part a pedagogical device for illustrating Galen.

Among the weapons of the ancients were the civil and the ecclesiastical censorship, and, as a last resort, the Inquisition. The party in opposition, the moderns, consisted of individuals here and there, dependent on their private means or the chance support of a liberal patron. They sought to gain strength by organizing themselves in societies or academies, which in turn required even more powerful patronage to survive attack.

Though the moderns in Italy lacked the stimulus and support of a rising and militant middle class, by the end of the seventeenth century they were well represented in most of the universities. By the middle of the eighteenth they had won the field. Two years a century apart may serve as symbols. In 1644, John Milton, pleading for unlicensed printing in England, said that he had sat among the learned men of other countries

> and had been counted happy to be born in such a place of philosophic freedom as they supposed England was, while themselves did nothing but bemoan the servile condition into which learning amongst them was brought; that this was it which had dampt the glory of Italian wits; that nothing had been there written now these many years but flattery and fustian. There it was [in 1638] that I found and visited the famous Galileo grown old a prisoner to the Inquisition for thinking otherwise than the Franciscan and Dominican licensers thought.[2]

A century later, in 1744, seven years after the removal of his body to a place of honour in Santa Croce, Galileo's Dialogue of 1632 was allowed to be reprinted. In the same year the third and definitive edition of Vico's *New Science* was published.

Of the Italian academies of the seventeenth century which led the fight for the moderns, the best known are the Lincei at Rome, of which Galileo was a member, and the Cimento at Florence, whose leading members were disciples of Galileo. If a third were to be named, it would be the much less familiar

---

[1] This essay is a delayed and partial fulfilment of the promise in Vico (1944), p. 217, note 147; cf. Vico (1948), p. vii, note 1. In an earlier form under the title 'The Quarrel of Ancients and Moderns at Naples', it was read before the Italian Group of the Modern Language Association at Chicago, Illinois, 27 December 1945. For aspects of the quarrel at Naples which are here slighted or omitted, see Berthé de Besaucèle, Cortese (1923), Cotugno, Maugain, Napoli-Signorelli, Nicolini (1928), Torraca, Zagaria. For parallel movements in England, see Jones. (Footnotes refer to the bibliography. When a page reference is not required, and when it is obvious from the text and the bibliography what work is being referred to, no footnote is supplied.)

[2] Milton, pp. 329 ff.

Investiganti of Naples.   Its most active period, roughly coinciding with that of
the Cimento, ended soon after Vico's birth, but its local influence continued
throughout his lifetime, and that is now its chief importance.

The earliest of all the societies for scientific research, the Segreti, was founded
at Naples about 1560 by Giambattista della Porta.   He says that this 'academy
of curious men' met in his home and helped him try the experiments described
in the later editions of his *Natural Magick*.[3]   The academy was dissolved by
order of the papal court, but the experiments continued.   Gassendi relates of
Peiresc's month at Naples in 1601 :

> As soon as ever he came to Naples, he could not contain himself, but he must visit
> the two Portas, those famous Bretheren . . . nor did he only see what ever they
> kept in their studies, and precious treasuries, but he was present at their Experiments
> of all kinds almost, intimating to them his earnest desires that way.[4]

Shortly after founding the Lincei at Rome, Federigo Cesi visited Naples in
1604 and conferred at length with Della Porta, from whose *Natural Magick* he
had taken the emblem of the lynx.   It was Cesi's plan to establish colonies of
the Lincei in the principal centres of learning, but the Liceo of Naples was the
first and apparently the only such colony, and Della Porta was its first president.[5]
After his death in 1615, he was succeeded by Fabio Colonna.   Another able
member was Stigliola, 'the first that discovered the ground of refraction'.
The Lincei published at least two of Della Porta's works and one of Stigliola's.
Neapolitan scientists were among Galileo's active correspondents, and several of
his most devoted disciples came to him from Naples.[6]

When Cesi died and Galileo bowed to the Inquisition, the moderns went
underground for a quarter of a century in northern Italy, until the Cimento was
established at Florence in 1657.   Meanwhile, however, experimental science
was kept alive at Naples by Marco Aurelio Severino and his disciples, of whom
the most distinguished in later life were the physicians Tommaso Cornelio
and Lionardo di Capoa and the brilliant lawyer Francesco d'Andrea.   Severino,
professor of anatomy and surgery, restored the use of knife and cautery and
practised refrigeration anaesthesia.   He wrote the first comprehensive treatise
on comparative anatomy[7] and the first text-book of surgical pathology.   His
fame as a teacher, it was said with pardonable exaggeration, emptied the
medical school at Padua.[8]   Accused before the Inquisition, he was ably
defended by d'Andrea.[9]

Di Capoa tells a story that may serve to illustrate the quarrel as it then stood :

> A company of curious and learned friends was gathered at the house of our
> Severino.   A diligent Danish anatomist showed us the lymphatic vessels in a dog
> he had dissected.   An obstinate Galenist, who had previously ridiculed similar
> findings as sophistries invented by the moderns to belittle Galen, at once arose to
> object.   With hair bristling, he adjusted his glasses on his nose and bobbed angrily
> about with a rapid *argumentor contra*.   He would never have made an end if it had

---

[3] Della Porta, preface.   But cf. Maylender, vol. iii, p. 432.   In this Academy the transition
from alchemy to modern science is still in progress.   On the cultural significance of the academies
see Fiorentino, vol. i, pp. 1 ff.

[4] Gassendi, pp. 36 ff.   Their villa was bought in 1715 by Giannone, who wrote a great part of
his *Civil history of the Kingdom of Naples* there.   Nicolini (1932), p. 90.

[5] Gabrieli (1927), *passim*.

[6] Spampanato, *passim*; Berthé de Besaucèle, p. 1; Gabrieli (1939), *passim*.

[7] Cole, pp. 132–49.   [8] Torraca, p. 349.   [9] Cortese (1923), p. 21.

not been for the laughter of the bystanders, and if the prudent anatomist had not then quietly and in a voice full of charity and modesty besought him not to remain on the defensive but to satisfy himself with what was evident to his own eyes and hands.[10]

In 1644, at the age of thirty, Cornelio, urged by his friend Di Capoa and preceded by letters from Severino, journeyed to northern Italy to study with the men who were quietly continuing Galileo's work there. He spent some time with Michelangelo Ricci in Rome, Torricelli in Florence, and Cavalieri in Bologna. He wished to apply the new physics to problems of physiology, and especially of respiration, to which he had been introduced by Severino. He composed the larger part of a system of the physical world, adjusted to recent discoveries in astronomy, which survives in a manuscript of 1646. At Rome in 1648 he published a Latin essay explaining motion in terms, not of nature's abhorrence of a vacuum, but of the circular thrust of Plato's *Timaeus*, to which Galileo had also resorted on occasion. This essay is noteworthy as containing the first account published in Italy of Torricelli's barometric experiments four years earlier. Viviani thought enough of it to make an Italian translation.[11] At Rome in 1649, shortly before returning to Naples, Cornelio addressed to Severino another essay on the air contained in water, apropos of the respiration of fishes.[12]

First Period (1649–1663)

Returning to Naples late in 1649, Cornelio brought with him the works of Galileo, Gassendi, Descartes, Bacon, Harvey, Boyle and other moderns.[13] He and his friends Di Capoa and d'Andrea became the leaders of a group of younger men who met in his home, read and discussed these writings critically, and sharpened their own views upon them. From time to time various members of the group read papers on topics they had been meditating and endeavoured to meet the objections that were raised. Cornelio, the dominant scientific thinker of the group, composed and read a series applying the new mathematical and experimental physics to the problems of physiology.[14]

Through d'Andrea's growing influence, Cornelio became professor of mathematics in the University of Naples in 1653.[15] This was the entering wedge by which modern physics, astronomy and medicine, and modern philosophy with them, found their way into the educational system. By the end of the century d'Andrea could say that Naples owed to Cornelio all that was then accepted as most probable in philosophy and medicine.[16]

[10] Di Capoa (1681), p. 86. The materials gathered by Amabile for a biography of Severino are in the Naples National Library (MS. XI. AA. 35–37). Such a biography is much to be desired. New light has recently been shed on Severino's relations with English physicians; see Trent, Fisch.

[11] Caverni, vol. i, pp. 207 ff., 454.

[12] A first draft had been sent to Severino in 1646. See Severino's letters to Cassiano dal Pozzo, 3 November 1646, 15 December 1646, 6 October 1647, transcribed by Amabile, in Severino (q.v.).

[13] Amenta, *Vita*, pp. 15 ff. Severino wrote Dal Pozzo in March 1650: 'I regret the death of Descartes. Tommaso Cornelio, his sworn friend and partisan, is in tears.' Contemporary with the scientific circle of Severino and the early years of the Cornelio–Di Capoa–d'Andrea group was the anti-peripatetic academy of Camillo Colonna, of which d'Andrea was a member. Cortese (1923), pp. 24 ff., 120 ff. Cornelio was a member of the Oziosi; cf. Cornelio (1652), the preface to which, perhaps by d'Andrea or Di Capoa, is important for Cornelio's biography.

[14] Di Capoa (1681), p. 3, and preface to Cornelio (1663).

[15] Cortese, p. 155; Torraca, p. 355.

[16] Cortese, p. 124.

Cornelio was urged by Severino and by his younger friends to publish his physiological essays, and they were in the printer's hands when the great plague of 1656 postponed all such enterprises.[17]   Severino died of the plague, and the work of the group of moderns was interrupted for a time, but it was resumed in 1657 or shortly thereafter.   The deaths from the plague included a fair share of the lawyers, and d'Andrea now came to the fore as the most learned, eloquent and influential jurist of the next forty years.   For the first time the new jurisprudence founded on philological and historical criticism came out of the study and entered the forum, in the city in which, more than anywhere else, the debates of the courts were the events of the day.[18]

Cornelio was again urged by his fellow innovators to collect and publish his essays on physiology and on more general topics of philosophy and scientific method.   With Severino's encouragement removed, however, he postponed publication from year to year.   The orthodox doctors of the college of physicians, he said, when they let slip a word of involuntary tribute, hastened to qualify it by adding that, as a physician, he was too fond of novelty, and given to prescribing dubious and dangerous cures.   He was reluctant to publish his scientific observations and theories until he had established a reputation for conscientious and successful practice.   He was gradually persuaded, however, that there was no remedy against a sycophant's bite, that he could not hope to escape envy and calumny.[19]   In 1661 he once more set about publishing his essays for the press, and introducing each of them with a letter to some member of his circle of friends.[20]   The book was printed at Venice in 1663 with an engraved frontispiece (Fig. 1) and a dedication to Prince Francesco Marino Caracciolo.[21]   The long delay in publication lost Cornelio the credit for discoveries in anatomy and physiology which Glisson and Willis had meanwhile published in England.[22]

At about the same time there were three other developments which, along with the publication of Cornelio's book, brought the quarrel of ancients and moderns to a head.   These were (i) the suppression of a book by Sebastian Bartoli, (ii) the attempt to suppress the study of chemistry, and (iii) the beginnings of the Lake Agnano controversy.

Bartoli, a younger physician than Cornelio and Di Capoa and a more militant modern, was not a member of their immediate circle.   He had 'emancipated himself from the tyranny of the schools' in 1654 in his twenty-fifth year.[23] He set about composing a series of 'paradoxical exercitations' attacking the tenets of the regular physicians.   In 1663 he resolved to publish some of these, along with his new 'system of microcosmic astronomy'—that is, of medicine. He obtained the ecclesiastical and civil imprimaturs, the book was printed at Naples (Fig. 2), and it was about to be issued, when the regular physicians got

---

[17] Cornelio (1663), dedication.   Cf. Giannone (1731), vol. ii, p. 777.

[18] Cortese, pp. 11 ff.

[19] Cornelio (1663), p. 52.

[20] These letters are undated in the 1663 edition but dated 1661 in the Venice 1683 edition.

[21] It was reprinted several times thereafter in Naples, Venice, Germany and Denmark.

[22] See his letter to Glisson and Willis: Cornelio (1663), pp. 191 ff.   On what is original in Cornelio's work, see also Di Capoa's preface; Amenta, *Rapporti*, p. 16, note 1; Caverni, vol. i, pp. 207 ff.; vol. ii, pp. 135 ff., 180; vol. iii, pp. 94, 99, 175, 197, 203, 247, 386; Napoli-Signorelli, pp. 304 ff.; Pandolfi, *passim*; Spiriti, p. 163, note 2.

[23] Bartoli (1666), p. 109.   He was born 20 January 1630; cf. Capone-Marano, p. 38.

PLATE XLV

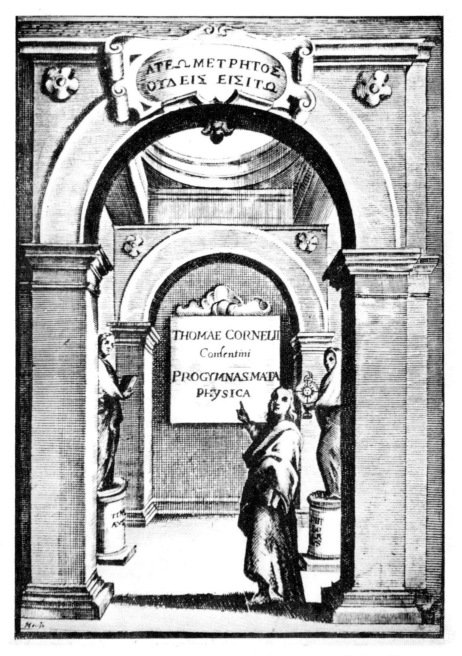

ΑΓΕΩΜΕΤΡΗΤΟΣ
ΟΥΔΕΙΣ ΕΙΣΙΤΩ

THOMAE CORNELII
Consentini

PROGYMNASMATA
PHYSICA

FIG. 1.   Engraved title-page of T. Cornelio, *Progymnasmata*, Venice, 1663

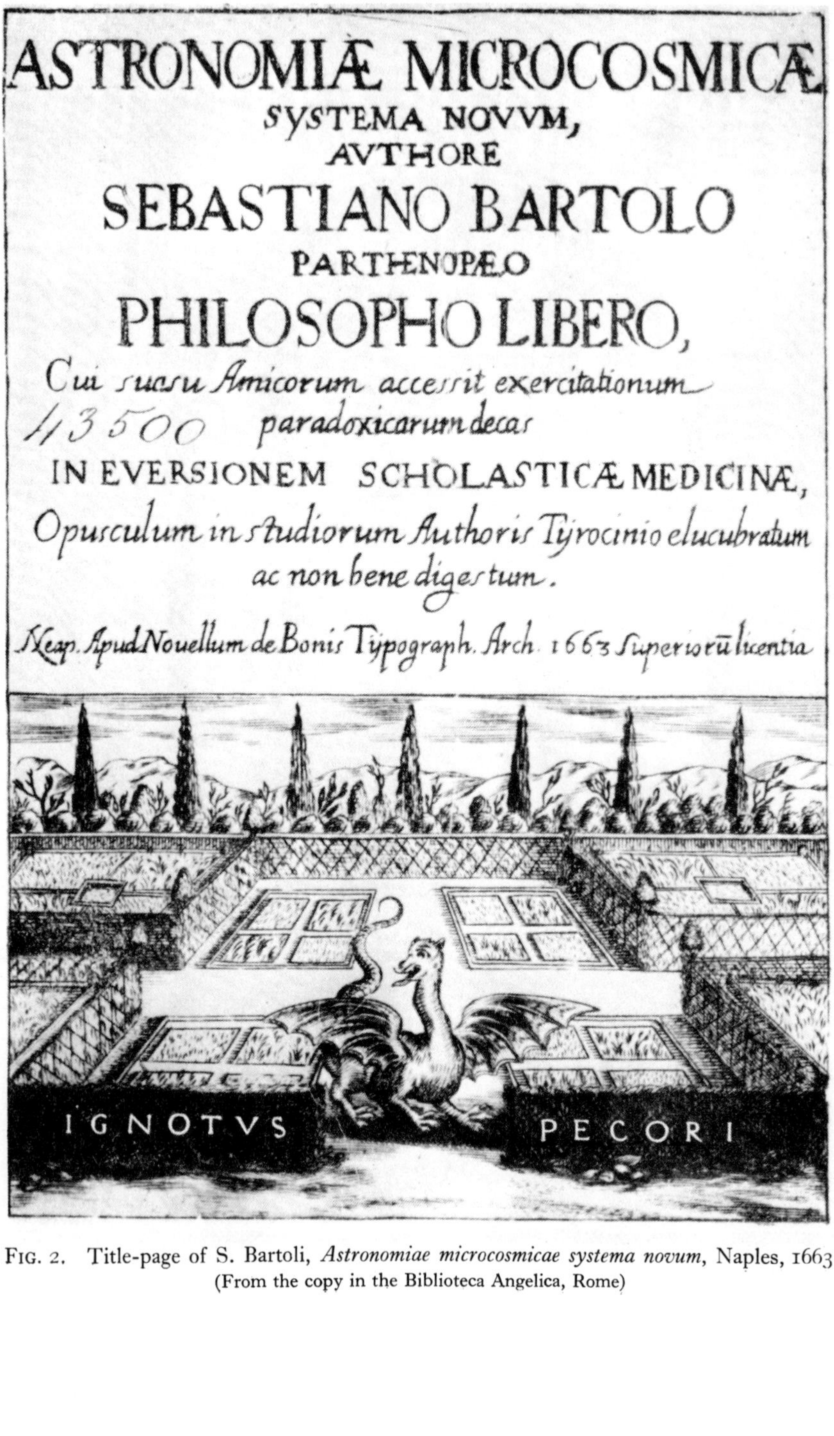

PLATE XLVI

ASTRONOMIÆ MICROCOSMICÆ
SYSTEMA NOVVM,
AVTHORE
SEBASTIANO BARTOLO
PARTHENOPÆO
PHILOSOPHO LIBERO,
Cui suasu Amicorum accessit exercitationum
43500 paradoxicarum decas
IN EVERSIONEM SCHOLASTICÆ MEDICINÆ,
Opusculum in studiorum Authoris Tyrocinio elucubratum
ac non bene digestum.

Neap. Apud Nouellum de Bonis Typograph. Arch. 1663 Superiorū licentia

IGNOTVS   PECORI

Fig. 2. Title-page of S. Bartoli, *Astronomiae microcosmicae systema novum*, Naples, 1663
(From the copy in the Biblioteca Angelica, Rome)

wind of it. At the instance of Carlo Pignataro, the protomedico or chief medical officer of the Kingdom of Naples, it was condemned by one of the ecclesiastical authorities as blasphemous, and nearly all the copies that had been printed were seized and destroyed.[24]

> I have brought upon myself [Bartoli said] the insults of the whole synagogue; for here the barbers have gathered, there the surgeons, yonder the pharmacists, in the homes the physicians, in the cloisters the scholastics—indeed the whole miserable corporation and their tributary following plies me with curses, because I do not let blood, because I use balsams, because I shrink from purgatives, because I subvert the medicine which has been accepted for so many centuries, because I do not admit the authority of Aristotle in physics, and finally because I exhort men to free themselves from these impostures.[25]

Since there was no provision for the teaching of chemistry in the University, and since it was necessary for the practice of medicine as the moderns conceived it, they offered private instruction. Among the teachers at Naples, Di Capoa was the acknowledged master. The ancients, not content with suppressing published attacks upon themselves, now obtained a decree, again apparently at the instance of Pignataro, forbidding such private teaching and study. The moderns challenged the legality of such a prohibition. They published an anonymous pamphlet—probably the work of d'Andrea, assisted perhaps by Di Capoa and Cornelio[26]—in the form of a remonstrance addressed to the Viceroy and the Collateral Council under the date 28 September 1663, and entitled, 'Discourse in defence of the art of chemistry and of its professors, in which it is demonstrated that, by the statutes of the University and by common law, the private reading of chemistry in vacation time is not subject to restraint'.[27] The ancients, 'after many consultations',[28] retorted, under the name of Moinerio di Giarbo, with a pamphlet entitled, 'Discourse in which it is demonstrated that the spagyric medicines are for the most part unreliable and dangerous and are not to be permitted without the approval of the Galenic physicians; and that the reading of chemistry, even privately, being useless, should remain prohibited, contrary to the recent allegation of the modern chemical physicians'.[29] The author of the defence did not deign to reply.[30]

While this skirmish was in progress, there arose a pressing problem of public health on which the two parties took opposite sides in a protracted war of decrees, court decisions, and pamphlets. In October and November 1663, there was an epidemic of 'malign fevers', accompanied by skin eruptions, with high mortality. Though it was by no means confined to the region of Naples, the ancients there alleged a local cause. The summer rains had been so heavy and so continuous that at near by Lake Agnano it had not been possible to remove at the proper time the great quantities of flax and hemp which, as usual,

---

[24] Bartoli (1663), fo. †1r; (1666), dedication, preface, pp. 25, 87, 100. Cf. *Il lago d'Agnano utile*, p. 13; *La morsa domatrice*, p. 15.

[25] Bartoli (1666), p. 52.

[26] Gimma (1703), vol. i, p. 125, says it was believed to be the joint work of d'Andrea, Cornelio and Di Capoa, but *Copia di una lettera* (p. 23) refers to 'the learned author' as a single 'member of our Academy'.

[27] *Discorso*.

[28] *Copia di una lettera*, p. 23.

[29] Di Giarbo. Perhaps a pseudonym for Federigo Meninni? Gimma (1703), vol. i, p. 125, says that Meninni, 'in his youth a partisan of the Galenic school, was given the task of replying, and his reply was published, though without his name'.

[30] *Copia*, p. 23.

were submerged there for retting; and these had remained in the lake. The theory proposed by the protomedico and adopted by the ancients generally was that the water of Agnano and thence the air of the region were thereby corrupted, and that this was the source of the epidemic. From this they moved rapidly to the view that even in normal years the retting itself, being a partial rotting, was injurious to the health of the inhabitants of the region, and ought to be stopped. The moderns rejected both positions and regarded the problem as one calling for extended investigation, pending which there was no ground for destroying an industry on which so many depended for their livelihood.[31]

Second Period (1663–1670)

It was under these circumstances—the suppression of Bartoli's book; the attempt to suppress the private study of chemistry; the publication of Cornelio's book at Venice; the need he and his supporters felt to gird themselves for its defence; and the first rumblings of the Lake Agnano controversy—that the leading Neapolitan moderns organized themselves as a formal academy in the autumn of 1663. They assumed the name of Investiganti 'to signify their intent to search out the truth in the things of nature, and at the same time their modesty in not professing to have found it already';[32] and they took a setting dog for their device, with a motto adapted from Lucretius, Vestigia lustrat (Fig. 6).[33] They put themselves under the protection, and held their meetings in the palace, of Andrea Concublet, Marquis of Arena, whose grandfather had been the patron of the philosopher Telesio.[34]

In the eyes of the regular medical profession, of course, and to a large extent of the general public, they were not inquirers but partisans; and they were ridiculed as 'chemists' or 'spagyrists'. In a Neapolitan diary for January 1664 we read:

> The chemical academy, whose principal protector is the Marquis of Arena, and which rejects Aristotle and Plato as well as Galen, Hippocrates and Avicenna, goes on growing in the Marquis's house. . . . They treat diseases with violent remedies that give rise to other diseases, or even kill the patients outright, as experience has shown.[35]

Meanwhile the new learning had begun to lift its head again in northern Italy. The Academy of the Cimento had been founded at Florence in 1657 by Prince

[31] Fuidoro, vol. i, pp. 200, 202 ff., and the pamphlets reviewed below; cf. Agnano.

[32] Copia, p. 5. Caramuel (1670), vol. i, p. 678, giving the Latin form of the Academy's name, Academia Indagatrix, says it was so called 'because, neglecting the opinions of ancient and modern philosophers, it tracks down the truth hidden in the book of nature'.

[33] The passage in the De rerum natura is in Bk. i, lines 402–9. Some members wished to use Lucretius' exact phrase, vestigia parva sagaci, according to Gimma (1703), vol. i, p. 145.

[34] Borelli (1670), dedication. (Caramuel [1668], p. 702, and [1670], vol. i, pp. 680, 712, says that the Academy was a revival of one founded a century before in the same palace by the then Marquis of Arena. It was a common fiction to confer antiquity on academies by affiliating them to earlier ones.) The archives of the Academy, including unpublished papers read by its members, were kept by the Marquis, and after his death in 1675 were inherited by Giovan Girolamo Acquaviva, Duke of Atri, who had studied under Cornelio and Di Capoa and was a poet after the manner of Buragna. As late as 1710, these archives were among the Duke's most cherished possessions. Cf. Amenta, Vita, p. 18; Crescimbeni, Notizie, vol. i, pp. 98–101. The Marquis's widow Ippolita Carafa in later years presided over a salon frequented by Vico; cf. Vico (1947), p. 171. It was to one of the Duke's sons, Cardinal Troiano Acquaviva d'Aragona, that Vico dedicated the definitive edition of his New Science; cf. note 144 below.

[35] Fuidoro, vol. i, p. 206. Fuidoro lists as frequenters 'the presumptuous Cornelio, Don Carlo de Ferrariis of Barletta, Francesco d'Andrea and his brother Gennaro, Don Antonio Gomez, Lionardo di Capoa the physician, Giuseppe Donzelli the Neapolitan chemist, and Sebastian Bartoli'. See note 61 below.

Leopold and provided with a well-equipped laboratory. On behalf of the Neapolitan Investigators the Marquis of Arena now made a trip to the north and brought back a stock of instruments for their experiments.[36]

The Cimento had as a corresponding member at Rome Michelangelo Ricci, who had been Cornelio's mentor. He acted as judge of publications for the society and conducted much of its foreign correspondence. Through him, as well as directly by Borelli, Redi and others, the Investigators were kept informed of the work of the Cimento and repeated many of its experiments at Naples.[37]

The relations were reciprocal. Among the visitors sent by Prince Leopold to Naples were Sir John Finch and his companion Thomas Baines.[38] Finch had taught anatomy at Pisa since 1659 and was intimately associated with Malpighi and Borelli. From Rome on 24 November 1663 he reported to Leopold that he had bought at Naples a part of the great library left by Severino.

We had very detailed particulars [he added] of Tommaso Cornelio, a mathematician and physician of great reputation and friend of Michelangelo Ricci. He has written a book entitled *Progymnasmata physica* which was printed at Venice and one part of which is dedicated to Alfonso Borelli. He is a follower of Descartes and a great favourer of things new, and on this account is hated in Naples by those who swear loyalty to their old teachers. In this book he says that before Pecquet or any other he was the inventor of the hypothesis of the compressibility and elastic force of the air. He is a Calabrian by birth, a lively acute man, and like most of his compatriots very hot tempered.[39]

Finch and Baines had been enrolled on 20 May 1663 as original Fellows of the Royal Society.[40] Fellows who travelled abroad were of course instructed to visit scientific academies, report on their organization and proceedings, and make arrangements for regular correspondence with them. Dr. Walter Pope,

[36] Mosca, p. 17. Gennaro d'Andrea, writing twenty years afterwards, says that the Academy was disbanded 'after some months' because of the Marquis's departure on a journey through Italy; but (if this is the journey in question) it was certainly resumed on his return; and the Marquis still presided over the Academy when the dedication of Borelli (1670) was written, probably as late as 1669. Perhaps d'Andrea is referring to a later journey.

[37] For descriptions of some of the experiments as performed in the Cimento, see Magalotti, *Saggi*; for many others, see Targioni Tozzetti. Redi's relations with the Neapolitan group are a story in themselves. See Baglivi; Redi, *Opere*, vol. i, pp. 4 ff., 60 ff.; vol. iv, pp. 83, 89; vol. viii, pp. 146-8, 173-6, 221, 351 ff. Typical though minor instances of Ricci's services: On 13 May 1664, he wrote to Leopold: 'Tommaso Cornelio, author of the *Progymnasmata* recently published, and hero, so to speak, of the Academy at Naples, writes me that he plans to come to Rome for an entire month. From him I shall hear in greater detail the story of the founding and the slight progress of the Academy, and if anything seems worthy of your curiosity I shall communicate it to you promptly.' Cornelio's plans were changed and he did not come to Rome on that occasion, but in the winter of 1668-9 he came with Cardinal Boncompagni to serve as consulting physician to Prince Borghese, and remained more than a month. Prince Leopold inquired through Ricci about Cornelio's not letting blood and received the reply that he had no repugnance to bloodletting, but abstained from it solely because he was able to cure his patients without it. See Ricci's letters of 13 May, 5 and 12 July, 1664, 25 December 1668, and 4 February and 2 April 1669, in the Galileo papers at the Florence National Library, vol. cclxxvii, and cf. Fabroni, vol. ii, p. 164.

[38] Malloch, pp. 40 ff. The secretary of the Cimento, Lorenzo Magalotti, had been sent still earlier, in March and April 1663; see Magalotti (1769), vol. i, p. 9, and his letters to Viviani, dated 27 March and 10 April in MS. 2487, cc. 59, 67 in the Biblioteca Riccardiana, Florence. Nicolaus Steno went in 1668; see Fabroni, vol. ii, p. 163.

[39] Fabroni, vol. i, p. 266; Malloch, p. 41. The greater part of Severino's library was bought by Lancisi and is preserved in the Biblioteca Lancisiana in Rome. Finch's numerous letters to Leopold and to other members of the Cimento, all in Italian, are among the Galileo papers in the Biblioteca Nazionale in Florence; for this one see vol. 276, fo. 224.

[40] Royal Society, *Record*, pp. 375 ff. Another original Fellow of the Royal Society, Sir Robert Southwell, had visited Rome and Naples in 1661-2. The notebook he kept is in the British Museum (Egerton MS. 1632). See also Magalotti (1769), vol. i, p. 2.

another original Fellow, wrote from Rome on 5 April 1664 that he would give a
detailed report of his visit to Naples if he were not sure that Finch and Baines
had already done so, or would be doing so on their return to England.[41]   Finch
was later English Resident at the court of Tuscany and Italian correspondent
for the Royal Society, chosen for his acquaintance with the virtuosi of Florence,
Naples and Rome.

Still another original Fellow of the Royal Society, Francis Willughby, was at
Naples in April 1664, accompanied by John Ray and Philip Skippon, who
became Fellows in 1667, and by a Nathaniel Bacon of whom little else is known.[42]
After a week in Naples, Ray and Skippon left for Sicily and Malta.   Willughby
and Bacon remained and probably attended at least one session of the Investigators before proceeding to Rome and parts north.   Ray and Skippon returned
to Naples in June 1664.   They visited Cornelio in his home, and they were
shown through San Domenico Maggiore, where they saw the cell of Thomas
Aquinas and the room where Cornelio lectured on 'mathematicks and physick'.[43]
They attended a meeting of the Investigators and each recorded his impressions.
Skippon's account, which is slightly more circumstantial than Ray's, is as
follows:[44]

> At the marquis of *Arena's* palace, 29 *June*, we were introduced into the room
> where the *Academici Investigantes* meet every *Wednesday* in the afternoon, when we
> observed about 60 persons present.   They discoursed about several things, and
> brought in the experiment of water ascending in glass *tubuli*, or small pipes; which
> they reasoned upon.   After that, *Leonardus à Capua* discoursed about heat and
> cold; then *Lucas Anton. Portius* seated himself in a chair at the upper end of the
> room, and read a discourse on the same subject; and when the company was pleased
> with anything, they cried *bene*.   (Note, none but those who are *Academici* may read
> in the chair.)   This done, *Caramuel*, a fryar of the *Benedictine* order, professor in
> *Salamanca*, and bishop of *Campania*, in elegant *Latin*, answered *extempore* the
> assertions of *Franciscus ab Andrea*, who most ingeniously defended the lord *Verulam's*
> opinion, that it is possible for a man to live for ever, if he can keep himself in one and
> the same condition of health.   The marquis of *Arena* moderated with great ingenuity
> and understanding; and he was particularly civil to us.   There are about 14
> *Academici.* . . .[45]

[41] Royal Society, Letter Books, P.1.43.   Pope describes the most frequent experiment at the
Cave of the Dogs near the shore of Lake Agnano, where a vapour rises from the floor to a height of
half a foot.   Two dogs had their heads held down in this vapour; they both became unconscious,
as if dead; one was dipped in the lake and revived immediately; the other was laid in the open air
and recovered in about an hour.

[42] Raven, pp. 131, 133 ff.

[43] Skippon, pp. 615, 620.

[44] Skippon, p. 620.

[45] Skippon's list of members, with Italian substituted for Latin forms of names, is as follows:
(i) The Marquis of Arena.   (ii) Tommaso Cornelio.   (iii) Giovanni Caramuel.   (iv) Lionardo
di Capoa.   (v) D. Michele Gentile.   (vi) Francesco d'Andrea.   (vii) Gennaro d'Andrea.   (viii)
Giovanni Battista Capucci.   (ix) D. Giuseppe de' Medici, Prince of Ottaiano.   (x) Lucantonio
Porzio.   (xi) Domenico Scutari, a young man but very learned for his years.   (xii) Francesco
Rossi.   (xiii) D. Domenico Emanuele Cioffi.   (xiv) Salvatore Scaglione.
    All but De' Medici and Rossi appear in other accounts: Amenta, *Vita*, p. 17; Gennaro d'Andrea;
Borelli (1670), dedication; Di Capoa (1681), p. 586; Fuidoro, vol. i, p. 206 (cf. note 35 above);
Gimma (1703), vol. i, p. 146; Gimma (1723), vol. ii, pp. 483 ff.; Mosca, pp. 10, 16; Carlo Susanna,
etc.   Rossi is unknown to me, but De' Medici is a prominent figure in Fuidoro's journals (see
also Crescimbeni, *Notizie*, vol. ii, pp. 1–5; Capone-Marano, p. 197; and note 76 below).
    Caramuel was the Spanish polymath Juan Caramuel Lobkowitz, bishop of Campagna from
1657 to 1673 and one of the most active, as he was certainly the most widely erudite and the most
prolific of all the Investigators.   So voluminous were the works that flowed from his pen that he
set up a press of his own to publish them.   At this time he was engaged on his *Mathesis Biceps*, a

PLATE XLVII

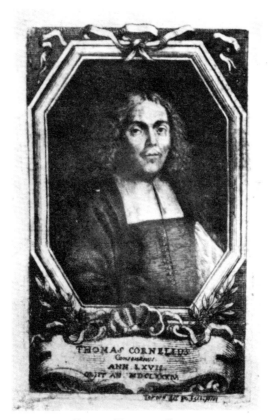

Fig. 3.   Tommaso Cornelio
(In his *Progymnasmata*, Naples, 1688)

They complained to us of the Inquisition, and their clergymens opposition to the new philosophy; and of the difficulty they met with in getting books out of *England, Holland*, &c.

To a substantially similar though less detailed account,[46] Ray adds the following observations:

A man could scarce hope to find such a knot of ingenious persons and of that latitude and freedom of judgment in so remote a part of *Europe*, and in the communion of such a Church. They are well acquainted with writings of all the learned and ingenious men of the immediately preceding age, as *Galileo, Cartes, Gassendus, Harvey, Verulam*; and of the present yet surviving, as Mr. *Boyle*, Sir George *Ent*, Dr. *Glisson*, Dr. *Willis*, Dr. *Wharton*, Mr. *Hobbs*, Mr. *Hook*, Monsieur *Pecquet*, &c. We were very much pleased and satisfied with the conversation and discourse of some of them. Amongst the rest Dr. *Thomas Cornelius* hath made himself known to the world by his writings.

Perhaps at the instance of Ray, a summary of Cornelio's *Progymnasmata* was published in one of the early numbers of the *Philosophical Transactions of the Royal Society*.[47] Ray also transcribed a long passage in his own *Observations*, apropos of the movements of Venetian glass *icunculae* (hollow perforated figurines) in water under changes of pressure or temperature.[48]

The subjects discussed during this first year of the Academy's formal existence are summarized by Di Capoa as follows:

The true method of philosophizing [i.e. of scientific enquiry]; the principles of natural things; the soul; motion; fluid and solid, hot and cold; light and colours and the other so-called sensible qualities; how the sensations arise; in what the life of animals consists and whether its functioning may be suspended for a space of time; whence comes that movement or flux which is called the ebb and flow of the sea; whence the fall of bodies called heavy, and how it comes that they all move

comprehensive treatise on the mathematical sciences in two volumes, printed 'Campaniae in officina episcopali' in 1667 and 1669 and issued in 1670. Like all his works it is more learned than original; apart from its accounts of the activities of the Investigators (see note 32 above and notes 46, 50, 54 and 63 below), it contains little of present interest except his argument for the superiority of the duodecimal over the decimal system. Cf. Tadisi, Croce (1925).

Three principal names in other lists are missing from Skippon's, for three quite different reasons: (i) Sebastian Bartoli, presumably because he was not yet a member (see note 61 below). (ii) Carlo Buragna, because he was at this time a member *in absentia* (see text to which note 82 below refers). (iii) Camillo Pellegrino, because he had already died on 9 November 1663. Pellegrino's work on the sources of south Italian history prepared the way for Muratori and also for Giannone, who (1731, vol. ii, p. 842, following Gennaro d'Andrea) calls him 'the so famous Camillo Pellegrino, who, though he had spent his whole life in different studies, to wit, of history, and searching into our antiquities, in his old age was so fond of the new discoveries and methods of this new philosophy that he found fault with his age, that would not allow him to apply himself to these studies'.

[46] Ray (1673), pp. 271 ff. 'While we staid in this City we were present at the meeting of the *Virtuosi* or Philosophic Academy, which is held weekly on Wednesdays in the Palace of that most civil and obliging, noble and vertuous person the Marquess *D'Arena*. There were of the academy but 15 or 16 admitted, but at the meeting were present at least three score. First there was shewed the experiment of the water's ascending above its level in slender tubes, upon which when they had discoursed a while, three of the Society recited discourses they had studied and composed about particular subjects, which were appointed them to consider the week before; and after some objections against what was delivered and reasonings to and fro about it, the company was dismist. . . '

It appears from other accounts also, as from Skippon's and Ray's, that there were usually many more invited guests than members. Caramuel (1670), vol. i, p. 712, writting to Prague in 1664, says that the meetings were frequented not only by the local nobility, clergy, politicians, physicians and philosophers, but also by distinguished visitors from abroad, Frenchmen, Germans, Poles, 'and a steady stream of Spaniards'.

[47] 1667, vol. ii, pp. 576–9. For a modern account see Berthé de Besaucèle, pp. 5 ff.
[48] Ray (1673), pp. 199 ff.

I   2 L

uniformly in the end; what is the cause of the overwhelming force of percussion; and how the splitting of solid bodies begins.[49]

Another principal member of the Academy, Lucantonio Porzio, whom we have met in Skippon's report and of whom there will be more to say presently, left manuscript records cited by his biographer to the effect that there were also many experiments on air pressure, filters, the elevation of liquids in capillary tubes, the expansion of glass rings by the action of warm water, and the shattering of glass bubbles when broken at any point.[50]

This programme of basic research, inspired in part by the investigations of Galileo and the Cimento and in part by the philosophy of Gassendi, was interrupted in the autumn of 1664 by a crisis in the Lake Agnano controversy. A medical commission of fourteen or more members, appointed by the protomedico, met with the city authorities of Naples on 31 July 1664.[51] The commission recommended, with four dissenting votes, that the retting of flax and hemp in Lake Agnano should be forbidden for that year. Of the four whom the protomedico could not win over,[52] the chief was Cornelio, the only Investigator on the commission. The city authorities adopted the majority's recommendation and there was no retting at Agnano that year, and no epidemic at Naples—or elsewhere in Italy.

The decision of the city authorities was subject to review by the Collateral Council of the Kingdom of Naples. The hundreds of peasants and workers who earned a living by the linen and hemp industry were without a voice; but not so the Jesuits, who, as chief proprietors of the land surrounding Lake Agnano, collected a thousand ducats a year from it. They instituted proceedings in the Collateral Council to protect this revenue. The Council at once asked for reports from members of the medical commission. A protégé of Pignataro named Nicolo Susanna, who had everything to gain and not much to lose, was pressed into publishing the report which, under the date 12 August 1664, he had addressed to the Duke of Girifalco (Fabrizio Caracciolo) in support of the majority recommendation.

Susanna's pamphlet seemed to the Investigators but little less hasty than the decision it supported.[53] The problems involved—the nature of the waters of Agnano, of their peculiar bleaching action, of the flax, of the process of retting, of the vapours given off, of the effects on the plant, on the water and on the air, whether these effects were properly described as a kind of corruption, and whether a causal connexion between them and the fevers could be made out— these were questions not for a session or a pamphlet but for prolonged inquiry, experimentation, and discussion. The Investigators addressed themselves to these questions. The discussion of the waters of Agnano and the effects of the

[49] Di Capoa (1683), pp. 3 ff.

[50] Mosca, pp. 17 ff. Cf. Caramuel (1670), vol. i, pp. 712 ff. for descriptions of several experiments and a general statement of the procedure followed. Avoiding theological disputes (he says), and treating only of physics, we investigate the nature and properties of material or corporeal substance. All assertions are tested by ocular experiment. The experiment is next discussed until there is agreement as to what has taken place. We then seek to account for the result and, lastly, to determine whether it confirms or discredits Peripatetic doctrine in the matter. (The Investigators might have made more effective contributions to modern science if they had been clearer as to the role of hypothesis in experimental inquiry.)

[51] Fuidoro, vol. i, p. 233.

[52] Tommaso Cornelio, Diego Ragusa, Francesco Liotta, Antonio Cappella. Cf. *Il lago d'Agnano utile*, p. 12; *La morsa domatrice*, p. 14.

[53] *Copia*, pp. 19 ff.

PLATE XLVIII

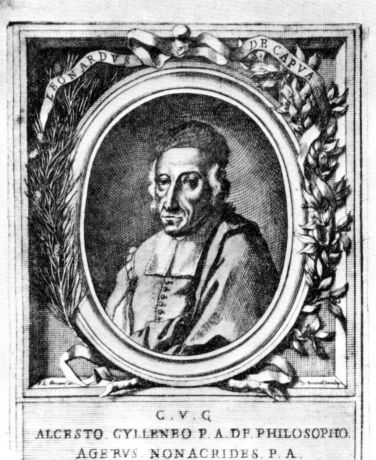

FIG. 4. LIONARDO DI CAPOA
(In G, M, Crescimbeni, *Vite*, vol. ii)

retting led on to an extensive study of the phenomena of the surrounding region, with its hot springs, fumaroles and mephitic vapours. Numerous experiments were performed on the flame-quenching and animal-asphyxiating properties of the damps in the Cave of the Dogs near the shore of Agnano.[54]

At the Academy's request, Lionardo di Capoa interrupted the series of papers he had been presenting on the sensory qualities to deliver a series on the phenomena of the Phlegrean Fields, beginning with 'two learned lectures . . . on the nature of the waters of this Lake, and on the marvellous effects which are experienced near by'[55]—'investigating impartially as a philosopher and according to the statutes of the Academy all the conditions of the Lake, and taking account of all the experiments which had been performed by the Academy in this connexion'.[56] Though he was careful not to pronounce directly on the dispute which then divided the physicians of Naples, it was sufficiently evident to those who attended the meetings 'that the Academicians were all of one mind in disapproving the prohibition of the infusion of the flax'.[57]

The negative conclusion on that point left standing the positive problem of the nature of the fevers—of which there were again some cases though no epidemic—and of the measures to be taken for their cure and prevention. The Marquis urged this as a question for discussion in the Academy. As usually happens when discussion is free, some proposed this and some that. The only view of which we have any particulars was that of Giovanni Battista Capucci. He compared these fevers with the petechial camp fevers, and especially with those which afflicted the soldiers of Hungary, and whose incidence fluctuated so widely from year to year. Capucci urged that the remedies which had been found effective in treating the latter should be adapted, with some improvements, to the treatment of the former.[58]

Meanwhile there appeared an anonymous reply to Susanna, in the form of a letter addressed to the viceroy under the date 25 September 1664,[59] but

[54] Mosca, p. 17, with reference to Porzio's lost memoirs, vol. i, pp. 51 ff. Porzio (1684), pp. 66–8; (1685), pp. 322–4, and cf. note 41 above. Caramuel (1670), vol. i, pp. 678 ff., gives the fullest surviving account: 'several even of the chief members of the Academy had visited the Cave, but they had reported many things so difficult of belief as not to be admitted without common examination; for, when we trusted neither ancient nor modern teachers, why should we give assent to fellow-students? We decided therefore to attack the matter by common study, so that, having ascertained the facts, we might investigate their causes. On Sunday, 26 October 1664, accordingly, a company of us betook ourselves thither, in the afternoon, so that the morning mists should not hinder our observations. By two hours before sunset there had arrived ten carriages and a great many horse. Besides the servants who attended *per accidens*, there were fifty or more nobles; that is, doctors, counts, marquises, dukes, princes, prelates, bishops. Never, I believe, was the Cave honoured with such a host of dignitaries or with such majesty of genius. Being thus gathered, we methodically set about examining the phenomena by common labour and study.' [Caramuel proceeds to describe in detail their numerous experiments with flaming torches, gunpowder trains, dogs, ducks, pigs and frogs. Cornelio, he adds, filled a flask with soil from the Cave to take home for chemical analysis. The Marquis would have collected some of the vapour itself, but his servants had forgotten the instruments he had ordered to be brought for the purpose.] 'The sun had already set when, because we were to return to Naples, our learned conference was concluded with a rich repast provided by order of the excellent Marquis of Arena; and there was such an abundance of everything that, after the masters were satisfied, there were costly sweets and chilled wines left over for the servants, so that they also had something to philosophize about on the return journey.'

[55] *Copia*, p. 20.

[56] *ibid.*, pp. 21 ff.

[57] *ibid.*, p. 20.

[58] Porzio (1685), pp. 322–47. Di Capoa probably began at this time a treatise on fevers on which he was working as late as 1693, as we learn from a letter of Bulifon on 10 March of that year in Magliabechi 632.

[59] *Il lago d'Agnano utile.*

apparently not published until two months later.[60]   It was rumoured that the author was Sebastian Bartoli,[61] and the rumour was probably correct.   Not only, the argument ran, did the retting not render the waters of Agnano injurious to health, but it kept them from being so—a paradox worthy of the author of the 'paradoxical exercitations'.   The protomedico's manœuvre was attributed to a desire to avenge himself on the Jesuits.[62]   (The previous viceroy's infant son had died under Pignataro's care; the viceroy had written to the provinces asking them to send some good doctors to Naples; Calabria had sent Diego Ragusa; the Jesuits, who had previously called in Pignataro when they needed a doctor, now called in Ragusa instead.   The epidemic had offered a pretext for stopping the retting in Agnano and thereby a large part of the Jesuits' income.   Ragusa, to make the story complete, had joined Cornelio in his dissent in the medical commission.)

In the calendar of the protomedico's benefactions [the author said]—such as forbidding the use of aqua vitae in the summer-time, eliminating the means of acquaintance with the spagyric art, co-operating in the suppression of the book Sebastian Bartoli was publishing—the most signal was this of having by his watchfulness freed the city from a perpetual contagious disease.   God grant that he may be content with this much and that he may not lay claim to the cult and the divine rites which Hippocrates deserved of Greece, when he has only deprived the people of a vital restorative by banning aqua vitae, impoverished medicine of its spagyric treasures, defrauded the studious of many new observations, and inflicted a clear loss of a hundred thousand scudi a year on the many poor farmers who lived by the linen of Agnano.[63]

Bartoli—if, as I think, it was he—briefly sketched an alternative explanation of the fevers, and promised to publish shortly a book on the subject.[64]   He concluded with an apology for the haste with which he had been obliged to write, and for the lack of finish in style, and begged his readers to 'think only that this crop was germinated in a HEAD of integrity, FREE OF DREAMS, and far from prejudices'.[65]

The phrase 'Free Head'—*Testa Libera*—offered an irresistible butt for counter-attacks.   Susanna replied with a still longer pamphlet dated 7 February 1665, and entitled, 'The innocence of Agnano found culpable in the deliriums of Free Head'.   Another member of Pignataro's following—probably Federigo Meninni—published a pamphlet in more satirical vein: 'A bit to break Free

---

[60] *L'innocenza d'Agnano*, p. 18.

[61] G. M. Lancisi's copy of this pamphlet has a MS. annotation on the title-page, 'Believed to be by the physician Sebastian Bartoli'.   The volume containing it (see Agnano) is labelled on the spine: 'Defence of the chemical art—Susanna & Bartoli on Lake Agnano.'   The annotations in other pamphlets in this volume were evidently made in Naples as the pamphlets appeared (see note 70 below), and that is probably true of this one.   (Lancisi was a friend of Porzio and perhaps obtained the pamphlets—or the bound volume—from him.)   The only apparent difficulty is that the author of this pamphlet, though a frequenter, was not at this time a member of the Investiganti, whereas according to Fuidoro (cf. note 35 above) Bartoli was attending as early as January 1664. But Fuidoro mentions other frequenters who do not appear in any list of members, and it is clear that he is making no distinction between members and non-members.   Furthermore, as we have seen (note 45 above), Bartoli's name does not appear in Skippon's list, from which it would appear that he was not yet a member in June 1664.

[62] *Il lago d'Agnano utile*, pp. 10 ff.

[63] *ibid.*, p. 13.   Caramuel (1670), vol. i, p. 684, deprecates the author's abusive language and rejects his paradox but reaches essentially the same conclusion.   In this he probably speaks for his fellow Investigators.

[64] *ibid.*, pp. 47 ff.

[65] *ibid.*, p. 48.

Head of his belief in the innocence of Agnano'[66]. These two pamphlets gave licence to the militant moderns for a barrage of satire directed against Pignataro's party. Perhaps it was Bartoli who wrote the pamphlet entitled 'Broken fragments of a brutal horse-doctor's bit, shattered on the anvil of truth by the insuperable force of free philosophy'.[67] (Meninni was a farrier's son.[68]) Then came two satiric poems, one in Latin, the other in Italian, in a four-page leaflet.[69] The former was called 'The Complaints of Jewbeard', a nickname for Pignataro suggested by the beards, the old-fashioned costumes, and the affected dignity of the orthodox physicians. The latter poem was called 'The undeceiving of the foreigner unfamilar with the ways of the town'.[70] There followed still another pamphlet entitled 'Claims laid before His Majesty Apollo by the bestial Signory of Arcadia for the jurisdiction usurped from them by certain physicians obstinately maintaining that the retting of flax in Lake Agnano is injurious. News received through the gazette of the Parnassus courier in these last days of Carnival'—more exactly 25 February 1665.[71]

So far none of the opposition pamphleteers had identified himself as a member of the Academy of the Investigators or made any reference to it. It was well understood, however, both by Pignataro's party and by the interested public, that the Academy was the stronghold of the opposition, and Susanna in his second pamphlet had kept shooting over the head of his ostensible adversary at the leaders of the Academy, and especially at Di Capoa and Cornelio. At last he drew fire from the Academy itself, deliberately aimed and deadly. It took the form of a pamphlet dated 1 April 1665 and entitled 'Copy of a letter written by an Academician Investigator to a noble friend concerning a writing printed in reply to an earlier one in defence of Lake Agnano'.[72] The author of the letter disclaimed any intention of defending Susanna's adversary, as he was perfectly capable of defending himself if he saw need.[73] There was one insinuation, however, concerning his relation to the Academy, which ought to be scotched; namely that he had intruded himself at one of its sessions and been heckled out. On the contrary, the Academy had sought him out as being 'a free spirit who applied himself to learn philosophy not from books but from experiments, which are the leaves one must turn to read it in the great book of nature'— and had invited him to its meetings. He had attended many of them, spoken at not a few, and been applauded. It was true that he had entered into controversy with a 'principal Academician' (probably Lucantonio Porzio) concerning the height to which mercury could rise in tubes, and the controversy had waxed hotter than it perhaps need have done; but he had desisted of his own accord in order not to give displeasure to the others who wished to turn from dispute to experiment.[74]

[66] *La morsa domatrice.*

[67] *Frantumi.*

[68] Fuidoro, vol. iii, p. 231 (for Meninti read Meninni); cf. note 122 below.

[69] *Barbaiudaei querimonia.*

[70] A MS. note in the Lancisi copy runs: 'Will C[arlo] P[ignataro] be the People's Elect? As long as the sodomitic crowd creates the People's Elect, the People's Elect will be Jewbeard.' This could only have been written in the last week of April or the first week of May 1665, between the resignation of Gennaro d'Amico and the election of Domenico Petrone. Cf. Fuidoro, vol. i, pp. 276 ff., 278.

[71] *Istanze.* This was in reply to the second pamphlet of Susanna, who is referred to throughout as SVSanna.

[72] *Copia.*   [73] *ibid.*   [74] *ibid.*, pp. 4 ff.

Without pronouncing on the main issue, the author of the letter—perhaps d'Andrea—presented a coolly devastating critique of Susanna's arguments, a dignified defence of the actions of the Investigators individually and as an Academy, and an eloquent tribute to Galileo and Gassendi as pioneers of the new science and philosophy. He announced that Di Capoa's lectures on Agnano would soon be published.[75] He appended to the letter a four-page 'Ode in praise of the famous Academy of the Investigators' by another of its members, probably Giuseppe de' Medici, Prince of Ottaiano.[76]

To this letter there was no reply. The retting of flax in Agnano was resumed and continued for two centuries longer—until the draining of the lake began in 1865—though with intermittent protests that the retting was a cause of malaria, offset by retorts that it was innocent or even beneficial.[77]

Just after the war of pamphlets subsided in 1665, Bartoli achieved an opportune cure. Domenico Caracciolo, Marquis of Brienza, had wasted away in April and May from a painful illness which the orthodox treatment failed to arrest. On 20 May, as he lay despaired of, unconscious, cold and pulseless, with preparations already proceeding for his funeral, one of his relatives induced Bartoli to try to save his life. By the end of August, Bartoli had brought him back to the good health he had previously enjoyed.

On the strength of this and other spectacular cures, in the following year Bartoli was appointed physician to the new viceroy, Pietro Antonio d'Aragona, who encouraged him to publish the book which had been suppressed four years before. Bartoli published it in the same year, 1666, not, to be sure, at Naples but at Venice—or at least with a Venetian imprint—under the title, *An examination of the commonly received dogmas of the art of medicine.* He omitted the 'new system of microcosmic astronomy', but added an appendix, 'The triumph of spagyric medicine', narrating his cure of the Marquis of Brienza.[78]

The phrase *Accademico Investigante* does not appear after Bartoli's name on the title-page of his book. The preface by Capucci, the most widely respected physician of the Academy, makes no mention of it. If, as these facts seem to indicate, Bartoli was not yet a member, he must have become one soon after the book was published, in recognition of its contribution and of Bartoli's other services to the cause for which the Academy stood. As Amenta, the biographer of Di Capoa, wrote long afterwards,

[75] *ibid.,* p. 21.

[76] De' Medici seems to be the only person to whom the phrase '*un nobilissimo nostro Accademico*' (*ibid.,* p. 36) could be applied. See note 45 above. Many of his poems were published here and there, but they seem never to have been collected.

[77] For a sample near the end of this two-century controversy, see Napoli-Pascale. The arguments are still the same.

[78] Bartoli (1666), pp. 140–52. The title of the Appendix was a retort to an attack upon Malpighi published at Cosenza the year before by Michele Lipari of Messina: 'The Triumph of the Galenists, completely uprooting the follies of the neoteric physicians, so that mortals may not die premature and even violent deaths in consequence of their doctrines, which are to be buried forever.' Among these doctrines was that of the circulation, which Malpighi had confirmed in his second epistle *De pulmonibus* to Borelli in 1661. On Borelli's recommendation, Malpighi had been invited to Messina in 1662 to take the chair vacated by the death of Pietro Castelli. He had stopped at Naples on his way south from Bologna in the autumn of that year, to visit Cornelio, Di Capoa and the other Investigators. Four years later, in May of 1666, on his return from Messina to Bologna, he stopped again at Naples, saw Cornelio and Di Capoa 'and the other scholars of that school, and refreshed my spirit by visiting with them as long as I could'. At the persuasion of his friends, Malpighi had himself written a reply to Lipari's attack, which he had addressed to Capucci, who was now editing Bartoli's *Examen.* Cf. Malpighi, pp. 24, 29. See also note 87 below.

Though Bartoli was not to be compared with Cornelio, Di Capoa or Capucci, or with Porzio or Tozzi among the living, he was nevertheless a very good talker, had a fine presence, was adventurous in treatment, and, what matters more, fortunate; so that, advancing in the favour of the viceroy and the nobles by reason of the happy outcome of his cures, particularly that of the Marquis of Brienza, he raised the esteem of many of the spagyrists who by themselves, either from excessive modesty or timidity, or from lack of spirit, or from distrust of medicaments, would have got nowhere.[79]

Medicinal baths were a prominent feature of Bartoli's practice. Probably at his suggestion, the new viceroy undertook the ambitious project of restoring the baths of Pozzuoli and vicinity, which had fallen into decay and disuse.[80] A medical commission was set up to consider the feasibility and desirability of the project. This was the first medical commission at Naples on which the moderns were in a majority. They reported favourably, and Bartoli played a prominent role in supervising the restoration. He composed the inscriptions which were set up at the various baths, and he wrote two books concerning the project. The first of these, a preliminary report, appeared in 1667. The second was published posthumously.

The year 1667 was marked by the appearance of two other works associated with the Academy. Lucantonio Porzio published at Venice the lecture on capillary action which he had delivered in the Academy in 1664; and Giuseppe Donzelli, Baron Dogliola (1596–1670), published at Naples his major work, *The pharmaceutic theatre, dogmatic and spagyric*, with a dedicatory epistle to Giovanni Battista Capucci, who had written the preface to Bartoli's *Examination*. Donzelli, if not a member, was at least a frequenter of the Academy,[81] and a sympathetic older friend and counsellor of its leading members. He had been a disciple of Galileo and friend of Severino, and was the author of the *Antidotario napoletano* and other pharmaceutical works. He had been a fervent republican during the revolution of 1647 and had also been its first historian in his 'Parthenope Liberated: an account of the heroic resolve of the people of Naples to shake off . . . the insupportable Spanish yoke'. In his epistle to Capucci he now took the most moderate position a modern could hold:

> Let no one think that by this discourse in praise of chemical medicine I mean to discredit the precepts of dogmatic medicine. But I do maintain that adding the former to the latter raises the physician's stature and makes him more useful to the sick. For dogmatic medicine by itself does not always suffice to cure diseases, because it does not have at its disposal such powerful remedies as those of chemical medicine, which even in small doses produce marvellous effects.

The *Theatre* was later revised and enlarged by Donzelli's son Tommaso, a friend of Vico. It went through twenty editions in sixty years, and continued to be printed thereafter.

The year 1667 was notable also for two other events which, together with the publications already mentioned, made it the Academy's climactic year. One was Borelli's sojourn in Naples and the other was Carlo Buragna's return after an absence of four years.

[79] Amenta, *Rapporti*, p. 17, note 1.
[80] Parrino, vol. iii, pp. 214–29.
[81] See Fuidoro, vol. i, p. 206 (cf. note 35 above).

Buragna had been a pupil of Cornelio and later an intimate of his circle and a friend of the Marquis of Arena. Just before the Academy was formally organized, he had left Naples, but he had been made a member *in absentia*, and had taken full advantage of the provision in the statutes that such members might send communications to be read and discussed at the meetings and subjected to experimental tests.[82]   He was now the Academy's chief poet, but he set little store by his poetry, being all intent on developing a new system of philosophy.[83]   He combined a grasp of mathematics and physics with facility in the three learned languages.[84]   He wrote a commentary on Plato's *Timaeus*, a preface to an edition of Lucretius, various essays on mathematics and musical theory, and a treatise on philosophy demonstrated in the geometrical manner. After his death in 1679 his friends projected an edition of his philosophical works, but for some reason it never appeared.   One of them reported that the treatise had been stolen and could not be found, but that it would have been difficult to get it published anywhere in Italy because of certain opinions expressed in it.[85]

Of all the scientific work with which the name of the Investigators was associated, the most enduring was that of Giovanni Alfonso Borelli on the principles of mechanics and hydrodynamics involved in animal motions.   Borelli had been born at Naples in 1608 and had taught for many years at Messina. Returning to Messina in 1667 after a decade at Pisa and Florence in the Academy of the Experiment, he spent part of the summer at Naples and repeated before the Investigators the experiments on animal motion which he had carried out in the Cimento.[86]   The Marquis of Arena provided for the publication of his treatise *On natural motions depending on gravity*, and accepted a dedication, in which Borelli addressed him as the patron of the Investigators and said:

> Since you have graciously received me among its members, and I do not wish to come with empty hands, I offer you this work of mine which expounds the scientific explanations of the many experiments which I supervised in the Medicean Academy of the Experiment at Florence, and which have been performed with equal pains in yours at Naples.[87]

[82] Carlo Susanna.

[83] Cesare di Capoa, preface to Buragna (1683).

[84] Gennaro d'Andrea.

[85] Bertani, pp. 85–90.

[86] He also repeated for his own satisfaction the experiments which the Investigators had performed at the Cave of the Dogs, adding others of his own contriving, and reported his results and conclusions to Prince Leopold in letters dated at Naples, 12 July, and at Messina, 4 October and 1 December 1667, which are preserved among the Galileo papers in the Florence National Library (vol. cclxxviii).   From a later letter (14 August 1669) we learn that Borelli used the facilities of the Marquis's office at Naples for forwarding mail, and from an undated draft of a letter from Leopold to Borelli (in vol. cclxxxii) that Leopold did also.   Porzio (1696), p. 194, gives 1669 as the year of Borelli's sojourn in Naples; but I assume that this is a typographical error or a slip of memory.

[87] Borelli (1670), dedication.   The first printed copies of Borelli's *De vi percussionis* reached him at Naples and were distributed thence in July 1667.   The volume had been dedicated to Giacopo Ruffo, Viscount Francavilla, who had been a member of Cornelio's circle and to whom he had addressed one of his *progymnasmata*.   (Ruffo had later been Malpighi's host at Messina for four years.   Malpighi had begun his study of the anatomy of plants in Ruffo's garden, and it was Ruffo who had urged him to address to Capucci his reply to Lipari's attack [note 78 above].)   Thus the first as well as the second of the two works that laid the foundations for Borelli's *De motu animalium* has associations with the Investigators.   It is a curious coincidence that a greater academy, the Royal Society of London, sought the privilege of publishing the *De motu animalium* (Birch, vol. iii, p. 457), as it had previously printed two works of Malpighi and was to print his posthumous works.   But the *De motu* was printed at Rome with a dedication to Christina of Sweden, whom we shall meet later as a patron of the Investigators.

By the time Borelli's book appeared in 1670, the Academy had been suspended. More than Cornelio's *Progymnasmata*, more than the 'defence of Agnano', the publication of Bartoli's *Examen* at Venice, after they had suppressed it at Naples, had aroused the ancients to battle. They had had it put on the Index and burned; it was never reprinted, and copies are extremely rare.[88] Carlo Pignataro, who had held since 1654 the chair of the practice of medicine in the University, and was vice-chancellor of the college of physicians as well as protomedico, had organized in 1666 a rival academy, the Discordanti. Its device was a seven-stringed zither and its motto *Discordia concors*.[89] Its president was a younger man, Luca Tozzi, who lived on into Vico's maturity as a respected champion of the ancients, and died in 1717. The sessions of the Discordanti were devoted to confrontations of the Galenic and modern doctrines in medicine, usually to the disadvantage of the latter. So hot was the rivalry between the two academies that the latest charges and countercharges became the news of the day in Naples. Finally, in 1669 or 1670, when the Marquis of Arena administered a public rebuke to Pignataro for speaking ill of the Investigators in public, the viceroy and the Collateral Council advised the disbanding of both academies.[90]

So runs the now accepted account of the closing of the Academy, based chiefly on a brief passage in Mosca's biography of Porzio, which in turn is based on Porzio's manuscript memoirs. It seems, however, that the creative energies of the Academy were exhausted for the time being, and that it would have lapsed from internal causes. Cornelio's health failed in the winter of 1669-70; he took a journey into Puglia; and his communications with the Royal Society were interrupted for about two years.[91] D'Andrea's health failed, and he spent four years in northern Italy. Porzio left to become professor of anatomy at Rome, and was absent from Naples for eighteen years. Giuseppe Donzelli, dean of the chemical moderns, died in 1670. Bartoli had become professor of anatomy and surgery at Naples in 1668, and this, along with the restoration of the baths of Pozzuoli, absorbed his attention. The Marquis of Arena was increasingly engrossed by his duties as *scrivano di ragione*, or secretary of the treasury, of the Kingdom of Naples. Michele Gentile, a guiding spirit in the Academy, died in February 1675. The Marquis was assassinated in April.[92] Bartoli died in the following year. A period of recuperation was needed.

Interlude (1670–1683)

The disbanding of the Investigators did not put a stop to informal private gatherings and mutual encouragement, or to the activity of individual members. Much of what they did and published in the next fifteen years and more—that is, in Vico's boyhood—was the fruit of the 1660's.

Bartoli's tenure of the chair of anatomy and surgery was short but distinguished. He brought from Padua the celebrated anatomist Antonio Manzoni

[88] Minieri Riccio (1877), p. 10.

[89] Gimma (1703), vol. i, p. 186, followed by Minieri Riccio (1879), pp. 44 ff.

[90] Mosca, p. 17. Mosca says on p. 16 that the Academy lasted 'about six years'. Minieri Riccio (1879), pp. 60–2, having started the Academy in 1662, a year too early, ended it in 1668. I believe 1663–9 or early 1670 fits the evidence better. Mosca does not say that the request of the viceroy and Collateral Council applied to the Discordanti as well as the Investiganti, but this has been generally assumed.

[91] Royal Society, Letter Books, C. 106–108; D. 16–29.

[92] Fuidoro, vol. iii, pp. 221, 241, 244 ff.

to conduct his dissections. A young disciple of Luca Tozzi, Gaetano Tremigliozzi, chanced in 1675 to attend a dissection in which the pancreatic and biliary ducts were exhibited in a human cadaver. His curiosity aroused, Tremigliozzi next day attended Bartoli's lecture on the circulation of the blood. He went to his former master Tozzi and complained of having been left in ignorance of so many new and important discoveries. He put himself under Cornelio and Bartoli to learn the new science of medicine and the philosophy of Gassendi, and he became a versatile and prolific defender of the new school.[93] When Carlo Celano wrote disparagingly of the moderns in 1676, Tremigliozzi replied under a pseudonym with his *Courier from Parnassus*, in which we are informed that, ever since his promotion from the chair of medicine to that of politics, Galen—that is, Pignataro—has been disturbing the philosophic peace of the true investigators of natural things.[94]

Among the subjects Ray and Skippon had discussed with Cornelio at Naples were tarantism and manna. At Ray's request, Cornelio had made a more careful study of the production and gathering of manna. To show that it was an exudation of the manna ash and refute the popular notion that it was a 'honey-dew' which condensed on the ash at night, he had tied cloths about the branches of an ash towards evening and removed them in the morning. He had found manna as usual on the branches and leaves but none on the cloths except what had adhered to them from the branches. He had reported his observations to Ray in a letter of 29 November 1664.[95] Ray incorporated them with due acknowledgment in his catalogue of the plants of England in 1670.[96] They were quoted thence by Dr. John Mapletoft at one of the Royal Society's sessions in 1678,[97] and by John Pechey in a tribute to the 'lithontriptick vertue' of manna in 1692.[98]

The tarantula's bite, as Ray relates, was commonly 'esteemed venemous, and thought to put people into phrenetick fits, enforcing them to dance to certain tunes of the musick, by which means they are cured, long and violent exercise causing a great evacuation by sweat. These fits they say do also yearly return at the same season the patient was bitten'. Cornelio, however, had been 'diligently enquiring into this generally received and heretofore unquestioned story, that he might satisfy himself and others whether it were really true in experience'.[99]

---

[93] Gimma (1703), vol. ii, pp. 156 ff. Bartoli left at his death an unpublished MS., 'Treatise on the Anatomy of the Liver with appendices on the Anatomy of the Spleen, Kidneys, and Urinary Bladder', which provides a fair sample of the anatomy lectures he delivered in the University. It was later owned by Domenico Cotugno and is now in the Naples National Library. See Bartoli (1673). Bartoli's death is mourned by his pupil Battista (1676), nephew of the poet Giuseppe Battista, who was a friend of the Investigators.

[94] Tremigliozzi (1676), pp. 5–9.

[95] Ray (1718), pp. 9 ff., where the year is mistakenly given as 1663.

[96] Ray (1670), pp. 117 ff.

[97] Birch, vol. iii, p. 381.

[98] Pechey, p. 146. The physician Tancred Robinson in the winter of 1683–4 'travelled from Capua to Naples in the company of an ingenious Neapolitan physican' (Cornelio?), whose account of the manna ash led him to suggest to Ray that the exudations were caused by insect punctures. Ray (1848), pp. 176 ff. Robinson, a Fellow of the Royal Society, published in the *Phil. Trans.*, vol. xv, pp. 922–5, 'Some observations on Boyling Fountains, and Subterraneous Steams', with extensive references to the Naples area.

[99] Ray (1673), pp. 410 ff. For a general account of tarantism based on other sources, see Sigerist.

In 1670 Cornelio's ill health gave him excuse for a trip into Puglia to study the matter at first hand. After the temporary breakdown of his communications with the Royal Society, indirect contact was re-established in 1671 by John Doddington, the King's Resident at Venice, through a friend in Naples who sent him a copy of Cornelio's *Progymnasmata*; and finally, in 1672, Cornelio himself carried on an extended correspondence with the Society through Doddington.[100] In a letter of 19 January to Doddington, he declared that 'the stories related of the odd effects of the tarantula's stinging were in his opinion fictitious; and that from many of his own observations he was induced to believe that without any preceding bite of that insect such symptoms befall many of those people who live in Apulia, a very dry country, and are often tormented with an excessive and long thirst'.[101] Oldenburg referred this letter to Martin Lister, who replied: 'We may well expect from the ingenuity and diligence of Signor Cornelio the full clearing of this matter; we being already beholden to him for that other rarity of his native soil, manna, which he hath put beyond exception to be a spontaneous exudation of the ash tree.' He reserved judgement, however, pending further details.[102]

On 5 March Cornelio wrote Doddington another letter which was transmitted to the Society, translated into English, and published in the *Philosophical Transactions*.[103] Cornelio had it on good authority, he said, that 'those that think themselves bitten by tarantulas (except such as for some ends fain themselves to be so) are for the most part young wanton girls . . . who by some particular indisposition falling into this melancholy madness, persuade themselves according to the vulgar prejudice, to have been stung by a tarantula'. He instanced parallel phenomena showing that 'of many strange effects we daily meet with, the true cause not being known, such an one is assigned, which is grounded upon some vulgar prejudice. . . . But why should not we rather think, that this distemper is caused by an inward disposition, like that which in some places of Germany is wont to produce that evil which they call . . . St. Vitus's dance?'.

Lionardo di Capoa had long been in the habit of noting down observations on the uncertainty of medical theory and practice, and on the frequency with which professed followers of Hippocrates and Galen deviated from their teachings and gave themselves the lie. In the autumn of 1678 an occasion arose for putting these notes to public use. Ottavio Caracciolo di Forino, a favourite of the viceroy, had died in the full vigour of manhood, and his death was attributed to a dose of 'antimony ill-prepared and inopportunely prescribed'.[104] His physician, Antonio Cappella, though a Galenist, was a dabbler in chemistry. He had been one of the dissenters with Cornelio in 1664. Perhaps at the instigation of the protomedico, the viceroy on 26 September 1678 laid before the Collateral Council this and other 'unhappy Accidents that had befaln some sick persons, and for which the Chimical Medicines were accused'. The Council asked the protomedico to appoint a

[100] Royal Society, Letter Books, C. 106–108; D. 16–29.

[101] Birch, vol. iii, pp. 9 ff.

[102] *ibid.*, pp. 17 ff.

[103] Vol. vii, pp. 4066 ff.

[104] Archivio di Stato, Naples, Consiglio Collaterale, Notamenti, vol. 73.2 (74 bis), fo. 141v. Cf. Francesco d'Andrea as quoted by Capone-Marano, pp. 16–18; cf. pp. 313, 318. Cf. Fuidoro, vol. iv, p. 230.

commission of leading physicians to devise measures 'for the putting of some stop to the abuses and errors daily committed in the practice of physick'.

They, after some discourse thereabout, judged it most convenient . . . that every one should set down his opinion in writing.   Signor Lionardo di Capoa, who was one of the aforesaid consult, was obliged therefore to write his opinion in this affair; and . . . he acquitted himself of his obligation with so much learning, eloquence and erudition, that his manuscript falling into the hands of certain learned men, and other friends of his, appeared to them rather composed for the universality of those that take delight in the sublime mysteries of literature, than to be kept up amongst a private and small company, as if the author in writing thereof had purposed to himself no other end, but to satisfie the command imposed upon him.   They . . . at last prevailed with him . . . to condescend, that this at least, of the many and different tracts, which he has lying by him, should be committed to the press.[105]

This most famous of all the productions of the Investigators, Di Capoa's *Parere* or 'Opinion', was published at Naples in 1681.   It employed a critical review of the entire history of medicine to support the conclusion that it was not 'possible for either the people, or magistrates, who, for the most part understand little or nothing thereof, to settle the practice of physick by firm and durable laws, when the wisest and skilfullest physicians, who with long study, and much practise have searched far into it, could never arrive thereunto'.[106]

Certain measures could, however, be taken.   Medical students should not only be trained in philosophy and medicine, and above all in chemistry, but they should have hospital experience before receiving their degrees.   Pharmacists should have some medical training, a thorough course in chemistry, and clinical observation of the action of drugs.   It was high time, moreover, that Naples, which had boasted so great a pharmacologist as Giuseppe Donzelli, should have its public 'garden of simples' like that at Padua, to improve the instruction of physicians and pharmacists and facilitate research.[107]

The last proposal was the first to take effect.   In 1682 Don Francesco Filomarino, 'being elected governor of the Hospital of the Annunciation of Naples, for the publick good, at his own charges, caused a garden without the walls of the city, in a place called Montagnuolo, to be planted with simples, of which Tommaso Donzelli, a famous physician in our time, took the direction, and inriched with many plants'.[108]   Above the gate was a Latin inscription composed by Cornelio.[109]

One of Di Capoa's most interested readers was Queen Christina of Sweden. At Stockholm, before her abdication, Christina had been the exhausting patroness of Descartes in his last months (1649–50).   Almost his last acts were planning an academy with her, and putting in order his physiological treatise, *L'Homme*.   At Rome she had established an academy of which at least two of the Naples Investigators—Borelli and Porzio—were distinguished members during their years of Roman residence.   Nowhere had Descartes been studied

[105] Di Capoa (1684), p. 3 and Buragna's preface.

[106] Di Capoa (1684), p. 23.

[107] Di Capoa (1681), pp. 579 ff.

[108] Giannone (1731), vol. ii, p. 843; cf. Bulifon, vol. iii, pp. 196–202.   Giannone follows Bulifon in linking this innovation with another reform proposed by Di Capoa, the revival of instruction in Greek, on which see the text to which note 116 below refers.   Burnet also links 'the Greek learning' and 'the new philosophy' in the quotation to which note 121 below refers.

[109] Bulifon, vol. iii, p. 201.

with greater enthusiasm, or received more sympathetic though searching criticism, than at Naples.[110] Christina entered into a correspondence with Di Capoa and urged him to publish his lectures of 1664 on the phenomena of the Phlegrean Fields. The book appeared in 1683 with a dedication to Christina written by his son Cesare. The long account of Lake Agnano, which had been the occasion for the series, was cut to two pages.[111]

Third Period (1683–1697)

It has become usual to say, without much show of evidence, that the Academy had a third period of life from 1683 to 1695. Certainly this was the period of greatest prestige of the leaders of the movement and greatest activity of their disciples. Unfortunately, there seems to be no contemporary record of a formal revival of the Academy as such, with a fixed meeting place and permanent patron.

Such a revival in 1683 may be inferred with some plausibility from the fact that the phrase *Accademico Investigante* does not occur on the title-page of Buragna's *Poesie* in the spring of 1683, but does occur on that of Di Capoa's lectures on the *Mofete* in the late summer or autumn of the same year and from the same press. But this fact is perhaps sufficiently accounted for by the further facts that the lectures had been delivered before the Investigators, whereas the poems had not, and that Di Capoa was still living, whereas Buragna had died in 1679.

In any case, early in the next century, when some of the members were still living, we encounter vague references to a 'revived Academy of the Investigators'[112] which we must assign to this period for the reason that some men are said to have been members who were too young in 1663–70 or not yet resident in Naples, but who were there and quite eligible in 1683–95. Yet in the hundreds of extant letters written to Cornelio's friend Magliabechi by these new members and by the survivors of the old Academy, there is no mention of it. And, as we shall see, the only contemporary documents which clearly imply its actual existence under the old name belong to 1696 and 1697, the years following that in which it is usually said to have lapsed again.

Perhaps all that happened in the 1680's was that the same group of men, with some losses by death and by removal from Naples, and with some accessions of younger men, began meeting again about 1683 with some regularity, now in one salon or library, now in another; and though they must have thought of themselves as resuming and continuing the work of the Investigators, they may not have reassumed the name and form of the old Academy until after the death of Di Capoa in 1695.

The men who are said to have belonged to the Academy were members in this period of an informal group which met most frequently in the library and museum of Giuseppe Valletta, but sometimes in the salon of Nicola Caravita. In the absence of evidence of more formal meetings, the 'revived Academy' is probably best identified—at least for the 1680's and the early 1690's—with

---

[110] Berthé de Besaucèle, pp. 1 ff., 37 ff. See also Maugain *passim*.
[111] Di Capoa (1683), pp. 32–4.
[112] Gimma (1703), vol. ii, p. 146.

this informal group. In that case, it is almost certain that Vico attended some of its later meetings, for Valletta and Caravita were his chief patrons.[113]

A tailor's son trained in law, Valletta had married wealth and acquired more, and had spent it in gathering the richest and best selected private library in Italy, along with a museum of art and antiquities.[114] He was a close friend of Francesco d'Andrea, who liked to say that between them, he by his tongue and Valletta by his pen, they maintained the splendour of the Neapolitan forum.[115] Valletta was also a staunch supporter of Di Capoa. The latter in his *Parere* had recommended instruction in Greek to emancipate physicians from imperfect Latin translations of the great sources of ancient medicine; and the chair of Greek, which had been suppressed half a century earlier, had been revived in 1681 by Valletta, who had brought Gregorio Messere from Brindisi to fill it.[116]

Messere was a man of universal culture, a great teacher, and much admired by the youth. A generation of younger men, such as Tommaso Donzelli and Agnello di Napoli, who had been trained in medicine by Cornelio, Di Capoa and Bartoli, now studied Greek with Messere, and the culture of Neapolitan physicians reached a level to which it has perhaps never returned. Messere, Donzelli, Di Napoli and the mathematician Monforte were the outstanding additions to the circle of the Investigators in this period. Di Napoli began teaching in 1683 as a militant modern, an experimentalist, and a follower of the philosophy of Gassendi who did not waver when the shift to Descartes took place in the next decade. It was through his influence chiefly that Giannone became a lifelong Gassendist.[117]

A second edition of Cornelio's *Progymnasmata* was published at Venice in 1683.[118] Cornelio died in the following year. Francesco d'Andrea spared no expense to provide a funeral and a monument worthy of the man who, after Severino, had done most to advance science and philosophy at Naples.[119] The memorial address was delivered by Luca Rinaldi, archdeacon of the cathedral at Capua, the sacred orator of the day and a friend of the moderns.[120]

In the autumn of 1685, when Vico was a lad of seventeen studying law, Gilbert Burnet, a Fellow of the Royal Society since 1664, later Bishop of Salisbury and author of the *History of His Own Time*, visited Naples. Shortly

[113] Vico (1944), pp. 33, 35, 148, 216 (note 133); Nicolini (1932), pp. 87, 92 ff., 100, 169 ff. 178–88.

[114] See Borzelli and Consoli Fiego.

[115] A. P. Berti in Crescimbeni, *Vite*, vol. iv, p. 42.

[116] G. Lombardo in Crescimbeni, *Vite*, vol. ii, pp. 47–51. Cf. note 108 above.

[117] Gimma (1703), pp. 197 ff.; Giannone, *Vita*, pp. 232 ff.

[118] It is noteworthy that there were three books published at Naples that year which contained accounts of the Investiganti: Buragna's poems with a life of Buragna by Carlo Susanna; Di Capoa's lectures on damps with a nostalgic preface by Gennaro d'Andrea; and Nicodemo's supplement to Toppi (see his account of Porzio, pp. 157 ff., and cf. his notices of works by Monforte, Di Capoa, Bartoli). Among other publications at Naples in that year which were associated with the Investigators were an edition of Fracastoro's poetical works published by Raillard with a dedication to Valletta; and Carlo Musitano's treatise on chemical medicine, with civil *parere* by Di Capoa.

[119] Carlo Cornelio in ded. epist. of Cornelio (1688).

[120] Spiriti, p. 164; Amenta, *Rapporti*, p. 16, note 1. Spiriti says the poetical compositions read at Cornelio's funeral, including some by former enemies, were published at Naples in 1685. On Rinaldi see the long quotation from Burnet on the following page. See also Rinaldi's letter on scientific method, dated 15 August 1685, in Bulifon, vol. i, pp. 335–9.

PLATE XLIX

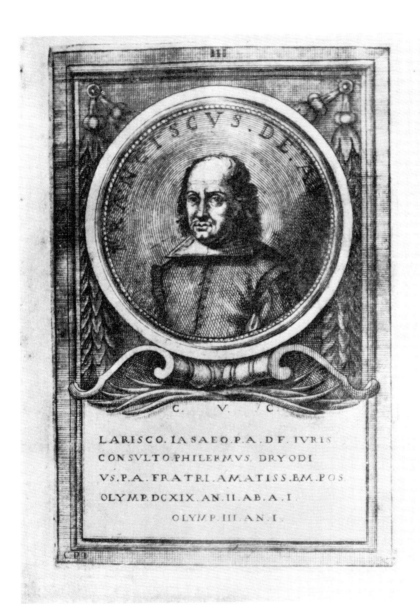

FIG. 5.   FRANCESCO D'ANDREA
(In G. M. Crescimbeni, *Vite*, vol. i)

afterwards, back in Rome, he wrote a letter to Robert Boyle which provides the most vivid contemporary English picture we have of Neapolitan life at the time—the swarming of the monks and their 'terrible' preachings on the one hand, the infiltration of French thought and customs on the other.

It is true that there are societies of men at Naples of freer thoughts than can be found in any other place of Italy: the Greek learning begins to flourish there, and the new philosophy is much studied; and there is an assembly that is held in Don Joseph Valletta's library (where there is a vast collection of well chosen books), composed of men that have a right taste of true learning and good sense. They are ill looked on by the clergy, and represented as a set of atheists and as the spawn of Pomponazzi's school; but I found no such thing among them (for I had the honour to meet twice or thrice with a considerable number of them during the short stay that I made among them). There is a learned lawyer, Francesco d'Andrea, that is considered as one of the most inquisitive men of the assembly; there is also a grandchild of the great Alciati who is very curious as well as learned. Few churchmen come into this attempt for the reviving of learning among them: on the contrary it is plain that they dread it above all things. Only one eminent preacher, Rinaldi, that is archdeacon of Capua, associates himself with them: he was once of the Jesuit order, but left it; and as that alone served to give a good character of him to me, so upon a longer conversation with him I found a great many things that possessed me with a high value for him. Some physicians in Naples are brought under the scandal of atheism. . . .[121]

In this period the high point was reached in the years 1687–9, under the encouragement of Queen Christina and with the co-operation of an enterprising bookseller and publisher, Jacques Raillard.

At the instance of his admirer Agnello di Napoli, the first Neapolitan edition of the works of Francesco Redi appeared in 1687, with dedications by the publisher Raillard to Francesco d'Andrea, Lionardo di Capoa, Tommaso Donzelli, Agnello di Napoli and Giuseppe Valletta.

In 1688 the same publisher produced at Naples a definitive edition of the works of Cornelio. A measure of the progress of the cause may be found in the fact that, a quarter of a century after the first edition of the *Progymnasmata* at Venice, it was now possible to print them at Naples, and that the civil imprimatur for this edition was written by Nicolo Susanna, who had apparently come over to the side of the moderns, as had also Federigo Meninni.[122]

Queen Christina had urged Di Capoa to round out his *Parere* on the uncertainty of medicine with a book on the uncertainty of medicaments. This was edited by Tommaso Donzelli and published at Naples in 1689 by Raillard, along with a revised edition of the *Parere*. It also would certainly have been dedicated to Christina if she had not died earlier in the year. Like the *Parere*, it was widely condemned for scepticism injurious to the dignity of the medical profession, and placed on the 'Index'.[123] At least until quite recently, the

[121] Burnet, pp. 195 ff. On Alciati, cf. note 124 below.

[122] On Meninni, cf. Fuidoro, vol. iii, pp. 230 ff., more accurately transcribed in Capone-Marano, pp. 24 ff. Cf. note 68 above. Tozzi also was now an admirer and friend of the moderns if he did not share their views. As early as 1681 he wrote of Cornelio and Di Capoa that 'nature had laid herself bare to them' (Nicodemo, p. 152); and in 1695 he wrote that Di Capoa had died with a generosity of spirit equal to the ingenuousness with which he had lived (letter of 23 July in Magliabechi 1095).

[123] Maugain, p. 45, note 4.

copy in the Biblioteca Beriana at Genoa was still marked on the back
a 'prohibited book'.[124]

The years 1688–93 were a period of intensified activity on the part of the
Roman Inquisition at Naples with a view to stamping out atomism and related
doctrines alleged to have been spread by Cornelio and Di Capoa.[125]   In
1691–4, at the request of the city authorities and with the help of his fellow
Investigators and other Neapolitan scholars, Valletta wrote a book-length
plea to Pope Innocent XII to remove the Roman Inquisition, leave matters of
faith and doctrine in the hands of the diocesan inquisition administered by
vicars of the bishops, and reinstate the canonical and time-honoured procedure
of the diocesan courts, so as not to permit their again becoming disguised tools
of the Roman Inquisition.   This book was never published, but it was widely
circulated in manuscript copies and was translated into Latin and French.[126]

The leader of the Anti-Capuists for a time was the Jesuit father De Benedictis
(1622–1701), author of a four-volume treatise on the peripatetic philosophy,
who in 1694 published under a pseudonym five *Apologetic Letters* 'in defence
of scholastic theology and peripatetic philosophy'—more exactly, an attack
on Di Capoa and the other moderns.   Francesco d'Andrea, who in his youth
had defended Severino before the Inquisition, now in his old age wrote a
defence of Di Capoa against the attack of De Benedictis.   It was never
published, but manuscript copies survive in the Naples National Library and
elsewhere.[127]

Valletta added another volume to his letter to the Pope, arguing the impiety
of the Aristotelian philosophy and the innocence of the atomic doctrine as
understood by Gassendi and the moderns.   This book, which he called his
'history of philosophy', was also circulated in manuscript.   For more than
a decade, however, Valletta was constantly on the point of publishing it, and
it was finally printed in 1709.[128]

---

[124] Benedicenti, vol. i, p. 2.   Paragallo's little book on the causes of earthquakes was published
at Naples in 1689 with civil *parere* by Giuseppe Alciati.   He sent ten copies to Magliabechi for
distribution (letter of 6 June 1690, in Magliabechi 556).   There were close relations throughout
this period between the Investigators and various survivors of the Cimento at Florence and Pisa,
including Alessandro Marchetti, the translator of Lucretius, a pupil of Borelli and continuer of
his work.   (See, e.g. Marchetti's letters of 21 October 1680 and 5 November 1688, in Magliabechi
748.)   In 1685 Valletta began negotiations for the purchase of Carlo Dati's library by a Neapolitan
bookseller (letters of 18 and 25 December in Magliabechi 1090).   In 1689 Raillard began printing
a Neapolitan edition of the *Saggi* of experiments performed in the Cimento.   Printing was far
advanced in December 1690.   (Letters of Bulifon, 15 November 1689, and 26 December 1690,
in Magliabechi 632.)   This edition seems not to have been published, probably because of the
appearance of the second Florentine edition in 1691, but Raillard published editions at Naples in
1701, 1704, and 1714.

[125] Nicolini in Vico (1947), pp. 209–18.   Cf. note 129 below.

[126] Berti in Crescimbeni, vol. iv, pp. 57 ff.   The alleged printed copy in the Naples National
Library, 149.Q.26, is in fact a copy of Valletta's *Istoria filosofica*, with an erroneous title supplied.
The minute of the Deputies in acknowledgment of Valletta's services, dated 19 October 1694, is
quoted on, fo. 336. of MS. 128 in the Biblioteca Angelica in Rome.

[127] Table of contents in Cotugno, p. 66, note 5; cf. pp. 54 ff.

[128] Valletta's intention to publish appears in the quotation from Silvestre below and in Vignoli,
p. 185.   That the book was printed in 1709 appears from a letter of 21 June quoted by Berti in
Crescimbeni *Vite*, vol. iv, p. 60, and from one of 14 December quoted by Nicolini (1934),
p. 302, in which it is described as 'a discourse in defence of the modern Democritean philosophy,
printed at Naples by Giuseppe Valletta, which will be followed by another in defence of the
Cartesian philosophy, to which the Neapolitans are now quite wedded'.   (The editor of the
posthumous edition of 1732, in ignorance of this previous edition, based his text on MS. copies.)
    Still another defence of atomism, written about the same time as d'Andrea's and Valletta's,

The Roman Inquisition, though shaken, was not finally dislodged until 1746,[129] but the activities of the moderns continued unabated.

A member of the Royal Society, the physician Peter Silvestre, who visited Italy in 1699–1700, reported that 'everything is very much cooled here since the death of Malpighi; there are scarce any who apply themselves to the study of nature': but

> I was mightily surpriz'd when I came to *Naples*, to find a great many persons applying themselves to the *Corpuscular Philosophy* and *Mathematicks*. They own'd to be oblig'd for it to *Tho. Cornelius Cosentinus*, who begun first to introduce them, and to *Leonado di Capoa*, who followed his steps. This great man died three [five] years ago. I was acquainted there with Signior *Joseph Valeta*, a Gentleman who has a very good library, and has learnt a little *English*, on purpose to understand *English* Books, for which he has a very great value. He lent me a Manuscript of his, that he will speedily publish. His design is to commend and encourage the *Experimental Philosophy*.[130]

The terminal year of this period of the Academy is usually set down as 1695 because it was in that year, on 17 June, that Lionardo di Capoa died. It is often said[131] that the memorial gathering at which Nicola Crescenzi delivered the oration[132] was a meeting of the Investigators, but this is a mistake; it was a meeting of the Adornati.[133] If the Investigators were already reorganized as a formal Academy, perhaps they preferred not to bring themselves forward as such at this time. In any case, the year of Di Capoa's death—a year in which Raillard published another edition of the discourses on the uncertainty of medicine and of medicaments, a year in which d'Andrea and Valletta and perhaps Porzio were composing defences of Di Capoa—has seemed a plausible terminal point for a period introduced by the publication in 1683 of the lectures on damps, a period in which, after the death of Cornelio, the dominant figure of the group of moderns at Naples was Lionardo di Capoa.

survives among some letters of Porzio and may have been composed by him: see Mandarini, pp. 285 ff.; Cotugno, p. 74.

   More thorough-going replies to De Benedictis were written by Constantino Grimaldi. See Mazzuchelli (1751); Maugain, pp. 153–63. Grimaldi in his autobiography acknowledges the assistance of Tommaso Donzelli, 'who revised his works as a trusty friend, to whom he had given licence to censure them freely'; Grimaldi, *Istoria*, fo. 9v. Musitano helped him to make arrangements for publication; *ibid.*, fo. 10r.

[129] On the inquisition at Naples, see Amabile, Monti, and the Appendix below.

[130] Royal Society, *Phil. Trans.*, vol. xxii, p. 629. Valletta was more than once offered membership of the Royal Society. He modestly declined but carried on a correspondence with the Society (Berti in Crescimbeni, *Vite*, vol. iv, p. 62). One of his letters was published in the *Phil. Trans.* The Valletta MS. Silvestre read was apparently a copy of his *Istoria philosophica*. Silvestre continues: 'I saw *Tho. Donzelli*, *Anello di Napoli*, *Ottavio Sandoro*, and several other learned Physicians', one of whom had several MSS. of Severino. Silvestre took back with him two works just published by members of the group: Sanguineti's *Dissertationes iatrophysicae* (with civil *parere* by Lucantonio Porzio) and Monforte's *De siderum intervallis*. The former was reviewed at length in the *Phil. Trans.* (vol. xxii, pp. 918–22); the latter, a more important book, was not. Silvestre also reported (*Phil. Trans.*, vol. xxii, p. 614) that 'They are printing at Venice another work of a Neapolitan, which has this Title, Dominici Aulisi Prodromus de origine & progressu medicinae'. On the strength of this report, it was included in the Boerhaave-Haller *Methodus*, but I can find no evidence that it was published, and Renzi's account (vol. iv, p. 562) was perhaps fabricated from notices of Aulisio's famous unpublished history of medicine, of which this *Prodromus* may have been a part. On the history itself see Nicolini (1942), pp. 408–12 where the *Prodromus* is not mentioned, and on Vico's relations with Aulisio see *ibid.*, 418–21.

[131] Following Minieri Riccio (1879), p. 61.

[132] Bulifon, vol. iv, pp. 270–310.

[133] As Minieri Riccio himself (1879, p. 6) correctly reports in his account of the Adornati.

There is evidence, however, that the third period of the Academy did not end with Di Capoa's death. Under the dates 1 August and 24 December 1696, Ferdinando Santanelli, a member *in absentia* practising medicine at Venice, addressed 'A' Signori Accademici Investiganti' two tracts in Italian, one on the use of vesicants, the other on the nature and causes of sleep. These were apparently written at the Academy's request, read at its meetings, and published at its initiative. Santanelli was a Neapolitan and had been a pupil of Cornelio; and in the first tract he gave an account, among other things, of the regimen by which Cornelio had finally cured himself of the hypochondria from which he had long suffered.[134] On 23 April 1697, Santanelli addressed to the Investigators a much longer and more ambitious tract, in Latin, on the 'mechanical organism' of the nervous, respiratory and circulatory systems. He proceeded to translate the two previous essays into Latin, added four others, and published the seven in book form at Venice in the following year. The first three essays retained their address to the Investigators, though the volume as a whole was dedicated by the publisher to Charles Montagu, Earl of Manchester, who was in Venice at the time, and though the preface in which Santanelli stated his general principles was addressed to the Royal Society of London.[135] A second edition, re-arranged and enlarged, including two further lucubrations and a treatise on fevers, was published at Naples in 1705, with the same three essays still addressed to the Investigators. It was perhaps on the strength of the Neapolitan edition of this his major work, a contribution to iatromechanics along Cartesian lines, that Santanelli became professor of medicine at Naples in 1708.[136]

It would appear, therefore, that 'the revived Academy of the Investigators' was still active in 1697 and perhaps in 1698. It is just possible, however, as we have suggested earlier, that it had not resumed the old form and name until after Di Capoa's death. In any case, it must have lapsed in about 1698, as the reform of the Spensierati and especially the organization of the Palatine Academy seemed to make it no longer necessary. The surviving Investigators became members of one or both of these academies, to which we now turn.

Interlude (1697–1735)

In the forty years that followed Di Capoa's death, there were at least three academies which were in some sense heirs of the Investigators. Vico was a member of the first two and in touch with the third.

The Academy of the Spensierati or Incuriosi of Rossano was reformed in 1696 by Giacinto Gimma. In 1703 Gimma published two volumes of biographical sketches of its members, for which Vico wrote an encomium.[137] There are biographies of Lucantonio Porzio and Gennaro d'Andrea, who were members of the Investiganti in the first and second periods as well as the third, and of Agnello di Napoli, Tommaso Donzelli, Antonio Monforte and others who were active in the third. One of the sketches is of Carlo Musitano, who had studied medicine under Cornelio, Di Capoa and Bartoli, and who

---

[134] *Galleria di Minerva*, vol. i, p. 98; Santanelli (1698), p. 9.

[135] Santanelli later dedicated his *Philosophia recondita* (1723) to the Royal Society.

[136] Torraca, p. 271.

[137] Vico, *Opere*, vol. v, p. 278.

had published at Naples in 1683 a treatise on chemical medicine, rumoured to have been put together from unpublished manuscripts of Bartoli;[138] a treatise for which Lionardo di Capoa had written the civil *parere*. There was also a sketch of Gaetano Tremigliozzi whom we have already met as a pupil of Bartoli. When Musitano's later *Trutina Medica* was attacked, the Academy undertook its defence and deputed Tremigliozzi to conduct it. Tremigliozzi published for the purpose his *New Courier from Parnassus concerning medical affairs*, which contains along with fresh matter a reprinting of his *Courier* of 1676 in defence of Bartoli and the other moderns. He also helped to prepare a collection of defences of Musitano by various physicians and scholars. One of these defences is in the form of a fake letter supposed to be addressed to Musitano by Bartoli from Parnassus.[139]

The Palatine Academy of Medinaceli was founded on 20 March 1698 by the viceroy, the Duke of Medinaceli, on the proposal of Federico Pappacoda and Nicola Caravita, and it continued until 1701. It met in the royal palace twice a month to discuss 'matters physical, astronomical, geographical and historical'. Among its members were Porzio, Messere, Monforte, Donzelli, Valletta and Vico. Copies of about 125 papers read to the Academy survive in five manuscript volumes in the Naples National Library.[140] The fifth volume begins with Vico's 'On the sumptuous dinners of the Romans'.[141] There is a slight predominance of historical over scientific papers, but more of the latter were published. Monforte's monograph on the intervals and magnitudes of the stars appeared as early as 1699. Some of Porzio's papers were published in 1711. Papers by Donzelli and others were published as late as 1743–4 in a Venetian miscellany.[142]

Celastino Galiani, prefect of the University, founded at Naples in 1732 an academy for which, with the help of Giannone at Vienna, he obtained in 1733 from Charles VI of Austria an imperial diploma constituting it the Academy of Sciences.[143] As its meeting place, the Duke of Gravina offered an apartment in his palace. Writing from Vienna on 15 November 1732 Giannone compared his hospitality with that of the Marquis of Arena in receiving the Academy of the Investigators under his protection, and predicted for the

[138] MS. note on end fly-leaf of British Museum copy of Musitano's *Pyrotechnia* (1033.K.16); cf. note 118 above.

[139] *Celeberr. virorum Apologiae*, pp. 40 ff. The Academy continued until after Gimma's death in 1735. His own academic dissertations on fabulous men and on fabulous animals (1714) carried its emblem on the title-page, and his treatise on 'subterranean physics' (1730) and another volume of dissertations (1732) also appeared under its auspices. Further volumes of biographical sketches of its members and various other publications were projected but did not appear for lack of patronage. Cf. *Galleria di Minerva*, vol. v, pp. 15 ff, 78–86, 264–7, 311–17, 322–38; vol. vii, pp. 25–44, 50–3, 68 ff., 74–9, 183–8; also Gimma (1723), vol. ii, pp. 467 ff.

[140] Cf. Naples.

[141] Cf. Vico, *Opere*, vol. vi, pp. 389–400, 440 ff.

[142] *Miscellanea*, vol. vi, pp. 245–344; vol. vii, pp. 221–70; vol. viii, pp. 269–425. Cf. Amodeo (1898); Rispoli; Nicolini (1932), pp. 185–8. Cf. also Porzio (1704), pp. 128 ff. If the belletristic pursuits of the Investigators were included in this essay, we should insert at this point an account of the Roman Arcadia and of its Neapolitan colony, Sebezia. Among the Arcadians who were also Investigators were Di Capoa, the d'Andrea brothers, Messere, Tremigliozzi, Valletta, Antonio Caraccio, and Vico. See Crescimbeni, *Vite* (from which our portraits of Di Capoa, and of d'Andrea, Figs. 4 and 5, were taken) and *Notizie*; see also Carini. Another work traceable to the Academy is that of Di Martino on the method for determining the forces of moving bodies.

[143] Amodeo (1905), pp. 65–7.

new Academy an even greater success.[144] Nicola Cirillo served as president until his death in the third year, and Francesco Serao as secretary. When the Kingdom of Naples was conquered by Charles of Bourbon in 1734, the Academy continued for a few years with his approval but apparently without his support. Galiani was elected a member of the Royal Society of London in 1735, and promised to communicate to it 'the experiments and observations of the Academy of Sciences recently established here'.[145] It was proposed, among other things, to gather the materials for a full description of the animals, plants, minerals and fossils of the Kingdom of Naples.[146] The members made chemical analyses of the mineral waters of the region about Naples, including the springs of Lake Agnano. They also made a study of the eruption of Vesuvius in 1737, and the results were published by Serao in the following year in a book which passed through several editions, Italian, Latin, bilingual Latin-Italian and English.[147] It contained references to Cornelio, Porzio, Borelli, Di Capoa and other Investigators. Serao also read three papers to the Academy on the tarantula, again with references to Cornelio and other Investigators, which he submitted to Vico for criticism before publishing them in 1742.[148]

Galiani's model was the Paris Academy of Sciences. This perhaps was the reason for the publication at Naples in 1739 of two volumes containing accounts of the work of that Academy in 1699 and 1700, and Italian translations of the papers in physics and mathematics read in those years.[149]

There is no evidence that Vico was a member of the Academy of Sciences, but it was perhaps its existence under the ostensible patronage of Charles of Bourbon which led him to think in 1736 or 1737 of dedicating to Charles his work 'on physical medicine'—probably a recasting of his *On the equilibrium of the living body*, which remained unpublished until the end of the century, and of which no copy can now be traced.[150]

The Academy died in 1744, the year of Vico's death, but was revived in 1780 as the Royal Academy of Sciences and Belles-Lettres, with Vico's son Gennaro as one of its four stipendiary fellows, representing the class of history and antiquities.[151]

[144] Giannone, *Epistolario*, vol. x, pp. 243 ff.; cf. vol. xi, pp. 226, 251.

[145] Royal Society, Letter Books, G.2.23–24, quoted by permission of the Society.

[146] Nicolini (1931), p. 309.

[147] Cf. Furchheim, pp. 180–2. The study and the book were subsidized by Cardinal Troiano Acquaviva d'Aragona, son of the Duke of Atri who had inherited the archives of the Investigators: Nicolini (1942), p. 56. It was to Acquaviva that Vico in 1744 dedicated the third and definitive edition of his New Science: *ibid.*, pp. 82–5, and refs. on p. 90. Cf. note 34 above.

[148] Vico, *Opere*, vol. v, pp. 275–7, 295. Another work traceable to the Academy is that of Di Martino on the method for determining the forces of moving bodies.

[149] *Istoria*. There had been Neapolitan editions of the Cimento's *Saggi* in 1701, 1704, and 1714. See Magalotti, and cf. note 124 above.

[150] Vico, *Opere*, vol. vii, pp. 255 ff., 299; vol. iii, pp. 276–80.

[151] Gentile, pp. 240–4. In the first quarter of the eighteenth century there were several important publications at Naples, not directly connected with any of the academies we have named, but indicative of the continuing influence of the Investigators. As we have seen (notes 124, 149 above), Raillard in 1689–91 was printing what would have been the second edition of the Cimento's *Saggi* if a second Florentine edition had not appeared in 1691. Raillard's edition could not compete with this, and it seems to have been withheld for the time being. In 1701, however, when the Florentine edition was exhausted, Raillard apparently used the sheets he had printed a decade earlier, with a fresh title-page, to bring out what must be counted as the third edition of the *Saggi*. It had scarcely appeared when the conspiracy of Macchia initiated a series of political disturbances as a result of which very few copies were sold and

Fourth Period (1735–1737)

After an interval of nearly forty years, the Academy of the Investigators was revived for the last time in 1735, probably by the jurist Stefano di Stefano, who was its first president. This time, if not in the third period, Vico was a member. On 31 July of that year the Academy met in Di Stefano's home to celebrate the return of Charles of Bourbon from Sicily by reciting poetical compositions, including a sonnet by Vico.[152]   These compositions were edited and published by the president's son Giuseppe di Stefano. The title-page carries a mediocre engraving of the Academy's emblem and motto (Fig. 6). The editor says: 'Indeed from our activity in this connection our most flourishing Academy will acquire such lustre that, for this fine work more than for the many studies by which it renders itself worthy of tribute, it will always and everywhere be most praised and prized'.[153] We seem to be back at the 'flattery and fustian' bemoaned to Milton a century before.

It was with slightly more promise that the Academy entered the third year of its reincarnation, under the presidency of Duke Annibale Marchese, for whose *Christian Tragedies* Vico had written the civil *parere* a few weeks earlier.[154] The inaugural address was delivered by G. G. Carulli on 5 August 1737, and was published with a dedication to Vico's old friend Paolo Mattia Doria, 'prize and honour of the Academicians Investigators'. One of the principal causes of the decline of letters, Carulli said, had been the multiplication of academies, so that they became filled with mediocrities who declaimed without investigating. The merit of the Investigators, and above all of their founders Cornelio and Di Capoa, was that they had restored that union of eloquence with genuine learning which the ancients had achieved. If the revived Academy will follow in their footsteps, he concluded,

> foreign nations will no longer be so inimical to our glory, and the generous sparks of ancient virtue in Italian souls will never be extinguished by the long circling of the heavens nor by our declining fortune; but, after we shall all have passed on, in the remotest future ages, beyond the seas and the mountains, there will resound forever living, safe from injury and vicissitude, the glorious memory and name of the Academicians Investigators.[155]

Raillard returned to France for several years. In 1704 the remaining copies were dressed with a new title-page and a dedication (dated at Paris) to Agnello di Napoli, 'the best philosopher, physician and scholar' of Naples, whom we have met as a leader of the Investigators in the third period. And finally, in 1714, after the death of Raillard, the still remaining copies were issued by his son Bernard-Michele with a fresh title-page and a dedication to Cesare Michelangelo d'Avalos, whose name is familiar to students of Vico (cf. *Opere*, vol. vii, pp. 229, 290, and vol. vi, index). The dedicatory epistle of the last issue was signed 'Cellenio Zacclori'. This was the anagram of Vico's friend the Abbé Lorenzo Ciccarelli, who in the same year edited the final edition of the works of Lionardo di Capoa, using the same anagram and (because the *Parere* had been prohibited since 1693) the false imprint 'In Cologna'. The first two volumes of this edition were dedicated by Ciccarelli to Nicola Gaetani, Duke of Laurenzano, and the third to the Duchess. Both were Vico's friends and fellow Arcadians. (Cf. Vico, *Opere*, vol. v, pp. 280, 289, and vol. vii, pp. 236, 279, 293 ff., 311.) In 1710 Ciccarelli had used the same anagram and the false imprint 'In Fiorenza' to publish at Naples the second edition of Galileo's still prohibited Dialogue of 1632; and in 1723–4 he used the same device to publish at Naples the edition of Boccaccio's works in the last two volumes of which the Commentary on Dante was printed for the first time. It was by 'the repeated and courteous pleading of Ciccarelli' that Vico was finally persuaded, in the spring of 1725, to write his Autobiography. (Vico, *Opere*, vol. v, p. 62; cf. pp. 124, 187, 285.)

[152] Vico, *Opere*, vol. viii, pp. 117, 147, 218.
[153] Di Stefano, pp. 12 ff.
[154] Vico, *Opere*, vol. vii, pp. 230 ff., 291 ff.
[155] Carulli (1737), fo. 6v.

On this burst of rhetoric the Academy seems to have expired, but Carulli himself lived on to deliver the inaugural oration for the Royal Academy of Sciences and Belles-Lettres in 1780.[156]

Long before this last revival began, all the original Investigators were dead. The cause for which they fought had finally triumphed, and they were no longer needed. Indeed, it was scarcely more than the name that was revived.

Review

It is just possible, however, that the moribund Academy had something to do with the publication at Naples in 1736 of the posthumously collected works of the last survivor of the original Academy, Lucantonio Porzio. In any case, a sketch of his long career will afford a review of the century we have been traversing, along with further examples of the ties between its scientific academies.

Porzio was a pupil of Cornelio, a member of his circle in the first period, and an original member of the formal Academy. He made a telescope which Cornelio admired, and gave private lessons in astronomy. In the winter of 1663–4, at the age of twenty-five, he conducted in the Academy a series of experiments on capillary action and surface tension, some of which, as we have seen, were repeated for the benefit of Ray and Skippon in the following June. Porzio published in 1667 the discourse to the Academy in which he had described these experiments and expounded their conclusions. Its title-page was apparently the first which bore beneath the author's name the proud phrase: *Accademico Investigante*.[157]

In 1670, after the formal dissolution of the Academy, Porzio began teaching medicine at Rome. He remained there for about twelve years. He was associated with Nazari and with Giovanni Giustino Ciampini in editing the *Giornale de' letterati*, the first Italian scientific review.[158] He was a member of at least three academies: that of Cardinal Flavio Chigi, in which he repeated with variations the vacuum experiments of the Cimento;[159] that of Christina of Sweden; and the Physico-Mathematical Academy founded by Girolamo Ciampini. He dedicated to Christina a Latin paraphrase of the Hippocratic tract *On Ancient Medicine*, published at Rome in 1681, with a preface in which he argued that the works contained in the Hippocratic Corpus were not by one author but by many; that among them all this tract was the one most likely to be by Hippocrates himself, because of the similarity between its doctrines and those of Democritus; that it was the best of all introductions to medicine, and that no advance in medical science was to be looked for along other lines than those there laid down. Porzio also dedicated to Christina his famous dialogue *Erasistratus*, published at Rome in 1682, in which he attacked the common practice of blood-letting as both superfluous and

---

[156] Carulli (1780).

[157] Since the *Copia* was published anonymously. Francesco d'Andrea, who may have been the author of the letter, revised Porzio's manuscript and 'lent his sweet eloquence to give better form to the matter which Lucantonio had briefly thought and expressed'. Mosca, p. 18.

[158] Melzi, vol. i, p. 452.

[159] Porzio (1736), vol. ii, p. 280.

PLATE L

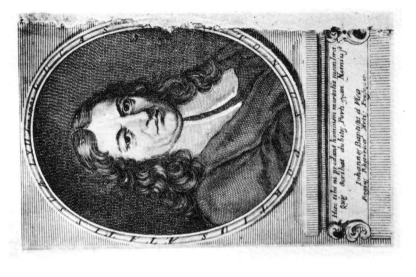

Fig. 7. Lucantonio Porzio

(In his *Opuscula*, 1701. The couplet is by Vico)

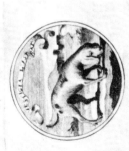

Fig. 6. Title-page of the *Componimenti*, 1735 with device
and motto of the Investiganti

harmful. It was perhaps he who interested Christina in the work of Di Capoa and the other Investigators at Naples.

In 1682-4 Porzio resided at Venice and was a member of the academy of Paolo Sarotti. Sarotti had been Venetian Resident at Naples from 1663 to 1669, the most active period of the Investigators, and had been admitted to their company.[160] He was then transferred to London, where he made the acquaintance of Robert Boyle. On Boyle's nomination, his son Giovanni Ambrosio Sarotti was elected a Fellow of the Royal Society in 1679.[161] On their return to Venice, the Sarottis took with them two young Englishmen who were adept at constructing apparatus for experimental work. With their assistance, the Sarottis founded and conducted at Venice an academy modelled on the Investigators of Naples and the Royal Society of London. Porzio there witnessed Giovanni Ambrosio's experiments showing 'what happened to fire and pigeons in "artificial air" ',[162] delivered and published a series of four dissertations,[163] and delivered at least two others on the cause and mechanism of the beginning of respiration in new-born infants.[164]

From Venice Porzio travelled through Bavaria and Austria and resided for three years at Vienna. The Austrian epidemic of dysentery in 1684-5, which swept the imperial armies and took more lives than did the Turkish invaders, provided the occasion for Porzio's best-known work, his *De militis in castris sanitate tuenda*, which was read by the Emperor in manuscript and published at Vienna in 1685.[165] It went through many editions and was translated into most of the languages of Europe. Porzio became a member of the Academia Naturae Curiosorum and contributed in 1687 a noteworthy essay on comparative anatomy, based on dissections of the male and female genitalia of the crayfish.[166]

Porzio returned to Naples in 1688 during the revival of the Investigators and taught there until his death in 1723; that is, until after Vico had conceived his New Science. The chair he held was that of anatomy and surgery, to which Ingrassias, Severino and Bartoli had lent distinction before him.[167] His most important publication during this period was an essay on the motion of bodies.[168] His frontispiece portrait in an edition of his *Opuscula* at Naples in 1701 (Fig. 7) was graced with a Latin couplet by Vico which may be freely rendered:

[160] Nicolini (1926), p. 271; (1928), p. 197.

[161] Birch, vol. iii, pp. 510 ff.

[162] Porzio (1684), pp. 63 ff.; (1736), vol. i, p. 311.

[163] Porzio (1684).

[164] Bulifon, vol. ii, p. 177.

[165] In pt. iv, ch. iv, Porzio gave a brief account of the Lake Agnano controversy, which we have summarized in the text to which note 58 above refers.

[166] Cole, pp. 344 ff.

[167] For the story of his appointment to this chair, for which he had been recommended by Malpighi, and for preceding episodes, see Mosca, pp. 53-7; Torraca, pp. 351, 391 (cf. *ibid.*, 233, note 2; 428, note 3); Confuorto, vol. ii, p. 142.

[168] Porzio (1704). This gave rise to a famous controversy, in which Porzio was attacked by Vico's friend Paolo Mattia Doria, and by Vitale Giordano and Guido Grandi, and was defended by Giambattista Balbi and Antonio Galeotta. For the literature (too extensive to be included in our bibliography), see Riccardi under these names. The view that prevailed was that expressed in Grandi's *Epistola mathematica* in reply to an inquiry from Vico's friend Bartolomio Intieri. Cf. Caverni, vol. iv, pp. 262-5.

True, this portrait shows a mortal,
     But the works that follow
Still must make us doubt who wrote them:
     Porzio or Apollo.[169]

'This last Italian philosopher of the school of Galileo', as Vico calls him in
his Autobiography, was Vico's counsellor and critic in the development of
the medical theory of his *On the equilibrium of living bodies*, and his lifelong
friend.[170]

Conclusion

The story of the Academy of the Investigators has a certain importance as
an integral and prominent part of the larger story of the quarrel of ancients and
moderns and of the inevitable triumph of the moderns. In the grand economy
of modern science, however, it was not much that was required of the
Neapolitan Investigators.   Reports on manna, on tarantulas and tarantism,
on eruptions of Vesuvius, on experiments in the Cave of the Dogs, and on
other phenomena of the Phlegrean Fields—that is about all. In the last third
of the seventeenth century and the first quarter of the eighteenth, as visitors
from abroad did not fail to remark, Naples was the one city of Italy, perhaps
even of Europe, in whose intellectual life natural science was pre-eminent.
It was the Investigators who had made it so. Yet neither their peculiar
combination of scepticism and speculative audacity nor their researches in
basic science seem to have contributed directly to the main movement of
European thought.   How far this was due to the economic backwardness and
isolation of the Kingdom of Naples, and how far to other factors, it is beyond
the scope of this essay to consider.

In the perspective of nearly three centuries, the Academy of the Investigators
is important chiefly as part of the Neapolitan background of Vico's New Science.
Of the ablest resident members of the Academy in its most flourishing period,
Bartoli died when Vico was eight, Cornelio when he was sixteen, Di Capoa
when he was twenty-seven, Francesco d'Andrea when he was thirty, and
Porzio when he was fifty-five. When the Academy finally ceased in 1737,
Vico was nearly seventy. It is not too much to say that he lived under the
shadow of the Investigators.[171]

APPENDIX

The Investigators and the Inquisition

The best account of the Academy of the Investigators hitherto available
in English is contained in two passages in the English translation of Giannone's
Civil History of the Kingdom of Naples, London, 1731, vol. ii, pp. 575–7,
840–3. The second of these passages has several times been quoted and

---

[169] Vico, *Opere*, vol. viii, pp. 91, 217. Vico's friend and printer Mosca published in 1728
a reprint of Porzio's work on military medicine with the same portrait and couplet, and it was
Mosca's son who printed Porzio's collected works in 1736.

[170] Vico, *Opere*, vol. v, p. 37.

[171] The French historian of 'la querelle des anciens et des modernes' concludes with a chapter
on Vico's New Science, as marking the end of this epoch in European culture and the beginning
of another. Rigault, pp. 449–60.

referred to in the preceding essay. The first passage occurs in the long chapter on the Inquisition (Bk. 32, ch. 5, sec. 3). It follows here, with a few corrections and with the addition in brackets of a paragraph included in all Italian editions after the first, from which the English translation was made. Giannone has just related how Piazza, a deputy from the Roman Inquisition, had come to Naples in 1661, and how popular commotion had forced the viceroy to expel him from the Kingdom. He continues:

M. Piazza's being chased out of Naples, put a Stop for some time to the coming of Inquisitors from Rome, but they did not give over their Pretensions, nor did they fail to make new Attempts when a proper Occasion offer'd, and which appeared plainly in the Reign of Charles II by reason of a new Philosophy introduced into Naples, which, running down the Scholastick Philosophy professed by the Monks, was very unacceptable at Rome.

The Academy set up at Naples, under the Name of *Investiganti*, of which the Marquis of Arena declared himself Protector, quite removed the Slavery commonly borne with hitherto, of swearing *in verba Magistri*; and having laid aside the Scholastick Philosophy, left its Members at more freedom to philosophize according to the Dictates of Reason. These Academists were all Learned Men, and the brightest Genius's of the City, which gained them great Reputation amongst Men of Knowledge, and especially among the Youth, to whom it was an easy Matter to demonstrate the Errors and Dreams of the Monkish Philosophy.

The Works of Pierre Gassendi had acquired great Fame, as well upon the Account of his great Learning and Eloquence, as for his having restored the Epicurean Philosophy, which, compar'd to that of Aristotle, and especially as taught in the Schools, had the Reputation of being more solid and true. These Books were brought to Naples, and when they were read there, the Youth was infinitely pleased with them, not only upon the Account of the Principles which they taught, but for the Variety of good Learning they contained: So that in a short Time they all became Gassendists; and this Philosophy was profess'd by the new Philosophers. And although Gassendi had adapted his Epicurean System to the Catholick Religion, which he himself professed, yet Titus Lucretius being the greatest Supporter of it, many were induced to read that Poet, hitherto known but to very few; however, the *Investiganti*, as well as Gassendi, having exposed the Errors of Lucretius, denounced them to the Youth, and taught that his Philosophy was not to be followed, save as it should submit itself to our Religion.

[In spite of all the prudence and precautions exercised by the *Investiganti*, the young Neapolitans could not avoid false reports being spread throughout Europe by the monks, charging that as a result of these studies they did not take seriously the immortality of human souls. So that Antoine Arnauld, in that accurate and learned book, *Difficultés proposées à Mr Steyaert*, declaiming against the abuse introduced in Rome of prohibiting books without discrimination, complains that Rome had prohibited the works of René Descartes by which the immortality of the soul had been demonstrated, whereas the books of Gassendi were permitted to circulate freely despite assurances from Naples that they had done great harm to the Neapolitan youth by reason of the contrary opinion to which the reading of the works of Lucretius and Gassendi had given rise.]

What made them likewise afraid, was the Fate of Galileo de' Galilei, who, notwithstanding his reverend gray Hairs, was obliged in Rome to abjure his Opinion concerning the Motion of the Earth.

But not many years after, the Works of René Descartes were likewise brought to Naples; and 'tis said, that Tommaso Cornelio, a famous Physician and Philosopher at that Time, was the first Introducer of them. The Youth therefore, and especially the Physicians, were very intent upon studying them, and very soon abandon'd the Epicurean Philosophy, and applied themselves to that of Descartes; and those who formerly were Gassendists, at last became most zealous Cartesians.

The Monks seeing, that by these new Studies, their Schools were not only forsaken, but themselves ridiculed for the many Fooleries which they taught, contracted such an implacable Hatred against the new Philosophers, that they ascribed many Errors in Religion to them, cavilling at all their Propositions, and treating themselves as Hereticks.

This was sufficient to give a Handle to the Inquisitors of Rome to arm themselves anew, and again endeavour to introduce their Commissaries into Naples, in order to watch the Proceedings of the new Philosophers. And they not only attempted, but actually establish'd an Inquisitor, who received Informations, put People in Prison, and, which was more, had his own Prison in the Convent of S. Domenico Maggiore. This Inquisitor was M. Gilberto, Bishop of Cava, who exercised this Office by secret Processes, and with such Rigour and Insolence, that he often forced many ignominiously to abjure, for no other Crime, but their holding Opinions in Matters purely Philosophical, contrary to those of the Schools, although no Taint of Infidelity could be found in them; which occasioned many Complaints and Disorders in Naples. . . .

In the remainder of the chapter Giannone carries the history of the Inquisition at Naples up to 1709. A brief account of some of the episodes may be found in Vico (1944), pp. 34 ff. For details see Amabile and Monti.

BIBLIOGRAPHY

(Locations of manuscripts and of copies of rare pamphlets and books are indicated as follows: A, Biblioteca Angelica, Rome; B, British Museum; Ca, Biblioteca Casanatense, Rome; Cr, library of Benedetto Croce, Naples; F, Biblioteca Nazionale, Florence; La, Biblioteca Lancisiana, Rome; Li, Biblioteca dei Lincei, Rome; M, Biblioteca Marucelliana, Florence; N, Biblioteca Nazionale, Naples; R, Biblioteca Nazionale, Rome; S, Biblioteca della Deputazione Napoletana di Storia Patria, Naples; V, Biblioteca Apostolica Vaticana, Rome.)

ACCIANO, GIULIO. See Capone–Marano.

ACETI, ANTONIO. *Reminiscenze virgiliane nelle opere del cosentino Tommaso Cornelio.* Cosenza, 1932. F.

—— *Un genio cosentino negletto* [Tommaso Cornelio]. Cosenza [1933]. F.

Affetti ossequiosi delle Muse di Perugia nella partenza del Sig. Francesco d'Andrea Napoletano. Perugia, 1672. Biblioteca Augusta, Perugia.

AGNANO, LAKE OF. (Bound volumes of pamphlets in Lake Agnano controversy: B, 33.d.18; La, XXIV.2.16; S, II.A.29. For titles see: Susanna, Nicolo; *Il lago d'Agnano utile; La morsa domatrice; Barbaiudaei querimonia; Istanze; Frantumi; Copia di una lettera.*)

ALETINO, BENEDETTO. See DE BENEDICTIS.

AMABILE, LUIGI. *Il Santo Ufficio della Inquisizione in Napoli.* 2 vols. Città di Castello, 1892.

AMENTA, NICCOLÒ. *Vita di Lionardo di Capoa.* Venice [Naples], 1710. (Also in Crescimbeni, *Vite,* vol. ii.)

—— *De' rapporti di Parnaso.* Naples, 1710.

AMODEO, FEDERIGO. *La prima data dell'Accademia Reale di Napoli.* Naples, 1898. (Reprinted from *Rend. della R. Accademia delle scienze fisiche e matematiche di Napoli.*)

AMODEO, FEDERIGO. *Vita matematica napoletana.* Naples, 1905. (Pt. ii, 1924.)

ARIANI, VINCENZO. *Commentarius de claris jurisconsultis neapolitanis.* Naples, 1769.

—— *Memorie della vita e degli scritti di Agostino Ariani.* Naples, 1782.

BAGLIVI, GIORGIO. MS. letter book in Osler Library, McGill University, *Bibliotheca Osleriana* 7516. (Letters 50, Cornelio to Malpighi, 18 September 1667; 53, Redi to d'Andrea, 6 November 1691, with a summary of d'Andrea's reply, 1692; 60, 56, 55, d'Andrea to Baglivi, 11 July, 2 August, 11 September 1692.)

Barbaiudaei querimonia; Disinganno del forestiere mal prattico del paese. 4 pp. in fol. (Satiric verses.) B, La.

BARBIERI, MATTEO. *Notizio storiche dei mattematici e filosofi del Regno di Napoli.* Naples, 1778.

BARTOLI, SEBASTIANO. *Astronomiae microcosmicae systema novum, authore Sebastiano Bartolo parthenopæo philosopho libero, cui suasu amicorum accessit exercitationum paradoxicarum decas in eversionem scholasticae medicinae, opusculum in studiorum authoris tyrocinio elucubratum ac non bene digestum.* Naples, Novello de Bonis, 1663. A. An imperfect copy, containing only the last two pages (49–50) of the first part (the *Systema*), and lacking the last few pages (113 ff.) of the separately paged second part (the *Exercitationes*). MS. note on p. 50 of first part: 'Qui termina il mio sistema, che va dedicato al Re di Spagna, seguitano poi immediatamente l'esercitationi paradoxiche . . .'

—— *Artis medicae dogmatum communiter receptorum examen in decem exercitationes paradoxicas distinctum.* Venice [Naples?], 1666. N.

—— *Breve ragguaglio de' bagni di Pozzuoli.* Naples, 1667.

—— *Tractatus anatomiae hepatis, cui accedit anatomes lienis, renum, et vesicae urinariae.* Naples, 1673. MS. N, XIV.D.38.

—— *Thermologia Aragonia.* Naples, 1679.

—— See also *Il lago d'Agnano utile.*

BATTISTA, SIMONE ANTONIO. *La gramaglia lagrimosa per la morte di Sebastiano Bartolo.* Naples, 1676. (No copy found. Cited from Toppi, p. 286.)

BENEDICENTI, ALBERICO. *Malati, medici e farmacisti.* 2 vols. Milan, 1924.

BERTANI, CARLO. *Il maggior poeta sardo, Carlo Buragna, e il petrarchismo del seicento.* Milan, 1905.

BERTHÉ DE BESAUCÈLE, LOUIS. *Les cartésiens d'Italie.* Paris, 1920.

BIRCH, THOMAS. *History of the Royal Society of London.* 4 vols. London, 1756–7.

BOCCACCIO, GIOVANNI. *Opere.* 6 vols. Florence [Naples], 1723–4.

BORELLI, GIOVANNI ALFONSO. *De vi percussionis.* Bologna, 1667.

—— *De motionibus naturalibus a gravitate pendentibus.* Reggio, 1670.

—— *De motu animalium.* 2 vols. Rome, 1680–1, and many later editions, including Naples, Felice Mosca, 1734.

BORZELLI, ANGELO. *Accuse in Giuseppe Valletta.* Naples, 1891. S.

BULIFON, ANTONIO. *Lettere memorabili.* 4 vols. Puzzuoli and Naples, 1685–98.

BURNET, GILBERT. *Some letters containing an account of what seemed most remarkable in travelling through Switzerland, Italy, some parts of Germany, &c., in the years 1685 and 1686.* Third edition. Rotterdam, 1687.

BURAGNA, CARLO. Preface to Di Capoa (1681).

—— *Poesie . . . colla vita del medesimo, scritta dal Signor Carlo Susanna.* Naples, Raillard, 1683.

CAPONE, GIULIO and MARANO, SALVATORE. *Un poeta satirico del XVII secolo* [Giulio Acciano]. Salerno, 1892.

CAPUCCI, GIOVANNI BATTISTA. Preface to Bartoli (1666).

—— Letter to Malpighi. In Malpighi, p. 109.

CARAMUEL LOBKOWITZ, JUAN. *Primus calamus*, vol. ii, *Rhythmica*. Second edition. Campagna, 1668.

—— *Mathesis biceps*. 2 vols. Campagna, 1670.

CARAVELLI, VITTORIO. *Pirro Schettini e l'antimarinismo*. Naples, 1889.

CARINI, ISIDORO. *L'Arcadia dal 1690 al 1890*. Rome, 1891.

CARULLI, GIOVANNI GIUSEPPE. *Orazione . . . detta nel riaprirsi l'Accademia degl' Investiganti il dì V. Agosto MDCCXXXVII*. [Naples, 1737?] N, S.

—— *Orazione recitata nell' aprirsi la Regale Accademia delle Scienze e delle Belle Lettere il dì 29 di Giugno 1780*. [Naples, 1780?] N.

CAVERNI, RAFFAELLO. *Storia del metodo sperimentale in Italia*. 5 vols. Florence, 1891-8.

CELANO, CARLO. *Avanzi delle poste*. 2 vols. Naples, 1676-81. N.

Celeberr. virorum Apologiae pro R. D. Carolo Musitano adversus Petrum Antonium de Martino medicum geofonensem qui Trutinam Medicam anno 1688 Venetiis typis editam, qua Harveana sanguinis circulatio aliaeque recentiorum medicorum sententiae statuminantur, temere, & inepte impugnare ausus est. Kruswick apud Petrum Antonium Martellum MDCC. B, 1166.e.10.3.

COLE, F. J. *A history of comparative anatomy from Aristotle to the eighteenth century*. London, 1944.

CONFUORTO, DOMENICO. *Giornali di Napoli dal 1679 al 1699*. 2 vols. Naples, 1930-1.

CONSOLI FIEGO, GIUSEPPE. 'Il Museo Valletta.' *Napoli Nobilissima*, 1922, n.s. iii, 105-10, 172-5. (Reprinted in his *Scritti vari di storia ed arte*, Naples, 1939.)

Copia di una lettera scritta da un Accademico Investigante ad un Cavaliero suo Amico, intorno ad una Scrittura, stampata in risposta di un' altra fatta prima, circa la difesa del Lago di Agnano. 36[+4] pp. in 4to. (The letter is dated at the end on p. 36: Nel dì 1. di Aprile 1665. It is followed by a four-page *Ode in lode della famosa Accademia de' Signori Investiganti*, which is referred to at the end of the letter as having been composed by one of the Academicians. B, La, S.)

CORNELIO, TOMMASO. *Meditationum de mundi structura liber primus continens physico-mathematicas de mundi partibus disquisitiones, phaenomenis nuper in cœlo observatis congruentis*. MS., Ca. 827. 53 leaves, illus. Dedication to Pompeo Colonna dated at Rome, 12 October 1646.

—— *Epistola qua motuum illorum qui vulgo ob fugam vacui fieri dicuntur, vera causa per circumpulsionem ad mentem Platonis explicatur*. Rome, 1648. Ca, R. Cf. Cornelio (1663), pp. 111 ff.

—— Letter to Severino, 28 August 1649. In Bulifon, vol. i, pp. 276-80. Cf. Cornelio (1663), pp. 141 ff.

—— *Discorso dell'eclissi detto nell' Accademia degli Otiosi nel dì 29 di Maggio 1652. Dato in luce per l'Accademico detto l'Arrestato*. Naples, 1652. 56 pp. in 8vo. V.

—— Consultation, 22 December 1661. In Bulifon, vol. iv, pp. 136 ff.

—— *Progymnasmata physica*. Venice, 1663. (Frankfurt, 1665; Leipzig and Jena, 1683, under title *Physiologia*; Venice, 1683; Copenhagen, 1685; Naples, 1688, best edition, with an added progymnasma 'De sensibus', and Cornelio's Latin poems, edited by Cornelio's nephew Carlo Cornelio, with dedication to Francesco d'Andrea.)

—— 'Relatione d'un gigante ritrovato a Tiriolo nel mese di Giugno dell' an. 1665.' *Giornale de' letterati*, vol. ii, pp. 23-5.

—— Letters to Doddington and Oldenburg, 19 January and 5 March 1672. Royal Society, Letter Books, C. 106-108. (Second letter to Doddington pub. in part in *Phil. Trans. Roy. Soc.*, 1672, viii, 4066 ff.)

—— Letter to Malpighi, 18 September 1677. In Baglivi (q.v.).

CORNELIO, TOMMASO. *De metempsychosi seu transmigratione pythagorica.* MS. Latin dialogue. Cf. Greco.

CORTESE, NINO. *I ricordi di un avvocato napoletano del seicento, Francesco d'Andrea.* Naples, 1923.

—— 'L'età spagnuola.' In Torraca, pp. 203-431.

COTUGNO, RAFFAELE. *La sorte di Giovan Battista Vico.* Bari, 1914.

CRESCIMBENI, GIOVANNI MARIA (ed.). *Le vite degli Arcadi illustri.* 4 vols. Rome, 1708-21. F.

—— (ed.). *Notizie istoriche degli Arcadi morti.* 3 vols. Rome, 1720-1. F.

CROCE, BENEDETTO. 'Giovanni Caramuel vescovo di Campagna.' *Archivio storico per le province napoletane,* 1925, l, 90-7.

—— 'La *Istoria filosofica* di Giuseppe Valletta.' *Quaderni della 'Critica',* 1947, no. viii, pp. 31-8. (Reprinted in his *La letteratura italiana del settecento, note critiche,* Bari, 1949, pp. 207-16.)

D'AFFLITTO, EUSTACHIO. *Memorie degli scrittori del Regno di Napoli.* 2 vols. Naples, 1782-94.

D'ANDREA, FRANCESCO. Letters to Baglivi and Redi. In Baglivi (q.v.).

—— *Difesa della filosofia di Lionardo di Capoa.* MS. N, two copies, I.D.4, I.C.12. (IX.A.66 is not a third copy but a continuation.)

—— *Avvertimenti ai nipoti.* In Cortese (1923), pp. 55-223. (MS. in S, XX.B.24, is preceded by letters of 1671 and 1672 to Porzio; cf. Cortese, pp. 15-18.)

—— See also *Discorso.*

D'ANDREA, GENNARO. Preface ('Il Volubile Accademico Investigante al lettore') to Di Capoa (1683).

DE BENEDICTIS, GIOVANNI BATTISTA. *Lettere apologetiche in difesa della teologia scolastica, e della filosofia peripatetica.* Naples, 1694. (Under pseudonym of Benedetto Aletino.)

DELLA PORTA, GIOVANNI BATTISTA. *Natural magick . . . in twenty books, . . . wherein are set forth all the riches and delights of the natural sciences.* London, 1669.

DE MARTINO, PIETRO ANTONIO. *Responsum Trutinae medicae Musitani.* Naples, 1699. N.

DE RENZI, SALVATORE. *Miasmi paludosi e luoghi del Regno di Napoli dove si sviluppano.* Naples, 1826.

—— *Storia della medicina in Italia.* 5 vols. Naples, 1845-8.

DE ROGATIS, GENEROSO. *Cenni biografici degli uomini illustri di Bagnoli Irpina.* Cavellino, 1914.

DI CAPOA, LIONARDO. Preface to Cornelio (1663).

—— *Parere . . . divisato in otto ragionamenti, ne' quali partitamente narrandosi l'origine e'l progresso della medicina, chiaramente l'incertezza della medesima si fa manifesta.* Naples, Bulifon, 1681. (Second edition, Naples, Raillard, 1689. Third edition, Naples, Raillard, 1695. Fourth edition, Cologne [Naples], 1714.)

—— *The uncertainty of the art of physick, together with an account of the innumerable abuses practised by the professors of that art, clearly manifested by a particular relation of the original and progress thereof ; also divers contests between the Greeks and Arabians concerning its authors.* Written in Italian by the famous Lionardo di Capoa, and made English by J[ohn] L[ancaster], Gent. London, printed by Fr. Clark, for Thomas Malthus at the Sun in the Poultrey, 1684. (Advertisement on p. 102: 'This is the first Discourse of Signor Lionardo di Capoa, who hath writ seven others upon the same subject; which according to the acceptance this meets with in Publick, shall likewise be Englished'.)

—— *Ragionamenti . . . intorno alla incertezza de' medicamenti.* Naples, Raillard, 1689. (Second edition, Naples, Raillard, 1695. Third edition, Cologne [Naples], 1714.)

Di Capoa, Lionardo. *Lezioni intorno alla natura delle mofete.* Naples, Castaldo, 1683. (Second edition, Cologne [Naples], 1714.)

Di Giarbo, Moinerio. *Discorso nel quale si dimostra, che i Medicamenti Spagirici sieno per lo più mal sicuri, e pericolosi, e da non permettersi senza l'approbazione de' Medici Galenisti: E che la lettura della chimica, benchè privatamente, come non utile, debba restare proibita. Contra la nuova pretenzione de' Moderni Chimici.* 10 leaves. La. (See footnote 29 above.)

Di Martino, Pietro. *De corporum quae moventur viribus, earumque aestimandarum ratione.* Naples, 1741.

Discorso per difesa dell'arte chimica, e de' professori di essa. Nel quale si dimostra, che il legger privatamente la chimica in tempo di vacanze, così per li statuti de gli Studi publici, come per legge comune, non possa esser cosa proibita . . . Al Sig. V.R. & al suo Consiglio Collaterale. 19 leaves. Dated at the end: In Napoli dì 28. di Settembre 1663. La. (See footnote 26 above.)

Di Stefano, Giuseppe (ed.). *Componimenti per lo faustissimo ritorno da Sicilia della Maesta di Carlo Re . . . recitati a XXXI. Luglio del MDCCXXXV. nell' Accademia degl' Investiganti nella casa del Presidente D. Stefano di Stefano.* In Parigi [Naples, 1735?]. N.

Doddington, John. Letters to Oldenburg. Royal Society, Letter Books, D.16–29.

Donzelli, Giuseppe. *Antidotario napoletano.* Naples, 1642, and later editions.

—— *Partenope liberata, overo, racconto dell'heroica risoluzione fatta dal popolo di Napoli per sottrarsi . . . dall'insopportabil giogo degli Spagnuoli.* Parte prima. Naples, Beltrano, 1647. N.

—— *Petitorio napoletano.* Naples, De Bonis, 1663.

—— *Teatro farmaceutico-dogmatico-spagirico.* Naples, Passero, 1667. (Revised and enlarged by Tommaso Donzelli, Naples, 1676; twentieth edition, Venice, 1728; and later editions.)

Donzelli, Tommaso. Preface to Di Capoa (1689).

—— 'Della figura e misura della terra.' In *Miscellanea di varie operette* (q.v.), vol. vii, pp. 221–70.

Fabroni, Angelo (ed.). *Lettere inedite di uomini illustri.* 2 vols. Florence, 1773.

Fiorentino, Francesco. *Bernardino Telesio.* 2 vols. Florence, 1872–4.

Fisch, Max H. 'John Houghton.' *Journ. Hist. Med. and Allied Sci.*, 1946, i, 338.

Fracastoro, Girolamo. *Opera poetica omnia.* Naples, Raillard, 1683. Li.

Frantumi della morsa di un bruto medico maniscalco, stritolata sù l'incudine delle verità dalla forza insuperabile della libera filosofia. 20 pp. in 4to. B, La.

Fuidoro, Innocenzo (Vincenzo d'Onofrio). *Giornali di Napoli dal 1660 al 1680.* 4 vols. Naples, 1934–43. (Cf. extracts in Capone-Marano, pp. 22 ff.)

Furchheim, Federigo. *Bibliografia del Vesuvio.* Naples, 1897.

Gabrieli, Giuseppe. 'Giovani Battista della Porta Linceo.' *Giornale critico della filosofia italiana*, 1927, viii, 360–97, 423–31.

—— 'Il "Liceo" di Napoli.' *R. Acc. Naz. dei Lincei (Rend. d. Cl. di Sci. mor., stor. e filol.)*, 1939, 6s., xiv, 499–565. (Also as separate publication, Rome, 1939.)

Galiani, Celestino. Letter to Cromwell Mortimer. Royal Society, Letter Books, G.2.23–24.

Galilei, Galileo. *Dialogo . . . sopra i due massimi sistemi del mondo . . . In questa seconda impressione accresciuta di una lettera dello stesso . . . e di varj Trattati di più autori . . .* Florence [Naples], 1710. F.

Galleria di Minerva. 7 vols. Venice, 1696–1717. F.

Gassendi, Pierre. *The mirrour of true nobility and gentility, being the life of the renowned Nicolaus Claudius Fabricius, Lord of Peiresk, Senator of the Parliament at Aix.* Englished by W. Rand. London, 1657.

GEMELLI-CARERI, GIOVANNI FRANCESCO. *Viaggio per Europa.* Naples, Raillard, 1693.

GENTILE, GIOVANNI. *Studi vichiani.* Second edition. Florence, 1927.

GIANNELLI, BASILIO. *Educazione al figlio.* Naples, 1781.

GIANNONE, PIETRO. *The civil history of the Kingdom of Naples.* Trans. by James Ogilvie. 2 vols. London, 1731.

—— *Epistolario inedito col fratello Carlo.* MS. copy in S, 12 vols., XXXI.B.4–15.

—— *Vita scritta da lui medesimo,* ed. Fausto Nicolini. *Archivio storico per le province napoletane,* 1904, xxix, 183–652. (Separate edition, Naples, 1905.)

GIMMA, GIACINTO. *Elogi accademici della Società degli Spensierati di Rossano.* 2 vols. Naples, 1703.

—— *Dissertationes academicae.* 2 vols. Naples, 1714, 1732.

—— *Idea della storia dell'Italia letterata.* 2 vols. Naples, 1723.

—— *Fisica sotterranea.* 2 vols. Naples, 1730.

Giornale de' letterati. Rome, 1668–81.

GIUSTI, DOMENICO. *Vita ed opere dell'abate Giacinto Gimma.* Bari, 1923.

GIUSTINIANI, LORENZO. *Breve contezza delle accademie istituite nel Regno di Napoli.* Naples, 1801.

GRADILONE, ALFREDO. 'L'Accademia degli Spensierati.' *Accademie e biblioteche d'Italia,* 1931, iv, 523–8.

GRECO, LUIGI MARIA. 'Nota intorno un autografo inedito di Tommaso Cornelio.' *Atti della Accademia Cosentina,* 1865, ix, 171–81.

GRIMALDI, COSTANTINO. *Risposta alla Lettera apologetica in difesa della teologia scolastica.* Cologne (Geneva), 1699.

—— *Risposta alla seconda lettera . . .* Cologne, 1702.

—— *Risposta alla terza lettera . . .* Cologne, 1703.

—— *Discussioni istoriche, teologiche, e filologiche . . . fatte per occasione della Risposta alle Lettere apologetiche di Benedetto Aletino.* 3 vols. Lucca [Naples], 1725. N. (MS. of unpublished fourth and fifth vols., N, XIII.D.114–5.)

—— *Istoria de' libri di D. Costantino Grimaldi scritta da lui medesimo.* MS., N, XV.B.32.

Il lago d'Agnano utile, et innocente con l'infusione de' lini, e senza quella dannosissimo alla cittadinanza di Napoli, & a'massari della Campagna Felice. 48 pp. in 4to. (Dated at the end: Napoli 25. Settembre 1664. B, La, S. La copy has MS. note on title-page: 'Si crede del Sig. Medico Sebastiano Bartolo'. See footnote 61 above.)

Istanze della Signoria Bestialissima di Arcadia fatte alla maestà di Apollo per la giurisdittione à quella usurpata da alcuni medici ostinati à sostenere dannosa l'infusione de' lini nel lago d'Agnano. Notizia havuta in questi ultimi giorni di carnevale per le gazzette del Corriero di Parnaso. 47 pp. in sm. 8vo. B, La.

Istoria dell'Accademia reale delle scienze dell'anno 1699, con le memorie di matematica, e di fisica dell'istesso anno. Naples, 1739.

Istoria dell'Accademia reale delle scienze dell'anno 1700, con le memorie di matematica e di fisica dello stesso anno. Naples, 1739.

JONES, RICHARD F. *Ancients and moderns.* St. Louis, 1936.

La morsa domatrice di Testa Libera nelle credenze d'Agnano innocente. 20 pp. in 4to. B, La, S.

MABILLON, JEAN. *Iter italicum litterarium.* In his *Museum italicum,* vol. i, Paris, 1724.

MAGALOTTI, LORENZO. *Lettere familiari.* 2 vols. Florence, 1769.

—— (ed.). *Saggi di naturali esperienze fatti nell'Accademia del Cimento.* Florence, 1666 [1667]. (Second Florentine edition, 1691; editions at Naples, Raillard, 1701, 1704, 1714; Eng. trans. by R. Waller: *Essayes of natural experiments made in the Academie del Cimento.* London, 1684.)

MAGLIABECHI, ANTONIO. MS. Carteggio. F. (Includes over six hundred letters from some fifty Neapolitan correspondents, 1675–1713. Refs. are to vols. of Cl. VIII.)

MALLOCH, ARCHIBALD. *Finch and Baines; a seventeenth century friendship.* Cambridge University Press, 1917.

MALPIGHI, MARCELLO. *Opera posthuma.* London, 1697, pp. 1–110: *Vita a seipso scripta.*

MANDARINI, ENRICO. *I codici manoscritti della Biblioteca Oratoriana di Napoli.* Naples, 1897.

MAUGAIN, GABRIEL. *Étude sur l'évolution intellectuelle de l'Italie de 1657 à 1750 environ.* Paris, 1909.

MAYLENDER, MICHELE. *Storia delle accademie d'Italia.* 5 vols. Bologna, 1929.

MAZZUCHELLI, GIAMMARIA. 'Notizie storiche e critiche intorno alla vita ed agli scritti di Costantino Grimaldi.' *Raccolta d'opuscoli scientifici e filologici*, Venice, 1751, xlv, i-lxxi.

—— *Gli scrittori d'Italia.* 6 vols. Brescia, 1753–63.

MELZI, GAETANO. *Dizionario di opere anonime e pseudonime di scrittori italiani.* 2 vols. Milan, 1848–9. (Supplements by Giambattista Passano, Ancona, 1887, and Emmanuele Rocco, Naples, 1888.)

MENINNI, FEDERIGO. See footnote 29 above.

MILTON, JOHN. *Areopagitica.* In his *Works*, vol. iv, New York, Columbia University Press, 1931.

MINIERI RICCIO, CAMILLO. *Notizie biografiche e bibliografiche degli scrittori napoletani fioriti nel secolo xvii.* Parts 1 and 2 (letters A and B), Naples, 1875, 1877. (No more published.)

—— *Cenno storico delle accademie fiorite nella città di Napoli.* Naples, 1879. (Reprinted from *Archivio storico per le province napoletane*, vols. iii–v, 1878–80.) *Miscellanea di varie operette.* 8 vols. Venice, Lazzaroni & Bettinelli, 1740–4.

MONFORTE, ANTONIO. *De syderum intervallis & magnitudinibus.* Naples, Abri, 1699. Cr.

MONTI, G. M. 'Nuovi documenti sull'Inquisizione a Napoli e sul suo procedimento nei secoli xvi–xviii.' In his *Dal duecento al settecento; studi storico-giuridici*, Naples, 1925, pp. 185–243.

MOSCA, GIUSEPPE. *Vita di Lucantonio Porzio.* Naples, 1755. Cr, N.

MUSITANO, CARLO. *Pyrotechnia sophica rerum naturalium.* Naples, 1683.

—— *Trutina medica.* Venice, 1688.

[Naples. Accademia Palatina.] *Delle lezioni accademiche de' diversi valentuomini de' nostri tempi recitate avanti l'ecc.mo sig.r Duca di Medinaceli . . . copiate dall' originale, che si conservava presso il sig.r D. Niccolò Sersale.* MS., 5 vols. N, XIII.B.69–73.

NAPOLI, RAFFAELE, and PASCALE, LODOVICO. *Relazione sul lago d'Agnano e sue influenze morbose.* Naples, 1867. S.

NAPOLI-SIGNORELLI, PIETRO. *Vicende della coltura nelle due Sicilie.* Vol. v. Naples, 1811.

NICODEMO, LEONARDO. *Addizioni copiose alla Biblioteca napoletana del Toppi.* Naples, Castaldo, 1683. (See Toppi.)

NICOLINI, FAUSTO. 'Frammenti veneto-napoletani.' In *Studi di storia napoletana in onore di M. Schipa*, Naples, 1926, pp. 247–74.

—— 'Sulla vita civile, letteraria e religiosa napoletana alla fine del seicento.' *Atti della R. Accademia di scienze morali e politiche di Napoli*, 1928, lii, 175–255.

—— 'Monsignor Celestino Galiani, saggio biografico.' *Archivio storico per le province napoletane*, 1931, n.s. xvii, 249–358.

NICOLINI, FAUSTO. *La giovinezza de Giambattista Vico.* Bari, 1932.

—— *Aspetti della vita italo-spagnuola nel cinque e seicento.* Naples, 1934.

—— *Uomini di spada, di chiesa, di toga, di studio, ai tempi di Giambattista Vico.* Milan, 1942.

ORIGLIA PAOLINO, GIOVANNI GIUSEPPE. *Istoria dello Studio di Napoli.* 2 vols. Naples, 1753–4.

PANDOLFI, EDOARDO. 'Brevi cenni intorno Tommaso Cornelio da Cosenza e la irritabilità Halleriana.' *Atti della Accademia Cosentina,* 1865, ix, 163–7.

PARAGALLO, GASPARE. *Ragionamento intorno alla cagione de' tremuoti.* Naples, 1689.

PARRINO, DOMENICO ANTONIO. *Teatro eroico e politico de' governi de' vicerè del Regno di Napoli.* 2 vols. Naples, 1692–4.

PECHEY, JOHN. *A collection of chronical diseases.* London, 1692.

PIGNATARO, CARLO. *Petitorium.* Naples, Castaldo, 1684. B.

POPE, WALTER. Letters to Wilkins. Royal Society, Letter Books, P.1.43–46.

PORZIO, LUCANTONIO. *Del sorgimento de' licori nelle fistole aperte d'ambidue gli estremi, & intorno a molti corpi che tocchino la loro superficie.* Venice (Naples?), 1667.

—— *In Hippocratis librum De veteri medicina . . . paraphrasis.* Rome, Bernabò, 1681.

—— *Erasistratus, sive de sanguinis missione.* Rome, 1682; Venice, 1683.

—— *Dissertationes variae.* Venice, 1684.

—— *De militis in castris sanitate tuenda; oder, Von dess Soldaten im Lager Gesundheit Behaltung.* Vienna, 1685. Li. (Naples, 1701, 1728; The Hague, 1739; Leyden, 1741; French trans., Paris, 1744; Eng. trans., *The soldier's vade mecum; or, the method of curing the diseases and preserving the health of soldiers.* London, 1747.)

—— 'De cancri fluviatilis partibus genitalibus.' In *Miscellanea medico-physica Academiae naturae curiosorum Germaniae,* ann. vi, 1687 (pub. 1688).

—— Letter to Vidania, 15 June 1696. In Bulifon, vol. iv, pp. 193–210.

—— *Opuscula & fragmenta varia.* Naples, Bulifon, 1701.

—— *De motu corporum nonnulla, & de nonnullis fontibus naturalibus.* Naples, Gessari, 1704. N.

—— *Lettere e discorsi accademici.* Naples, 1711. N, S.

—— *Opera omnia,* ed. Francesco Porzio. 2 vols. Naples, Felice Carlo Mosca for Gaetano Elia, 1736.

RAVEN, CHARLES E. *John Ray, naturalist.* Cambridge University Press, 1942.

RAY, JOHN. *Catalogus plantarum Angliae.* London, 1670.

—— *Observations topographical, moral, & physiological, made in a journey through part of the Low-Countries, Germany, Italy, and France.* London, 1673.

—— *Philosophical letters,* ed. W. Derham. London, 1718.

—— *Correspondence,* ed. E. Lankester. London, 1848.

REDI, FRANCESCO. (Various works reprinted separately under their several titles.) 6 vols. Naples, Raillard, 1687.

—— *Opere.* 9 vols. Milan, 1809–11.

RICCARDI, PIETRO. *Biblioteca matematica italiana.* 3 vols. Modena, 1878–93.

RIGAULT, HIPPOLYTE. *Histoire de la querelle des anciens et des modernes.* Paris, 1856.

RISPOLI, GUIDO. *L'Accademia Palatina del Medinaceli.* Naples, 1924. N, S.

ROYAL SOCIETY OF LONDON. *Philosophical Transactions.* London, 1665–.

—— *The Record of the Royal Society.* Fourth edition. London, 1940.

—— Letter Books. (MSS.)

SANGUINETI, DOMENICO. *Dissertationes iatro-physicae.* Naples, 1699. F.

SANTANELLI, FERDINANDO. 'Dell'uso de'vessicanti'; 'Parere del modo di farsi il sonno'. *Galleria di Minerva,* vol. i, pp. 93–102, 190–202. (Two letters addressed 'A' Signori Accademici Investiganti', dated at Venice, 1 August and 24 December 1696.)

SANTANELLI, FERDINANDO. *Lucubrationes physico-mechanicae . . . in septem tractatus divisae.* Venice, 1698. A, B.

—— *Lucubrationes physico-mechanicae . . . in novem tractatus divisae . . . quibus in fine additus fuit completissimus tractatus de febribus.* Naples, Dom. Ant. Parrino, 1705. N.

—— *Philosophiae reconditae . . . explanatio . . .* Cologne, 1723. B, M.

SCHIPA, MICHELANGELO. 'Il Muratori e la coltura napoletana del suo tempo.' *Archivio storico per le province napoletane,* 1901, xxvi, 553–649.

Scritture varie mss. e stampate sull'Iride di Lionardo di Capoa. MS. N, XIV.G.18.3.

SERAO, FRANCESCO. *Istoria dell'incendio del Vesuvio, accaduto nel mese di Maggio dell'anno 1737, scritta per l'Accademia delle scienze.* Naples, 1738. (Other editions, Latin, Latin–Italian, Naples, 1738, 1740, 1778; Eng. trans.: *The Natural history of Mount Vesuvius.* London, E. Cave, 1743.)

—— *Lezioni accademiche sulla tarantola o falangio di Puglia.* Naples, 1742.

—— *Opuscoli di vario argomento.* Naples, 1767.

[SEVERINO, MARCO AURELIO]. *Documenti per Marco Aurelio Severino raccolti da Luigi Amabile.* MS. N, XI.AA.35–37.

SIGERIST, HENRY E. *Civilization and disease.* Ithaca, Cornell University Press, 1943. (Ch. xi, 'Disease and music', reprinted with a few changes as 'The story of tarantism' in *Music and medicine,* ed. Schullian & Schoen, New York, Schuman, 1948, pp. 96–116.)

SKIPPON, PHILIP. *An account of a journey made thro' part of the Low-Countries, Germany, Italy and France.* In *A collection of voyages and travels,* ed. A. & J. Churchill, London, vol. vi, 1752, pp. 373–749.

SPAMPANATO, VINCENZO. *Quattro filosofi napoletani nel carteggio di Galileo.* Portici, [1907].

SPIRITI, SALVATORE. *Memorie degli scrittori cosentini.* Naples, 1750.

SUSANNA, CARLO. 'Caroli Buragna Vita.' In Buragna (1683).

SUSANNA, NICCOLO. *All'illustriss. et eccellentiss. signore, e padrone mio osservandissimo il Sig. Duca di Girifalco del Consiglio Collaterale di sua maestá in questo Regno.* 6 leaves. Dated at the end: Nap. 12 d'Ag. 1664. B, La.

—— *L'innocenza d'Agnano trovata colpevole ne' delirij di Testa Libera.* 66 pp. in 4to. Ded. epist. dated: Napoli a dì 7. Febraro 1665. B, La, S.

TADISI, GIACOPO ANTONIO. *Memorie della vita di monsignor Giovanni Caramuel di Lobkowitz.* Venice, 1760. F.

TAFURI, GIOVANNI BERNARDINO. *Istoria degli scrittori nati nel Regno di Napoli.* Vol. ii. Naples, 1748.

TARGIONI TOZZETTI, GIOVANNI. *Notizie degli aggrandimenti delle scienze fisiche accaduti in Toscana nel corso di anni LX. del secolo XVII.* 3 vols. Florence, 1780.

TOPPI, NICOLA. *Biblioteca napoletana.* Naples, Bulifon, 1678. (See Nicodemo.)

TORRACA, FRANCESCO, et al. *Storia della Università di Napoli.* Naples, 1924. (Especially pp. 203–431, 'L'età spagnuola', by Nino Cortese.)

TREMIGLIOZZI, GAETANO. *Staffetta da Parnaso.* Rome, 1676. Cr.

—— *Nuova staffetta da Parnaso circa gli affari della medicina . . . dirizzata all'illustrissima Accademia degli Spensierati di Rossano.* Frankfurt, 1700.

TRENT, JOSIAH C. 'Five letters of Marcus Aurelius Severinus to "The Very Honourable English Physician, John Houghton".' *Bull. Hist. Med.,* 1944, xv, 306–23.

VALLETTA, GIUSEPPE. *Al nostro santissimo padre Innocenzio XII, Intorno al procedimento ordinario e canonico nelle cause che si trattano nel tribunale del Santo*

Uficio nella città e regno di Napoli [fo. 1–138]; *Al nostro santissimo padre Innocenzio XII, Discorso filosofico in materia d'Inquisizione et intorno al corregimento della filosofia di Aristotele* [fo. 140–256]. MS., Naples, 1697, N, XV.B.4. Other copies, with variations, of the first letter: I.C.72; I.E.12.1; I.E.20; XI.C.8, 9, 10. Another copy of the second: V.H.180.

—— [*Istoria filosofica.* Naples, 1709?] Two incomplete copies in N: 23.E.41 and 149.Q.26. Neither copy has a printed title-page. The former contains pp. 1–208, the latter 1–240 with 233–40 repeated. The latter has an erroneous MS. title.

—— 'De incendio et eruptione montis Vesuvii, anno 1707.' Royal Society, *Phil. Trans.*, 1713, xxviii, 22–5. (Original in Letter Books, V.51.)

—— *Lettera . . . in difesa della moderna filosofia, e de' coltivatori di essa, indirizzata alla Santità di Clemente XI, aggiuntavi in fine un'osservazione sopra la medesima.* In Rovereto, nella stamperia di Pierantonio Berno libr., 1732. Ca, Li.

VENTIMIGLIA, MARIANO. *Degli uomini illustri del regal convento del Carmine Maggiore di Napoli.* Naples, 1756. N.

VICO, GIAMBATTISTA. *Opere*, ed. Fausto Nicolini *et al.* 8 vols. Bari, Laterza, 1914–42; vol. iv, second edition, 1942; vol. v, second edition, 1929.

—— *Autobiografia*, ed. Fausto Nicolini. Milan, 1947.

—— *Autobiography*, trans. Fisch and Bergin. Ithaca, Cornell University Press, 1944.

—— *The New Science*, trans. Bergin and Fisch. Ithaca, Cornell University Press, 1948.

VIGNOLI, GIOVANNI. *De columna imperatoris Antonini Pii dissertatio. Accedunt antiquae inscriptiones ex quamplurimis, quae apud auctorem extant, selectae.* Rome, 1705. (Inscriptions obtained from Valletta, pp. 185 ff., 196, 286–301, 309.)

ZAGARIA, RICCARDO. *Vita e opere di Niccolò Amenta.* Bari, 1913.

ZAVARRONE, ANGELO. *Bibliotheca Calabria.* Naples, 1753.

HISTORY, PHILOSOPHY AND
SOCIOLOGY OF SCIENCE

Classics, Staples and Precursors

An Arno Press Collection

Aliotta, [Antonio]. **The Idealistic Reaction Against Science.** 1914

Arago, [Dominique François Jean]. **Historical Eloge of James Watt.** 1839

Bavink, Bernhard. **The Natural Sciences.** 1932

Benjamin, Park. **A History of Electricity.** 1898

Bennett, Jesse Lee. **The Diffusion of Science.** 1942

[Bronfenbrenner], Ornstein, Martha. **The Role of Scientific Societies in the Seventeenth Century.** 1928

Bush, Vannevar. **Endless Horizons.** 1946

Campanella, Thomas. **The Defense of Galileo.** 1937

Carmichael, R. D. **The Logic of Discovery.** 1930

Caullery, Maurice. **French Science and its Principal Discoveries Since the Seventeenth Century.** [1934]

Caullery, Maurice. **Universities and Scientific Life in the United States.** 1922

Debates on the Decline of Science. 1975

de Beer, G. R. **Sir Hans Sloane and the British Museum.** 1953

Dissertations on the Progress of Knowledge. [1824]. 2 vols. in one

Euler, [Leonard]. **Letters of Euler.** 1833. 2 vols. in one

Flint, Robert. **Philosophy as Scientia Scientiarum and a History of Classifications of the Sciences.** 1904

Forke, Alfred. **The World-Conception of the Chinese.** 1925

Frank, Philipp. **Modern Science and its Philosophy.** 1949

The Freedom of Science. 1975

George, William H. **The Scientist in Action.** 1936

Goodfield, G. J. **The Growth of Scientific Physiology.** 1960

Graves, Robert Perceval. **Life of Sir William Rowan Hamilton.** 3 vols. 1882

Haldane, J. B. S. **Science and Everyday Life.** 1940

Hall, Daniel, et al. **The Frustration of Science.** 1935

Halley, Edmond. **Correspondence and Papers of Edmond Halley.** 1932

Jones, Bence. **The Royal Institution.** 1871

Kaplan, Norman. **Science and Society.** 1965

Levy, H. **The Universe of Science.** 1933

Marchant, James. **Alfred Russel Wallace.** 1916

McKie, Douglas and Niels H. de V. Heathcote. **The Discovery of Specific and Latent Heats.** 1935

Montagu, M. F. Ashley. **Studies and Essays in the History of Science and Learning.** [1944]

Morgan, John. **A Discourse Upon the Institution of Medical Schools in America.** 1765

Mottelay, Paul Fleury. **Bibliographical History of Electricity and Magnetism Chronologically Arranged.** 1922

Muir, M. M. Pattison. **A History of Chemical Theories and Laws.** 1907

National Council of American-Soviet Friendship. **Science in Soviet Russia: Papers Presented at Congress of American-Soviet Friendship.** 1944

Needham, Joseph. **A History of Embryology.** 1959

Needham, Joseph and Walter Pagel. **Background to Modern Science.** 1940

Osborn, Henry Fairfield. **From the Greeks to Darwin.** 1929

Partington, J[ames] R[iddick]. **Origins and Development of Applied Chemistry.** 1935

Polanyi, M[ichael]. **The Contempt of Freedom.** 1940

Priestley, Joseph. **Disquisitions Relating to Matter and Spirit.** 1777

Ray, John. **The Correspondence of John Ray.** 1848

Richet, Charles. **The Natural History of a Savant.** 1927

Schuster, Arthur. **The Progress of Physics During 33 Years (1875-1908).** 1911

Science, Internationalism and War. 1975

Selye, Hans. **From Dream to Discovery: On Being a Scientist.** 1964

Singer, Charles. **Studies in the History and Method of Science.** 1917/1921. 2 vols. in one

Smith, Edward. **The Life of Sir Joseph Banks.** 1911

Snow, A. J. **Matter and Gravity in Newton's Physical Philosophy.** 1926

Somerville, Mary. **On the Connexion of the Physical Sciences.** 1846

Thomson, J. J. **Recollections and Reflections.** 1936

Thomson, Thomas. **The History of Chemistry.** 1830/31

Underwood, E. Ashworth. **Science, Medicine and History.** 2 vols. 1953

Visher, Stephen Sargent. **Scientists Starred 1903-1943 in American Men of Science.** 1947

Von Humboldt, Alexander. **Views of Nature: Or Contemplations on the Sublime Phenomena of Creation.** 1850

Von Meyer, Ernst. **A History of Chemistry from Earliest Times to the Present Day.** 1891

Walker, Helen M. **Studies in the History of Statistical Method.** 1929

Watson, David Lindsay. **Scientists Are Human.** 1938

Weld, Charles Richard. **A History of the Royal Society.** 1848. 2 vols. in one

Wilson, George. **The Life of the Honorable Henry Cavendish.** 1851